QM 451 .M27 2003

Martin, John H. 1951-

Neuroanatomy

D0209939

Neuroanatomy
TEXT AND ATLAS

Third Edition

John H. Martin, PhD

Center for Neurobiology & Behavior
Department of Psychiatry
College of Physicians & Surgeons of Columbia University
New York

MEDICAL PHOTOGRAPHY BY

Howard J. Radzyner, RBP, AIMBI, FRMS

ILLUSTRATED BY

Michael E. Leonard, MA, CMI, FAMI

McGraw-Hill
MEDICAL PUBLISHING DIVISION

New York   Chicago   San Francisco   Lisbon   London   Madrid   Mexico City   Milan
New Delhi   San Juan   Seoul   Singapore   Sydney   Toronto

The McGraw·Hill Companies

Neuroanatomy: Text and Atlas, Third Edition

Copyright © 2003 by The **McGraw-Hill Companies, Inc.** All rights reserved. Printed in the United States of America. Except as permitted under the United States Copyright Act of 1976, no part of this publication may be reproduced or distributed in any form or by any means, or stored in a data base or retrieval system, without the prior written permission of the publisher.

Previous editions copyright © 1996, 1989 by Appleton & Lange.

Photographs copyright © 1988 Howard J. Radzyner (unless otherwise credited).

1 2 3 4 5 6 7 8 9 0   KGP/KGP   0 9 8 7 6 5 4 3

ISBN 0-07-138183-X

NOTICE

Medicine is an ever-changing science. As new research and clinical experience broaden our knowledge, changes in treatment and drug therapy are required. The author and the publisher of this work have checked with sources believed to be reliable in their efforts to provide information that is complete and generally in accord with the standards accepted at the time of publication. However, in view of the possibility of human error or changes in medical sciences, neither the author nor the publisher nor any other party who has been involved in the preparation or publication of this work warrants that the information contained herein is in every respect accurate or complete, and they disclaim all responsibility for any errors or omissions or for the results obtained from use of the information contained in this work. Readers are encouraged to confirm the information contained herein with other sources. For example and in particular, readers are advised to check the product information sheet included in the package of each drug they plan to administer to be certain that the information contained in this work is accurate and that changes have not been made in the recommended dose or in the contraindications for administration. This recommendation is of particular importance in connection with new or infrequently used drugs.

This book was set in Palatino by The Clarinda Company.
The editors were Janet Foltin, Harriet Lebowitz, and Nicky Fernando.
The production supervisor was Catherine H. Saggese.
The interior text designer was Patrice Sheridan.
The cover designer was Janice Bielawa.
The index was prepared by Jerry Ralya.
Illustrations created by Michael E. Leonard, Dragonfly Media Group, and Charissa Baker.
The illustration manager was Charissa Baker.
Quebecor World, Kingsport was the printer and binder.

This book is printed on acid-free paper.

Library of Congress Cataloging-in-Publication Data

Martin, John H. (John Harry), 1951–
    Neuroanatomy: text and atlas/John H. Martin; medical photography by Howard J.
Radzyner; illustrated by Michael E. Leonard.—3rd ed.
    p.; cm.
    ISBN 0-07-138183-X (alk. paper)
    1. Neuroanatomy. 2. Neuroanatomy—Atlases. I. Title.
    [DNLM: 1. Central Nervous System—anatomy & histology. 2. Central Nervous
System—anatomy & histology—Atlases. WL 300 M381n 2003]
    QM451 .M27 2003
    611´.8—dc21
                                                                                    2002035061

INTERNATIONAL EDITION ISBN: 0-07-121237-X
Copyright © 2003. Exclusive rights by The McGraw-Hill Companies, Inc., for manufacture and export. This book cannot be re-exported from the country to which it is consigned by McGraw-Hill. The International edition is not available in North America.

TO CAROL, FOR HER SUPPORT AND UNDERSTANDING

Box Features

Contents

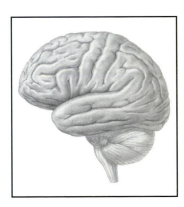

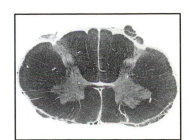

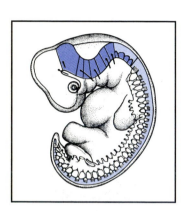
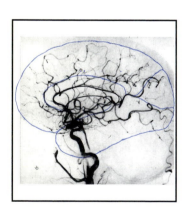

II *Sensory Systems* 105

5 Spinal Somatic Sensory Systems 107

6 Cranial Nerves and the Trigeminal and Viscerosensory Systems 135

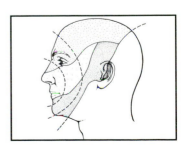

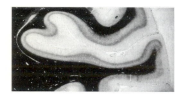

7 The Visual System 161

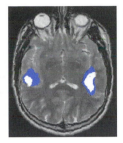
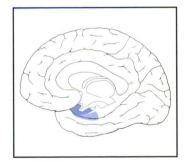

III   *Motor Systems*   227

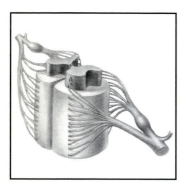

10 Descending Motor Pathways and the Motor Function of the Spinal Cord   229

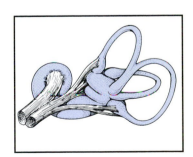

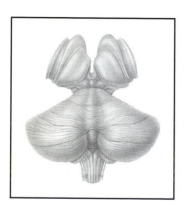

13 The Cerebellum 301

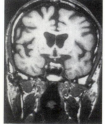 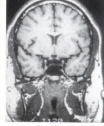

14 The Basal Ganglia 327

IV   Integrative Systems   349

15 The Hypothalamus and Regulation of Endocrine and Visceral Functions   351

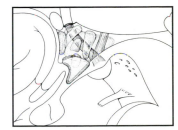

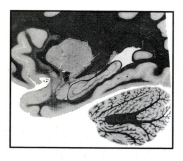

V   Atlas   407

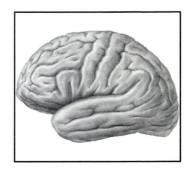
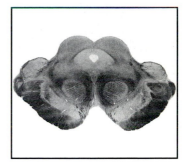

Preface

Neuroanatomy plays a crucial role in the health science curriculum, particularly as a means of preparing students for understanding the anatomical basis of clinical neurology. The routine use of the high-resolution brain imaging technique magnetic resonance imaging further underscores the importance of studying human neuroanatomy.

Neuroanatomy is the basic science for localizing function in the human brain. Imaging helps to identify, in the living brain, the particular brain regions where drugs may be acting to produce their neurological and psychiatric effects. Various experimental approaches in animals—including pathway tracing, localization of neuroactive chemicals using immunological techniques, and the effects of lesions—provide a rigorous scientific basis for localization of function that can be correlated with imaging data in humans. Thus, human brain imaging and experimental approaches in animals provide the neuroscientist and clinician with the means to elucidate and localize function in the human brain, to study the biological substrates of disordered thought and behavior, and to identify traumatized brain regions with unprecedented clarity. Nevertheless, to interpret the information obtained requires a high level of neuroanatomical competence.

Since the second edition of *Neuroanatomy: Text and Atlas,* clinical neuroscience has become significantly more dependent on localization of brain structures for treatments. Interventional electrophysiological procedures, such as deep brain stimulation for Parkinson disease and other movement disorders, is almost routine in many major medical centers. Surgical intervention is now the treatment of choice for many patients with temporal lobe epilepsy. These innovative approaches clearly require that the clinician have greater knowledge of functional neuroanatomy to carry out these tasks.

Neuroanatomy helps to provide key insights into disease by providing a bridge between molecular and clinical neural science. We now know the distribution of many different gene products, such as neurotransmitter receptor subtypes, in the normal human brain. By knowing how this distribution changes in the brains of patients with neurological and psychiatric disease, neuroanatomy helps to further our understanding of how pathological changes in brain structure alter brain function.

While always important for students of systems neuroscience, neuroanatomy is also becoming a key discipline for students of molecular neuroscience. This is because our understanding of basic neuronal processes has advanced at such a rapid pace that it is now necessary in many fields of study to move from the single neuron to the neural circuit. Learning and memory and drug addiction are two clear examples where molecular models are now being applied to diverse sets of brain regions that are interconnected by complex circuits.

An important goal of *Neuroanatomy: Text and Atlas* is to prepare the reader for interpreting a new wealth of images by developing an understanding of the anatomical localization of brain function. To provide a workable focus, this book is restricted to a treatment of the central nervous system. It takes a traditional approach to gaining neuroanatomical competence: Because the basic imaging picture is a two-dimensional slice through the brain, the locations of structures are examined on two-dimensional myelin-stained sections through the human central nervous system.

What is new for the third edition of *Neuroanatomy: Text and Atlas?* In addition to expanded coverage of important underrepresented topics, all chapters have been revised to reflect advances in neural science since the last edition; there are also several new features. Important to instructors and students alike, the overall length of the book has not increased significantly.

The order of the introductory chapters has been changed to better reflect how the chapters are typically used.

There are two somatic sensory chapters, one on the ascending spinal pathways and the organization of the somatic sensory thalamic and cortical areas, and the other on the trigeminal system. This approach was taken because the organization of the spinal and trigeminal somatosensory systems is remarkably similar.

The auditory and vestibular systems are covered in separate chapters. Audition is covered in its own chapter, and the vestibular system is addressed along with balance and eye movement control. This organization is both practical and efficient because the vestibular system is so tightly linked to balance and eye movement control, and it is also clinically relevant because vestibular functions are routinely tested in physical and neurological examinations.

A glossary of key terms and structures is intended to provide salient information about function and location.

Many new boxes have been added that augment clinical topics and demonstrate how recent research findings are being applied to solve clinical problems. For example, one box discusses how scientists are using brain mapping to promote functional recovery after brain injury and another examines innovative approaches to axonal regeneration after spinal injury.

Several boxes have been added that describe research that is beginning to elucidate the functional circuits for important public health issues such as drug addiction and the control of feeding.

The organization of *Neuroanatomy: Text and Atlas* parallels that of *Principles of Neural Science,* edited by Eric R. Kandel, James H. Schwartz, and Thomas Jessell (McGraw-Hill). Like *Principles of Neural Science, Neuroanatomy: Text and Atlas* is aimed at medical, dental, physical therapy, and other allied health science students, as well as graduate students in the neurosciences and psychology. Designed as a self-study guide and resource for information on the structure and function of the human central nervous system, this book could serve as both text and atlas for an introductory laboratory course in human neuroanatomy. Here at the College of Physicians and Surgeons, we use this book in conjunction with a series of weekly neuroanatomy laboratory exercises during a single semester.

John H. Martin, PhD

Acknowledgments

I take this opportunity to recognize the help I received in the preparation of the third edition of *Neuroanatomy: Text and Atlas.* I am grateful to the following friends and colleagues who have read portions of the manuscript or have provided radiological or histological materials: David Amaral, Jim Ashe, Richard Axel, Bertil Blok, Bud Craig, Mike Crutcher, Christine Curcio, Adrian Danek, Aniruddha Das, Sam David, John Dowling, Gary Duncan, Susan Folstein, Peter Fox, Stephen Frey, Apostolos Georgopoulos, Lice Ghilardi, Mickey Goldberg, James Goldman, Pat Goldman-Rakic, Suzanne Haber, Shaheen Hamdy, Jonathan Horton, David Hubel, Sharon Juliano, Joe LeDoux, Marge Livingstone, Randy Marshall, Bill Merigan, Etienne Olivier, Jesús Pujol, Josef Rauschecker, Patricia Rodier, David Ruggiero, Neal Rutledge, Brian Somerville, Bob Vassar, Bob Waters, Torsten Wiesel, and Semir Zeki. I also would like to thank Alice Ko for help with the three-dimensional reconstructions that provided the basis for various illustrations.

I would like to extend a special note of thanks to members of the neuroanatomy teaching faculty at the College of Physicians and Surgeons for many helpful discussions. For the text, I am grateful to Amy Marks for editorial assistance. For the illustrations carried over from the second edition, I thank Michael Leonard, the original illustrator, and the folks at Dragonfly Media Group, for their fine modifications of many figures of this edition. I also thank Howard Radzyner for the superb photographs of myelin-stained brain sections. At McGraw-Hill, I am indebted to Charissa Baker for her careful management of the art program. I appreciate the hard work of Harriet Lebowitz, Senior Development Editor, Nicky Fernando, Editorial Supervisor, and Catherine Saggese, Production Supervisor. Finally, I would like to thank my Editor Janet Foltin for her support, patience, and guidance—not to mention timely pressure—in the preparation of the third edition. Last, and most important, I thank Carol S. Martin for untiring support during the preparation of this edition and all previous editions of the book, and to Caitlin E. Martin, Rachel A. Martin, and Emma V. Martin for help with the many tasks incurred in preparing the book.

Guide to Using This Book

Neuroanatomy: Text and Atlas takes a combined regional and functional approach to teaching neuroanatomy: Knowledge of the spatial interrelations and connections between brain regions is developed in relation to the functions of the brain's various components. The book first introduces the major concepts of central nervous system organization. Subsequent chapters consider neural systems subserving particular sensory, motor, and integrative functions. At the end of the book is an atlas of surface anatomy of the brain and histological sections stained for the presence of the myelin sheath that surrounds axons, and a glossary of key terms and structures.

Overview of Chapters

The general structural organization of the mature central nervous system is surveyed in Chapter 1. This chapter also introduces neuroanatomical nomenclature and fundamental histological and imaging techniques for studying brain structure and function. The three-dimensional shapes of key deep structures are also considered in this chapter. The functional organization of the central nervous system is introduced in Chapter 2. This chapter considers how different neural circuits, spanning the entire central nervous system, serve particular functions. The circuits for touch perception and voluntary movement control are used as examples. The major neurotransmitter systems are also discussed. Development of the central nervous system is taken up in Chapter 3. The complex shapes of brain structures are better understood by considering their development.

Central nervous system vasculature and cerebrospinal fluid are the topics of Chapter 4. By considering vasculature early in the book, the reader can better understand why particular functions can become profoundly disturbed when brain regions are deprived of nourishment. These four chapters are intended to provide a synthesis of the basic concepts of the structure of the central nervous system and its functional architecture. A fundamental neuroanatomical vocabulary is also established in these chapters.

The remaining 12 chapters examine the major functional neural systems: sensory, motor, and integrative. These chapters reexamine the views of the surface and internal structures of the central nervous system presented in the introductory chapters, but from the perspective of the different functional neural systems. As these latter chapters on functional brain architecture unfold, the reader gradually builds a neuroanatomical knowledge of the regional and functional organization of the spinal cord and brain, one system at a time.

These chapters on neural systems have a different organization from that of the introductory chapters: Each is divided into two parts, functional and regional neuroanatomy. The initial part, on functional neuroanatomy, considers how particular brain regions work together to produce their intended functions. This part of the chapter presents an overall view of function in relation to structure before considering the detailed anatomical organization of the neural system. Together with descriptions of the functions of the various components, diagrams illustrate each system's anatomical organization, including key connections that help to show how the particular system accomplishes its tasks. Neural circuits that run through various divisions of the brain are depicted in a standardized format: Representations of myelin-stained sections through selected levels of the spinal cord and brain stem are presented with the neural circuit superimposed.

Regional neuroanatomy is emphasized in the latter part of the chapter. Here, structures are depicted on myelin-stained histological sections through the brain. These sections reveal the locations of major pathways and neuronal integrative regions. Typically, this part examines a sequence of myelin-stained sections ordered according to the flow of information processing in the system. For example, coverage of regional anatomy of the auditory system begins with the ear, where sounds are received and initially processed, and ends with the cerebral cortex, where our perceptions are formulated. In keeping with the overall theme of the book, the relation between the structure and the function of discrete brain regions is emphasized.

To illustrate the close relationship between neuroanatomy and radiology, magnetic resonance imaging (MRI) scans and positron emission tomography (PET) scans are included in many of the chapters. These scans are intended to facilitate the transition from learning the actual structure of the brain, as revealed by histological sections, to the "virtual structure," as depicted on the various imaging modalities. This is important in learning to "read" the scans, an important clinical skill. However, there is no substitute for actual stained brain sections for developing an understanding of three-dimensional brain structure.

Atlas of the Central Nervous System

This book's atlas, in two parts, offers a complete reference of anatomical structure. The first part presents key views of the surface anatomy of the central nervous system. This collection of drawings is based on actual specimens but emphasizes features shared by each specimen. Thus, no single brain has precisely the form illustrated in the atlas. The second part of the atlas presents a complete set of photographs of myelin-stained sections through the central nervous system in three anatomical planes.

With few exceptions, the same surface views and histological sections used in the chapters are also present in the atlas. In this way, the reader does not have to cope with anatomical variability and is thus better able to develop a thorough understanding of a limited, and sufficiently complete, set of materials. Moreover, brain views and histological sections shown in the chapters have identified only the key structures and those important for the topics discussed. In the atlas, all illustrations are comprehensively labeled. The atlas also serves as a useful guide during a neuroanatomy laboratory.

Didactic Boxes

Selected topics that complement material covered in the chapters are presented in boxes. Neuroradiological and functional circuitry are two topics that are emphasized. In many of the boxes, a new perspective on neuroanatomy is presented, one that has emerged only recently from research. The neuroscience community is enthusiastic that many of these new perspectives may help explain changes in brain function that occur following brain trauma or may be used to repair the damaged nervous system.

Glossary

The glossary contains a listing of key terms and structures. Typically, these terms are printed in boldface. Key terms are defined briefly in the context of their usage in the chapters. Key structures are identified by location and function.

Study Aids

This book offers three features that can be used as aids in learning neuroanatomy initially as well as in reviewing for examinations, including professional competency exams:

- Summaries at the end of each chapter, which present concise descriptions of key structures in relation to their functions.
- A glossary of key terms.
- The atlas of key brain views and myelin-stained histological sections, which juxtapose unlabeled and labeled views. The unlabeled image can also be used for self-testing, such as for structure identification.

These study aids are designed to help the reader assimilate efficiently and quickly the extraordinary amount of detail required to develop a thorough knowledge of human neuroanatomy.

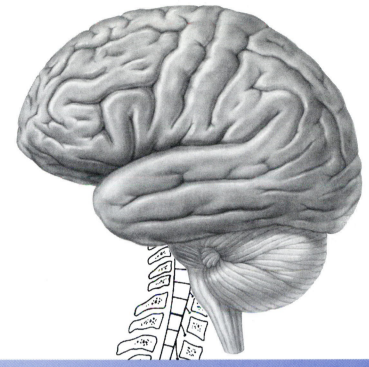

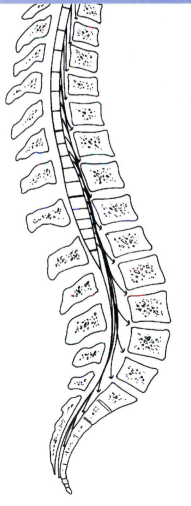

I The Central Nervous System

1

Introduction to the Central Nervous System

THE HUMAN NERVOUS SYSTEM CARRIES OUT an enormous number of functions by means of many subdivisions. Indeed, the brain's complexity has traditionally made the study of neuroanatomy a demanding task. This task can be greatly simplified by approaching the study of the nervous system from the dual perspectives of its regional and functional anatomy. **Regional neuroanatomy** examines the spatial relations between brain structures within a portion of the nervous system. Regional neuroanatomy defines the major brain divisions as well as local, neighborhood, relationships within the divisions. In contrast, **functional neuroanatomy** examines those parts of the nervous system that work together to accomplish a particular task, for example, visual perception. Functional systems are formed by specific neural connections within and between regions of the nervous system, connections that form complex neural circuits. A goal of functional neuroanatomy is to develop an understanding of the neural circuitry underlying behavior. By knowing regional anatomy together with the functions of particular brain structures, the clinician can determine the location of nervous system damage in a patient who has a particular neurological or psychiatric impairment. Combined knowledge of what structures do and where they are located is essential for a complete understanding of nervous system organization. The term *neuroanatomy* is therefore misleading because it implies that knowledge of structure is sufficient to master this discipline. Indeed, in the study of neuroanatomy, structure and function are tightly interwoven, so much so that they should not be separated. The interrelationships between structure and function underlie **functional localization,** a key principle of nervous system organization.

This chapter examines the organization of the nervous system and the means to study it by developing the vocabulary to describe its functional and regional anatomy. First, the cellular constituents of the nervous

3

system are described briefly. Then the chapter focuses on the major regions of the nervous system and the functions of these regions. This background gives the reader insight into functional localization. Box 1–1 discusses techniques for examining human brain structure. This material prepares the reader for a detailed exploration of the nervous system's functional and regional organization in the chapters that follow.

Neurons and Glia Are the Two Principal Cellular Constituents of the Nervous System

The nerve cell, or **neuron,** is the functional cellular unit of the nervous system. Neuroscientists strive to understand the myriad functions of the nervous system partly in terms of the interconnections between neurons. The other major cellular constituent of the nervous system is the neuroglial cell, or **glia.** Glia provide structural and metabolic support for neurons during development and in the mature brain.

All Neurons Have a Common Morphological Plan

Although neurons come in different shapes and sizes, each has four morphologically specialized regions with particular functions: dendrites, cell body, axon, and axon terminals (Figure 1–1A). **Dendrites** receive information from other neurons. The **cell body** contains the nucleus and cellular organelles critical for the neuron's vitality. The cell body also receives information from other neurons and serves important integrative functions. The **axon** conducts information, which is encoded in the form of action potentials, to the **axon terminal.** Connections between two neurons in a neural circuit are made by the axon terminals of one and the dendrites and cell body of the other.

Despite a wide range of morphology, we can distinguish three classes of neurons based on the configuration of their dendrites and axons: unipolar, bipolar, and multipolar. Figure 1–1B shows examples of the three neuron types. These neurons were drawn by the distinguished Spanish neuroanatomist Santiago Ramón y Cajal at the beginning of the twentieth century.

Unipolar neurons are the simplest in shape (Figure 1–1B1). They have no dendrites; the cell body of unipolar neurons receives and integrates incoming information. A single axon, which originates from the cell body, gives rise to multiple processes at the terminal. In the human nervous system, unipolar neurons

control exocrine gland secretions and smooth muscle contractility.

Bipolar neurons have two processes that arise from opposite poles of the cell body (Figure 1–1B2). The flow of information in bipolar neurons is from one of the processes, which functions like a dendrite, across the cell body to the other process, which functions like an axon. A morphological subtype of bipolar neuron is a pseudounipolar neuron (see Figure 5–1A). During development the two processes of the embryonic bipolar neuron fuse into a single process in the pseudounipolar neuron, which bifurcates a short distance from the cell body. Many sensory neurons, such as those that transmit information about odors or touch to the brain, are bipolar and pseudounipolar neurons.

Multipolar neurons feature a complex array of dendrites on the cell body and a single axon (Figure 1–1B3). Most of the neurons in the brain and spinal cord are multipolar. Multipolar neurons that have long axons, with axon terminals located in distant sites, are termed **projection neurons.** Projection neurons mediate communication between brain regions, and much of the study of human neuroanatomy focuses on the origins, paths, and terminations of these neurons. The neuron in Figure 1–1B3 is a particularly complex projection neuron. The terminals of this neuron are not shown because they are located far from the cell body. For this type of neuron in the human, the axon may be up to 1 meter long, about 50,000 times the width of the cell body! The long axons of projection neurons are particularly vulnerable to trauma: When an axon is cut because of an injury, the portion isolated from the cell body degenerates. This is because the neuron's cell body provides nutritional and other support for the axon. A specialized projection neuron is the motor neuron, which projects to peripheral targets, such as striated muscle cells. Other multipolar neurons, commonly called **interneurons,** have short axons that remain in the same brain region in which the cell body is located. Interneurons help to process neuronal information within a local brain region.

Neurons Communicate with Each Other at Synapses

Information flow along a neuron is polarized. The dendrites and cell body receive and integrate incoming information, which is transmitted along the axon to the terminals. Communication of information from one neuron to another also is polarized and occurs at specialized sites of contact called **synapses.** The neuron that sends information is the **presynaptic neuron** and the one that receives the information is the **post-**

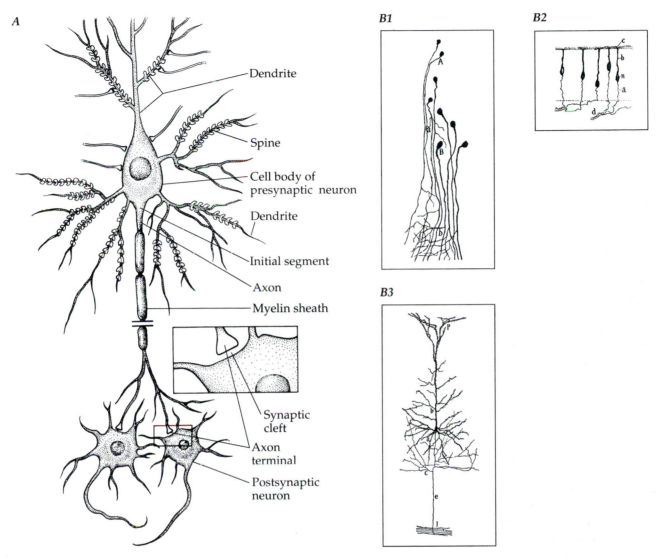

A

Dendrite

Spine

Cell body of
presynaptic neuron

Dendrite

Initial segment

Axon

Myelin sheath

Synaptic
cleft

Axon
terminal

Postsynaptic
neuron

B1

B2

B3

Figure 1–1. Neurons are the functional cellular unit of the nervous system. *A.* A schematic nerve cell is shown, illustrating the dendrites, cell body, and axon. Dendritic spines are located on the dendrites. These are sites of excitatory synapses. Inhibitory synapses are located on the shaft of the dendrites, the cell body, and the initial segment. The axon can be seen to emerge from the cell body. The presynaptic terminals of the neuron are shown synapsing on the cell bodies of the postsynaptic neurons. The inset shows the spatial relations of three components of the synapse: the presynaptic axon terminal, the synaptic cleft, and the postsynaptic neuron. *B.* Selected examples of three neuron classes: (*B1*) unipolar, (*B2*) bipolar, and (*B3*) multipolar. (*A, Adapted from Kandel ER, Schwartz JH, Jessell TM (editors): Principles of Neural Science, 4th ed. McGraw-Hill, 2000. B, Reproduced from Cajal SR: Histologie du système nerveux de l'homme et des vertébres. 2 vols. Maloine, 1909, 1911.)*

synaptic neuron. The information carried by the presynaptic neuron is transduced at the synapse into a chemical signal that is received by the dendrites and cell body of the postsynaptic neuron.

The synapse consists of three distinct elements: (1) the **presynaptic terminal,** the axon terminal of the presynaptic neuron, (2) the **synaptic cleft,** the narrow intercellular space between the neurons, and (3) the

receptive membrane of the postsynaptic neuron. Synapses are present on dendrites; the cell body; the **initial segment,** or the portion of the axon closest to the cell body; and the presynaptic terminal. Synapses located on different sites can serve different integrative functions.

To send a message to its postsynaptic target neurons, a presynaptic neuron releases **neurotransmitter,** packaged into vesicles, into the synaptic cleft. Neurotransmitters are small molecular weight compounds; among these are amino acids (eg, glutamate; glycine; and γ-aminobutyric acid, or GABA), acetylcholine, and monoaminergic compounds such as norepinephrine and serotonin. Larger molecules, such as peptides (eg, enkephalin and substance P), also can function as neurotransmitters. After release into the synaptic cleft, the neurotransmitter molecules diffuse across the cleft and bind to receptors on the postsynaptic membrane. The various postsynaptic actions of a particular neurotransmitter are mediated through distinct receptor populations. Neurotransmitters have two principal postsynaptic actions. First, by changing the permeability of particular ions, a neurotransmitter can either excite or inhibit the postsynaptic neuron. For example, excitation can be produced by a neurotransmitter that increases the flow of sodium ions into a neuron (ie, depolarization), and inhibition can be produced by a neurotransmitter that increases the flow of chloride ions into a neuron (ie, hyperpolarization). Glutamate and acetylcholine typically excite neurons, whereas GABA and glycine typically inhibit neurons. Many neurotransmitters, like dopamine and serotonin, have more varied actions, exciting some neurons and inhibiting others. They can even excite or inhibit the same neuron depending on which receptor the neurotransmitter engages. Second, most neurotransmitters also influence the function of the postsynaptic neuron through somewhat slower actions on second messengers and other intracellular signaling pathways. This action can have short-term effects, such as changing membrane ion permeability, or long-term effects, such as gene expression. Several compounds that produce strong effects on neurons are not packaged into vesicles; they are thought to act through diffusion. These compounds, for example, nitric oxide, are produced in the postsynaptic neuron and are thought to act as retrograde messengers that serve important regulatory functions, including maintaining and modulating the strength of synaptic connections.

Although chemical synaptic transmission is the most common way of sending messages from one neuron to another, purely electrical communication can occur between neurons. At such **electrical synapses** there is direct cytoplasmic continuity between the presynaptic and postsynaptic neurons.

Glial Cells Provide Structural and Metabolic Support for Neurons

Glial cells comprise the other major cellular constituent of the nervous system; they outnumber neurons by about 10 to 1. Given this high ratio, the structural and metabolic support that glial cells provide for neurons must be a formidable task! There are two major classes of glia: microglia and macroglia. **Microglia** subserve a phagocytic or scavenger role, responding to nervous system infection or damage. They are rapidly mobilized in response to minor pathological changes. Activated microglial cells can destroy invading microorganisms, remove debris, and promote tissue repair. **Macroglia,** of which there are four separate types—oligodendrocytes, Schwann cells, astrocytes, and ependymal cells—have a variety of support and nutritive functions. **Schwann cells** and **oligodendrocytes** form the **myelin sheath** around peripheral and central axons, respectively (Figures 1–1A and 1–2). The myelin sheath increases the velocity of action potential conduction. It is whitish in appearance because it is rich in a fatty substance called **myelin.** Schwann cells also play important roles in organizing the formation of the connective tissue sheaths surrounding peripheral nerves during development and in axon regeneration following damage in maturity. Oligodendrocytes may help guide developing axons to targets. **Astrocytes** have important structural and metabolic functions. For example, in the developing nervous system astrocytes act as scaffolds for growing axons. Astrocytes and the neurons for which they provide support may communicate directly: Changes in intracellular calcium in an astrocyte can modulate neuronal activity, and neural activity can trigger astrocytes to produce trophic substances. The last class of macroglia, **ependymal cells,** line fluid-filled cavities in the central nervous system (see below). They play an important role in regulating the flow of chemicals from these cavities into the brain.

The Nervous System Consists of Separate Peripheral and Central Components

Neurons and glial cells of the nervous system are organized into two anatomically separate but functionally interdependent parts: the **peripheral** and the **central nervous systems** (Figure 1–3A). The peripheral nervous system is subdivided into **somatic** and **autonomic** divisions. The somatic division contains the sensory neurons that innervate the skin, muscles, and joints. These neurons detect and, in turn, inform the central nervous system of all stimuli. This division also contains the axons of motor neurons that innervate skeletal muscle, although the cell bodies of motor neurons lie within the central nervous system. These axons transmit control signals to muscle to regulate the force of contraction. The autonomic division

Figure 1–2. Astrocytes and oligodendrocytes are the most ubiquitous types of glial cells in the central nervous system. Parts *A* and *B* are histological sections from the rat brain. *A.* An astrocyte from the cerebral cortex with multiple processes that end up on cerebral capillaries. *B.* Two oligodendrocytes from the subcortical white matter showing the fine processes connecting the cell bodies to the myelin sheaths surrounding several axons. *C.* Schematic diagram of an oligodendrocyte with processes surrounding multiple axons, similar to *B.* The node corresponds to the node of Ranvier, which is the gap between the myelin sheaths over adjacent segments of an axon. *(Parts A and B, courtesy of Dr. James Goldman, Columbia University. Part A, adapted from Kakita and Goldman, Neuron 23: 461–472, 1999. Part B, adapted from Levinson and Goldman, Neuron 10: 201–212, 1993. Part C, adapted from Kandel ER, Schwartz JS, Jessell TM (editors): Principles of Neural Science, 4th ed. McGraw-Hill, 2000.)*

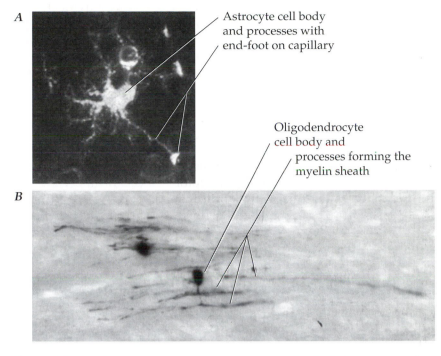

Astrocyte cell body and processes with end-foot on capillary

Oligodendrocyte cell body and processes forming the myelin sheath

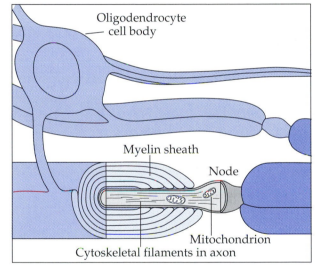

Oligodendrocyte cell body

Myelin sheath

Node

Cytoskeletal filaments in axon

Mitochondrion

contains the neurons that innervate glands and the smooth muscle of the viscera and blood vessels (see Chapter 15). This division, with its separate **sympathetic, parasympathetic,** and **enteric** subdivisions, regulates body functions based, in part, on information about the body's internal state. The autonomic nervous system was once thought not to be under conscious control. We now know that many autonomic functions can indeed be controlled but with greater difficulty than that required to control skeletal muscles.

The central nervous system consists of the **spinal cord** and **brain** (Figure 1–3A), and the brain is further subdivided into the medulla, pons, cerebellum, mid-brain, diencephalon, and cerebral hemispheres (Figure 1–3B). Within each of the seven central nervous system divisions resides a component of the **ventricular system,** a labyrinth of fluid-filled cavities that serve various supportive functions (see Figure 1–11).

Neuronal cell bodies and axons are not distributed uniformly within the nervous system. In the peripheral nervous system, cell bodies collect in peripheral **ganglia** and axons are contained in **peripheral nerves.** In the central nervous system, neuronal cell bodies and dendrites are located in **cortical** areas, which are flattened sheets of cells (or laminae) located primarily on the surface of the cerebral hemispheres, and in **nuclei,** which are clusters of neurons located beneath

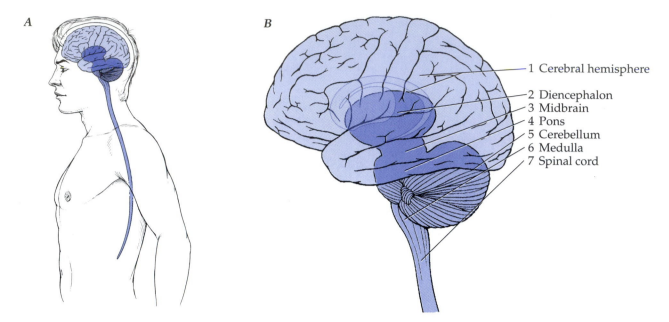

A

B

1 Cerebral hemisphere
2 Diencephalon
3 Midbrain
4 Pons
5 Cerebellum
6 Medulla
7 Spinal cord

Figure 1–3. *A.* Location of the central nervous system in the body. *B.* There are seven major divisions of the central nervous system: (1) cerebral hemispheres, (2) diencephalon, (3) midbrain, (4) pons, (5) cerebellum, (6) medulla, and (7) spinal cord. The midbrain, pons, and medulla comprise the brain stem.

the surface of all of the central nervous system divisions. Nuclei come in various sizes and shapes; they are commonly spherical and oval but sometimes occur in complex three-dimensional configurations (see Figure 1–8B). Regions of the central nervous system that contain axons have an unwieldy number of names, the most common of which is **tract**. In fresh tissue, nuclei and cortical areas appear grayish and tracts appear whitish, hence the familiar terms **gray matter** and **white matter.** The whitish appearance of tracts is caused by the presence of the myelin sheath surrounding the axons (Figure 1–1A). The gray and white matter can be distinguished in fixed tissue using anatomical methods and in the living brain using radiological methods (see Box 1–1).

The Spinal Cord Displays the Simplest Organization of All Seven Major Divisions

The spinal cord participates in processing sensory information from the limbs, trunk, and many internal organs; in controlling body movements directly; and in regulating many visceral functions (Figure 1–4). It also provides a conduit for the transmission of both sensory information in the tracts that ascend to the brain and motor information in the descending tracts. The spinal cord is the only part of the central nervous system that has an external **segmental** organization,

reminiscent of its embryonic (see Chapter 3) and phylogenetic origins (Figure 1–4B, C). The spinal cord has a modular organization, in which every segment has a similar basic structure (Figure 1–4C).

Each spinal cord segment contains a pair of nerve roots (and associated rootlets) called the **dorsal** and **ventral roots.** (The terms *dorsal* and *ventral* describe the spatial relations of structures; these and other anatomical terms are explained later in this chapter.) Dorsal roots contain only **sensory axons,** which transmit sensory information into the spinal cord. By contrast, ventral roots contain **motor axons,** which transmit motor commands to muscle and other body organs. Dorsal and ventral roots exemplify the separation of function in the nervous system, a principle that is reexamined in subsequent chapters. These sensory and motor axons, which are part of the peripheral nervous system, become intermingled in the **spinal nerves** en route to their peripheral targets (Figure 1–4C).

The Brain Stem and Cerebellum Regulate Body Functions and Movements

The next three divisions—medulla, pons, and midbrain—comprise the **brain stem** (Figure 1–5). The brain stem has three general functions. First, it receives sensory information from cranial structures and controls the muscles of the head. These functions are simi-

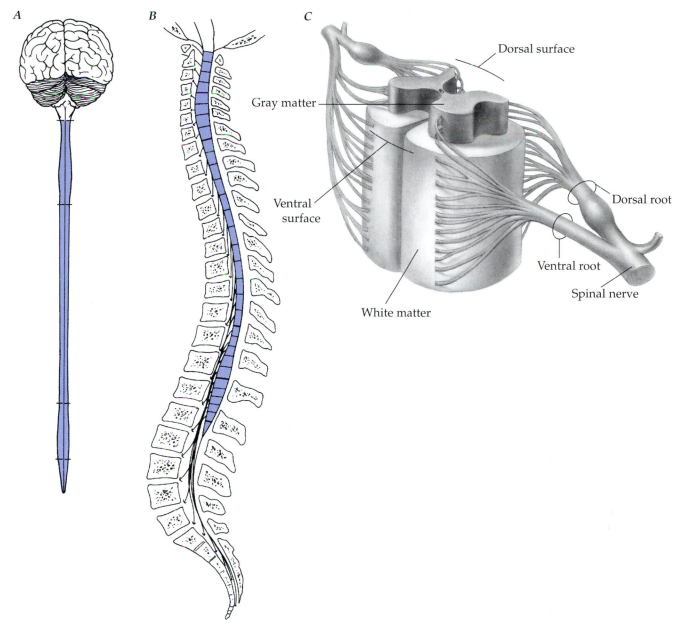

A

B

C

Dorsal surface

Gray matter

Ventral surface

White matter

Dorsal root

Ventral root

Spinal nerve

Figure 1–4. Spinal cord organization. *A.* A dorsal view of the central nervous system. *B.* A lateral view of the spinal cord and the vertebral column. *C.* Surface topography and internal structure of the spinal cord.

lar to those of the spinal cord. **Cranial nerves,** the sensory and motor nerve roots that enter and exit the brain stem, are parts of the peripheral nervous system and are analogous to the spinal nerves (Figure 1–5). Second, similar to the spinal cord, the brain stem is a conduit for information flow because ascending sensory and descending motor tracts travel through it. Finally, nuclei in the brain stem integrate information from a variety of sources for arousal and other higher brain functions.

In addition to these three general functions, the various divisions of the brain stem each subserve specific sensory and motor functions. For example, portions of the **medulla** participate in essential blood pressure and respiratory regulatory mechanisms. Indeed, damage to these parts of the brain is almost always life threatening. Parts of the **pons** and **midbrain** play a key role in the control of eye movement.

The principal functions of the **cerebellum** are to regulate eye and limb movements and to maintain

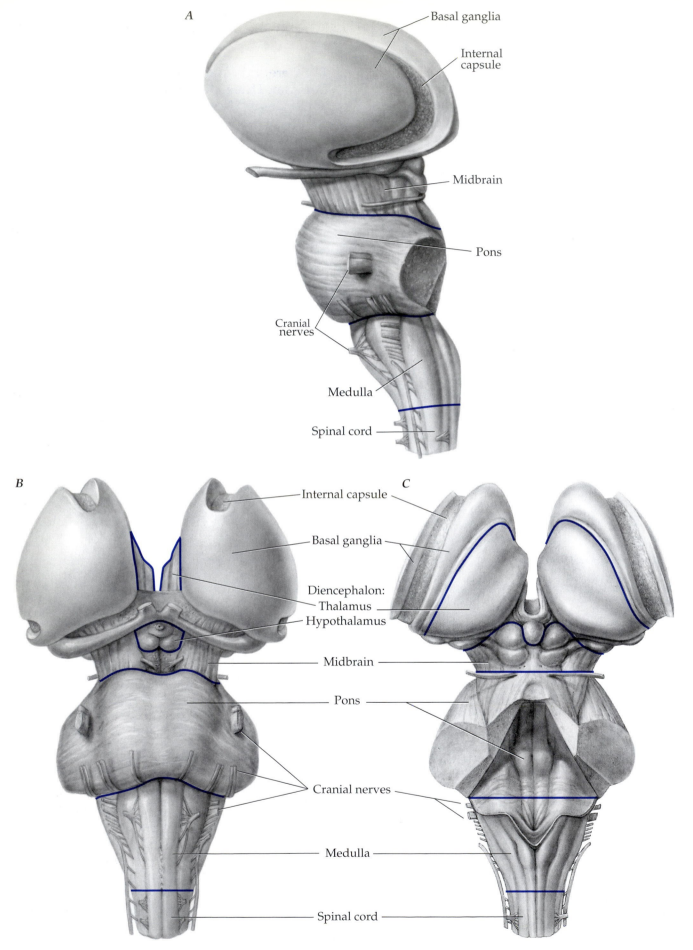

Figure 1–5. Lateral (*A*), ventral (*B*), and dorsal (*C*) surfaces of the brain stem. The thalamus and basal ganglia are also shown.

posture and balance (Figure 1–6). Limb movements become erratic and poorly coordinated when the cerebellum is damaged. The cerebellum also plays a role in more complex aspects of movement control, such as in motor decision making.

The Diencephalon Consists of the Thalamus and Hypothalamus

The two principal components of the **diencephalon** participate in diverse sensory, motor, and integrative functions. One component, the **thalamus** (Figure 1–7), is a key structure for transmitting information to the cerebral hemispheres. Neurons in separate thalamic nuclei transmit information to different cortical areas. In most brains, a small portion of the thalamus in each half adheres at the midline, the **thalamic adhesion.** The other component of the diencephalon, the **hypothalamus** (Figure 1–7; see also Figure 1–10A), integrates the functions of the autonomic nervous system and controls endocrine hormone release from the pituitary gland.

The Cerebral Hemispheres Have the Most Complex Three-Dimensional Configuration of All Central Nervous System Divisions

The **cerebral hemispheres** are the most highly developed portions of the human central nervous system. Each hemisphere is a distinct half, and each has four major components: cerebral cortex, hippocampal formation, amygdala, and basal ganglia. Together, these structures mediate the most sophisticated of human behaviors, and they do so through complex anatomical connections.

The Subcortical Components of the Cerebral Hemispheres Mediate Diverse Motor, Cognitive, and Emotional Functions

The **hippocampal formation** is important in learning and memory, whereas the **amygdala** not only participates in emotions but also helps to coordinate the body's response to stressful and threatening situations, such as preparing to fight (Figure 1–8A). These two

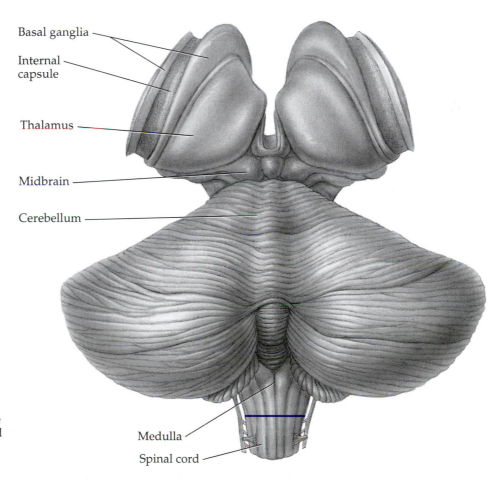

Basal ganglia

Internal capsule

Thalamus

Midbrain

Cerebellum

Medulla

Spinal cord

Figure 1–6. Dorsal view of the brain stem, thalamus, and basal ganglia, together with the cerebellum.

A

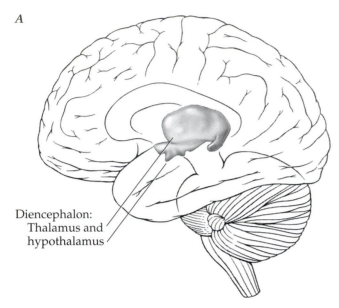

Diencephalon:
Thalamus and
hypothalamus

B

Thalamic
adhesion

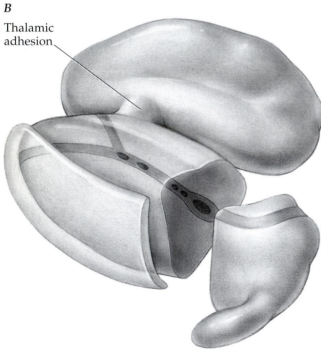

Figure 1–7. **A.** Lateral surface of the cerebral hemispheres and brain stem, illustrating the location of the thalamus and hypothalamus. **B.** Three-dimensional structure of the thalamus.

structures are part of the **limbic system** (see Chapter 16), which includes other parts of the cerebral hemispheres, diencephalon, and midbrain. Because parts of the limbic system play a key role in mood, it is not surprising that psychiatric disorders are often associated with limbic system dysfunction.

The **basal ganglia** are another deeply located collection of neurons. The portion of the basal ganglia that has the most complex shape is called the **striatum** (Figure 1–8B). The role of the basal ganglia in the control of movement is clearly revealed when they become damaged, as in Parkinson disease. Tremor and a slowing of movement are some of the overt signs of this disease. The basal ganglia also participate in cognition and emotions in concert with the cerebral cortex and are key brain structures involved in addiction.

The Four Lobes of the Cerebral Cortex Each Have Distinct Functions

The **cerebral cortex,** which is located on the surface of the brain, is highly convoluted (Figures 1–9 and 1–10). Convolutions are an evolutionary adaptation to fit a greater surface area within the confined space of the cranial cavity. In fact, only one quarter to one third of the cerebral cortex is exposed on the surface. The elevated convolutions on the cortical surface, called **gyri,** are separated by grooves called **sulci** or **fissures** (which are particularly deep sulci). The cerebral hemispheres are separated from each other by the **sagittal** (or interhemispheric) **fissure** (Figure 1–10B).

The four **lobes** of the cerebral cortex are named after the cranial bones that overlie them: frontal, parietal, occipital, and temporal (Figure 1–9, inset). The functions of the different lobes are remarkably distinct, as are the functions of individual gyri within each lobe.

The **frontal lobe** serves diverse behavioral functions, although most of the lobe is devoted to the planning and production of body and eye movements, speech, cognition, and emotions. The **precentral gyrus** contains the **primary motor cortex,** which participates in controlling the mechanical actions of movement, such as the direction and speed of reaching. Many projection neurons in the primary motor cortex have an axon that terminates in the spinal cord. The superior, middle, and inferior frontal gyri form most of the remaining portion of the frontal lobe. The premotor areas, which are important in motor decision making and planning movements, are adjacent to the primary motor cortex in these gyri. The inferior frontal gyrus in the left hemisphere in most people contains Broca's area, which is essential for the articulation of speech. Much of the frontal lobe is **association cortex.** Association cortical areas are involved in the complex processing of sensory and other information for higher brain functions, including emotions, organizing behavior, thoughts, and memories. Areas closer to the frontal pole comprise the **prefrontal association**

A

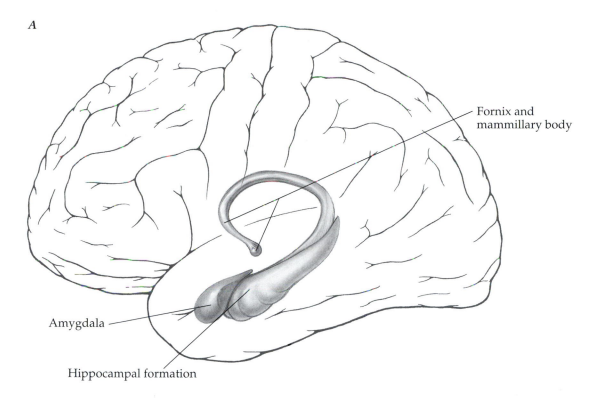

B

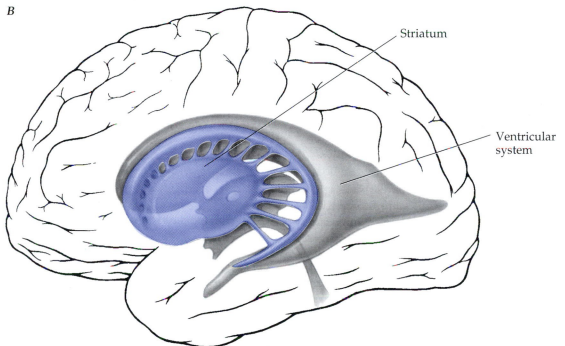

Figure 1–8. Three-dimensional views of deep structures of the cerebral hemisphere. *A.* The hippocampal formation and amygdala. The fornix and mammillary body are structures that are anatomically and functionally related to the hippocampal formation. *B.* Striatum, a component of the basal ganglia. The ventricular system is also illustrated. Note the similarity in overall shapes of the striatum and the lateral ventricle.

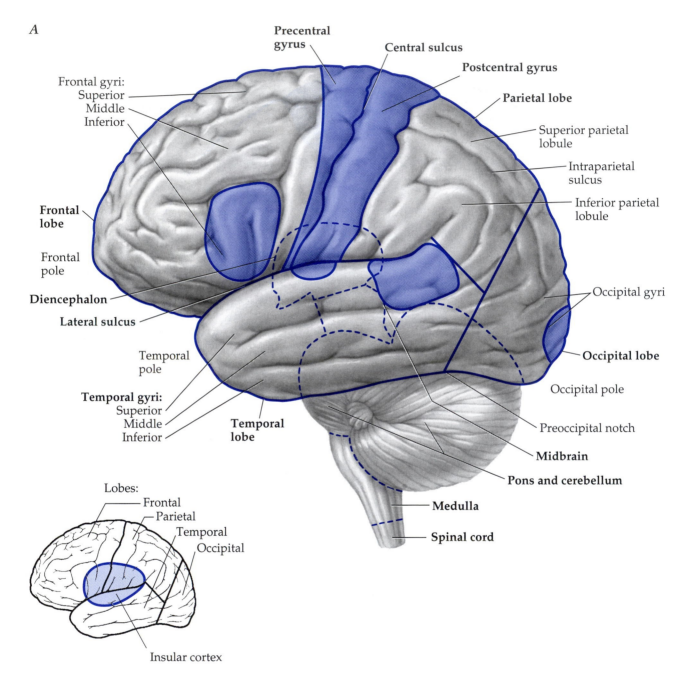

A

Precentral gyrus

Central sulcus

Postcentral gyrus

Parietal lobe

Frontal gyri:
Superior
Middle
Inferior

Superior parietal lobule

Intraparietal sulcus

Inferior parietal lobule

Frontal lobe

Frontal pole

Occipital gyri

Diencephalon

Lateral sulcus

Occipital lobe

Temporal pole

Occipital pole

Temporal gyri:
Superior
Middle
Inferior

Preoccipital notch

Temporal lobe

Midbrain

Pons and cerebellum

Medulla

Spinal cord

Lobes:
Frontal
Parietal
Temporal
Occipital

Insular cortex

Figure 1–9. *A.* Lateral surface of cerebral hemisphere and brain stem and a portion of the spinal cord. The blue regions correspond to distinct functional cortical areas. The primary motor and somatic sensory areas are located in the pre- and postcentral gyri, respectively. The primary auditory cortex lies in the superior temporal gyrus adjacent to the sensory and motor areas. Broca's area comprises most of the inferior frontal gyrus and Wernicke's area is in the posterior part of the superior temporal gyrus. Boldface labeling indicates key structures. The inset shows the four lobes of the cerebral cortex.

B

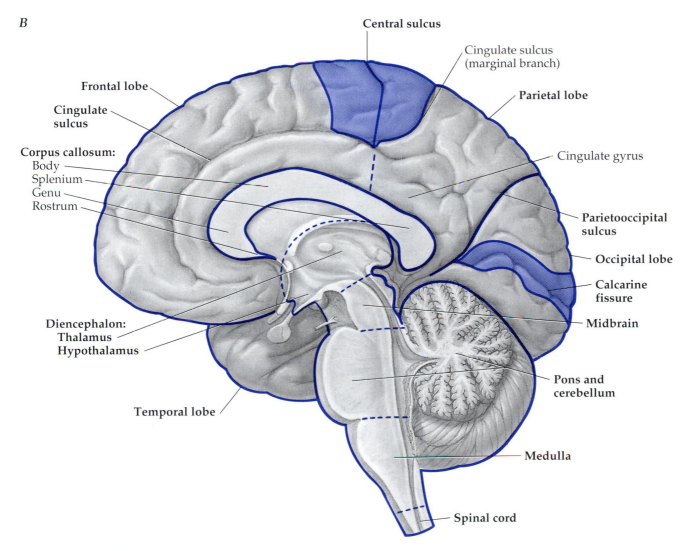

Figure 1–9 (continued).   *B.* Medial surface. The primary visual cortex is in the banks of the calcarine fissure.

A

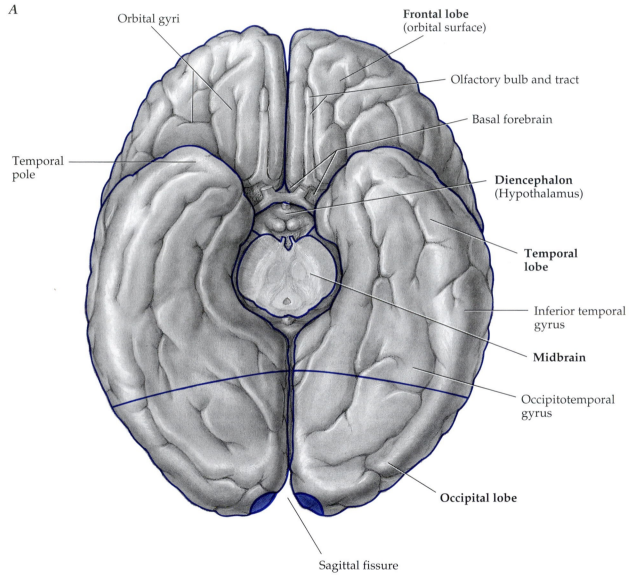

Orbital gyri

Frontal lobe
(orbital surface)

Olfactory bulb and tract

Basal forebrain

Temporal pole

Diencephalon
(Hypothalamus)

Temporal lobe

Inferior temporal gyrus

Midbrain

Occipitotemporal gyrus

Occipital lobe

Sagittal fissure

Figure 1–10. *A.* Ventral surface of the cerebral hemisphere and diencephalon; the midbrain is cut in cross section. The primary visual cortex is shown at the occipital pole.

B

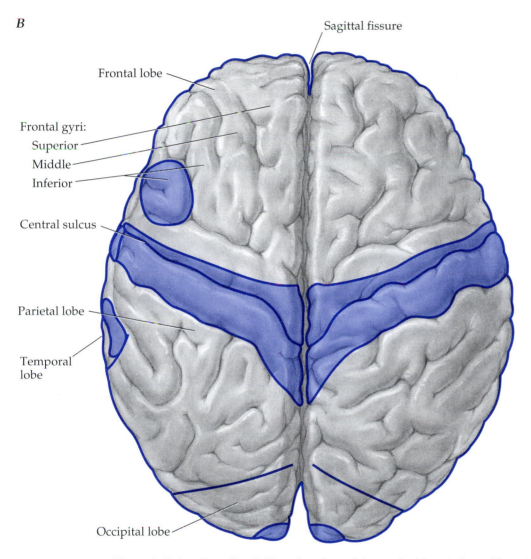

Sagittal fissure

Frontal lobe

Frontal gyri:
Superior
Middle
Inferior

Central sulcus

Parietal lobe

Temporal lobe

Occipital lobe

Figure 1–10 (continued). **B.** Dorsal surface of the cerebral hemisphere. The primary motor and somatic sensory cortical areas are located anterior and posterior to the central sulcus. Broca's area is in the inferior frontal gyrus and Wernicke's area is located in the posterior temporal lobe. The primary visual cortex is shown at the occipital pole.

cortex, which is important in cognition and emotions. The **cingulate gyrus** (Figure 1–9B) and most of the **orbital gyri** (Figure 1–10A) are important for emotional functions. The **basal forebrain,** which is on the ventral surface of the frontal lobe, contains a special population of neurons that use acetylcholine to regulate cortical excitability. These neurons are examined further in Chapter 2. Although the olfactory sensory organ, the **olfactory bulb,** is located on the ventral surface of the frontal lobe, its connections are predominantly with the temporal lobe (Figure 1–10A).

The **parietal lobe,** which is separated from the frontal lobe by the **central sulcus,** mediates our perceptions of touch, pain, and limb position. These functions are carried out by the **primary somatic sensory cortex,** which is located in the **postcentral gyrus.** Primary sensory areas are the initial cortical processing stages for sensory information. The remaining portion of the parietal lobe on the lateral brain surface consists of the superior and inferior parietal lobules, which are separated by the intraparietal sulcus. The **superior parietal lobule** contains higher-order somatic sensory areas, for further processing of somatic sensory information, and other sensory areas. Together these areas are essential for a complete self-image of the body, and they mediate behavioral interactions with the world around us. A lesion in this portion of the parietal lobe in the right hemisphere, the side of the brain that is specialized for spatial awareness, can produce bizarre neurological signs that include neglecting a portion of the body on the side opposite the lesion. For example, a patient may not dress one side of her body or comb half of her hair. The **inferior parietal lobule** is involved in integrating diverse sensory information for perception and language, mathematical thought, and visuospatial cognition. Interestingly, the inferior parietal lobule was greatly enlarged in Albert Einstein's brain. It is intriguing to speculate that Einstein's intellectual gifts reflect this structural difference.

The **occipital lobe** is separated from the parietal lobe on the medial brain surface by the **parietooccipital sulcus** (Figure 1–9B). On the lateral and inferior surfaces there are no distinct boundaries, only an imaginary line connecting the **preoccipital notch** (Figure 1–9A) with the parietooccipital sulcus. The occipital lobe is the most singular in function, subserving visual perception. The **primary visual cortex** is located in the walls and depths of the **calcarine fissure** on the medial brain surface (Figure 1–9B). Whereas the primary visual cortex is important in the initial stages of visual processing, the surrounding higher-order visual areas play a role in elaborating the sensory message that enables us to see the form and color of objects. For example, on the ventral brain surface is a portion of the occipitotemporal gyrus in the occipital lobe (also termed the fusiform gyrus) that is important for recognizing faces (Figure 1–10A). Patients with a lesion of this area can confuse faces with inanimate objects.

The **temporal lobe,** separated from the frontal and parietal lobes by the **lateral sulcus** (or **Sylvian fissure**) (Figure 1–9A), mediates a variety of sensory functions and participates in memory and emotions. The **primary auditory cortex,** located on the **superior temporal gyrus,** works with surrounding areas on the superior temporal gyrus within the lateral sulcus and on the middle temporal gyrus for perception and localization of sounds (Figure 1–9A). The superior temporal gyrus on the left side is specialized for speech. Lesion of the posterior portion of this gyrus, which is the location of Wernicke's area, impairs the understanding of speech. The **inferior temporal gyrus** mediates the perception of visual form and color (Figures 1–9A and 1–10A). The cortex located at the **temporal pole** (Figure 1–10A), together with adjacent portions of the medial temporal lobe and inferior and medial frontal lobes, are important for emotions.

Deep within the lateral sulcus are portions of the frontal, parietal, and temporal lobes. This territory is termed the **insular cortex** (Figure 1–9, inset). It becomes buried late during prenatal development (see Chapter 3). Portions of the insular cortex are important in taste, internal body senses, and some aspects of pain.

The **corpus callosum** contains axons that interconnect the cortex on the two sides of the brain (Figure 1–9B). Tracts containing axons that interconnect the two sides of the brain are called **commissures,** and the corpus callosum is the largest of the brain's commissures. To integrate the functions of the two halves of the cerebral cortex, axons of the corpus callosum course through each of its four principal parts: rostrum, genu, body, and splenium (Figure 1–9B). Information between the occipital lobes travels through the splenium of the corpus callosum, whereas information from the other lobes travels through the rostrum, genu, and body.

Cavities Within the Central Nervous System Contain Cerebrospinal Fluid

The central nervous system has a tubular organization. Within it are cavities, collectively termed the **ventricular system,** that contain **cerebrospinal fluid** (Figure 1–11). Cerebrospinal fluid is a watery fluid that cushions the central nervous system from physi-

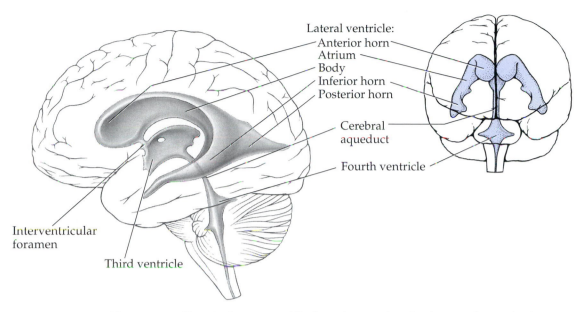

Lateral ventricle:
Anterior horn
Atrium
Body
Inferior horn
Posterior horn

Cerebral aqueduct

Fourth ventricle

Interventricular foramen

Third ventricle

Figure 1–11. Ventricular system. The lateral ventricles, third ventricle, cerebral aqueduct, and fourth ventricle are seen from the lateral brain surface (left) and the front (right). The lateral ventricle is divided into four main components: anterior (or frontal) horn, body, inferior (or temporal) horn, and the posterior (or occipital) horn. The interventricular foramen (of Monro) connects each lateral ventricle with the third ventricle. The cerebral aqueduct connects the third and fourth ventricles.

cal shocks and is a medium for chemical communication. An intraventricular structure, the **choroid plexus,** secretes most of the cerebrospinal fluid. Cerebrospinal fluid production is considered in Chapter 4.

The ventricular system consists of ventricles—often with bizarre shapes—where cerebrospinal fluid accumulates, and narrow communication channels. There are two **lateral ventricles,** and each is located within one cerebral hemisphere. They are further subdivided into a body and three compartments termed horns: anterior, posterior, and inferior (Figure 1–11). The confluence of the three horns is termed the **atrium.** Between the two halves of the diencephalon is the **third ventricle,** forming a midline cavity. (The two lateral ventricles were formerly termed the first and second ventricles.) The **fourth ventricle** is located between the brain stem and cerebellum: The medulla and pons form the floor of the fourth ventricle and the cerebellum, the roof. The ventricles are interconnected by narrow channels: The **interventricular foramina** (of Monro) connect each of the lateral ventricles with the third ventricle, and the **cerebral aqueduct** (of Sylvius), in the midbrain, connects the third and fourth ventricles. The ventricular system extends into the spinal

cord as the **central canal.** Cerebrospinal fluid exits the ventricular system through several apertures in the fourth ventricle and bathes the surface of the entire central nervous system.

The Central Nervous System Is Covered by Three Meningeal Layers

The **meninges** consist of the dura mater, the arachnoid mater, and the pia mater (Figure 1–12). The **dura mater** is the thickest and outermost of these membranes and serves a protective function. (*Dura mater* means "hard mother" in Latin.) Ancient surgeons knew that patients could survive even severe skull fractures if bone fragments had not penetrated the dura.

The portion of the dura mater overlying the cerebral hemispheres and brain stem contains two separate layers: an outer **periosteal layer** and an inner **meningeal layer** (Figure 1–12). The periosteal layer is attached to the inner surface of the skull. Two important partitions arise from the meningeal layer and separate different components of the cerebral hemispheres and brain stem (Figure 1–12B): (1) The **falx**

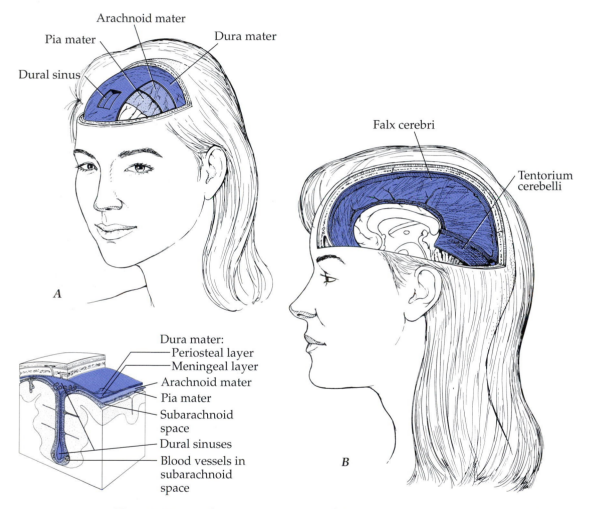

Pia mater

Arachnoid mater

Dura mater

Dural sinus

A

Falx cerebri

Tentorium cerebelli

Dura mater:
Periosteal layer
Meningeal layer
Arachnoid mater
Pia mater
Subarachnoid space
Dural sinuses
Blood vessels in subarachnoid space

B

Figure 1–12. ***A.*** The meninges consist of the dura mater, arachnoid mater, and pia mater. ***B.*** The two major dural flaps are the falx cerebri, which incompletely separates the two cerebral hemispheres, and the tentorium cerebelli, which separates the cerebellum from the cerebral hemisphere. The inset shows the dural layers. (***A,*** *Adapted from Snell RS: Clinical Neuroanatomy for Medical Students. Little, Brown, 1987.*)

cerebri separates the two cerebral hemispheres, and (2) the **tentorium cerebelli** separates the cerebellum from the cerebral hemispheres. The dura mater that covers the spinal cord is continuous with both the meningeal layer of the cranial dura and the epineurium of peripheral nerves.

The **arachnoid mater** adjoins but is not tightly bound to the dura mater, thereby allowing a potential space, the **subdural space,** to exist between them. This space is important clinically. Because the dura mater contains blood vessels, breakage of one of its vessels due to head trauma can lead to subdural bleeding and to the formation of a blood clot (a **subdural hematoma**). In this condition the blood clot pushes the arachnoid mater away from the dura mater, fills the subdural space, and compresses underlying neural tissue.

The innermost meningeal layer, the **pia mater,** is very delicate and adheres to the surface of the brain and spinal cord. (*Pia mater* means "tender mother" in Latin.) The space between the arachnoid mater and pia mater is the **subarachnoid space.** Filaments of arachnoid mater pass through the subarachnoid space and connect to the pia mater, giving this space the appearance of a spider's web. (Hence the name *arachnoid,* which derives from the Greek word *arachne,* meaning "spider.") After leaving the fourth ventricle, cerebrospinal fluid circulates over the surface of the brain and spinal cord within the subarachnoid space. Chapter 4 examines the path through which cerebrospinal fluid is returned to the venous circulation.

The meninges also serve an important circulatory function. The veins and arteries that overlie the surface of the central nervous system are located in the subarachnoid space. Moreover, within the dura mater are large, low-pressure blood vessels that are part of the return path for cerebral venous blood. These vessels are termed the **dural sinuses** (Figure 1–12, inset; see also Chapter 4). (The meninges are more commonly called the dura, arachnoid, and pia, without using the term *mater.*)

An Introduction to Neuroanatomical Terms

The terminology of neuroanatomy is specialized for describing the brain's complex three-dimensional organization. The central nervous system is organized along the **rostrocaudal** and **dorsoventral** axes of the body (Figure 1–13). These axes are most easily understood in animals with a central nervous system that is simpler than that of humans. In the rat, for example, the rostrocaudal axis runs approximately in a straight line from the nose to the tail (Figure 1–13A). This axis

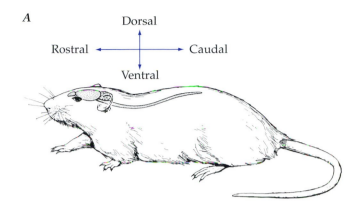

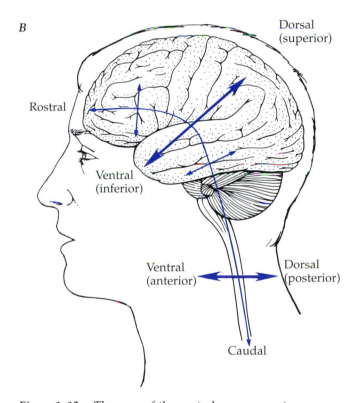

Figure 1–13. The axes of the central nervous system are illustrated for the rat (***A***), an animal whose central nervous system is organized in a linear fashion, and the human (***B***), whose central nervous system has a prominent flexure at the midbrain. (*Adapted from Kandel ER, Schwartz JH, Jessell TM (editors): Principles of Neural Science, 4th ed. McGraw-Hill, 2000.*)

is the **longitudinal axis** of the nervous system and is often termed the **neuraxis** because the central nervous system has a predominant longitudinal organization. The dorsoventral axis, which is perpendicular to the rostrocaudal axis, runs from the back to the abdomen. The terms **posterior** and **anterior** are synonymous with dorsal and ventral, respectively.

The longitudinal axis of the human nervous system is not straight as it is in the rat (Figure 1–13B). During development the brain—and therefore its longitudinal axis—undergoes a prominent bend, or **flexure,** at the midbrain. Instead of describing structures located rostral to this flexure as dorsal or ventral, we typically use the terms **superior** and **inferior.**

We define three principal planes relative to the longitudinal axis of the nervous system in which anatom-ical sections are made (Figure 1–14). **Horizontal** sections are cut parallel to the longitudinal axis, from one side to the other. **Transverse** sections are cut perpendicular to the longitudinal axis, between the dorsal and ventral surfaces. Transverse sections through the cerebral hemisphere are roughly parallel to the coronal suture and, as a consequence, are also termed **coronal** sections. **Sagittal** sections are cut parallel both to the longitudinal axis of the central nervous system and to the midline, between the dorsal and ventral surfaces. A **midsagittal** section divides the central nervous system into two symmetrical halves, whereas a **parasagittal** section is cut off the midline. Radiological images are also obtained in these planes. Box 1–1 shows an example of a magnetic resonance image in the sagittal plane (see Figure 1–16B).

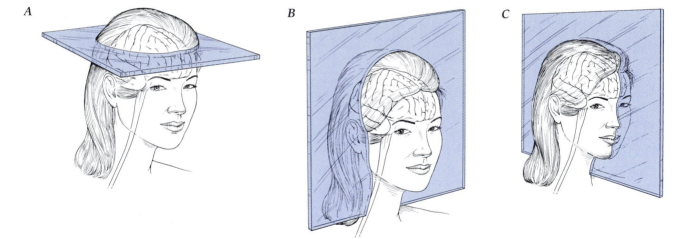

A *B* *C*

Figure 1–14. The three main anatomical planes: (*A*) horizontal, (*B*) coronal, and (*C*) sagittal. Note that the horizontal plane is shown through the cerebral hemispheres and diencephalon. A section in the same plane but through the brain stem or spinal cord is called a transverse section because it cuts the neuraxis at a right angle (see Figure 1–13B). The coronal plane is sometimes termed transverse because it is also at a right angle to the neuraxis (see Figure 1–13B). Unfortunately the terminology becomes even more confusing. A coronal section through the cerebral hemispheres and diencephalon will slice the brain stem and spinal cord parallel to their long axis. Strictly speaking this would be a horizontal section. However, this term is not useful for the human brain because such a "horizontal" section is oriented vertically.

Box 1–1. Anatomical and Radiological Techniques for Studying the Regional Anatomy of the Human Central Nervous System

There are two principal anatomical methods for studying normal regional human neuroanatomy using postmortem tissue. **Myelin stains** use dyes that bind to the myelin sheath surrounding axons. Unfortunately, in myelin-stained material the white matter of the central nervous system stains black and the gray matter stains light. (The terms white matter and gray matter derive from their appearance in fresh tissue.) **Cell stains** use dyes that bind to components within a neuron's cell body. Tissues prepared with either a cell stain or a myelin stain have a characteristically different appearance (Figure 1–15). The various staining methods are used to reveal different features of the nervous system's organization. For example, cell stains are used to characterize the cellular architecture of nuclei and cortical areas, and myelin stains are used to reveal the general topography of brain regions. Myelin staining is also used to reveal the location of damaged axons because, after such damage, the myelin sheath degenerates. This results in unstained tissue that otherwise ought to stain darkly (see Figure 2–4). Other staining methods reveal the detailed morphology of neurons—their dendrites, cell body, and axon (see Figure 13–12)—or the presence of specific neuronal chemicals such as neurotransmitters, receptor molecules, or enzymes (see Figure 14–9). Certain lipophilic dyes that diffuse preferentially along neuronal membranes can be applied directly to a postmortem brain specimen. This technique allows a limited amount of tracing of neural connections in the human brain.

Several radiological techniques are routinely used to image the living human brain. **Computerized tomography** (CT) produces scans that are images of a single plane, or "slice," of tissue. The image produced is a computerized reconstruction of the degree to which different tissues absorb

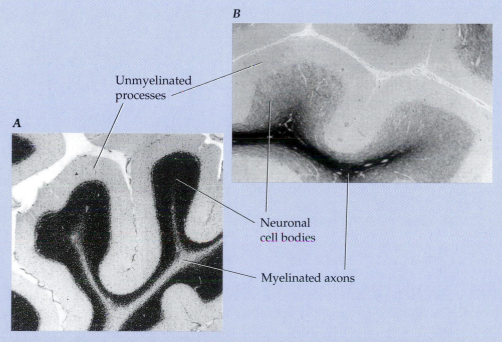

Figure 1–15. **A.** Section through the human cerebellar cortex, stained to indicate the location of neuronal cell bodies. The Nissl method was used for this tissue. This staining method uses a dye that binds to acid groups, in particular to ribonucleic acids of the ribosomes, located within cell bodies. The portion of the gray matter with the highest density of neuronal cell bodies stains the darkest. **B.** Myelin-stained section through the human cerebellar cortex. The white matter of the cerebellar cortex stains the darkest.

Box 1–1 (continued).

transmitted x-rays. Although CT scans are commonly used clinically to reveal intracranial tumors and other pathological changes, the overall level of anatomical resolution is poor. **Magnetic resonance imaging** (MRI) probes the regional anatomy of the brain in remark-ably precise detail. Magnetic resonance images reveal primarily differences in the water content of tissue. Figure 1–16A shows a magnetic resonance image, in the sagittal plane, close to the midline. The gyri and cerebrospinal fluid in the sulci look like the drawn image of the medial surface of the brain (Figure 1–16B). The image of the brain stem and cerebellum is a "virtual slice." MRI mechanisms are described in more detail in Box 2–1, and functional imaging methods are described in Box 2–2.

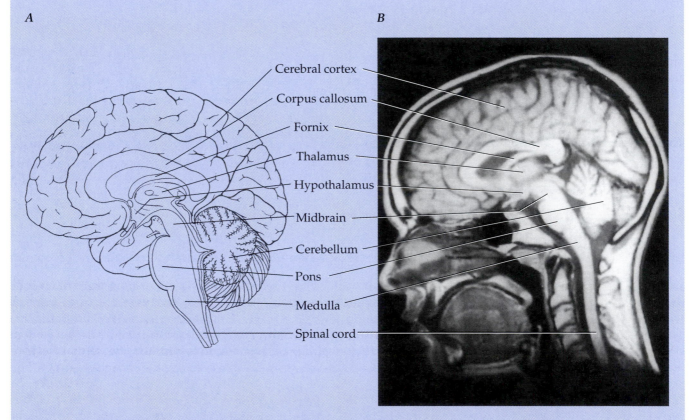

A

B

Cerebral cortex

Corpus callosum

Fornix

Thalamus

Hypothalamus

Midbrain

Cerebellum

Pons

Medulla

Spinal cord

Figure 1–16. **A.** Drawing of the medial surface of the cerebral hemisphere. **B.** Magnetic resonance imaging (MRI) scan of the midsagittal human central nervous system. (*B, Courtesy of Dr. Neal Rutledge, University of Texas at Austin.*)

Summary

Cellular Organization of the Nervous System

The cellular constituents of the nervous system are **neurons** (Figure 1–1) and **glia** (Figure 1–2). Neurons have four specialized regions: (1) the **dendrites,** which receive information, (2) the **cell body,** which receives and integrates information, and (3) the **axon,** which transmits information from the cell body to (4) the **axon terminals.** There are three neuron classes: **unipolar, bipolar,** and **multipolar** (Figure 1–1B). Intercellular communication occurs at **synapses,** where a **neurotransmitter** is released. The glia include four types of **macroglia. Oligodendrocytes** and **Schwann cells** form the myelin sheath in the central and peripheral nervous systems, respectively. **Astrocytes** serve as structural and metabolic support for neurons. **Ependymal cells** line the ventricular system. The glia also consist of the **microglia,** which are phagocytic.

Regional Anatomy of the Nervous System

The nervous system contains two separate divisions, the **peripheral nervous system** and the **central nervous system** (Figure 1–3). Each system may be further subdivided. The **autonomic** division of the peripheral nervous system controls the glands and smooth muscle of the viscera and blood vessels, whereas the **somatic** division provides the sensory innervation of body tissues and the motor innervation of skeletal muscle. There are seven separate components of the central nervous system (Figures 1–3 through 1–10): (1) **spinal cord,** (2) **medulla,** (3) **pons,** (4) **cerebellum,** (5) **midbrain,** (6) **diencephalon,** which contains the **hypothalamus** and **thalamus,** and (7) **cerebral hemispheres,** which contain the **basal ganglia, amygdala, hippocampal formation,** and **cerebral cortex.** The external surface of the cerebral cortex is characterized by **gyri** (convolutions), **sulci** (grooves), and **fissures** (particularly deep grooves). The cerebral cortex consists of four lobes: **frontal, parietal, temporal,** and **occipital.** The **insular cortex** is buried beneath the frontal, parietal, and temporal lobes. The **corpus callosum,** a **commissure,** interconnects each of the lobes. Three sets of structures lie beneath the cortical surface: the **hippocampal formation,** the **amygdala,** and the **basal ganglia.** The **limbic system** comprises a diverse set of cortical and subcortical structures. The olfactory bulbs lie on the orbital surface of the frontal lobes.

Ventricular System

Cavities comprising the **ventricular system** are filled with **cerebrospinal fluid** and are located within the central nervous system (Figure 1–11). One of two **lateral ventricles** is located in each of the cerebral hemispheres, the **third ventricle** is located in the diencephalon, and the **fourth ventricle** is between the brain stem (pons and medulla) and the cerebellum. The **central canal** is the component of the ventricular system in the spinal cord. The **interventricular foramina** connect the two lateral ventricles with the third ventricle. The **cerebral aqueduct** is in the midbrain and connects the third and fourth ventricles.

Meninges

The central nervous system is covered by three meningeal layers, from outermost to innermost: **dura mater, arachnoid mater,** and **pia mater** (Figure 1–12). Arachnoid mater and pia mater are separated by the **subarachnoid space,** which also contains cerebrospinal fluid. Two prominent flaps in the dura separate brain structures: **falx cerebri** and the **tentorium cerebelli** (Figure 1–12). Also located within the dura are the **dural sinuses,** low-pressure blood vessels (Figure 1–12).

Axes and Planes of Section

The central nervous system is oriented along two major axes (Figure 1–13): the **rostrocaudal axis,** which is also termed the **longitudinal axis,** and the **dorsoventral axis,** which is perpendicular to the longitudinal axis. Sections through the central nervous system are cut in relation to the rostrocaudal axis (Figure 1–14). **Horizontal** sections are cut parallel to the rostrocaudal axis, from one side to the other. **Transverse,** or **coronal,** sections are cut perpendicular to the rostrocaudal axis, between the dorsal and ventral surfaces. **Sagittal** sections are cut parallel to the longitudinal axis and the midline, also between the dorsal and ventral surfaces.

Related Sources

Kandel ER, Schwartz JH, Jessell TM (editors): Principles of Neural Science, 4th ed. McGraw-Hill, 2000.

Selected Readings

Duvernoy HM: The Human Hippocampus. J. F. Bergmann Verlag, 1988.

Jessen KR, Mirsky R: Schwann cells and their precursors emerge as major regulators of nerve development. Trends Neurosci 1999;22:402–410.

Sigal R, Doyon D, Halimi P, Atlan H: Magnetic Resonance Imaging. Springer-Verlag, 1988.

Steinhauser C, Gallo V: News on glutamate receptors in glial cells. Trends Neurosci 1996;19:339–345.

References

Cajal SR: Histologie du système nerveux de l'homme et des vertèbres. 2 vols. Maloine, 1909, 1911.

Kreutzberg GW: Microglia: A sensor for pathological events in the CNS. Trends Neurosci 1996;19:312–318.

Nieuwenhuys R, Voogd J, Van Huijzen C: The Human Central Nervous System: A Synopsis and Atlas, 3rd ed. Springer-Verlag, 1988.

Ridet JL, Malhotra SK, Privat A, Gage FH: Reactive astrocytes: Cellular and molecular cues to biological function. Trends Neurosci 1997;20:570–577.

Rolls ET: The orbitofrontal cortex. Philos Trans R Soc Lond B Biol Sci 1996;351:1433–1443; discussion 1443–1444.

St George-Hyslop PH: Piecing together Alzheimer's. Sci Am 2000;283:76–83.

Witelson SF, Kigar DL, Harvey T: The exceptional brain of Albert Einstein. Lancet 1999;353:2149–2153.

Verkhratsky A, Kettenmann H: Calcium signalling in glial cells. Trends Neurosci 1996;19:346–352.

2

Structural and Functional Organization of the Central Nervous System

CHAPTER 1 FOCUSED ON THE LOCATIONS of the major divisions and components of the central nervous system (ie, regional anatomy) along with the functions in which these structures are engaged (ie, functional anatomy). From this consideration of regional and functional anatomy the principle of **functional localization** emerged. Each major division of the central nervous system, each lobe of the cortex, and even the gyri within the lobes perform a limited and often unique set of functions. For a thorough understanding of neuroanatomy, two essential features of nervous system organization—the specific patterns of connections between structures and the neural systems that regulate neuronal excitability—must also be understood.

By considering the patterns of **neural connections** between specific structures, this chapter begins to explain how the various components of the spinal cord and brain acquire their particular sensory, motor, or integrative functions. In addition to the specific connections between structures, neural circuits with widespread connections modulate the actions of neural systems with particular functions. Consider how the quiescent state of a mother's brain can be mobilized by the sound of her infant's cry during the night. The neural systems mediating arousal and other generalized functions involve the integrated actions of different parts of the brain stem, as well as populations of neurons that use particular neurotransmitters such as serotonin and dopamine. These neurotransmitter-specific regulatory systems are also particularly important in human behavioral dysfunction because many of their actions go awry in psychiatric disease.

This chapter explores brain connectivity and the internal structure of the central nervous system. First, it examines the overall organization of the neural systems for touch and for voluntary movement control and the different modulatory systems. Then it examines key anatomical sections through the spinal cord and brain. An understanding of the different neural systems is reinforced by identifying the locations of these systems in the central nervous system. Knowledge of the location of nuclei and tracts in these anatomical sections is important not only for understanding neuroanatomy but also for learning to identify brain structure on radiological images, the topics of Boxes 2–1 and 2–2.

The Dorsal Column–Medial Lemniscal System and Corticospinal Tract Have a Component at Each Level of the Neuraxis

The **dorsal column–medial lemniscal system,** the principal pathway for touch, and the **corticospinal tract,** the key pathway for voluntary movement, each have a longitudinal organization, spanning virtually the entire neuraxis. These two pathways are good examples of how particular patterns of connections between structures at different levels of the neuraxis produce a circuit with a limited number of functions.

The dorsal column–medial lemniscal system is termed an **ascending pathway** because it brings information from sensory receptors in the periphery to lower levels of the central nervous system, such as the brain stem, and then to higher levels, such as the thalamus and cerebral cortex. In contrast, the corticospinal tract, a **descending pathway,** carries information from the cerebral cortex to a lower level of the central nervous system, the spinal cord.

The dorsal column–medial lemniscal system (Figure 2–1A) consists of a three-neuron circuit that links the periphery with the cerebral cortex. In doing so it traverses the spinal cord, brain stem, diencephalon, and cerebral hemispheres. Even though there are minimally three neurons linking the periphery with the cortex, many thousands of neurons at each level are typically engaged during normal tactile experiences. The first neurons in the circuit are the dorsal root ganglion neurons, which translate stimulus energy into neural signals and transmit this information directly to the spinal cord and brain stem. This component of the system is a fast transmission line that is visible on the dorsal surface of the spinal cord as the **dorsal column** (see Figure 2–5B).

The first synapse is made in the **dorsal column nucleus,** a relay nucleus in the medulla. A relay nu-

---

A   Dorsal column – medial lemniscal system

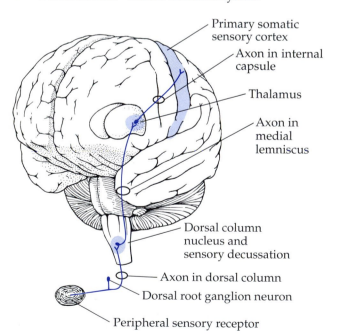

- Primary somatic sensory cortex
- Axon in internal capsule
- Thalamus
- Axon in medial lemniscus
- Dorsal column nucleus and sensory decussation
- Axon in dorsal column
- Dorsal root ganglion neuron
- Peripheral sensory receptor

B   Corticospinal tract

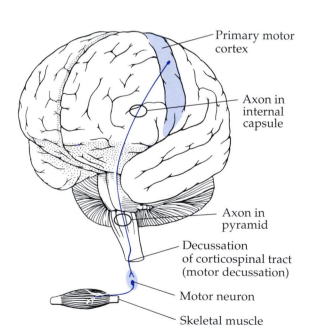

- Primary motor cortex
- Axon in internal capsule
- Axon in pyramid
- Decussation of corticospinal tract (motor decussation)
- Motor neuron
- Skeletal muscle

Figure 2–1. The dorsal column–medial lemniscal system (*A*) and the corticospinal tract (*B*) are longitudinally organized.

cleus processes incoming signals and transmits this information to the next component of the circuit. The cell bodies of the second neurons in the pathway are located in the dorsal column nucleus. The axons of these second-order neurons cross the midline, or **decussate.** Because of this decussation, sensory information from the right side of the body is processed by the left side of the brain. Most sensory (and motor) pathways decussate at some point along their course. Surprisingly, we do not know why neural systems decussate.

After crossing the midline the axons ascend in the brain stem tract, the **medial lemniscus,** to synapse in a relay nucleus in the **thalamus.** From here, third-order neurons send their axons through the white matter underlying the cortex, in the **internal capsule.** These axons synapse on neurons in the **primary somatic sensory cortex,** which is located in the postcentral gyrus of the parietal lobe (Figure 2–1A). Each sensory system has a primary cortical area and several higher-order areas. The primary area receives input directly from the thalamus and processes basic sensory information. The higher-order areas receive input predominantly from the primary and other cortical areas and participate in the elaboration of sensory processing leading to perception.

Axons of the corticospinal tract descend from the cerebral cortex to terminate on motor neurons in the spinal cord (Figure 2–1B). In contrast to the dorsal column–medial lemniscal system, in which fast transmission lines are interrupted by series of relay nuclei in the brain stem and thalamus, the corticospinal tract consists of single neurons that link the cortex directly with the spinal cord. The cell bodies of many corticospinal tract neurons are located in the primary motor cortex on the **precentral gyrus** of the frontal lobe, just rostral to the primary somatic sensory cortex. The axons of these neurons leave the motor cortex and travel down in the internal capsule, near the thalamic axons transmitting information to the somatic sensory cortex.

The corticospinal tract emerges from the internal capsule in the cerebral hemisphere to course ventrally within the brain stem. In the medulla the corticospinal axons form the **pyramid,** a prominent landmark on the ventral surface. In the caudal medulla, most corticospinal axons decussate (pyramidal, or motor, decussation) and descend into the spinal cord. These cortical axons travel within the white matter before terminating on motor neurons in the gray matter. These motor neurons innervate skeletal muscle; hence, the motor cortex can directly control limb and trunk movements. For example, patients with corticospinal tract damage,

commonly caused by interruption of the blood supply to the internal capsule, demonstrate arm muscle weakness and impaired fine motor skills.

The Modulatory Systems of the Brain Have Diffuse Connections and Use Different Neurotransmitters

Specificity of neural connections characterizes the somatic sensory and motor pathways. The dorsal column–medial lemniscal system can mediate our sense of touch because it specifically connects touch receptors in the skin with the cerebral cortex. Similarly, the corticospinal tract's role in controlling movement is conferred by its particular connections with motor circuits in the spinal cord. Several major exceptions exist in which systems of neurons have more widespread projections, and in each case these systems are thought to serve more generalized functions, such as motivation, arousal, or facilitation of learning and memory. The cell bodies of **diffuse-projecting neurons** are located throughout the brain stem, diencephalon, and basal forebrain; some are clustered into distinct nuclei and others are scattered. They terminate throughout the central nervous system. The reticular formation, which forms the central core of the brain stem, also has neurons with widespread connections that are important in regulating the overall level of arousal. Many neurons of the reticular formation project to neurons in the thalamus that, in turn, have diffuse projections (see below).

Four systems of diffuse-projecting neurons are highlighted here because of their importance in the sensory, motor, and integrative systems examined in subsequent chapters. Dysfunction of these systems can result in devastating psychiatric or neurological diseases. Each system uses a different neurotransmitter: acetylcholine, dopamine, noradrenalin (norepinephrine), or serotonin. Many of the neurons that use one of these neurotransmitters also contain other neuroactive compounds, such as peptides, that are released at the synapse at the same time.

Neurons in the Basal Nucleus of Meynert Contain Acetylcholine

The axons of **acetylcholine-**containing neurons in the basal forebrain (ie, at the base of the cerebral hemispheres) project throughout the cerebral cortex and hippocampal formation (Figure 2–2A). Acetylcholine

A

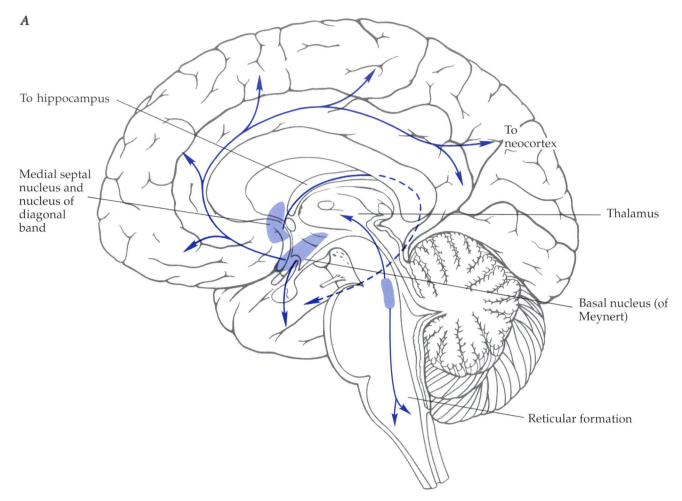

To hippocampus

Medial septal nucleus and nucleus of diagonal band

To neocortex

Thalamus

Basal nucleus (of Meynert)

Reticular formation

Figure 2–2. Groups of brain stem and forebrain neurons have diffuse projections throughout the central nervous system. *A.* Schematic illustration of the diffuse projection pattern of acetylcholine-containing neurons in the basal nucleus (of Meynert), septal nuclei, and nucleus of the diagonal band (of Broca). Many of the axons projecting to the hippocampal formation course in the fornix (dashed line).

augments the excitability of cortical neurons, especially in association areas. The **basal nucleus** (of Meynert) contains the cholinergic neurons that project to the cortex (Figure 2–2A), both on the medial surface (eg, the cingulate gyrus) and laterally (not shown). The cholinergic projection to the hippocampus and adjoining regions, located medially in the temporal lobe, originates from neurons in the medial septal nucleus and the nucleus of the diagonal band (of Broca). In **Alzheimer disease,** a neurological disease in which individuals lose memories and cognitive functions, these cholinergic neurons degenerate. There are also cholinergic neurons in the pedunculopontine nucleus, which is located in the pons. These cholinergic neurons are implicated in disordered movement control in Parkinson disease.

Neurons in the Substantia Nigra and Ventral Tegmental Area Contain Dopaminergic Neurons

The cells of origin of the dopaminergic system are located mostly in the midbrain (Figure 2–2B1), in the **substantia nigra** and **ventral tegmental area;** the major targets of these dopaminergic neurons are the striatum and portions of the frontal lobe. Dopamine strongly influences brain systems engaged in organizing behavior and planning movements. There are at least five major dopamine receptor types, which have different distributions within the central nervous system and different cellular actions. More is known of the clinical consequences of damage to brain dopamine systems than of the other neurotransmitter-specific

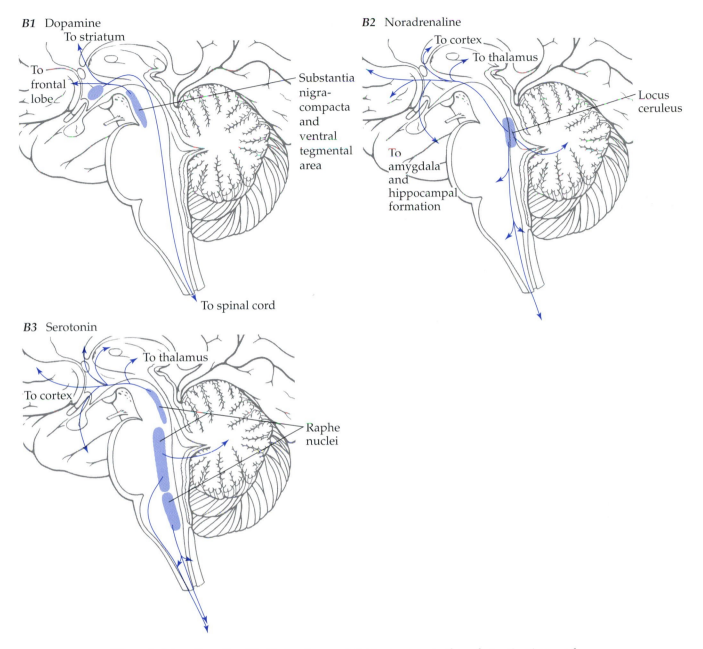

Figure 2–2 (continued). ***B1.*** Dopamine-containing neurons in the substantia nigra and ventral tegmental area. ***B2.*** Norepinephrine-containing neurons in the locus ceruleus. ***B3.*** Serotonin-containing neurons in the raphe nuclei.

systems. In **Parkinson disease,** for example, there is a loss of the dopamine-containing neurons in the substantia nigra. Movements become slowed in patients with Parkinson disease, and they develop tremor (see Chapter 14). These motor signs improve with dopamine replacement therapy. Dopamine is also implicated in schizophrenia, through the actions of the ventral tegmental area. The hypothalamus also contains dopaminergic neurons that are important in neuro-

endocrine control and regulation of the autonomic nervous system.

Neurons in the Locus Ceruleus Give Rise to a Noradrenergic Projection

Although there are numerous brain stem nuclei with noradrenergic neurons (Figure 2–2B2), the **locus** ceruleus has the most widespread projections. Based on the connections and the physiological properties of locus ceruleus neurons, this noradrenergic projection is thought to play an important role in the response of the brain to stressful stimuli, particularly those that evoke fear. The locus ceruleus, through its widespread noradrenergic projections to the cerebral cortex, has been implicated in depression and in panic attacks, an anxiety disorder. Additional noradrenergic cell groups are located in the caudal pons and medulla; these neurons are critically involved in maintaining the function of the sympathetic nervous system, especially in blood pressure regulation.

Neurons of the Raphe Nuclei Use Serotonin as Their Neurotransmitter

The **raphe nuclei** (Figure 2–2B3) consist of numerous distinct groups of brain stem neurons located close to the midline. Neurons in the raphe nuclei use serotonin as a neurotransmitter. The actions of the serotonin systems are diverse because there are many different serotonin receptor types. The raphe nuclei from the rostral pons and midbrain give rise to ascending projections. Dysfunction of the ascending serotonergic projection to the diencephalon and telencephalon has been implicated in disorders of thought and mood. Projections from the raphe nuclei in the medulla target other brain stem regions and the spinal cord. One function of the serotonergic projection to the spinal cord is to control the transmission of information about pain from the periphery to the central nervous system.

Guidelines for Studying the Regional Anatomy and Interconnections of the Central Nervous System

The rest of this chapter focuses on central nervous system organization from the perspective of its internal structure. In this and subsequent chapters, myelin-stained sections are used to help illustrate the structural and functional organization of the central nervous system. Many structures are distinguished clearly from their neighbors on these sections because of morphological changes at boundaries. For example, the lightly stained dorsal horn of the spinal cord (Figure 2–3A), which contains primarily neuronal cell bodies, can be distinguished from the darkly stained white matter, which contains myelinated axons. However, locating other structures on myelin-stained sections can be dif-

ficult because neighboring structures stain similarly. Thus, on a section from a person without corticospinal damage we can localize the corticospinal tract only to a general region in the white matter, because it is surrounded by other myelinated axons that stain the same. As we see in the next section, the location of such a structure in humans is determined by examining tissue from a person who sustained damage to the corticospinal tract during life. This is because after an axon has been damaged, such as by a physical injury or stroke, consistent structural changes occur. The portion of the axon distal to the cut, now isolated from the neuronal cell body, degenerates because it is deprived of nourishment. This process is termed **Wallerian** (or **anterograde**) **degeneration.** In the central nervous system, when a myelinated axon degenerates, the myelin sheath around the axon also degenerates. The tissue can be stained for the presence of myelin, in which case the territory with the degenerated axons will remain unstained, creating a negative image of their locations (Figure 2–4). Magnetic resonance imaging (MRI) is also used to illustrate brain structures, both in healthy patients and in those with neurological disease. Unfortunately, MRI does not provide sufficient detail for learning anatomy. We therefore use a combination of radiological and histological images throughout this book. In this chapter, radiological and histological images of the spinal cord, brain stem (five levels), and diencephalon and telencephalon (two levels) are used to illustrate the functions and locations of nuclei and tracts.

The Spinal Cord Has a Central Cellular Region Surrounded by a Region That Contains Myelinated Axons

The slice through the spinal cord shown in Figure 2–3A is stained for myelinated axons. The gray matter of the spinal cord contains two functionally distinct regions, the **dorsal** and **ventral horns.** The dorsal horn is the receptive, or sensory, portion of the spinal gray matter, and the ventral horn, the motor portion. The white matter of the spinal cord, which surrounds the gray matter, contains three rostrocaudally oriented columns in which axons ascend or descend: the dorsal, lateral, and ventral columns. Between the gray matter on the two sides of the spinal cord is the **central canal,** a component of the ventricular system. Portions of the central canal become closed in the adult.

Somatic sensory receptor neurons, **dorsal root ganglion neurons,** innervate peripheral tissue and trans-

A

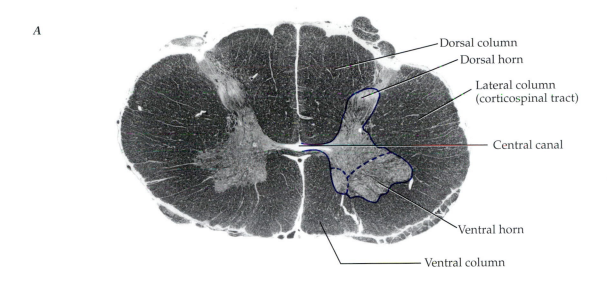

B

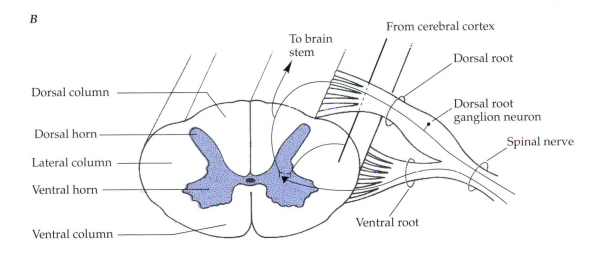

Figure 2–3. **A.** Myelin-stained transverse section through the cervical spinal cord. The three parts of the spinal gray matter—the dorsal horn, intermediate zone, and ventral horn—are distinguished. **B.** Three-dimensional schematic view of a spinal cord segment showing key spinal cord structures and the circuit for the knee-jerk reflex.

mit this sensory information to neurons in the central nervous system (Figure 2–3B). Different classes of dorsal root ganglion neurons sense different kinds of stimuli (eg, thermal or mechanical). The axons of the ganglion neurons enter the spinal cord through the **dorsal root.** Dorsal root ganglion neurons project their axons directly into the spinal gray and white matter. The ganglion neurons that synapse in the dorsal horn (not shown in the figure) are part of a circuit for protective senses: pain, temperature sense, and itch. The dorsal root ganglion neurons that branch into the white matter enter the dorsal column (Figure 2–3B). These neurons transmit to the brain stem sensory information about touch and limb position sense

Corticospinal tract

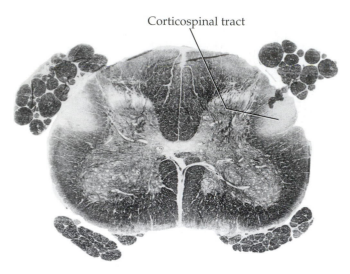

Figure 2–4. Myelin-stained section of pathological material from a patient who sustained damage to the corticospinal tract in the brain. The lightly stained region in the white matter is the region containing degenerated axons.

and are part of the dorsal column–medial lemniscal system.

Neurons of the ventral horn subserve limb and trunk movements. Motor neurons located here have axons that exit the spinal cord through the **ventral root.** Monosynaptic connections occur between a certain type of dorsal root ganglion neuron that innervates stretch receptors in muscles and motor neurons (Figure 2–3B). In certain segments of the spinal cord, this circuit mediates the **knee-jerk reflex.** A tap to the patella tendon stretches the quadriceps muscle, thereby stretching the receptors in the muscle. The central branches of dorsal root ganglion cells that innervate these receptors synapse on quadriceps motor neurons. Because this synapse is excitatory, the quadriceps motor neurons are discharged and the muscle contracts. Many leg and arm muscles have similar stretch reflexes.

Motor neurons also receive direct connections from the corticospinal tract, whose axons course in the **lateral column** of the white matter (Figure 2–3B). Whereas in healthy tissue the location of the corticospinal tract can only be inferred (Figure 3–3A), its location in tissue from a person who had a lesion involving the tract is clearly revealed as the lightly stained region in Figure 2–4. The ventral column contains the axons of both ascending sensory and descending motor pathways and is considered in later chapters.

For spinal circuits the terms *afferent* and *efferent* are often used in place of *sensory* and *motor* to describe the

direction of information flow. The term **afferent** means that axons transmit information toward a particular structure. For the dorsal root ganglion neurons, information flow is from the periphery to the central nervous system. Dorsal root ganglion neurons are often called primary afferent fibers. The term **efferent** indicates that the axons carry information away from a particular structure. For motor neurons, information flow is from the central nervous system to muscle fibers. The terms *afferent* and *efferent* are also commonly used to describe direction of information flow within the central nervous system in relation to a particular target. For example, with respect to the motor neuron, both dorsal root ganglion axons and axons in the corticospinal tract carry afferent information. There is a distinction, however, because only the former transmit sensory information.

Surface Features of the Brain Stem Mark Key Internal Structures

The rostral spinal cord merges with the brain stem, as can be seen in Figure 2–5, which illustrates the dorsal and ventral surfaces of these structures. On the dorsal brain stem surface (Figure 2–5B) are four major landmarks: dorsal columns, dorsal column tubercles, the fourth ventricle, and the colliculi. The dorsal columns and **tubercles** are part of the dorsal column–medial lemniscal system and are discussed further later in this chapter. With the cerebellum removed, the floor of the **fourth ventricle** can be identified by its rhomboid shape. The **colliculi** are four bumps located on the dorsal surface of the midbrain. The rostral pair of bumps, termed the superior colliculi, are important in controlling eye movements. The caudal pair, called the inferior colliculi, are involved in the processing of sounds.

Four major landmarks also can be identified on the ventral surface (Figure 2–5A): pyramids, olives, base of the pons, and basis pedunculi. Remarkably, all four are key components of the motor system. In the medulla the axons of the corticospinal tract are located in the **pyramids** and, just lateral to them, the **olives.** Neurons in the olives together with those in the **base of the pons,** the large basal surface of the pons, are major sources of afferent information to the cerebellum. Using this information the cerebellum controls the accuracy of movement. Finally, many of the axons immediately beneath the ventral midbrain surface in the **basis pedunculi** are part of the corticospinal tract. These axons descend through the base of the pons and emerge on the medullary surface in the pyramid.

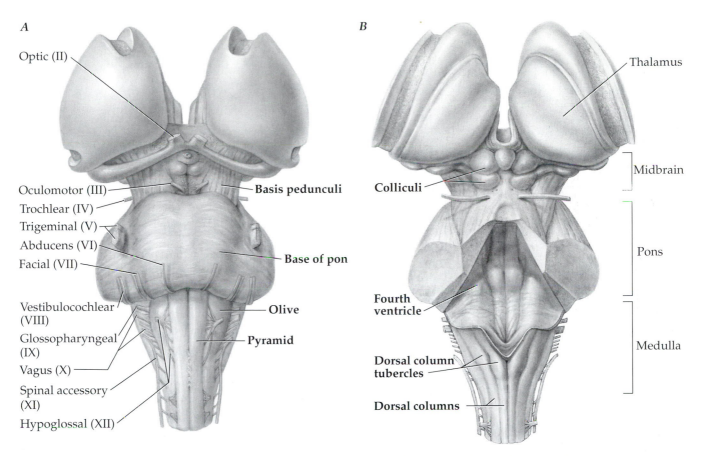

A

Optic (II)

Oculomotor (III)
Trochlear (IV)
Trigeminal (V)
Abducens (VI)
Facial (VII)

Basis pedunculi

Base of pon

Vestibulocochlear
(VIII)
Glossopharyngeal
(IX)
Vagus (X)
Spinal accessory
(XI)
Hypoglossal (XII)

Olive

Pyramid

B

Thalamus

Midbrain

Colliculi

Pons

**Fourth
ventricle**

Medulla

**Dorsal column
tubercles**

Dorsal columns

Figure 2–5. Ventral (*A*) and dorsal (*B*) surfaces of the brain stem, diencephalon, and telencephalon.

Another characteristic of the brain stem is the presence of the **cranial nerves** (Figure 2–5). Knowledge of their locations helps develop a general understanding of brain stem anatomy. There are 12 pairs of cranial nerves, which, like the spinal nerves, mediate sensory and motor function, but of cranial structures.

The next several sections address brain stem anatomy by examining transverse sections through five key levels: (1) the spinal cord–medullary junction, (2) the caudal medulla, (3) the middle medulla, (4) the caudal pons, and (5) the rostral midbrain. Knowledge of the surface features of the brain stem helps in recognizing the level of a particular section.

*The Organization of the Medulla Varies
From Caudal to Rostral*

There are three characteristic levels through the medulla. The caudal-most level is at the junction with the spinal cord. The key feature of this level is the

pyramidal (or motor) **decussation** (Figure 2–6C), which is where the corticospinal tract decussates. This decussation is also visible on the ventral brain stem surface (Figure 2–5A). Because of this decussation, one side of the brain controls muscles of the opposite side of the body (see Figure 2–1B).

The next level is in the midmedulla, through the dorsal column nuclei (Figure 2–6B), which relay information about touch to the thalamus. At this level the dorsal column nuclei bulge to form the dorsal surface landmarks, the dorsal column tubercles (Figure 2–5B). The second-order neurons of the dorsal column–medial lemniscal system originate in these nuclei. Their axons decussate and ascend to the thalamus in the medial lemniscus (Figure 2–6A and B). Because of this decussation, sensory information from one side of the body is processed by the other side of the brain (see Figure 2–1A). The corticospinal tract is located ventral to the medial lemniscus, in the medullary pyramid (Figure 2–5A). The medullary section in Figure 2–7 is from a person who sustained a corticospinal system injury.

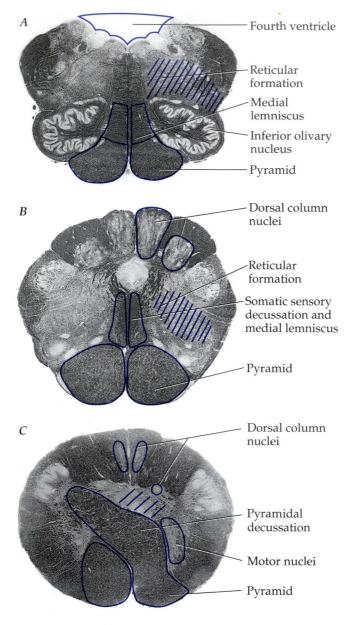

A — Fourth ventricle

Reticular formation

Medial lemniscus

Inferior olivary nucleus

Pyramid

B — Dorsal column nuclei

Reticular formation

Somatic sensory decussation and medial lemniscus

Pyramid

C — Dorsal column nuclei

Pyramidal decussation

Motor nuclei

Pyramid

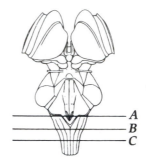

Figure 2–6. Myelin-stained sections through three levels of the medulla. From rostral to caudal through the: inferior olivary nucleus (*A*), dorsal column nuclei (*B*), and pyramidal decussation (*C*). Planes of the sections are indicated in the inset. Key medullary structures are highlighted.

Axons in the pyramid on one side have degenerated. Because of the absence of staining of that pyramid, the ventral border of the medial lemniscus is apparent.

The **reticular formation** comprises the central core of the brain stem. Although the reticular formation begins in the caudal medulla, it is a large structure in the midmedulla as well as farther rostrally in other brain divisions. Neurons in this region regulate arousal by influencing the excitability of neurons throughout the central nervous system. Some neurons of the modulatory systems described above are located in the reticular formation. Receiving input from all of the sensory modalities, neurons of the reticular formation can

affect neuronal excitability directly through diffuse projections rostrally and caudally, or indirectly by contacting other neurons with diffuse projections. An important path by which the reticular formation affects the excitability of cerebral cortical neurons is through connections with thalamic nuclei that have diffuse cortical projections (see below).

The third key medullary level is through the olive, a bulge located on the ventral medullary surface lateral to the medullary pyramid (Figure 2–5A), which marks the position of the **inferior olivary nucleus** (Figure 2–6A). This nucleus contains neurons whose axons project to the cerebellum, where they form one of the

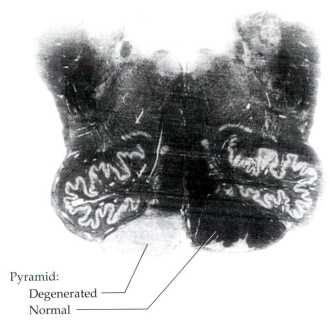

Pyramid:

Degenerated ———

Normal ———

Figure 2–7. Myelin-stained transverse section through the medulla from someone who had a large lesion of the internal capsule that destroyed the corticospinal tract on one side. Compare this section to the one in Figure 2–6A. The border between the medial lemniscus and the pyramid is estimated in Figure 2–6A but is revealed clearly in this figure.

strongest excitatory synapses in the entire central nervous system (see Chapter 13).

The rostral medulla provides a clear view of the ventricular system. The central canal, which is a microscopic structure in the spinal cord, expands to form the fourth ventricle in the rostral medulla. Whereas the ventricular floor is formed by the dorsal medulla, the roof consists of a thin tissue formed by the apposition of two glial layers during development: pia and ependyma.

Many of the nuclei of the brain stem are analogous in connections and functions to regions of spinal cord gray matter. For example, nuclei in the brain stem receive sensory input directly from the receptor neurons innervating cranial structures. These are the cranial nerve sensory nuclei, which have general functions similar to neurons of the dorsal horn. Similarly, cranial nerve motor nuclei in the brain stem innervate cranial muscles and are similar to motor nuclei of the ventral horn (see Figure 2–6A–C).

The Pontine Nuclei Surround the Axons of the Corticospinal Tract in the Base of the Pons

The dorsal surface of the pons forms part of the floor of the fourth ventricle; the cerebellum forms the roof (Figure 2–8A). The medial lemniscus, which is less distinct than in the medulla because neighboring myelinated fibers obscure its borders, is displaced dorsally by the **pontine nuclei.** Neurons in the pontine nuclei, which transmit information from the cerebral cortex to the cerebellum, participate in skilled movement control. The pontine nuclei surround the corticospinal axons; both nuclei and axons are located within the base of the pons (Figure 2–5A). The MRI scan of a similar pontine level in Figure 2–8B is from another patient who sustained injury to the corticospinal system (where it is located in the cerebral hemisphere; see below). The region containing degenerating fibers is revealed by a bright signal. The MRI scan also shows the cerebellum, which is attached to the dorsal pons.

The Dorsal Surface of the Midbrain Contains the Colliculi

The midbrain can be divided into three regions, moving from the dorsal surface to the ventral surface (Figure 2–9A): (1) the **tectum** (Latin for "roof"), (2) the **tegmentum** (Latin for "cover"), and (3) the **basis pedunculi** (Latin for "base stalk or support"). The tegmentum and basis pedunculi comprise the **cerebral peduncle.** The colliculi are located in the tectum. The superior colliculi (Figure 2–9) play an important role in controlling saccadic eye movement, and the inferior colliculi (located more caudally) are important in hearing.

The **cerebral aqueduct (of Sylvius),** which connects the third and fourth ventricles, is located at the border of the tectum and tegmentum. This ventricular conduit is surrounded by a nuclear region, termed the **periaqueductal gray,** which contains neurons that are part of the circuit for endogenous pain suppression. For example, pain may be perceived as less severe during intense emotional experiences such as childbirth or military combat, and this neural system participates in this pain diminution. The medial lemniscus is located within the tegmentum.

The corticospinal tract is located in the basis pedunculi. This pathway is therefore seen on the ventral surfaces of the midbrain and the medulla (as the pyramid). The substantia nigra, which contains dopaminergic neurons important in movement control (see Figure 2–2B1), separates the corticospinal fibers and the medial lemniscus. The **red nucleus** is another midbrain nucleus that helps control movement. The companion MRI in Figure 2–9B is from the same patient as in Figure 2–8B and shows the location of degenerating corticospinal axons in the midbrain. It should be noted

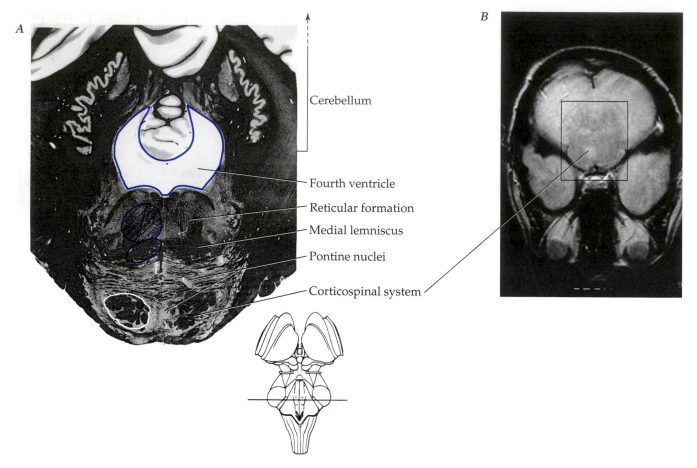

Figure 2–8. Myelin-stained section (*A*) and MRI scan (*B*) through the pons. The inset shows the planes of the section and the MRI scan. The reticular formation, medial lemniscus, and corticospinal system are outlined in *A*. The leader in *B* points to the light region, which contains degenerated descending cortical axons. (*B, Courtesy of Dr. Jesús Pujol; from Pujol J, Martí-Vilalta JL, Junqué C, Vendrell P, Fernández J, Capdevila A: Wallerian degeneration of the pyramidal tract in capsular infarction studied by magnetic resonance imaging. Stroke 1990;21:404–409.*)

that the imaging plane of this MRI scan is slightly different from that of the myelin midbrain section. As a consequence, the borders of the midbrain are blurred because of adjacent parts of the cerebellum, diencephalon, and cerebral hemispheres.

The Thalamus Transmits Information From Subcortical Structures to the Cerebral Cortex

Most sensory information reaches the cortex indirectly by relay neurons in the thalamus (Figure 2–10). This is also the case for neural signals controlling movements, learning and memory, and emotions. Neurons in each half of the thalamus project to the cerebral cortex on the same (ipsilateral) side. Thalamic neurons are clustered into discrete nuclei. The organization of thalamic nuclei can be approached from anatomical and functional perspectives. Based on their locations, six nuclear groups are distinguished in the thalamus (Figure 2–10). The four major groups are named according to their locations with respect to bands of myelinated axons, called the **internal medullary laminae:** (1) anterior nuclei, (2) medial nuclei, (3) lateral nuclei, and (4) intralaminar nuclei, which lie within the laminae. The two other nuclear groups are (5) the midline nuclei and (6) the reticular nucleus.

On the basis of the extent and functions of their cortical connections, we divide the various thalamic

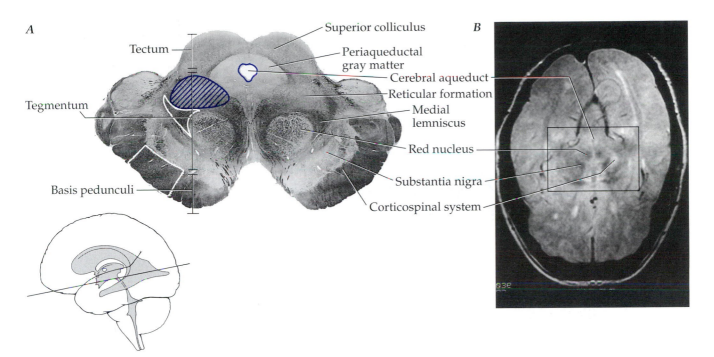

Figure 2–9. Myelin-stained section (***A***) and MRI scan (***B***) through the midbrain. The inset shows the planes of the section and the MRI scan. The reticular formation, medial lemniscus, and corticospinal system are outlined in ***A.*** Note that the descending cortical axons in ***B*** have degenerated. (***B,*** *Courtesy of Dr. Jesús Pujol; from Pujol J, Martí-Vilalta JL, Junqué C, Vendrell P, Fernández J, Capdevila A: Wallerian degeneration of the pyramidal tract in capsular infarction studied by magnetic resonance imaging. Stroke 1990;21:404–409.)*

nuclei into two major functional classes: (1) relay nuclei and (2) diffuse-projecting nuclei. Table 2–1 lists the major thalamic nuclei. **Relay nuclei** transmit information from particular subcortical inputs to a restricted portion of the cerebral cortex. Because of this specificity of connections, each relay nucleus serves a distinct role in perception, volition, emotion, or cognition. By contrast, the **diffuse-projecting nuclei** are thought to function in arousal and in regulating the excitability of wide regions of the cerebral cortex.

The cortical projections of some of the major thalamic relay nuclei are shown in Figure 2–11. Relay nuclei that mediate sensation and movement are located in the lateral portion of the thalamus and project their axons to the sensory and motor cortical areas. For each sensory modality, there is a different relay nucleus. The only exception is olfaction, in which information from the periphery is transmitted directly to the cortex on the medial temporal lobe (see Chapter 16). Each sensory modality has a primary area, which receives input directly from the thalamic relay nucleus for that modality. For example, the ventral posterior lateral nucleus is the relay nucleus for

the dorsal column–medial lemniscal system. It transmits somatic sensory information from the medial lemniscus to the primary somatic sensory cortex for touch and other mechanical sensations (Figure 2–11, dark gray). The different motor areas of the frontal lobe also receive input directly from motor relay nuclei. An important nucleus for controlling voluntary movement, the ventral lateral nucleus, transmits signals from the cerebellum to the motor cortex (Figure 2–11, dark blue stipple), which gives rise to the corticospinal tract.

Relay nuclei located in the anterior, medial, and other parts of the lateral thalamus project to the **association cortex,** the cortical regions that lie outside the sensory and motor areas. There are three major regions of association cortex, which subserve distinct sets of functions: the parietal-temporal-occipital cortex, the prefrontal cortex, and the limbic cortex. The **parietal-temporal-occipital association cortex,** located at the juncture of these lobes (Figure 2–11, blue), receives information primarily from the pulvinar nucleus as well as from different sensory cortical areas. This area is crucial for perception. The **prefrontal association**

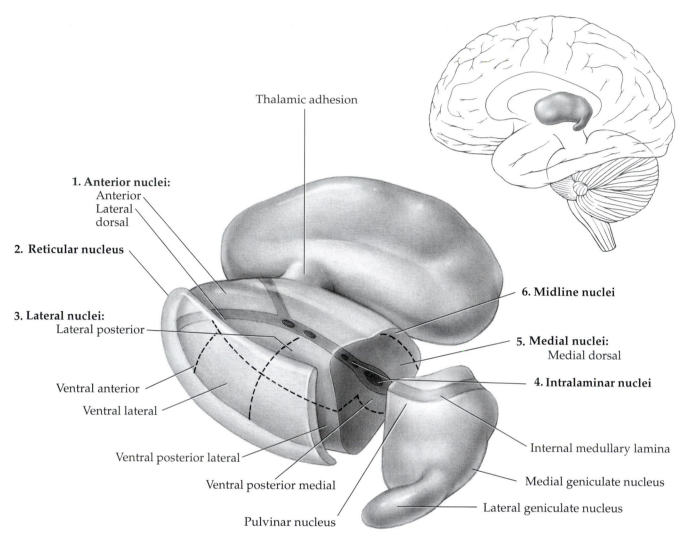

Thalamic adhesion

1. Anterior nuclei:
Anterior
Lateral
dorsal

2. Reticular nucleus

3. Lateral nuclei:
Lateral posterior

Ventral anterior

Ventral lateral

Ventral posterior lateral

Ventral posterior medial

Pulvinar nucleus

6. Midline nuclei

5. Medial nuclei:
Medial dorsal

4. Intralaminar nuclei

Internal medullary lamina

Medial geniculate nucleus

Lateral geniculate nucleus

Figure 2–10. A three-dimensional view of the thalamus as well as its approximate location in the cerebral hemispheres. The major nuclei are labeled. Nuclei of the lateral group of nuclei are numbered.

cortex is important for cognitive functions and for organizing behavior, including the memories and motor plans necessary for interacting with the environment (Figure 2–11, light stipple). For example, patients with damage to the prefrontal cortex blindly repeat motor acts irrespective of their efficacy. The prefrontal association cortex receives a major projection from the medial dorsal nucleus, with a smaller input from the pulvinar nucleus. The **limbic association cortex** is essential for emotions as well as for learning and memory. It is located primarily on the medial brain surface, in the cingulate gyrus and medial frontal lobe, and on the orbital surface of the frontal lobe (Figure 2–11). Patients with structural or func-

tional abnormalities of the limbic cortex, such as temporal lobe epilepsy, often also have mood disorders such as depression. The limbic association cortex receives input from the anterior nucleus, medial dorsal nucleus, and pulvinar nucleus.

Diffuse-projecting nuclei of the thalamus receive input from many converging sources and, in turn, project widely to the cerebral cortex. The **intralaminar** and **midline thalamic nuclei** are the nuclei in this class (Table 2–1). The patterns of termination of neurons in diffuse-projecting nuclei are described as **regional** because they may cross functional boundaries in the cortex. By contrast, the terminations of an individual relay nucleus are confined to a **single func-**

Table 2–1. Thalamic nuclei: major connections and functions.

Nucleus	Functional class	Major imputs	Major outputs	Functions
Anterior Group				
Anterior	Relay	Hypothalamus (mammillary body), hippocampal formation	Cingulate gyrus (limbic association cortex)	Learning, memory, and emotions
Lateral dorsal	Relay	Hippocampal formation; pretectum	Cingulate gyrus	?
Medial Group				
Medial dorsal	Relay	Basal ganglia, amygdala, olfactory system, hypothalamus	Prefontal association cortex	Emotions, cognition, learning, and memory
Lateral Group				
Ventral anterior	Relay	Basal ganglia	Supplementary motor cortex	Movement planning
Ventral lateral	Relay	Cerebellum	Premotor and primary motor cortex	Movement planning and control
Ventral posterior	Relay	Spinal cord, brain stem, medial lemniscus, trigeminal lemniscus	Primary somatic sensory cortex	Touch, limb position sense, pain, and temperature sense
Lateral geniculate	Relay	Retina	Primary visual cortex	Vision
Medial geniculate	Relay	Inferior colliculus	Primary auditory cortex	Hearing
Pulvinar	Relay	Superior colliculus; parietal, temporal, occipital lobes	Parietal, temporal, occiptal association cortex	Sensory integration, perception, language
Lateral posterior	Relay	Superior colliculus, pretectum, occipital lobe	Posterior parietal association cortex	Sensory integration
Intralaminar Nuclei				
Centromedian	Diffuse-projecting	Brain stem, basal ganglia, spinal cord	Cerebral cortex, basal ganglia	Regulation of cortical activity
Central lateral	Diffuse-projecting	Spinal cord, brain stem	Cerebral cortex, basal ganglia	Regulation of cortical activity
Parafascicular	Diffuse-projecting	Spinal cord, brain stem	Cerebral cortex, basal ganglia	Regulation of cortical activity
Midline Nuclei	Diffuse-projecing	Reticular formation, hypothalamus	Cerebral cortex, basal forebrain allocortex	Regulation of forebrain neuronal excitability
Reticular Nucleus		Thalamus, cortex	Thalamus	Regulation of thalamic neuronal activity

tional cortical area. The thalamic **reticular nucleus** does not project axons to the cortex. Rather, it sends its axons to other thalamic nuclei. It coordinates the activity of neurons within the thalamus and may play a role, together with the intralaminar nuclei, in regulating arousal.

The Internal Capsule Contains Ascending and Descending Axons

The internal capsule (Figure 2–12) is a tract, but unlike the medial lemniscus and corticospinal tract, it is a two-way path for transmission of information

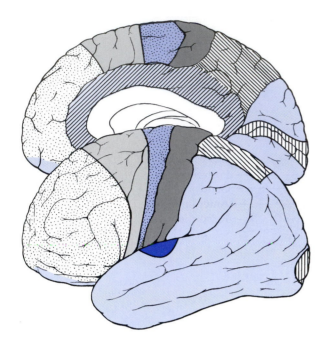

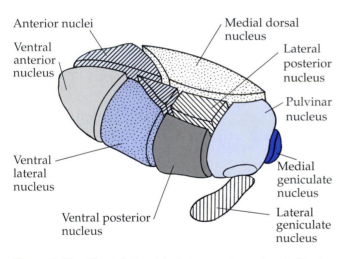

Anterior nuclei

Medial dorsal nucleus

Ventral anterior nucleus

Lateral posterior nucleus

Pulvinar nucleus

Ventral lateral nucleus

Medial geniculate nucleus

Ventral posterior nucleus

Lateral geniculate nucleus

Figure 2–11. The relationship between the major thalamic nuclei and the cortical regions to which they project.

from the thalamus to the cerebral cortex and from the cerebral cortex to subcortical structures. The axons of the thalamic neurons that receive input from the medial lemniscus pass through the internal capsule en route to the primary somatic sensory cortex. The corticospinal axons descend through the internal capsule. The descending fibers of the internal capsule that project into the brain stem, or farther into the spinal cord, form the basis pedunculi in the midbrain. The internal capsule looks like a curved fan (Figure 2–12). Although it appears as though the axons of the internal capsule

condense as they course toward the brain stem, their numbers actually decrease: The contingent of ascending axons is not present in the basis pedunculi, accounting for a large reduction, and descending axons terminate in the brain stem and spinal cord, resulting in further decreases in numbers.

When the cerebral hemispheres are sliced horizontally (Figure 2–13A), the internal capsule resembles an arrowhead with the tip pointing medially. This configuration gives the internal capsule three divisions: anterior limb, genu (Latin for "knee"), and posterior limb. The thalamus is located medial to the posterior limb. The internal capsule also separates various components of the basal ganglia. Two components of the striatum, the caudate nucleus and putamen (see Figure 14–2A), are split by the internal capsule, with the caudate nucleus located laterally and the putamen located medially. The putamen, together with the globus pallidus—another part of the basal ganglia important in movement control—is termed the lenticular nucleus because it has a lens-like shape. The corresponding MRI scan from a healthy person (Figure 2–13B) shows many of the structures present on the myelin-stained section. The path of the descending fibers of the internal capsule, from the cerebral hemispheres to the pons, can be followed on a myelin-stained coronal section (Figure 2–14A) and on the corresponding MRI scan from the patient with the corticospinal tract lesion (Figure 2–14B). Box 2–1 briefly describes magnetic resonance imaging and the characteristics of different types of images.

Cerebral Cortex Neurons Are Organized Into Layers

The dorsal column–medial lemniscal system projects to the cerebral cortex, which is also the origin of the corticospinal tract. Its neurons are organized into layers. Lamination is a feature of all cortical regions, although different cortical regions characteristically contain different numbers of layers (Figures 2–16 and 2–17). Approximately 95% of the cerebral cortex contains at least six cell layers; this cortex is commonly called **neocortex** because it dominates the cerebral cortex of phylogenetically higher vertebrates such as mammals. The remaining 5% of cortex, which is termed **allocortex,** is morphologically distinct. Allocortex is involved in olfaction and aspects of learning and memory.

Each region of neocortex that subserves a different function has its own microscopic anatomy: The thickness of the six principal cell layers varies, as does the

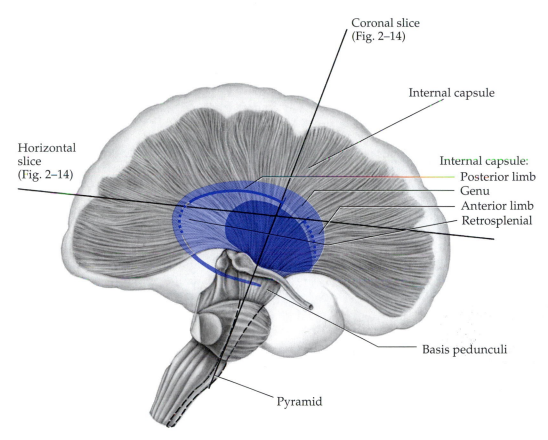

Figure 2–12. Three-dimensional view of the internal capsule. The descending cortical axons collect into a discrete tract in the brain stem. Lines indicate planes of horizontal (eg, Figure 2–13) and coronal (eg, Figure 2–14) sections. *(Adapted from Carpenter MB, Sutin J: Human Neuroanatomy. Williams & Wilkins, 1983.)*

density of neurons in each layer. Areas that subserve sensation (eg, primary visual cortex) have a thick layer IV (Figure 2–16). This is the layer in which axons from most thalamic sensory neurons synapse. In contrast, the primary motor cortex has a thin layer IV and a thick layer V (Figure 2–16). Layer V contains the neurons that project to the spinal cord, via the corticospinal tract. Association areas of the cerebral cortex, such as prefrontal and parietal-temporal-occipital association cortex, have a morphology that is intermediate between those of sensory cortex and motor cortex (Figure 2–16).

The Cerebral Cortex Has an Input-Output Organization

The cerebral neocortex, of which the somatic sensory cortical areas are part, has six principal cell lay-

ers. Thalamic neurons that project to the cortex send their axons primarily to layer IV (Figure 2–17). This is the input layer of cortex. There they synapse on dendrites of layer IV neurons, as well as neurons whose cell bodies are located in other layers, but they have dendrites in layer IV. Neurons in layer IV distribute this incoming information to neurons in other layers. Layers II, III, V, and VI are the output layers of cortex. Pyramidal neurons in these layers project to other cortical areas as well as to subcortical structures. Layer I does not contain many neurons in the mature brain, only dendrites of neurons located in deeper layers and elsewhere.

The cortex contains three kinds of efferent projections from the output layers, mediated by three separate classes of pyramidal neurons: corticocortical association, callosal, and descending projection. The efferent projection neurons with different targets are located in different cortical layers:

A

B

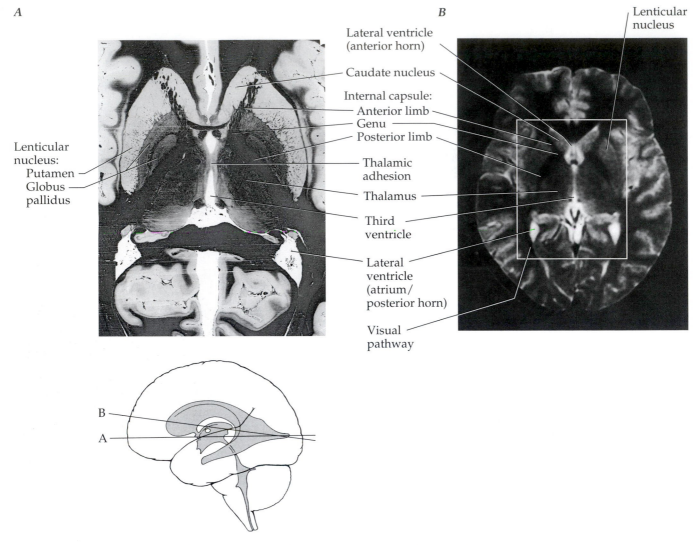

Lenticular
nucleus

Lateral ventricle
(anterior horn)

Caudate nucleus

Internal capsule:
Anterior limb
Genu
Posterior limb

Thalamic
adhesion

Thalamus

Third
ventricle

Lateral
ventricle
(atrium/
posterior horn)

Visual
pathway

Lenticular
nucleus:
Putamen
Globus
pallidus

B

A

Figure 2–13. Myelin-stained section (*A*) and MRI scan (*B*) through the cerebral hemi-sphere, at the level of the thalamus. The inset shows the planes of the section and the MRI scan.

- **Corticocortical association neurons,** located predominantly in layers II and III, project to cortical areas on the same side.
- **Callosal neurons** are also located in layers II and III. They project their axons to the contralateral cortex via the **corpus callosum** (see Figure 1–9B).
- **Descending projection neurons** are separate classes of projection neurons whose axons descend to (1) the striatum (the caudate nucleus and putamen), (2) the thalamus, (3) the brain stem, or (4) the spinal cord. Descending projec-

tion neurons that terminate in the striatum, brain stem, and spinal cord are found in layer V, whereas those projecting to the thalamus are located in layer VI.

The Cytoarchitectonic Map of the Cerebral Cortex Is the Basis for a Map of Cortical Function

Based primarily on differences in the thickness of cortical layers and on the sizes and shapes of neurons,

Text continues on page 50

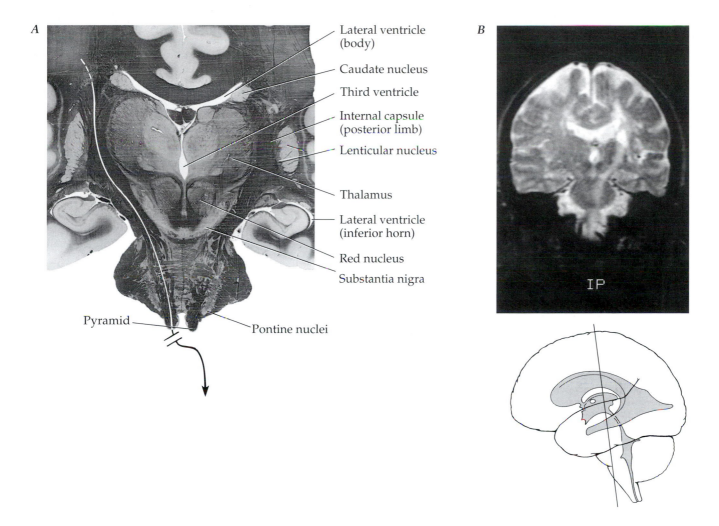

A

Lateral ventricle
(body)

Caudate nucleus

Third ventricle

Internal capsule
(posterior limb)

Lenticular nucleus

Thalamus

Lateral ventricle
(inferior horn)

Red nucleus

Substantia nigra

Pyramid

Pontine nuclei

B

IP

Figure 2–14. Myelin-stained section (***A***) and MRI scan (***B***) through the cerebral hemisphere, at the level of the thalamus. The path of the descending cortical axons is drawn
on ***A***. The inset shows the planes of the section and the MRI scan. The light region in ***B***
contains degenerated descending cortical axons in the posterior limb of the internal capsule, basis pedunculi, and pyramid. *(Courtesy of Dr. Jesús Pujol; from Pujol J, Martí-Vilalta
JL, Junqué C, Vendrell P, Fernández J, Capdevila A: Wallerian degeneration of the pyramidal
tract in capsular infarction studied by magnetic resonance imaging. Stroke 1990;21:404–409.)*

Box 2–1.   *Magnetic Resonance Imaging*

Routine magnetic resonance imaging (MRI) of the nervous system reveals the proton constituents of neural tissues and fluids; most of the protons are contained in water. Protons in different tissue and fluid compartments, when placed in a strong **magnetic field,** have slightly different properties. MRI takes advantage of such differences to construct an image of brain structure or even function.

MRI relies on the simple property that protons can be made to emit signals that reflect the local tissue environment. Hence, protons in different tissues or fluids emit different signals. This is achieved by exciting protons with low levels of energy, which is carried by electromagnetic waves emitted from a coil placed over the tissue. Once excited, protons emit a signal with three components, or parameters, that depend on tissue characteristics. The first parameter is related to **proton density** (ie, primarily a measure of water content) in the tissue. The second and third parameters are related to proton **relaxation times;** that is, the times it takes protons to return to the energy state they were in before excitation by electromagnetic waves. The two relaxation times are termed T1 and T2 (Figure 2–15). **T1 relaxation time**

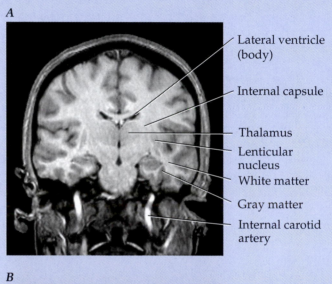

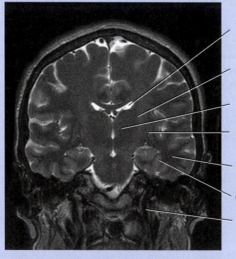

Figure 2–15. T1 *A* and T2 *B* MRI scans produce negative images. Cerebrospinal fluid appears white on T1 weighted MRI scans and dark on T2 weighted images. T1 weighted images look like a brain slice because gray matter appears dark and white matter appears white. The imaging planes for the two MRI scans are the same, and similar to Figure 2–19. *(Courtesy of Brian Somerville, Columbia University.)*

Box 2–1 (continued).

(or spin-lattice relaxation time) is related to the overall tissue environment, and **T2 relaxation time** (or spin-spin relaxation time), to interactions between protons. When an MRI scan is generated, it can be made to be dominated by one of these parameters. This differential dependence is accomplished by fine-tuning the electromagnetic waves used to excite the tissue. The choice of whether to have an image reflect proton density, T1 relaxation time, or T2 relaxation time depends on the purpose of the image. For example, in T2-weighted images, which are dominated by T2 relaxation time, watery constituents of the brain produce a stronger signal than fatty constituents (eg, white matter). These images can be used to distinguish an edematous region of the white matter after stroke, for example, from a normal region.

Four constituents of the central nervous system are distinguished using MRI: cerebrospinal fluid, blood, white matter, and gray matter. The exact appearance of these central nervous system con-stituents depends on whether the image reflects proton density, T1 relaxation time (Figure 2–15A), or T2 relaxation time (Figure 2–15B). For T1 images the signals produced by protons in cerebrospinal fluid are weak, and, on this image, cerebrospinal fluid is shaded black. Cerebrospinal fluid in the ventricles and overlying the brain surface, in the subarachnoid space, has the same dark appearance. On T2 images, cerebrospinal fluid appears white, because the signal it generates is strong. In T1 images, protons in blood in arteries and veins produce a strong signal, and these tissue constituents appear white. In T2 images, blood produces a weak signal. This weak signal derives from two factors: tissue motion (ie, normally blood flows) and the presence of hemoglobin, an iron-containing protein that attenuates the MRI signal because of its paramagnetic properties. The gray and white matter are also distinct because their protons emit signals of slightly different strengths. For example, on the T1-weighted image (Figure 2–15A), white matter appears white and gray matter appears dark.

Several major deep structures can be seen on MRI scans: the thalamus, the striatum, the lenticular nucleus, and the internal capsule. A fine structure also is present in the subcortical white matter. Portions, including the internal capsule and the visual pathway (see Figure 2–13B), are darker. The weak signal produced by these parts of the white matter is due to the presence of iron (probably as ferritin), which attenuates the MRI signal (Figure 2–15A).

There have been two major modifications of the basic MRI technique. **Diffusion-weighted MRI** takes advantage of a component of the MRI signal that depends on the direction of diffusion of water protons with the tissue, which is highly restricted within white matter tracts. This approach can be used to examine different fiber pathways in the brain. The other approach is **functional MRI,** which is considered in Box 2–2.

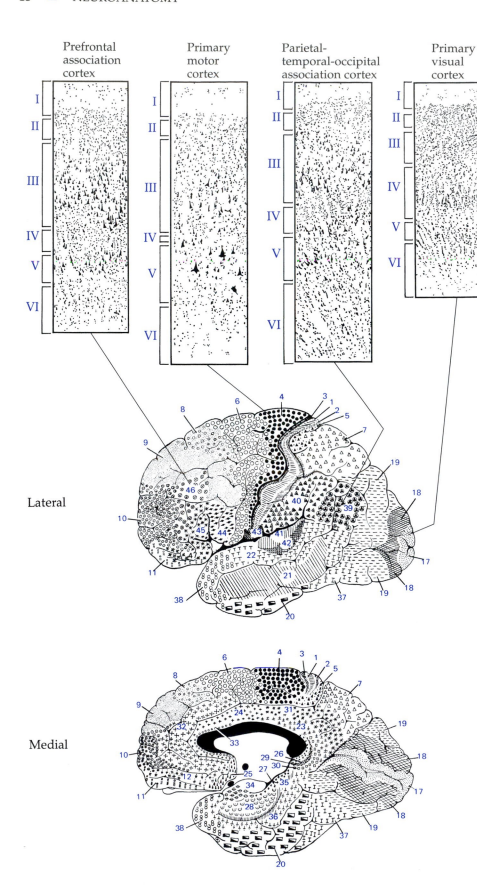

Prefrontal association cortex

Primary motor cortex

Parietal-temporal-occipital association cortex

Primary visual cortex

Lateral

Medial

Figure 2–16. Different regions of the cerebral cortex have a different cytoarchitecture. (*Top*) Nissl-stained sections through various portions of the cerebral cortex. (*Bottom*) Brodmann's cytoarchitectonic areas of the cerebral cortex. (*Top, Adapted from Campbell AW: Histological Studies on the Localisation of Cerebral Function. Cambridge University Press, 1905. Bottom, Adapted from Campbell 1905 and Brodmann K: Vergleichende Lokalisationslehre der Grosshirnrinde in ihren Prinzipien dargestellt auf Grund des Zellenbaues. Barth, 1909.)*

Table 2–2. Brodmann's areas.

Brodmann area	Functional area	Location	Function
1, 2, 3,	Primary somatic sensory cortex	Postcentral gyrus	Touch proprioception
4	Primary motor cortex	Precentral gyrus	Voluntary movement control
5	Higher-order somatic sensory cortex; posterior parietal association area	Superior parietal lobule	Sterognosia
6	Supplementary motor cortex; supplementary eye field; premotor cortex; frontal eye fields	Precentral gyrus and rostral adjacent cortex	Limb and eye movement planning
7	Posterior parietal association area	Superior parietal lobule	Visuomotor, spatial awareness, perception
8	Frontal eye fields	Superior, middle frontal gyri, medial frontal lobe	Saccadic eye movements
9, 10, 11, 12	Prefrontal association cortex; frontal eye fields	Superior, middle frontal gyri, medial frontal lobe	Thought, cognition, movement planning
17[1]	Primary visual cortex	Banks of calcarine fissure	Vision
18	Secondary visual cortex	Medial and lateral occipital gyri	Vision, depth
19	Higher-order visual cortex, middle temporal visual area	Medial and lateral occipital gyri	Vision, color, motion, depth
20	Visual inferotemporal area	Inferior temporal gyrus	Form vision
21	Visual inferotemporal area	Middle temporal gyrus	From vision
22	Higher-order auditory cortex	Superior temporal gyrus	Hearing, speech
23, 24, 25, 26, 27	Limbic association cortex	Cingulate gyrus, subcallosal area, retrosplenial area, and parahippocampal gyrus	Emotions, learning and memory
28	Primary olfactory cortex; limbic association cortex	Parahippocampal gyrus	Smell, emotions, learning and memory
29, 30, 31, 32, 33	Limbic association cortex	Cingulate gyrus and retrosplenial area	Emotions
34, 35, 36	Primary olfactory cortex; limbic association cortex	Parahippocampal gyrus	Smell, emotions
37	Parietal-temporal-occipital association cortex; middle temporal visual area	Middle and inferior temporal gyri at junction temporal and occipital lobes	Perception, vision, reading, speech
38	Primary olfactory cortex; limbic association cortex	Temporal pole	Smell, emotions
39	Parietal-temporal-occipital association cortex	Inferior parietal lobule (angular gyrus)	Perception, vision, reading, speech
40	Parietal-temporal-occipital association cortex	Inferior parietal lobule (supramarginal gyrus)	Perception, vision, reading, speech
41	Primary auditory cortex	Heschl's gyri and superior temporal gyrus	Hearing
42	Secondary auditory cortex	Heschl's gyri and superior temporal gyrus	Hearing
43	Gustatory cortex (?)	Insular cortex, frontoparietal operculum	Taste
44	Broca's area; lateral premotor cortex	Inferior frontal gyrus (frontal operculum)	Speech, movement planning
45	Prefrontal association cortex	Inferior frontal gyrus (frontal operculum)	Thought, cognition, planning behavior
46	Prefrontal association cortex (dorsolateral prefrontal cortex)	Middle frontal gyrus	Thought, cognition, planning behavior, aspects of eye movement control
47	Prefrontal association cortex	Inferior frontal gyrus (frontal operculum)	Thought, cognition, planning behavior

[1]Areas 13, 14, 15, and 16 are part of the insular cortex. The relationship between cytoarchitecture and function is not established for the insular cortex.

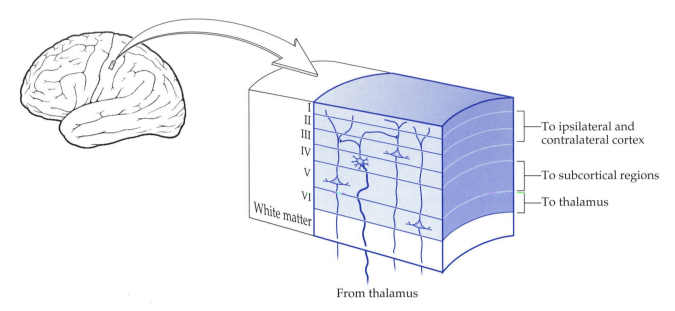

Figure 2–17. Three-dimensional schematic of a portion of the cerebral cortex. The piece is from the postcentral gyrus (see inset). Within the cortex are six layers in which cells and their processes are located. Neurons whose cell bodies are located in layers II and III project to other cortical areas, those in layer V project their axons to subcortical regions, and those in layer VI project to the thalamus.

the German anatomist Korbinian Brodmann identified over 50 divisions (now termed **Brodmann's areas;** Figure 2–16, bottom). These divisions are based only on the neuronal architecture, or **cytoarchitecture,** of the cortex, such as the size and shapes of neurons in the different laminae and their packing densities. It is remarkable that research on the functions of the cerebral cortex has shown that different functional areas of

the cortex have a different cytoarchitecture. In humans, by noting the particular behavioral changes that follow discrete cortical lesions and using functional imaging approaches, such as positron emission tomography (PET) and functional MRI, we have gained some insight into the functions of most of the cytoarchitectonic divisions identified by Brodmann (Table 2–2). Functional imaging approaches are described briefly in Box 2–2.

Box 2–2.   Human Functional Neuroanatomy

There are two radiological techniques for imaging brain function: **functional magnetic resonance imaging** (fMRI) and **positron emission tomography** (PET). fMRI provides an image of brain function by measuring changes in the oxygenated state of hemoglobin within local brain regions (Figure 2–18A). Active neurons consume more oxygen and more glucose and demand more blood flow than silent ones. Typically, fMRI scans reflect the difference in oxygenation state of hemoglobin between the resting condition and while the individual is engaged in a particular task. Like conventional MRI, fMRI has high spatial resolution. When an fMRI scan, which shows the locations of hemoglobin oxygenation values, is combined with a conventional scan, local brain function is shown in relation to structure.

The second technique for imaging brain function is PET, which can provide an image of brain function by computing the distribution of radiolabeled compounds involved in neuronal metabolism or cerebral blood flow (Figure 2-18B). PET also is used to provide an image of the distribution of administered radioactive membrane ligands. This application can be used to examine the density of neurotransmitter membrane receptors in patients with neurological and psychiatric disease.

A

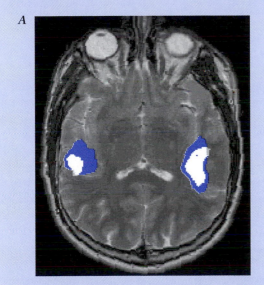

B1

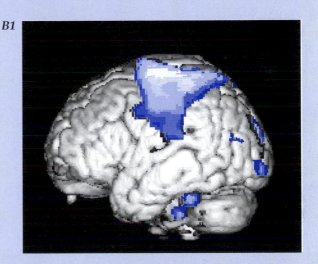

Figure 2–18.   Functional imaging techniques. *A.* A functional magnetic resonance image (fMRI) is shown through the auditory cortical areas in the superior temporal gyrus. The image was obtained while the subject listened to tones of different characteristics. The white areas corresponds to regions of neural activation in the primary auditory cortex, and the blue areas correspond to activation of the higher-order auditory areas. *(Courtesy of Dr. Josef Rauschecker, Georgetown University; adapted from Wessinger CM, et al: Hierarchical organization of the human auditory cortex revealed by functional magnetic resonance imaging. J Cogn Neurosci 2001;13:1–7.)* *B.* Positron emission tomography (PET) images obtained while the subject performed a motor task that involved positioning a joystick to control a computer cursor. A lateral view of the cortex is shown in *B1.* Regions of activation include the motor and somatic sensory cortical areas. The horizontal slice in *B2* is through the tips of the temporal lobes, the brain stem, and cerebellum. Three distinct portions of the cerebellum are activated. For the PET scan, the intensity of activation is shown according to a color scale from dark to light. *(Courtesy of Dr. Lice Ghilardi, Columbia University; adapted from Ghilardi M-F, et al: Patterns of regional brain activation associated with different forms of motor learning. Brain Research 2000;871:127–145.)*

B2

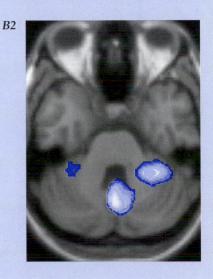

Summary

Ascending and Descending Projection Systems

Ascending pathways (ie, the dorsal column–medial lemniscal system) transmit **sensory** information to the brain. The pathways are interrupted by **relay nuclei.** Information **decussates** from one side to the other. Most sensory systems relay through the thalamus. **Descending pathways** (ie, the corticospinal tract) convey **motor** control signals from the brain to the spinal cord. Descending pathways also decussate.

Diffuse-Projecting Neurotransmitter-Specific Systems

Four neurotransmitter-specific systems have diffuse projections throughout the central nervous system: (1) **Cholinergic** neurons in the basal nucleus (of Meynert), on the ventral telencephalic surface, and in neurons on the ventromedial telencephalic surface project throughout the neocortex and allocortex (Figure 2–2A). (2) Midbrain **dopaminergic** neurons, located mostly in the **substantia nigra** and **ventral tegmental area,** project to the basal ganglia and frontal lobes (Figure 2–2B1). (3) The **locus ceruleus** contains **noradrenalin** and projects throughout all central nervous system divisions (Figure 2–2B2). (4) The **raphe nuclei** contain serotonin and have ascending projections to the cerebral hemispheres and diencephalon and descending projections to the spinal cord (Figure 2–2B3).

Spinal Cord Organization

The spinal cord, the most caudal of the major central nervous system divisions, has a central region that contains predominantly cell bodies of neurons (gray matter), surrounded by a region that contains mostly myelinated axons (white matter) (Figures 2–2 and 2–3). Both of these regions can be further subdivided. The **dorsal horn** of the gray matter subserves somatic sensation, and the **ventral horn,** skeletal motor function. The **dorsal column** of the white matter carries somatic sensory information to the brain; the **lateral** and **ventral columns** carry both sensory and motor information (Figures 2–3 and 2–4).

Brain Stem Organization

The caudal medulla (Figure 2–6C) is similar in its organization to the spinal cord. At a more rostral level (Figure 2–6B), the medulla contains nuclei on its dorsal surface—the **dorsal column nuclei**—that subserve tactile sensation, and a pathway on its ventral surface—the corticospinal tract, located in the **pyramid**—that subserves voluntary movement. The **medial lemniscus** is located dorsal to the pyramid. At the level of the **inferior olivary nucleus** (Figure 2–6A), the fourth ventricle forms the dorsal surface of the medulla. The pons (Figure 2–8) contains nuclei in its ventral portion—the **pontine nuclei**—that transfer information from the cerebral cortex to the cerebellum. The midbrain (Figure 2–9) contains the **colliculi** on its dorsal surface and the **basis pedunculi** on its ventral surface (Figures 2–5B and 2–9).

Organization of the Diencephalon and Cerebral Hemispheres

The **diencephalon** and the **cerebral hemispheres** have a more complex organization than that of the brain stem or spinal cord. The **thalamus,** which relays information from subcortical structures to the cerebral cortex, contains two different functional classes of nuclei: **relay** and **diffuse-projecting** (Table 2–1). Three of the four main anatomical divisions of the thalamus serve relay functions (Figure 2–10): (1) **anterior nuclei,** (2) **medial nuclei,** and (3) **lateral nuclei.** The fourth main anatomical division of the thalamus, the **intralaminar nuclei,** contains diffuse-projecting nuclei. The anatomical divisions are based on the spatial location of nuclei with respect to the **internal medullary lamina,** bands of myelinated fibers in the thalamus. A **topographical relationship** exists between the projections of the different thalamic nuclei and the cerebral cortex (Figure 2–11). Thalamocortical projections (as well as descending cortical projections) course through the **internal capsule** (Figures 2–12, 2–13, and 2–14).

Two types of cortex can be identified, based on the number of cell layers. **Neocortex** (or isocortex) has six layers (Figures 2–16 and 2–17), and the different layers have different thicknesses depending on the function of the particular cortical area. Layer IV is the principal input layer (Figure 2–17). Layers II and III contain corticocortical association and callosal neurons and project to other cortical areas. Layer V contains descending projection neurons that terminate in the striatum, brain stem, and spinal cord. Layer VI contains descending projection neurons that terminate in the thalamus. Based on cortical layering patterns as well as the sizes and shapes of cortical neurons, or **cytoarchitecture,** about 50 different areas of the cerebral cortex have been identified (Figure 2–16; Table 2–2). These are termed **Brodmann's areas.**

Related Sources

Brust JCM: The Practice of Neural Science. McGraw-Hill; 2000. (See ch. 16, case 79.)

Kandel ER, Schwartz JH, Jessell TM (editors): Principles of Neural Science, 4th ed. McGraw-Hill, 2000.

Selected Readings

Jones EG: The Thalamus. Plenum Press, 1985.

Sigal R, Doyon D, Halimi P, Atlan H: Magnetic Resonance Imaging. Springer-Verlag, 1988.

Rye DB: Tracking neural pathways with MRI. Trends Neurosci 1999;22:373–374.

References

Axer H, Berks G, Keyserlingk DG: Visualization of nerve fiber orientation in gross histological sections of the human brain. Microsc Res Tech 2000;51:481–492.

Basser PJ, Pajevic S, Pierpaoli C, Duda J, Aldroubi A: In vivo fiber tractography using DT-MRI data. Magn Reson Med 2000;44:625–632.

Brodmann K: Vergleichende Lokalisationslehre der Grosshirnrinde in ihren Prinzipien dargestellt auf Grund des Zellenbaues. Barth, 1909.

Campbell AW: Histological Studies on the Localisation of Cerebral Function. Cambridge University Press, 1905.

Carpenter MB, Sutin J: Human Neuroanatomy. Williams & Wilkins, 1983.

Gorman DG, Unützer J: Brodmann's missing numbers. Neurology 1993;43:226–227.

Hassler R: Architectonic organization of the thalamic nuclei. In Shaltenbrand G, Warhen WW (editors): Stereotaxy of the Human Brain. G. Thieme Verlag; 1982:140–180.

Hirai T, Jones EG: A new parcellation of the human thalamus on the basis of histochemical staining. Brain Res Rev 1989;14:1–34.

Jones EG: Organization of the thalamocortical complex and its relation to sensory processes. In Darian-Smith I (editor): Handbook of Physiology, Section 1: The Nervous System, Vol. 3: Sensory Processes. American Physiological Society; 1984:149–212.

Macchi G, Jones EG: Toward an agreement on terminology of nuclear and subnuclear divisions of the motor thalamus. J Neurosurg 1997;86:670–685.

Markowitsch HJ, Emmans D, Irle E, Streicher M, Preilowski B: Cortical and subcortical afferent connections of the primate's temporal pole: A study of rhesus monkeys, squirrel monkeys, and marmosets. J Comp Neurol 1985; 242:425–458.

Mesulam MM, Mufson EJ: Insula of the old world monkey. III: Efferent cortical output and comments on function. J Comp Neurol 1982;212:38–52.

Nieuwenhuys R, Voogd J, van Huijzen C: The Human Central Nervous System: A Synopsis and Atlas, 3rd ed. Springer-Verlag, 1988.

Pearson J, Halliday G, Sakamoto N, Michel J-P: Catecholaminergic neurons. In Paxinos G (editor): The Human Nervous System. Academic Press; 1990:1022–1049.

Pujol J, Martí-Vilalta JL, Junqué C, Vendrell P, Fernández J, Capdevila A: Wallerian degeneration of the pyramidal tract in capsular infarction studied by magnetic resonance imaging. Stroke 1990;21:404–409.

Rexed B: The cytoarchitectonic organization of the spinal cord in the cat. J Comp Neurol 1952;96:415–495.

Rodriguez EM, Rodriguez S, Hein S: The subcommissural organ. Microsc Res Tech 1998;41:98–123.

Romanski LM, Giguere M, Bates JF, Goldman-Rakic PS: Topographic organization of medial pulvinar connections with the prefrontal cortex in the rhesus monkey. J Comp Neurol 1997;379:313–332.

Saper C: Cholinergic system. In Paxinos G (editor): The Human Nervous System. Academic Press; 1990;1095–1113.

Saper CB: Diffuse cortical projection systems: Anatomical organization and role in cortical function. In Plum F (editor): Handbook of Physiology. The Nervous System, Vol. 5. American Physiological Society; 1987:169–210.

Saunders NR, Habgood MD, Dziegielewska KM: Barrier mechanisms in the brain: I. Adult brain. Clin Exp Pharmacol Physiol 1999;26:11–19.

Soares JG, Gattass R, Souza AP, Rosa MG, Fiorani M Jr., Brandao BL: Connectional and neurochemical subdivisions of the pulvinar in Cebus monkeys. Vis Neurosci 2001;18:25–41.

Törk I, Hornung J-P: Raphe nuclei and the serotonergic system. In Paxinos G (editor): The Human Nervous System. Academic Press; 1990:1001–1022.

Yeterian EH, Pandya DN: Corticothalamic connections of extrastriate visual areas in rhesus monkeys. J Comp Neurol 1997;378:562–585.

Zilles K: Cortex. In Paxinos G (editor): The Human Nervous System. Academic Press; 1990:757–802.

3

Development of the Central Nervous System

T*HE KEY TO UNDERSTANDING THE COMPLEX* anatomy of the mature brain is to understand how it develops. Principles that govern the regional anatomy of the brain are more easily appreciated in its simpler, embryonic form. Knowing how the central nervous system develops also is essential for understanding how congenital abnormalities and intrauterine trauma, such as fetal drug exposure, affect brain function. In fact, early defects in the formation of the central nervous system are a common cause of perinatal mortality, and babies who survive often have multiple cognitive and motor handicaps.

This chapter examines central nervous system development in order to provide insight into the complex three-dimensional structure of the mature brain. First, the chapter considers how the nervous system forms from the ectoderm of the embryo. Then it examines how key components of each major division of the central nervous system and the ventricular system develop from their earliest stages through maturity.

The Neurons and Glial Cells Derive From Cells of the Neural Plate

Similar to all vertebrates, the human embryo has three principal cell layers: **ectoderm,** the outer layer; **mesoderm,** the middle layer; and **endoderm,** the inner layer. The cellular constituents of the central nervous system—neurons and glial cells—are formed from a specialized region of the ectoderm called the **neural plate.** The neural plate is induced to form the nervous system by signaling molecules that diffuse from the nearby mesoderm. This is the process of **neural induction.**

The neural plate lies along the dorsal midline of the embryo (Figure 3–1). Proliferation of cells is greater

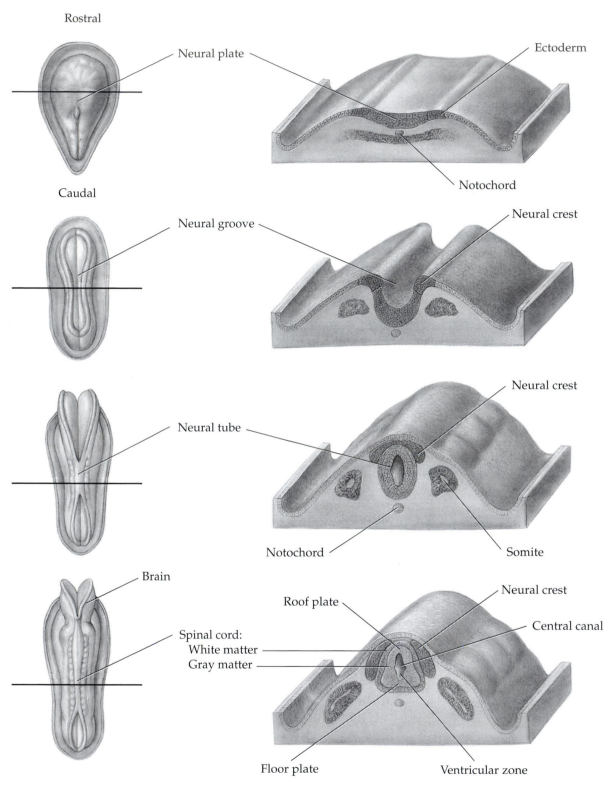

Figure 3–1. The neural tube forms from the dorsal surface of the embryo. The left side of the figure presents dorsal views of the developing embryo during the 3rd and 4th weeks after conception. The right side illustrates transverse sections through the developing nervous system. The bold lines on the left indicate the planes of the sections. The notochord is first present at about the 4th gestational week. Before then, it exists as the notochordal plate, which is less well organized than the notochord. *(Adapted from Cowan WM: The development of the brain. Sci Am 1979;241:112–133.)*

along the margin of the neural plate than along the midline, resulting in the formation of the **neural groove.** This midline indentation deepens gradually and closes (see below) to form a hollow structure, the **neural tube.** Lining the neural tube is the **ventricular zone,** which consists of the epithelial cells that generate virtually all the neurons and glial cells (astrocytes, oligodendrocytes, and Schwann cells; see Chapter 1) of the **central nervous system.** In most areas of the central nervous system, developing neurons migrate from the ventricular zone to other sites before forming functional neural circuits. Although it previously had been thought that neurogenesis occurred only during early development, a remarkable series of experiments has shown that neurons are generated in adults of various species, including humans. This finding offers hope for devising ways to restore function to the damaged nervous system.

Whereas the central nervous system develops from the epithelial cells lining the neural tube, many of the key components of the peripheral nervous system develop from a population of cells called the **neural crest** (Figure 3–1). This collection of cells emerges from the dorsal region of the neural tube to migrate peripherally and give rise to the neurons whose cell bodies lie outside of the central nervous system. These neurons include the sensory neurons that innervate body tissues and peripheral components of the autonomic nervous system. The neural crest also gives rise to certain nonneural cells, including the chromaffin cells of the adrenal medulla and the **Schwann cells,** which form the myelin sheath of peripheral nerves. The two inner meningeal layers, the arachnoid and pia mater, also derive from the neural crest (see Figure 1–12). However, the outermost (and toughest) meningeal layer, the dura mater, derives from the mesoderm.

After neural tube formation, important developments occur that establish the normal structure of the nervous system. The caudal portion of the neural tube forms the spinal cord, and the rostral portion becomes the brain. The cavity within the neural tube forms the **ventricular system.** Closure of the neural plate to form the neural tube occurs first at the location where the neck will form and then proceeds both caudally and rostrally. The location at which the rostral end of the neural tube closes is termed the **lamina terminalis,** a landmark that will form the rostral wall of the ventricular system (see Figure 3–16D). Neural tube closure has important clinical implications. For example, when the caudal portion of the neural plate fails to close, the functions of the caudal spinal cord are severely disrupted. This disruption results in varying degrees of lower limb paralysis and defective bladder control. This developmental abnormality is one of a wide range of neural tube defects, collectively termed **spina bifida,** that are often associated with herniation of the meninges and neural tissue to the body surface. When the rostral neural plate fails to close, **anencephaly** may occur, resulting in gross disturbance of the overall structure of the brain.

The Neural Tube Forms Five Brain Vesicles and the Spinal Cord

The inductive signals that lead to the formation of the neural plate, together with other signals secreted from adjacent nonneural cells, are also important in establishing the coarse rostrocaudal plan of the central nervous system. Very early in development the rostral portion of the neural tube forms the three primary brain vesicles, or hollow swellings (Figure 3–2A): (1) the **prosencephalon,** or **forebrain,** (2) the **mesencephalon,** or **midbrain,** and (3) the **rhombencephalon,** or **hindbrain.** The caudal portion of the neural tube remains relatively undifferentiated and forms the **spinal cord.** Two secondary vesicles emerge from the prosencephalon later in development, the **telencephalon** (or cerebral hemisphere) and the **diencephalon** (or thalamus and hypothalamus). Whereas the mesencephalon remains undivided throughout further brain development, the rhombencephalon gives rise to the **metencephalon** (or pons and cerebellum) and the **myelencephalon** (or medulla). The five brain vesicles and primitive spinal cord, already identifiable by the 5th week of fetal life, give rise to the seven major divisions of the central nervous system (see Figure 1–3B).

This rostrocaudal morphological plan of the developing central nervous system is accompanied by developmental control genes that are expressed in particular locations along the neuraxis. Genetic manipulations in animals and mutations in humans show that these control genes play a key role in determining both that a particular brain region or nucleus develops in the correct location and the organization of the brain regions and local nuclei (see Box 3–1).

The Longitudinal Axis of the Developing Brain Bends at the Midbrain-Diencephalic Juncture

The complex configuration of the mature brain is determined in part by how the developing brain bends, or **flexes.** Flexures occur because proliferation

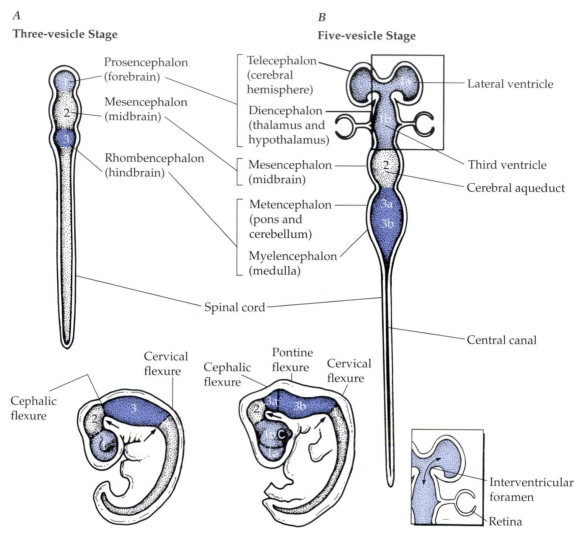

Figure 3–2. Schematic illustration of the three- and five-vesicle stages of the neural tube. The top portion of the figure shows dorsal views of the neural tube drawn without flexures. The bottom portion of the figure presents lateral views. *A.* Three-vesicle stage. *B.* Five-vesicle stage. The inset shows the location of the intraventricular foramen on one side in the five-vesicle stage. *(Adapted from Kandel ER, Schwartz JH, Jessell TM (editors): Principles of Neural Science, 3rd ed. Elsevier, 1991.)*

of cells in the brain stem and cerebral hemispheres is enormous, and the space that the developing brain occupies in the cranium is constrained. At the three-vesicle stage there are two prominent flexures: the **cervical flexure,** at the junction of the spinal cord and the caudal hindbrain (or future medulla), and the **cephalic flexure,** at the level of the midbrain (Figure 3–2). At the five-vesicle stage a third flexure becomes prominent, the **pontine flexure.** By birth the cervical and pontine flexures have straightened out. The cephalic flexure, however, remains prominent and causes the longitudinal axis of the forebrain to deviate from that of the midbrain, hindbrain, and spinal cord.

The Ventricular System Develops From the Cavities in the Neural Tube

The large cavities within the cerebral vesicles develop into the ventricular system of the brain, and the caudal cavity becomes the central canal of the spinal cord (Figure 3–2). The ventricular system contains **cerebrospinal fluid,** which is produced mainly by the **choroid plexus.** This section examines how the entire ventricular system develops. The section on the c-shaped development of the cerebral cortex considers development of the complex three-dimensional structure of the lateral ventricle.

As the five brain vesicles develop, the forebrain cavity divides into the two **lateral ventricles** (formerly termed the first and second ventricles) and the **third ventricle** (Figure 3–2). The lateral ventricles, which develop as outpouchings from the rostral portion of the third ventricle, are each interconnected with the third ventricle by an **interventricular foramen** (of Monro) (Figure 3–2, inset). The **fourth ventricle,** the most caudal ventricle, develops from the cavity within the hindbrain. It is connected to the third ventricle by the **cerebral aqueduct** (of Sylvius) and merges caudally with the **central canal** (of the caudal medulla and spinal cord).

Cerebrospinal fluid normally exits from the ventricular system into the subarachnoid space through foramina in the fourth ventricle (see Chapter 4). (The central canal does not have such an aperture for the outflow of cerebrospinal fluid.) Pathological processes can prevent flow of cerebrospinal fluid from the ventricular system. For example, later in development the cerebral aqueduct becomes narrowed because of cell proliferation in the midbrain. Its narrow diameter makes it vulnerable to the constricting effects of tumors or swelling from trauma, and occlusion can occur. Cerebrospinal fluid continues to be produced despite occlusion. If occlusion occurs before the bones of the skull are fused (ie, in embryonic life or in infancy), ventricular volume will increase, the brain will enlarge rostral to the occlusion, and head size will increase. This condition is called **hydrocephalus.** If occlusion occurs after the bones of the skull are fused, ventricular size cannot increase without increasing intracranial pressure. This is a life-threatening condition.

The Choroid Plexus Forms When Blood Vessels Penetrate the Ventricular Roofs

As the neural tube thickens, the nutritional requirements of the central nervous system are supplied by the vasculature rather than by diffusion. At this time the blood vessels that overlie the pia (Figure 3–3A) penetrate the brain surface, carrying the pia into the brain. In most locations this pial sheath over the vasculature disappears close to the surface (see Figure 4–17).

At the roofs of the developing ventricles, neural and glial cells do not proliferate. Here, the pia remains apposed to the penetrating blood vessels (Figure 3–3). At these sites the **choroid plexus** develops. The cellular constituents of embryonic, as well as mature, choroid plexus are, from the central core to the ventricular surface: **blood vessels, pia,** and **choroid epithelium.** This epithelium is specialized to secrete cerebrospinal fluid. The choroid plexus is present only in the ventricles. In the mature brain the choroid plexus

remains in the roof of the third and fourth ventricles. In the lateral ventricles the choroid plexus is located in the ventricular roof and floor.

The Spinal Cord and Brain Stem Have a Segmented Structure

The spinal cord receives sensory information from the limbs and trunk and provides motor innervation of the muscles of these structures via the **spinal nerves.** The sensory and motor innervation of the head is provided by the cranial nerves, which enter and exit from the brain stem. The developing spinal cord and brain stem comprise a rostrocaudal series of modules, or **segments,** each of which has a similar basic structure. Whereas segmentation in the spinal cord also is present in maturity, segmentation in the brain stem is apparent only during early development.

Spinal segmentation is dependent on mesodermal tissue, which breaks up into 38 to 40 pairs of repeating units, called **somites.** The muscles, bones, and other structures of the neck, limbs, and trunk develop from these somites, which also have a rostrocaudal organization. There are 8 cervical, 12 thoracic, 5 lumbar, 5 sacral, and 8 to 10 coccygeal somites. For each of these somites, there is a corresponding vertebra and spinal cord segment. Each spinal cord segment provides the sensory and motor innervation of the skin and muscle of the body part derived from its associated somite. Neural connections between the developing somite and spinal cord are made by the axons of primary sensory neurons and motor neurons (ie, peripheral nervous system). Traveling together in spinal nerves (Figure 3–4A), the sensory and motor axons enter and leave the spinal cord via the **dorsal** and **ventral roots,** respectively, as shown for a mature segment (Figure 3–4B). The mature spinal cord is shown in Figure 3–4C; its segmentation is apparent as the series of dorsal and ventral roots emerging from its surface. The cervical segments innervate the skin and muscles of the back of the head, neck, and arms. The thoracic segments innervate the trunk, and the lumbar and sacral segments innervate the legs and perineal region. (Most of the coccygeal segments disappear later in development.)

Throughout the first 3 months of development, the spinal cord grows at about the same rate as the vertebral column (Figure 3–5A). During this period, the spinal cord occupies the entire **vertebral canal,** the space within the vertebral column. The dorsal and ventral roots associated with each segment pass directly through the intervertebral foramina to reach their target structures. Later, the growth of the vertebral column exceeds that of the spinal cord. In the adult the most caudal spinal cord segment is located

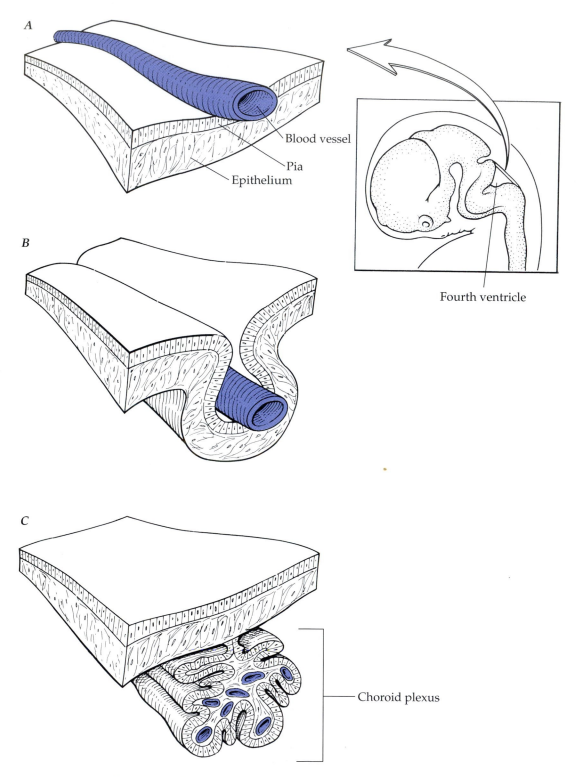

Figure 3–3. Development of the choroid plexus in the fourth ventricle. *A.* A blood vessel is shown apposing the pia, which adheres to the epithelium lining the ventricle. *B.* The blood vessel invaginates the ventricle, carrying with it the pia. *C.* Later in development the choroid plexus proliferates within the ventricle.

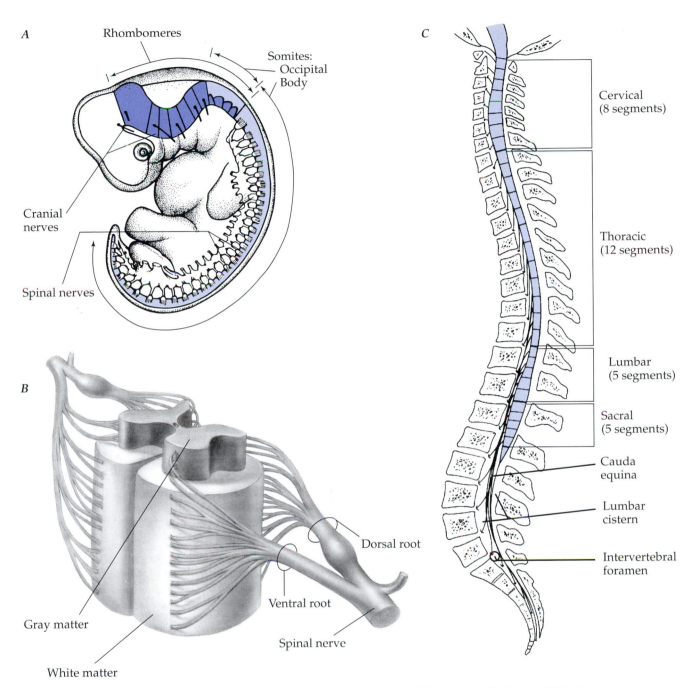

A

Rhombomeres

Somites:
Occipital
Body

Cranial
nerves

Spinal nerves

C

Cervical
(8 segments)

Thoracic
(12 segments)

Lumbar
(5 segments)

Sacral
(5 segments)

Cauda
equina

Lumbar
cistern

Intervertebral
foramen

B

Dorsal root

Ventral root

Spinal nerve

Gray matter

White matter

Figure 3–4. The hindbrain and spinal cord are segmented structures. In the caudal brain stem the segments are called rhombomeres; in the spinal cord they are called body somites. Four occipital somites form structures of the head. These are shown in the caudal medulla. *A.* The position of the developing nervous system in the embryo is illustrated as well as the segmental organization of rhombomeres and somites. The cranial nerves that contain the axons of brain stem motor neurons are also shown. From rostral to caudal the following cranial nerves are illustrated: IV, V, VI, VII, IX, X, and XII. The two mesencephalic segments and the segment between the metacephalon and mesencephalon are not shown. *B.* Drawing of a single spinal cord segment from the mature nervous system. *C.* Lateral view of the mature spinal cord in the vertebral canal. Note that the spinal nerves exit from the vertebral canal through intervertebral foramina. *(A, Adapted from Lumsden A: The cellular basis of segmentation in the developing hindbrain. Trends Neurosci 1990;13:329–335.)*

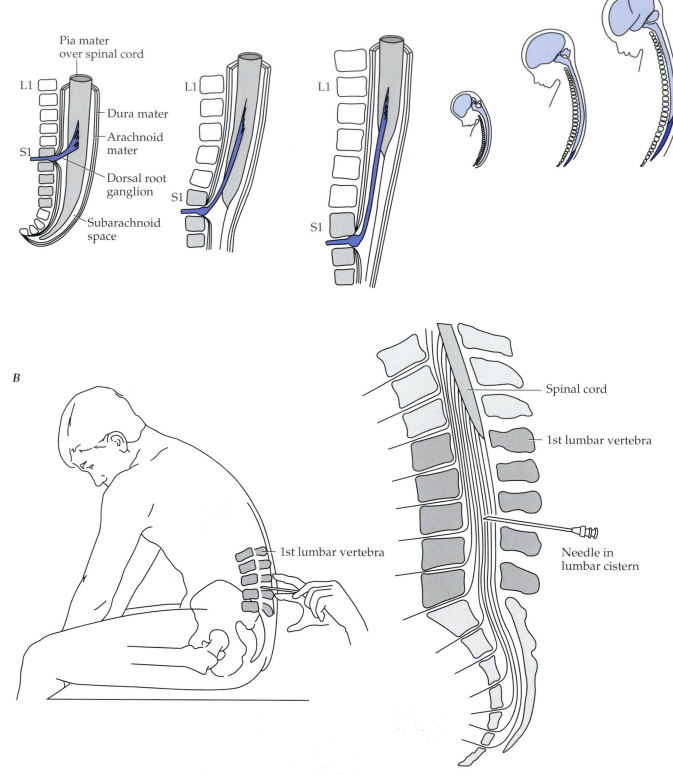

Figure 3–5. The lumbar cistern forms because the vertebral column grows in length more than the spinal cord. ***A.*** Side view of the lumbosacral spinal cord and vertebral column at three developmental stages: 3 months, 5 months, and in the newborn. The inset (right) shows the fetus at these stages. ***B.*** Withdrawal of cerebrospinal fluid from the lumbar cistern (lumbar puncture). The needle is inserted into the subarachnoid space of the lumbar cistern. The view on the right shows the relationship between the needle and the roots in the cistern. Note that the lumbar puncture is performed with the patient lying on his or her side. In this figure the patient is sitting upright to simplify visualization of the procedure. *(Adapted from Kandel ER, Schwartz JA: Principles of Neural Science. Elsevier, 1985.)*

at the level of the **first lumbar vertebra.** This differential growth produces the **lumbar cistern,** an enlargement of the subarachnoid space in the caudal portion of the spinal canal (Figures 3–4C and 3–5). The dorsal and ventral roots from the lumbar and sacral segments, which subserve sensation and movement of the legs, travel within the lumbar cistern before exiting the vertebral canal (Figure 3–5B). These roots resemble a horse's tail in gross dissection, hence the name **cauda equina.** Cerebrospinal fluid can be withdrawn from the lumbar cistern without risk of damaging the spinal cord by inserting a needle through the intervertebral space between the third and fourth (or fourth and fifth) vertebrae (Figure 3–5B). The roots are displaced by the needle rather than being pierced. This procedure is known as a **spinal** or **lumbar tap.**

The developing brain stem is also segmented. The eight hindbrain segments, termed **rhombomeres,** provide the sensory and motor innervation for most of the head through the peripheral projections of the cranial nerves. In contrast to the spinal cord, where each segment contains a pair of dorsal and ventral roots, each rhombomere is not associated with a single pair of sensory and motor cranial nerve roots. More rostral brain stem segments are termed **neuromeres.** A rhombomere between the metencephalon and mesencephalon, sometimes termed the **isthmus,** plays a critical role in organizing development of the two neuromeres of the mesencephalon. In maturity the isthmus is typically considered part of the pons. Segmentation may be a mechanism for establishing a basic plan of organization for the various parts of the spinal cord and hindbrain. This segmental plan is maintained into maturity for the spinal cord. In the mature brain stem, however, segmentation is obscured by later elaboration of neural interconnections. Box 3–1 considers the genetic determinants of the rostrocaudal pattern of rhombomeres.

The Location of Developing Spinal Cord and Brain Stem Nuclei Determine Their Functions and Connections

The developmental plans of the spinal cord and brain stem are similar. Spinal and brain stem neurons develop from precursor cells in the ventricular zone of the neural tube cavity. They migrate locally to form two zones of developing neurons, which are separated by the **sulcus limitans:** the alar plate and the basal plate. Initially the **alar plate** (Figure 3–7A) is located in the dorsal portion of the neural tube wall and mediates **sensory** functions. The **basal plate** (Figure 3–7A) is located in the ventral portion of the

neural tube wall and mediates **motor** functions. Diffusion of molecular signals from the **roof** and **floor plates** (Figures 3–1, 3–7A1, and 3–8A1), and adjacent tissues, is important in establishing this dorsoventral pattern of functional organization. Signals from the roof plate and nearby ectoderm help to establish the organization of the dorsal neural tube. Signals from the floor plate and **notochord** (Figure 3–1) are important for organizing the ventral neural tube. These early developmental events set the stage for development of the distinctive circuits formed by neurons of the dorsal and ventral neural tube.

Dorsal and Ventral Regions of the Spinal Cord Mediate Somatic Sensation and Motor Control of the Limbs and Trunk

Developing neurons from the alar plate form the interneurons and projection neurons of the **dorsal horn** of the mature spinal cord (Figure 3–7B). Dorsal horn neurons are important primarily in pain and visceral sensations. These neurons receive sensory information directly from the dorsal root ganglion neurons (see Figure 2–3). Many dorsal horn neurons project to the brain stem or diencephalon; others are interneurons. Most of the developing neurons of the basal plate give rise to the interneurons and motor neurons of the **ventral horn** of the mature spinal cord (Figure 3–7B). The motor neurons project their axons to the periphery via the ventral roots (Figure 3–7A). Although a clear functional distinction exists between the dorsal and ventral horns, the functions of axons in different locations of the white matter, especially in the lateral and ventral columns, are more heterogeneous. Because the spinal cord has a longitudinal organization, the alar and basal plates form columns of developing neurons that run rostrocaudally (see Figure 3–4B).

Dorsal root ganglion neurons that innervate skin, skeletal muscles, and joints (ie, somatic structures) synapse in different parts of the dorsal horn than do neurons that innervate blood vessels and body organs (ie, visceral structures). Similarly, somatic motor neurons controlling striated muscle are located in different parts of the ventral horn than are neurons controlling visceral structures.

Nuclear Columns in the Brain Stem Are Further Differentiated From Those in the Spinal Cord

The cranial nerve sensory and motor nuclei of the brain stem are analogous to the dorsal and ventral

Box 3–1.   Development of the Regional Anatomy of the Brain Stem and Autism

The *Hox* genes have been implicated in brain stem development through their role in determining the identity of the different rhombomeres (Figure 3–6A). *Hox* genes encode transcription factors that regulate development in many different species through their actions on other genes. The *Hox* genes, as well as other transcription factors, have complex patterns of expression in the brain stem (Figure 3–6B). Many have a rhombomere-specific pattern. It is thought that the formation of a particular rhombomere could be determined by interactions between the products of *Hox* genes. Genetically engineered mice that have had one of the *Hox* genes deleted show an abnormal brain stem anatomy. For example, after a *Hox* gene deletion, particular nuclei, cranial nerves, and peripheral

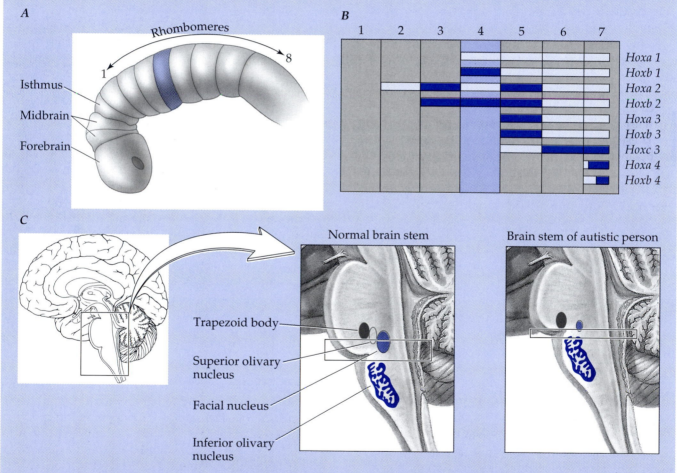

Figure 3–6.   A. Schematic side view of the developing central nervous system showing the forebrain, the midbrain, the isthmus, and the eight rhombomeres of the hindbrain. The fourth rhombomere is highlighted. **B.** The pattern of *Hox* gene expression. **C.** A slice of the pons is missing in a person that had autism. This resulted in several anatomical changes in the pons, including the loss of the superior olivary nucleus and a reduction in the size of the facial motor nucleus. (**A,** *Adapted from O'Rahilly R, Müller F: The Embryonic Human Brain. Wiley-Liss, 1999.* **B,** *Adapted from Lumsden A, Krumlauf R: Patterning of the vertebrate neuraxis. Science 1996;274:1109–1115.* **C,** *Adapted from Rodier PM: The early origins of autism. Sci Am 2000;282:56–63.*)

Box 3–1 (continued).

somatic structures may not develop normally or may be absent.

Although our understanding of the precise role of *Hox* genes in shaping brain stem anatomy is incomplete, mounting evidence indicates that *Hox* gene mutations cause birth defects in humans. A particularly intriguing example is the role of *Hoxa1* in autism. Autism is a developmental disorder characterized by a wide range of behavioral impairments including disorders in interpreting emotions and in language and communication skills and preoccupation with a single event or subject. These complex integrative behaviors are associated with the functions of the forebrain. However, autistic individuals also have impaired motor control, which involves both the forebrain and the hindbrain. Two such motor impairments involve defective control of eye movement and facial expressions.

Although patients with autism have many brain abnormalities, researchers discovered that two brain stem nuclei were virtually absent in an autistic patient. This finding has provided an important clue to the genetic determinants of the disease. It also helps explain development of the fine structure of the central nervous system. One of the missing nuclei is the **facial motor nucleus,** which contains motor neurons that innervate muscles of facial expression. The other is the **superior olivary nucleus,** which is important in sound localization. Autistic patients lack facial expressions, although it is not yet known if they have hearing localization impairments. The researchers described the pons as if a slice had been removed (Figure 3–6C). This structural deletion is reminiscent of the proposed role for *Hox* genes in specifying features of hindbrain segmentation. Genetic analysis in humans has revealed that

allelic variants of the *Hoxa1* gene are much more common in people with autism. This genetic defect may confer susceptibility to autism. Transgenic mice, in which the *Hoxa1* gene is not expressed, show similar anatomical changes in the brain stem.

Multiple biological and environmental factors contribute to autism. A heritable component exists, although it is more complex than a single dominant or recessive mutation. There are also many risk factors, such as in utero exposure to rubella or various teratogens. Recent research suggests that the events that trigger autism occur early during development, soon after neurogenesis. This is because autism is 30 times more common among patients exposed to the motion-sickness drug thalidomide, which causes birth defects at the time of neural tube closure, during the first few weeks of pregnancy.

horn, respectively. Cranial nerve sensory nuclei contain neurons that receive sensory information directly from cranial structures via cranial sensory nerves. Cranial nerve motor nuclei contain the cell bodies of motor neurons, whose axons course through cranial motor nerves to innervate their peripheral targets. Despite these similarities, three important differences exist between the developmental plans of the spinal cord and the brain stem. These differences make brain stem neuroanatomy more complicated than that of the spinal cord. First, the alar and basal plate cell columns of the hindbrain (ie, the developing medulla and pons) are aligned roughly from the lateral surface to the midline rather than being oriented in the dorsoventral axis, as in the spinal cord. This is because the cavity in

the neural tube of the hindbrain "opens up" at its dorsal surface to form the fourth ventricle (Figure 3–8). Second, in brain stem development, immature neurons migrate more extensively from the ventricular floor to distant sites than in the spinal cord (see next section). Extensive neuronal migration also characterizes the developmental plan of the cerebellum and forebrain. Third, as a consequence of the greater diversity of sensory and motor structures of the head, there is further differentiation of cranial nerve nuclei. For example, the inner ear has a structural complexity greater than that of somatic sensory receptors projecting to the spinal cord, and its functions are mediated by distinct nuclei. Moreover, cranial striated muscle develops either from the occipital somites or from the branchial

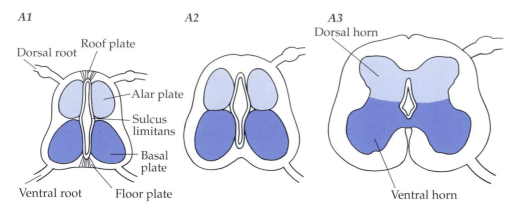

A1

Dorsal root
Roof plate
Alar plate
Sulcus limitans
Basal plate
Ventral root
Floor plate

A2

A3
Dorsal horn
Ventral horn

Figure 3–7. ***A.*** Schematic drawing of transverse sections of the spinal cord at three stages of development. ***B.*** Myelin-stained section through spinal cord of mature nervous system.

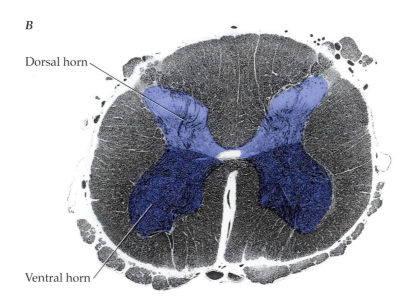

B

Dorsal horn

Ventral horn

arches (ie, tissue corresponding to gills that is present early in human development and corresponds to evolutionary derivatives of aquatic vertebrates). The locations of motor neurons innervating muscles of different origins—**somatic** or **branchiomeric**—is distinct.

This diversity in the innervation of cranial structures creates a large number of functional nuclear groups in which sensory fibers synapse and motor neurons are located (Table 3–1). With the exception of the olfactory and optic nerves (the first and second cranial nerves), which mediate smell and sight but do not enter the brain stem, there are seven distinct functional categories of cranial nerve sensory and motor nuclei. Nuclei within each category form a column. Some columns are more contiguous than others (see Figure 3–12).

The sensory columns are lateral to the sulcus limitans, with the somatic sensory and hearing and balance columns tending to be lateral to the viscerosensory and taste columns. The motor columns are medial to the sulcus limitans, with the somatic skeletal motor

medial to the autonomic motor column. The branchiomeric column contains neurons that are located in the region of the reticular formation. In the adult the sulcus limitans remains as a landmark on the floor of the fourth ventricle (see Figure AI–7).

The Complex Morphology of the Brain Stem Is Determined by the Migratory Patterns of Developing Neurons

Cranial nerve nuclei have relatively simple roles in processing afferent information or transmitting motor control signals. However, most brain stem nuclei have more complex integrative functions. Whereas brain stem integrative nuclei also derive from developing neurons of the alar and basal plates in the ventricular floor, the immature neurons that give rise to these structures migrate to their destinations in more dorsal or ventral regions (Figures 3–9 through 3–11).

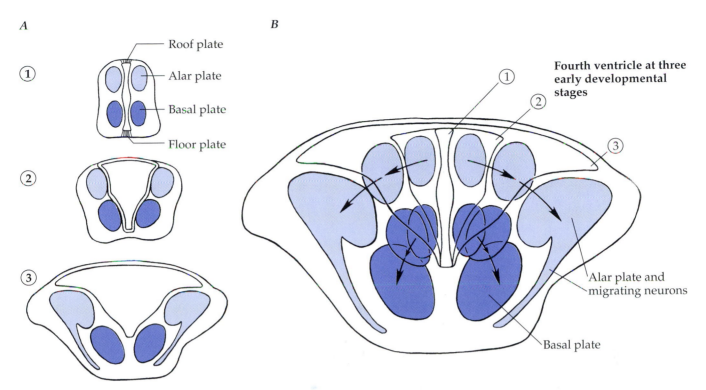

A

B

Fourth ventricle at three early developmental stages

Figure 3–8. At the junction of the spinal cord and medulla, it is as if the central canal opens along its dorsal margin. This has the effect of transforming the dorsoventral nuclear organization of the spinal cord into the lateromedial organization of nuclei in the caudal brain stem (the future medulla and pons).

Table 3–1. Functional classes of peripheral nerves.

Function	Structure innervated	Spinal nerves	Cranial nerves
Sensory Fibers			
Somatic sensory (mechanosensory, pain, temperature, itch)	Skin mucous membranes, skeletal muscles	All spinal nerves	V, VII, IX, X
Viscerosensory	Visceral structures	Thoracic, sacral spinal nerves	V, VII, IX, X
Hearing, balance	Cochlea, labyrinth		VIII
Taste	Taste buds		VII, IX, X
Olfaction[1]	Olfactory epithelium		I
Vision[1]	Eye		II
Motor Fibers			
Somatic skeletal motor	Limb and axial muscles	All spinal nerves	
	Extraocular muscles and tongue		III, IV, VI, XII
Branchiomeric skeletal motor	Facial, jaw, pharyngeal, and laryngeal		V, VII, IX, X, XI
Autonomic	Sweat, tear, and salivary glands; gut; smooth muscle	Thoracic and sacral (3–5 segments)	VII, IX, X

[1]The olfactory and optic nerves enter the cerebral hemispheres and diencephalon, respectively.

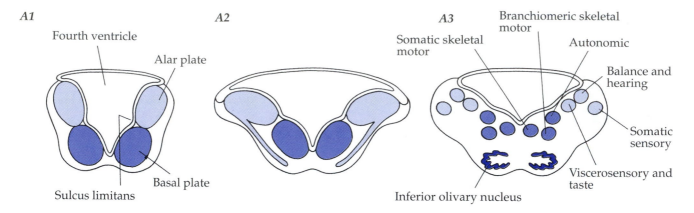

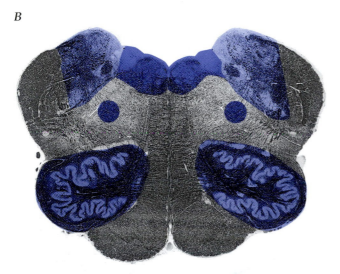

Figure 3–9. The alar and basal plates are subdivided in the medulla. *A.* Schematic drawing of transverse sections of the medulla at three stages of development. *B.* Myelin-stained section through medulla of mature nervous system.

Most neurons migrate radially (ie, at right angle to the neuraxis) along local paths established by astrocytes, which are a class of glial cells. Some of the more prominent nuclei that develop from migrating neurons include the inferior olivary nucleus in the medulla (Figure 3–9A3) and the pontine nuclei (Figure 3–10A3). These nuclei integrate sensory information and motor control signals from diverse brain areas and transmit this information to the cerebellum. The inferior olivary and pontine nuclei, together with the cerebellum, form important circuits for motor skill learning and producing movements. In the midbrain the red nucleus and substantia nigra (Figure 3–11A3) also develop from immature neurons that migrate from more dorsal portions. These two midbrain structures are also part of the motor control systems.

Schematic sections through the developing medulla, pons, and midbrain (parts A in Figures 3–9 through

3–11) can be compared with myelin-stained sections through the same divisions of the mature brain stem (parts B in Figures 3–9 through 3–11). Note that the midbrain has a dorsoventral organization, like the spinal cord. This is because the fourth ventricle does not extend into the midbrain.

Knowledge of how the brain stem alar and basal plates are organized provides an essential framework for understanding the mature brain stem. During development the various cranial nerve nuclear columns maintain similar relative positions with respect to the midline and the floor of the fourth ventricle. Because cranial nerve nuclei that serve similar functions are aligned in the same rostrocaudal columns, knowledge of the locations of these columns aids in understanding their function. Figure 3–12 shows the longitudinal organization of the cell columns forming the cranial nerve nuclei in the mature brain stem.

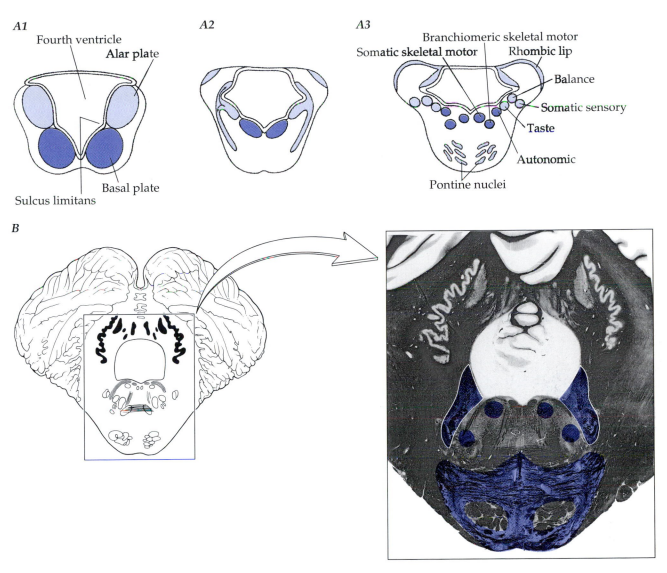

Figure 3–10. Immature neurons migrate from the alar plate and form the pontine nuclei. *A.* Schematic drawing of transverse sections of the pons at three stages of development. *B.* Myelin-stained section through pons of mature nervous system. The inset shows a slice through the pons and cerebellum. The rectangle corresponds approximately to the section in *B.*

The Cerebellum Develops From the Rhombic Lips

The cerebellum plays a key role in controlling movement and posture. Without the cerebellum, even simple and routine motor behaviors are uncoordinated. Indeed, patients with damage to the cerebellum reach inaccurately and display a characteristically unsteady gait. Most of the cerebellum develops from neurons located in the **rhombic lips,** specialized regions of the alar plate of the dorsolateral metencephalon (or future pons) (Figure 3–10A3). Migration of developing cerebellar neurons is extensive, much more so than for brain stem or spinal cord neurons. Initially the cerebellar surface is smooth, but later in development, fissures form that are oriented from one side to the other. Chapter 13 addresses the organization of the cerebellum.

The Rostral Portion of the Neural Tube Gives Rise to the Diencephalon and Cerebral Hemispheres

Between the two halves of the diencephalon is the third ventricle. Early in development, at the five-vesicle stage, the major components of the diencephalon are

A1 *A2* *A3*

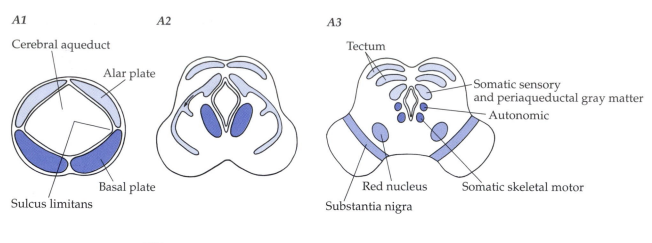

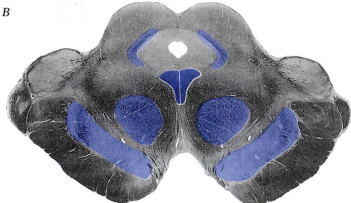

Figure 3–11. The tectum of the midbrain develops from the alar plate. *A.* Schematic drawing of transverse sections of the midbrain at three stages of development. *B.* Myelin-stained section through midbrain of mature nervous system.

present (Figure 3–2B): the **thalamus,** a collection of nuclei that communicate directly with the cerebral cortex; and the **hypothalamus,** a major brain structure for regulating visceral functions and their emotional counterparts (Figure 3–13A). The thalamus and hypothalamus are separated by the hypothalamic sulcus. (The retina also develops from the diencephalon [Figure 3–2, inset]. Despite its peripheral location, the retina is actually a portion of the central nervous system.)

The developing cerebral hemispheres are located anterior to the diencephalon, and each contains a lateral ventricle (Figures 3–2 and 3–13A2). The structure of the cerebral hemispheres is transformed markedly during development, in contrast to the spinal cord, brain stem, and diencephalon, which largely retain their longitudinal organization (Figure 3–14). This transformation is primarily the result of the enormous proliferation of cells of the **cerebral cortex,** the principal component of the cerebral hemispheres. The striatum and the amygdala, other cerebral hemisphere

components, develop from the **corpus striatum,** in the floor of the lateral ventricle.

The Cerebral Cortex Has an Inside-First Outside-Last Developmental Plan

Most of the neurons of the cerebral cortex originate from the ventricular zone lining the lateral ventricles (Figure 3–15A). Cortical development follows an inside-first outside-last program of neurogenesis (Figure 3–15B). Neurons born during early developmental stages migrate from the ventricular zone to form the deepest layers of cortex, whereas those born later migrate to form more superficial layers. **Radial glia** (a special class of astrocyte) provide the scaffold for these migrating neurons.

In addition to local migration from the ventricular zone along radial glial paths, there also is extensive longitudinal neuronal migration in the developing

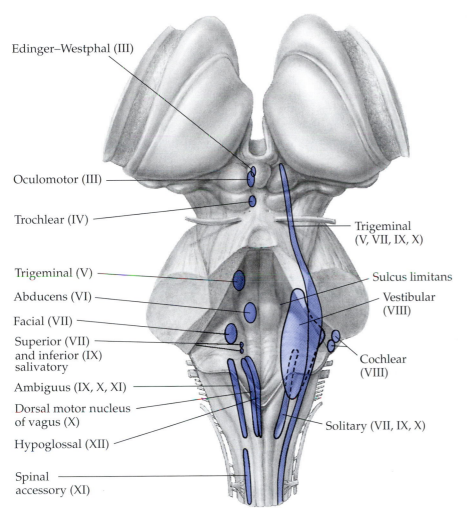

Edinger–Westphal (III)

Oculomotor (III)

Trochlear (IV)

Trigeminal (V)

Abducens (VI)

Facial (VII)

Superior (VII)
and inferior (IX)
salivatory

Ambiguus (IX, X, XI)

Dorsal motor nucleus
of vagus (X)

Hypoglossal (XII)

Spinal
accessory (XI)

Trigeminal
(V, VII, IX, X)

Sulcus limitans

Vestibular
(VIII)

Cochlear
(VIII)

Solitary (VII, IX, X)

Figure 3–12. The cranial nerve nuclei have a longitudinal organization. A dorsal view of the brain stem of the mature central nervous system is illustrated, with the locations of the various cranial never nuclei indicated.

cortex, which may depend on contact with other neurons and not just glial cells. Many cortical interneurons that use γ-aminobutyric acid (GABA) as their neurotransmitter migrate from the developing corpus striatum to their final cortical location (Figure 3–15A). In humans, but apparently not in animals, these migrating GABA-ergic neurons follow a path to the dorsal thalamus (Figure 3–15A), specifically to nuclei that are disproportionately large, the pulvinar and medial dorsal nuclei. This may be a special mechanism in the human brain to populate certain important nuclei with more neurons.

The Cerebral Cortex and Underlying Structures Have a C-Shape

The surface area of the cerebral cortex increases enormously during development. As the cerebral cortex develops, it encircles the diencephalon and takes on a c-shape. First, the surface area of the parietal lobe increases, followed by an increase in the frontal lobe. Next, the cortex expands posteriorly and inferiorly, forming the occipital and temporal lobes (Figure 3–14, 50–100 days). Because the cranial cavity does not increase in size in proportion to the increase in cortical surface area, this expansion is accompanied by tremendous infolding. Apart from the lateral sulcus, the cerebral cortex remains smooth, or lisencephalic, until the 6th or 7th month, when it develops gyri and sulci, becoming gyrencephalic. About one third of the cerebral cortex is exposed, and the remainder is located within sulci.

As the cerebral cortex grows, it also forces many of the underlying subcortical structures to assume a c-shape (Figure 3–16). One such structure is the **caudate nucleus,** which plays a key role in such diverse higher brain functions as cognition and eye movement control. In maturity it consists of three components: The **head** is located within the frontal lobe, the **body** is mostly within the parietal lobe, and the **tail** is located in the temporal lobe. The other portions of

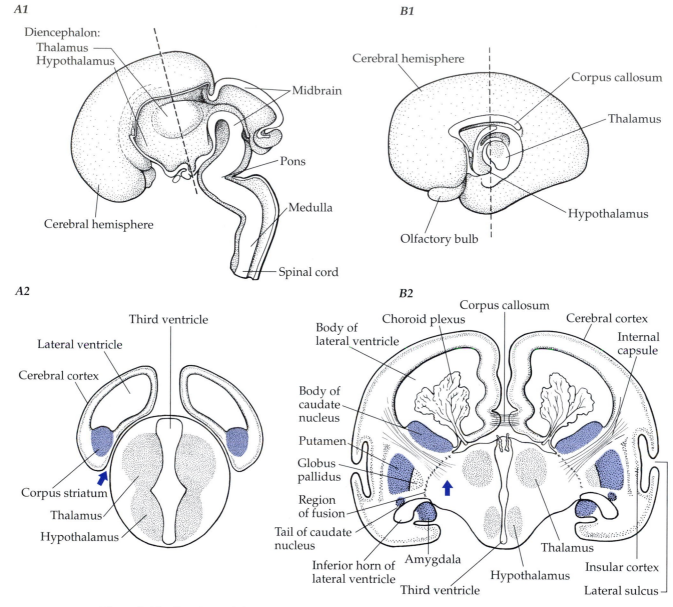

Figure 3–13. Portions of the cerebral hemispheres fuse with the diencephalon. The top portions of this figure illustrate medial views of brain during an early (*A*) and a later (*B*) stage of development. The bottom portion of the figure shows schematic transverse sections through the brain in the planes indicated on top (dashed lines). The arrow in *A2* marks the space separating the caudate nucleus (and other telencephalic structures) and diencephalon. Later in development, these regions fuse (arrow, *B2*) thereby allowing axons to cross at the point of attachment. (*Adapted from Patten BM: Human Embryology. McGraw-Hill [Blackston Division], 1968.*)

the striatum—the putamen and nucleus accumbens—comprise a more spherical mass. The putamen is important in limb and trunk movement control and the nucleus accumbens in emotions. Later chapters consider other c-shaped nuclear structures of the cerebral hemisphere.

The lateral ventricle is roughly spherical in shape at 2 months and is later transformed into a c-shape

(Figures 3–14 and 3–16). By about 5 months the lateral ventricle expands anteriorly to form the **anterior (or frontal) horn,** caudally to form the body and **posterior (or occipital) horn,** and inferiorly to form the **inferior (or temporal) horn.** The **atrium** is the region of confluence of the body, posterior horn, and inferior horn. The anterior horn and body of the two lateral ventricles remain close to the midline. The medial walls of each

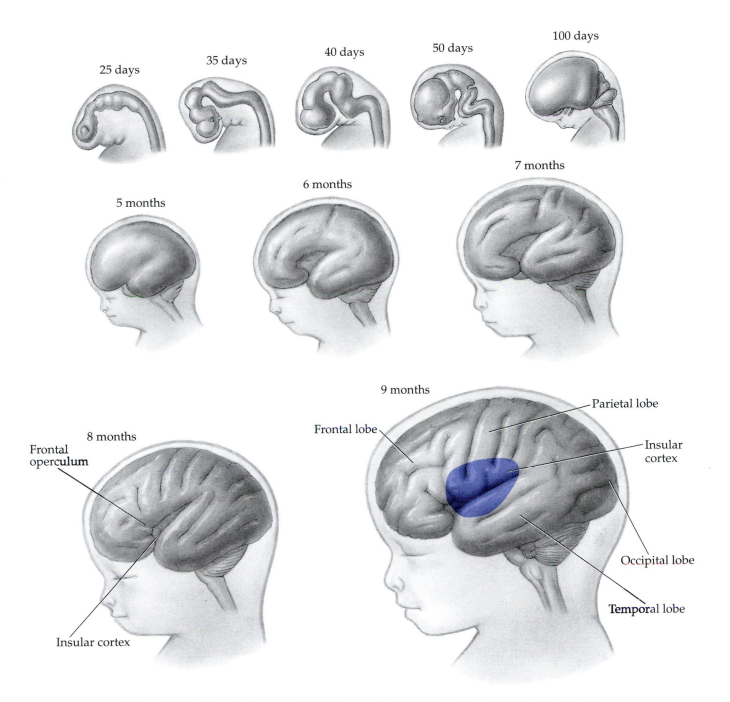

Figure 3–14. The development of the human brain is shown from the lateral surface in relation to the face and the general shape of the cranium. *(Adapted from Cowan WM: The development of the brain. Sci Am 1979;241:112–133.)*

lateral ventricle are formed by the **septum pellucidum,** which is a nonneural structure (Figure 3–16E, right). The choroid plexus, located in the lateral ventricle, also has a c-shape (Figure 3–17): It runs along the floor of the body of the lateral ventricle and then along the roof of the inferior horn. The choroid plexus in each lateral ventricle is continuous with that in the third ventricle, running through the interventricular foramina.

The lateral ventricle and caudate nucleus are important landmarks throughout most of the mature cerebral hemispheres. The key to understanding their locations in two-dimensional slices is in knowing that they are each located dorsally and ventrally. Myelin-stained transverse sections through the mature brain are shown in Figure 3–18. The body of the lateral ventricle is revealed in the dorsal portion of each

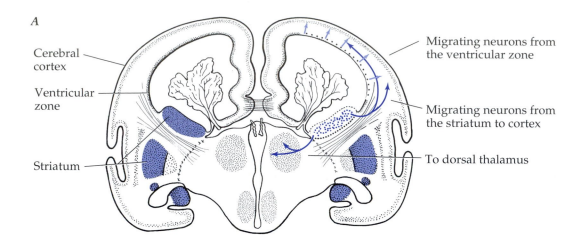

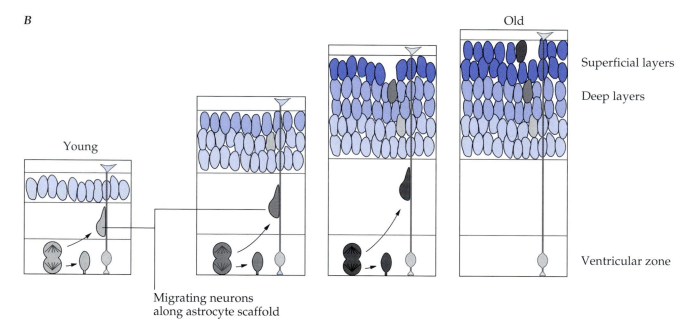

Figure 3–15. ***A.*** Schematic drawing of a section through the developing cerebral cortex and diencephalon. The two paths of migrating neurons are shown radially from the ventricular zones and longitudinally from the ganglionic eminence. ***B.*** Inside-first, outside-last development of cortical neurons. Schematic drawings of developing cortex at various developmental stages. The top of each rectangle indicates the pial surface; the bottom indicates the ventricular zone. (***A,*** *Adapted from Lumsden A, Gulisano M: Neocortical neurons: Where do they come from? Science 1997;274:1109–1115.* ***B,*** *Adapted from Kandel ER, Schwartz JS, Jessell TM (editors): Principles of Neural Science, 4th ed. McGraw-Hill; 2000:1019–1040.)*

section, in the frontal lobe; ventrally, the inferior horn of the lateral ventricle is seen in the temporal lobe. The caudate nucleus is also present in two locations: dorsally, in the lateral wall of the body of the lateral ventricle, and ventrally, in the roof of the inferior horn.

The Lateral Margin of the Diencephalon Fuses With the Telencephalon

Further development of the cerebral cortex results initially in the apposition and subsequent fusion of parts of the telencephalic and diencephalic surfaces

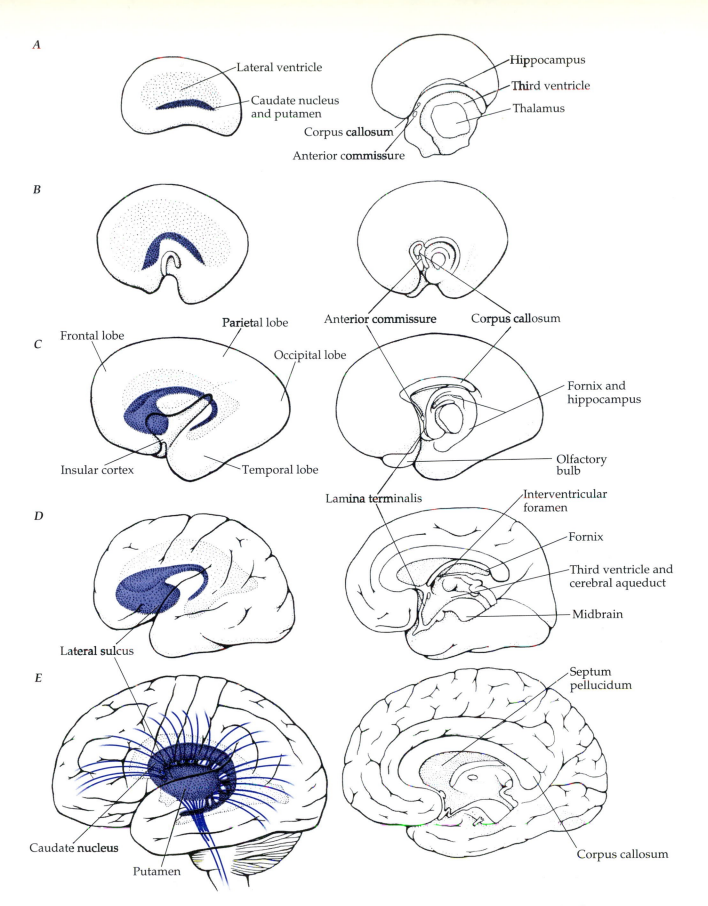

A

Lateral ventricle

Caudate nucleus and putamen

Hippocampus

Third ventricle

Thalamus

Corpus callosum

Anterior commissure

B

Parietal lobe

Anterior commissure

Corpus callosum

C

Frontal lobe

Occipital lobe

Fornix and hippocampus

Insular cortex

Temporal lobe

Olfactory bulb

Lamina terminalis

Interventricular foramen

D

Fornix

Third ventricle and cerebral aqueduct

Midbrain

Lateral sulcus

Septum pellucidum

E

Caudate nucleus

Putamen

Corpus callosum

Figure 3–16. Various components of the telencephalon acquire a c-shape during development. Lateral views of the cerebral hemisphere, with the lateral ventricle lightly stippled and the striatum tinted blue, are shown on the left; medial views are shown on the right. Five stages of development are illustrated: 2, 3, 5, 7, and 9 months. Ascending and descending axons of the internal capsule are shaded dark blue. They course between the caudate nucleus and the putamen. The descending axons in the internal capsule project into the brain stem. Many of these axons project farther caudally into the spinal cord. *(Adapted from Keibel F, Mall FP (editors): Manual of Human Embryology. 2 vols. Lippincott, 1910–1912.)*

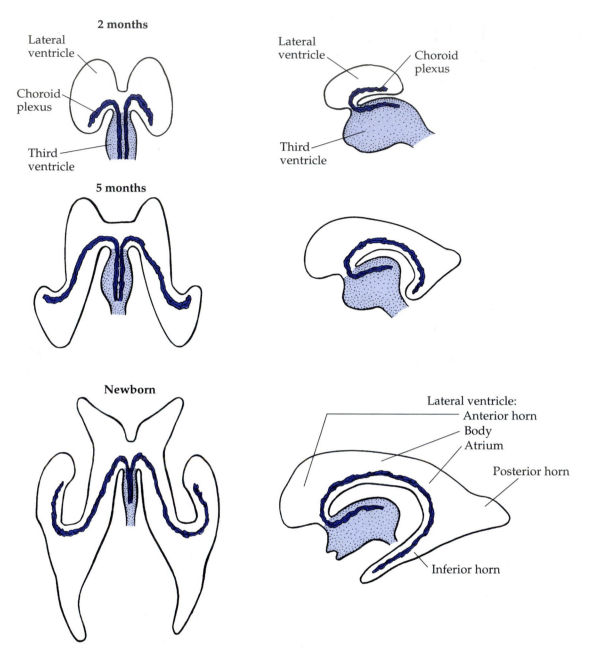

2 months

Lateral
ventricle

Choroid
plexus

Third
ventricle

Lateral
ventricle

Choroid
plexus

Third
ventricle

5 months

Newborn

Lateral ventricle:
Anterior horn
Body
Atrium

Posterior horn

Inferior horn

Figure 3–17. Development of the c-shape of the choroid plexus in the lateral ventricle. Three stages of development are shown: 2 months (***top***), 5 months (***middle***), and newborn (***bottom***). The left column illustrates a dorsal view of the lateral ventricles and third ventricle; the right column, the lateral view.

(Figure 3–13B2). This fusion has two important consequences. First, despite separation early in development (Figure 3–13A2, arrow), the caudate nucleus and the thalamus later become adjacent (Figure 3–13B2, arrow), an arrangement that continues into brain maturity. Second, after fusion there is a proliferation of ascending projections from the thalamus to the cor-

tex and of descending projections from the cortex to subcortical structures, including the thalamus, brain stem, and spinal cord. These axons connecting the cortex with other parts of the central nervous system form the **internal capsule** (Figure 3–13B2; see also Figure 2–12). The caudate nucleus and the putamen, which develop from the corpus striatum, are incom-

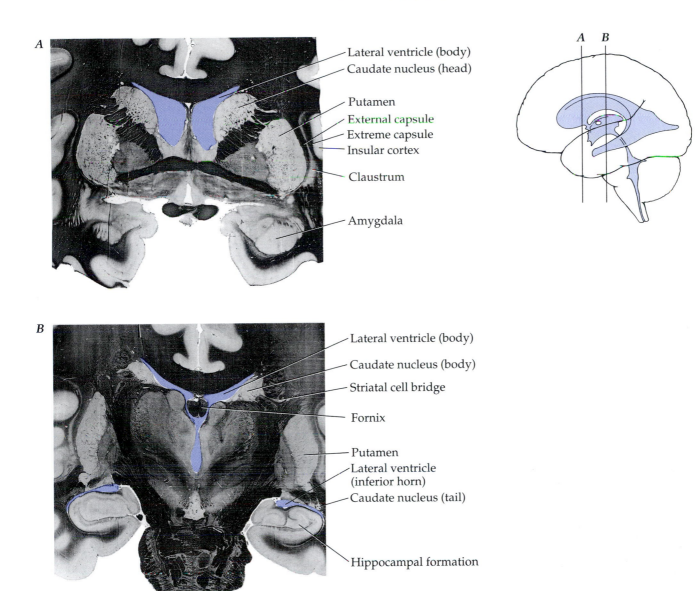

A

Lateral ventricle (body)
Caudate nucleus (head)

Putamen
External capsule
Extreme capsule
Insular cortex

Claustrum

Amygdala

B

Lateral ventricle (body)

Caudate nucleus (body)

Striatal cell bridge

Fornix

Putamen
Lateral ventricle
(inferior horn)
Caudate nucleus (tail)

Hippocampal formation

Figure 3–18. Coronal sections (myelin-stained) through the cerebral hemisphere of the mature brain illustrate that portions of the lateral ventricle and caudate nucleus are located dorsally and ventrally. The inset shows the shape of the lateral ventricle and the planes of section. The caudate nucleus follows the c-shaped course of the lateral ventricle. *A.* Rostral section through the anterior horn of the lateral ventricle and the head of the caudate nucleus. *B.* Caudal section through the body of the lateral ventricle and caudate nucleus (dorsomedially), the inferior horn of the lateral ventricle, and the tail of the caudate nucleus (ventrolaterally).

pletely separated by axons of the internal capsule (Figure 3–16E). The partial separation of the caudate nucleus and putamen by the fibers of the internal capsule also is reflected in the thin cell bridges that link these two structures (Figure 3–18).

Another major component of the basal ganglia is the **globus pallidus,** which is of diencephalic origin

(Figure 3–13B). The figure shows it at a slightly later stage of development. The globus pallidus works with the caudate nucleus and putamen in cognition and movement control. The constituent parts of the caudate nucleus are examined in Chapter 14. The **amygdala** (Figure 3–13B2) is another deep nuclear structure that develops from the corpus striatum. It plays a key role in the experience of emotions and in the behavioral expression of emotions, such as increased heart rate during a fearful experience. As development of the ascending and descending connections of the cerebral cortex proceeds, so too does that of the **corpus callosum,** the commissure interconnecting the cerebral cortex of the two hemispheres (Figure 3–16, right).

The Insular Cortex Is Hidden Beneath the Operculum of the Frontal, Parietal, and Temporal Lobes

Before most of the gyri and sulci are present on the cortical surface, a lateral region becomes buried by the developing frontal, parietal, and temporal lobes (Figures 3–13B2 and 3–14). This region, the **insular cortex** (see Figure 3–14, 9 months), is located deep within the lateral sulcus, one of the earliest grooves to form on the lateral surface. In the mature brain the insular cortex is revealed only when the banks of the lateral sulcus are partially separated or when the brain is sectioned, as in Figure 3–13 (see Figure 8–8). The portions of the frontal, parietal, and temporal cortices that cover the insular cortex are termed the **opercula.** The frontal operculum of the dominant hemisphere (typically the left hemisphere in right-handed individuals) contains Broca's area, which is important in speech articulation. The parietal and temporal opercular regions and the insular cortex have important sensory functions. Deep inside the insular cortex is the **claustrum** (Figure 3–18A), a thick sheet of neurons thought to derive from migrating neurons in the overlying cortex. The claustrum is separated from the cortex by the **extreme capsule** and from the putamen by the **external capsule** (Figure 3–18A). Although much is known about the anatomical connections of the claustrum, little is known of its function.

Summary

Early Development of the Central Nervous System

Nerve cells and glial cells are derived from a specialized portion of the ectoderm termed the **neural plate** (Figure 3–1). The edges of the neural plate fold, ultimately appose, and form the **neural tube** (Figure 3–1). The cerebral hemispheres and the brain stem develop from the rostral and intermediate portions of the neural tube, and the spinal cord develops from the

caudal portions. The **ventricular zone** (Figure 3–1) lines the neural tube and forms the cellular constituents of the central nervous system. Immature neurons arise from the ventricular zone. The cavity within the neural tube forms the **ventricular system** (Figure 3–1).

Development of Major Central Nervous System Divisions

Three brain vesicles first form from the rostral neural tube (Figure 3–2): (1) **prosencephalon (forebrain),** (2) **mesencephalon (midbrain),** and (3) **rhombencephalon (hindbrain).** The prosencephalon divides into the **telencephalon (cerebral cortex, hippocampal formation, basal ganglia,** and **amygdala)** and **diencephalon (thalamus** and **hypothalamus),** and the rhombencephalon divides into the **metencephalon (pons** and **cerebellum)** and **myelencephalon (medulla).** The **spinal cord,** like the mesencephalon, remains undivided throughout development. A persistent bend called the **cephalic flexure** occurs at the juncture of the mesencephalon and diencephalon (Figure 3–2). The **choroid plexus** is formed first by the apposition of brain vasculature overlying the ventricles and the **pia.** Then the blood vessels and pia invaginate into the ventricle (Figure 3–3).

Spinal Cord and Brain Stem Development

The spinal cord is segmented, both during development and in maturity. There are **8 cervical, 12 thoracic, 5 lumbar,** and **5 sacral segments.** During development the vertebral column grows more than the spinal cord, resulting in the formation of a cavity, the **lumbar cistern** (Figure 3–5). The hindbrain is segmented only during development. The eight hindbrain segments, termed **rhombomeres,** provide the sensory and motor innervation of most of the cranium. Immature neurons in the developing brain stem and spinal cord organize into rostrocaudally oriented columns of cells (Figures 3–4 and 3–12). There are two such columns in the spinal cord: the **alar plate** forms the **dorsal horn,** and the **basal plate** forms the **ventral horn** (Figures 3–4 and 3–6). In the brain stem the alar and basal plates become oriented mediolaterally (Figure 3–8) as if the central canal opens up to form the fourth ventricle. The alar and basal plates are divided into separate **somatic** and **visceral** columns, from which the cranial nerve nuclei derive (Figures 3–8 through 3–12). Other sensory and motor nuclei of the brain stem derive from immature neurons that migrate from the alar and basal plates. The cerebellum forms from a particular portion of the alar plate, the **rhombic lip** (Figure 3–10).

Development of the Diencephalon and Cerebral Hemispheres

The diencephalon (Figure 3–13) remains roughly spherical in shape throughout development. The cerebral cortex develops a laminar structure (Figure 3–15). Neurons in the deeper layers develop before those in the superficial layers. Some cortical interneurons develop from neurons that migrate from the ventricular zone near the developing striatum (Figure 3–15). Structures of the cerebral hemispheres, including the **cerebral cortex** and the **caudate nucleus,** take on a **c-shape** (Figures 3–14 and 3–16). The **lateral ventricle,** which is located within the cerebral hemisphere, and **choroid plexus** have a c-shape as well (Figure 3–17). c-shaped structures appear both dorsally and ventrally on transverse sections through the cerebral hemisphere (Figure 3–18).

Related Source Selections

Jessell TM, Sanes JR: The induction and patterning of the nervous system. In Kandel ER, Schwartz JH, Jessell TM (editors): Principles of Neural Science, 4th ed. McGraw-Hill; 2000:1019–1040.
Jessell TM, Sanes JR: The generation and survival of nerve cells. In Kandel ER, Schwartz JH, Jessell TM (editors): Principles of Neural Science, 4th ed. McGraw-Hill; 2000:1041–1062.

Selected Readings

Bonner-Fraser M: Crest density. Curr Biol 1993;3:201–203.
Copp AJ: Neural tube defects. Trends Neurosci 1993;16:381–383.

Dodd J, Jessell TM, Placzek M: The when and where of floor plate induction. Science 1998;282:1654–1657.
Jacobson M: Developmental Neurobiology, 2nd ed. Plenum Press, 1978.
Lumsden A: The cellular basis of segmentation in developing hindbrain. Trends Neurosci 1990;13:329–335.
Lumsden A, Gulisano M: Neocortical neurons: Where do they come from? Science 1997;278:402–403.
O'Rahilly R: The Embryonic Human Brain, 2nd ed. Wiley-Liss, 1999.
Puelles L, Rubenstein LR: Expression patterns of homeobox and other putative regulatory genes in the embryonic mouse forebrain suggest a neuromeric organization. Trends Neurosci 1993;16:472–479.
Rodier PM: The early origins of autism. Sci Am 2000;282:56–63.

References

Hemmati-Brivanlou A, Melton D: Vertebrate neural induction. Annu Rev Neurosci 1997;20:43–60.
Kandel ER, Schwartz JA: Principles of Neural Science. Elsevier, 1985.
Keibel F, Mall FP (editors): Manual of Human Embryology. 2 vols. Lippincott, 1910–1912.
Keynes RJ, Stern CD: Mechanisms of vertebrate segmentation. Development 1990;103:423–429.
Letinic K, Rakic P: Telencephalic origin of human thalamic GABAergic neurons. Nat Neurosci 2001;4:931–936.
Levitt P, Barbe MF, Eagleson KL: Patterning and specification of the cerebral cortex. Annu Rev Neurosci 1997;20:1–24.
Lumsden A, Keynes R: Segmental patterns of neuronal development in the chick hindbrain. Nature 1989;337:424–428.
O'Rahilly R, Müller F: Ventricular system and choroid plexuses of the human brain during the embryonic period proper. Am J Anat 1990;189:285–302.
Pansky B: Review of Medical Embryology. Macmillan, 1982.
Patten BM: Human Embryology. McGraw-Hill (Blackston Division), 1968.
Rodier PM, Ingram JL, Tisdale B, Nelson S, Romano J: Embryological origin for autism: Developmental anomalies of the cranial nerve motor nuclei. J Comp Neurol 1996;370:247–261.
Shuangoshoti S, Netsky MG: Histogenesis of choroid plexus in man. Am J Anat 1966;188:283–315.
Tuchmann-Duplessis H, Auroux M, Haegel P: Illustrated Human Embryology, Vol. 3: Nervous System and Endocrine Glands. Springer-Verlag, 1974.

Vasculature of the Central Nervous System and the Cerebrospinal Fluid

BRAIN VASCULATURE DISORDERS CONSTITUTE a major class of nervous system disease. The principal source of nourishment for the central nervous system is glucose, and because neither glucose nor oxygen is stored in appreciable amounts, when the blood supply of the central nervous system is interrupted, even briefly, brain functions become severely disrupted.

Much of what is known about the arterial supply to the central nervous system derives from three approaches. First, in fixed, postmortem tissue, colored dye can be injected into a blood vessel, thereby identifying the areas it supplies. Second, in postmortem tissue or on radiological examination, the portion of the central nervous system supplied by an artery can be inferred by observing the extent of damage that occurs when a particular artery is occluded or ruptures. Third, radiological techniques, such as cerebral angiography and magnetic resonance angiography, make it possible to view the arterial and venous circulation in the living brain (see Box 4–1). These important clinical tools permit localization of a vascular obstruction or other pathology.

As discussed in previous chapters, brain vasculature is closely related to the ventricular system and the watery fluid contained within it, the cerebrospinal fluid. This is because most cerebrospinal fluid is produced by active secretion of ions from blood plasma by the choroid plexus. Moreover, to maintain a constant brain volume, cerebrospinal fluid is returned to the blood through valves between the subarachnoid space and the dural sinuses.

This chapter initially focuses on arterial supply because of the importance of oxygenated blood to nor-

Table 4–1. Blood supply of the central nervous system.

Structure	Level	System	Major artery[1]
Spinal Cord		P	Anterior spinal artery
		P	Posterior spinal artery
		S	Radicular arteries
Medulla	Caudal	P	Anterior spinal artery
		P	Posterior spinal artery
	Rostral	P	Vertebral
		P	Vertebral: PICA
Pons	Caudal and	P	Basilar
	middle	P	Basilar: AICA
	Rostral	P	Basilar: SCA
Cerebellum	Caudal	P	Vertebral: PICA
	Middle	P	Basilar: AICA
	Rostral	P	Basilar: SCA
Midbrain	Caudal	P	Basilar
	(inferior colliculi)	P	Basilar: SCA
	Rostral	P	Posterior cerebral
	(superior colliculi)		
Diencephalon			
Thalamus		A	Posterior communicating
		P	Posterior cerebral: posterior choroidal
		P	Posterior cerebral: thalamogeniculate
		P	Posterior cerebral: thalamoperforating
Hypothalamus		A	Anterior cerebral
		A	Anterior communicating
		A	Posterior communicating
		P	Posterior cerebral
Subthalamus		A	Anterior choroidal
		A	Posterior communicating
		P	Posterior choroidal
		P	Posterior cerebral

mal brain function. Next it considers venous drainage and, finally, the blood-brain barrier and cerebrospinal fluid.

Neural Tissue Depends on Continuous Arterial Blood Supply

Local regions of the central nervous system receive blood from small sets of penetrating arteries that receive their blood from the major arteries (Table 4–1). Cessation or reduction of the arterial supply to an area results in decreased delivery of oxygenated blood to the tissue, a condition termed **ischemia.** Decreased blood supply occurs when an artery becomes occluded or when systemic blood pressure drops substantially, such as during a heart attack. Occlusion commonly occurs because of an acute blockade, such as from

an embolus, or the gradual narrowing of the arterial lumen (stenoses), as in atherosclerosis.

A brief reduction in blood flow produces transient neurological signs, attributable to lost functions of the blood-deprived area. This event is termed a transient ischemic attack, or TIA. If ischemia is persistent and is uncorrected for several minutes, it can produce tissue death, termed an **infarction.** This can result in more enduring or even permanent impairments. These events describe an **ischemic stroke.** Under special circumstances the local reduction in arterial blood flow may not produce an ischemic stroke and infarction because the tissue receives a redundant supply from another artery. This is termed **collateral circulation** (see below).

Hemorrhagic stroke can occur when an artery ruptures, thereby releasing blood into the surrounding tissue. A hemorrhagic stroke not only produces a loss of downstream flow but also can damage brain tissue

Table 4–1. *(continued.)*

Structure	Level	System	Major artery[1]
Basal Ganglia			
Globus pallidus	Superior	A	Middle cerebral: lenticulostriate
	Middle, inferior	A	Anterior choroidal
Striatum	Superior	A	Middle cerebral: lenticulostriate
	Inferior	A	Anterior cerebral: lenticulostriate
Septal Nuclei		A	Anterior cerebral
		A	Anterior communicating
		A	Anterior choroidal
Amygdala		A	Anterior choroidal
Hippocampal Formation		A	Posterior cerebral
Internal Capsule			
Anterior limb	Superior	A	Middle cerebral
	Middle	A	Anterior cerebral
	Inferior	A	Internal capsule
	Inferior	A	Anterior choroidal
Genu	Superior	A	Middle cerebral
	Middle	A	Anterior cerebral
	Inferior	A	Anterior choroidal; anterior cerebral
Posterior limb	Superior	A	Middle cerebral
	Inferior	A	Anterior choroidal
Retrolenticular		A	Anterior choroidal
Cerebral Cortex			
Frontal lobe		A	Anterior cerebral
		A	Middle cerebral
Parietal lobe		A	Anterior cerebral
		A	Middle cerebral
Occipital lobe		P	Posterior cerebral
Temporal lobe		P	Posterior cerebral

Abbreviation key: A, anterior circulation; AICA, anterior inferior cerebellar artery; P, posterior circulation; PICA, posterior inferior cerebellar artery; S, systemic circulation; SCA, superior cerebellar artery.
[1]Artery distributions based on radiological and dye-fill data; artery supplying more than approximately 80% of structure.

at the rupture site because of the volume now occupied by the blood outside of the vessel. A common cause of a hemorrhagic stroke is when an aneurysm, or ballooning of an artery due to weakening of the muscular wall, ruptures.

The Vertebral and Carotid Arteries Supply Blood to the Central Nervous System

The principal blood supply for the brain comes from two arterial systems that receive blood from different systemic arteries: the **anterior circulation,** fed by the **internal carotid arteries,** and the **posterior circulation,** which receives blood from the **vertebral arteries** (Figure 4–1, inset; Table 4–1). The vertebral arteries join at the junction of the medulla and pons (or pontomedullary junction) to form the **basilar artery,** which lies unpaired along the midline (Figure 4–1). The anterior circulation is also called the **carotid circulation,** and the posterior circulation, the **vertebral-basilar circulation.** The anterior and posterior circulations are not independent but are connected by networks of arteries on the ventral surface of the diencephalon and midbrain and on the cortical surface (see below).

Whereas the cerebral hemispheres receive blood from both the anterior and posterior circulations, the brain stem receives blood only from the posterior circulation. The arterial supply for the spinal cord is provided by the systemic circulation—which also supplies muscle, skin, and bones—and, to a lesser degree,

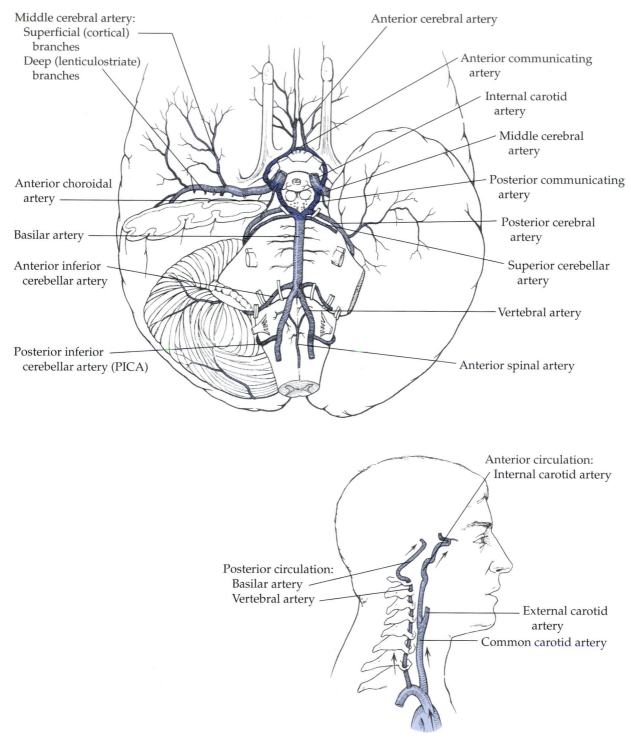

Middle cerebral artery:
Superficial (cortical) branches
Deep (lenticulostriate) branches

Anterior choroidal artery

Basilar artery

Anterior inferior cerebellar artery

Posterior inferior cerebellar artery (PICA)

Anterior cerebral artery

Anterior communicating artery

Internal carotid artery

Middle cerebral artery

Posterior communicating artery

Posterior cerebral artery

Superior cerebellar artery

Vertebral artery

Anterior spinal artery

Anterior circulation:
Internal carotid artery

Posterior circulation:
Basilar artery
Vertebral artery

External carotid artery
Common carotid artery

Figure 4–1. Diagram of the ventral surface of the brain stem and cerebral hemispheres, illustrating the key components of the anterior (carotid) circulation and the posterior (vertebral-basilar) circulation. The anterior portion of the temporal lobe of the right hemisphere is removed to illustrate the course of the middle cerebral artery through the lateral (Sylvian) fissure and the penetrating branches (lenticulostriate arteries). The circle of Willis (dark blue) is formed by the anterior communicating artery, the two posterior communicating arteries, and the three cerebral arteries. The inset (**bottom**) shows the extracranial and cranial courses of the vertebral, basilar, and carotid arteries.

by the vertebral arteries. Cerebral and spinal arteries drain into veins. Although spinal veins are part of the general systemic circulation and return blood directly to the heart, most cerebral veins drain first into the **dural sinuses,** a set of large venous collection channels in the dura mater.

The Spinal and Radicular Arteries Supply Blood to the Spinal Cord

The spinal cord receives blood from two sources. First are the **anterior** and **posterior spinal arteries** (Figure 4–1), branches of the vertebral arteries. Second are the **radicular arteries** (Figure 4–2), which are branches of segmental vessels, such as the cervical, intercostal, and lumbar arteries. Neither anterior nor posterior spinal arteries typically form a single continuous vessel along the entire length of the ventral or dorsal spinal cord. Rather, each forms a network of communicating channels oriented along the rostrocaudal axis of the spinal cord. The radicular arteries feed into this network along the entire length of the spinal cord.

Although the spinal and radicular arteries supply blood to all spinal cord levels, different spinal cord segments are preferentially supplied by one or the other set of arteries. The cervical spinal cord is supplied by both the vertebral and radicular arteries (the ascending cervical artery). In contrast, the thoracic, lumbar, and sacral segments are nourished primarily by the radicular arteries (the intercostal and lumbar arteries). When spinal cord segments are supplied by a single artery, they are particularly susceptible to injury after arterial occlusion. In contrast, segments that receive a redundant (or collateral) blood supply tend to fare better following single vessel occlusion. For example, individual rostral thoracic segments are supplied by fewer radicular arteries than are more caudal segments. When a radicular artery that serves the rostral thoracic segments becomes occluded, serious damage is more likely to occur because there is no backup system for perfusion of oxygenated blood. Interruption of the blood supply to critical areas of the spinal cord can produce sensory and motor control impairments similar to those produced by traumatic mechanical injury, such as that resulting from an automobile accident.

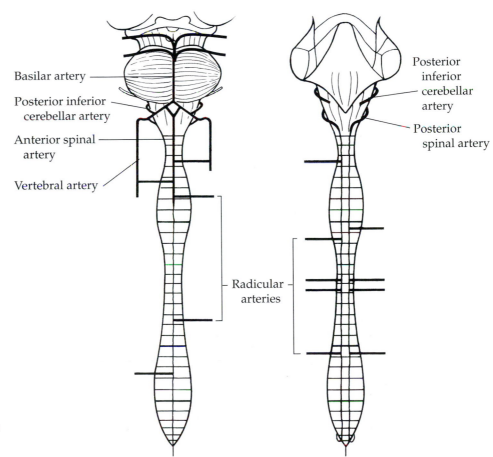

Figure 4–2. Schematic ventral (*left*) and dorsal (*right*) views of the spinal cord and brain stem are illustrated with the arterial circulation of the spinal cord. (*Adapted from Carpenter MB, Sutin J: Human Neuroanatomy. Williams & Wilkins, 1983.*)

The Vertebral and Basilar Arteries Supply Blood to the Brain Stem

Each of the three divisions of the brain stem and the cerebellum receives its arterial supply from the posterior circulation (Figure 4–3A). In contrast to the spinal arteries, which are located both ventrally and dorsally, arteries supplying most of the brain stem arise from the ventral surface only. Branches emerge from these ventral arteries and either penetrate directly or run around the circumference of the brain stem to supply dorsal brain stem structures and the cerebellum. Three groups of branches arise from the vertebral and basilar arteries: paramedian, short circumferential, and long circumferential. The **paramedian branches** supply regions close to the midline. The **short circumferential branches** supply lateral, often wedge-shaped regions, and the **long circumferential branches** supply the dorsolateral portions of the brain stem and cerebellum.

Even though the spinal arteries primarily supply the spinal cord, they also supply a small portion of the caudal medulla. The spinal arteries lie close to the dorsal and ventral midline and nourish the most medial areas (Figure 4–3B4). The more lateral area is served by the vertebral arteries, which are equivalent to the more rostral short circumferential branches.

Most of the medulla is supplied by the vertebral arteries on the ventral surface. Small (unnamed) branches that exit from the main artery supply the medial medulla (ie, paramedian and short circumferential branches). Because these arteries supply axons of the corticospinal tract and the medial lemniscus (see Figure 2–1), when the arteries become occluded patients develop impairments in voluntary limb movement and mechanosensation. The major laterally emerging (long circumferential) branch from the vertebral artery, the **posterior inferior cerebellar artery** (PICA), nourishes the most dorsolateral region (Figure 4–3B3). This region of the medulla does not receive blood from any other artery. The absence of a collateral arterial supply makes the posterior inferior cerebellar artery particularly important because occlusion almost always results in tissue damage. When this occurs, patients commonly develop characteristic sensory and motor impairments due to destruction of nuclei and tracts in the dorsolateral medulla. Common neurological signs include loss of facial pain sensation and uncoordinated limb movements, both on the side of the occlusion.

The vertebral arteries join to form the basilar artery at the pontomedullary junction (Figure 4–3A), from which paramedian and short circumferential arteries supply the base of the pons, where corticospinal fibers are located. The dorsolateral portion of the caudal pons is supplied by a long circumferential branch of the basilar artery, termed the **anterior inferior cere-**bellar artery (AICA). The region in the pons rostral to that supplied by the anterior inferior cerebellar artery is nourished by the **superior cerebellar artery,** another long circumferential branch of the basilar artery (Figure 4–3A).

The **posterior cerebral artery** nourishes most of the midbrain (Figure 4–3B1). Paramedian and short circumferential branches supply the base and tegmentum, whereas long circumferential branches supply the tectum. The colliculi, the most dorsal portion of the tectum, also receive a small supply by the superior cerebellar artery.

Long circumferential branches of the vertebral and basilar arteries supply the cerebellum. The posterior inferior cerebellar artery supplies the caudal portion of the cerebellum. More rostral portions are supplied by the anterior inferior cerebellar artery and the superior cerebellar artery (Figures 4–1 and 4–3A).

The Internal Carotid Artery Has Four Principal Portions

The **internal carotid artery** consists of four segments (Figure 4–4A): (1) The **cervical segment** extends from the bifurcation of the common carotid (into the external and internal carotid arteries; see Figure 4–1) to where it enters the carotid canal; (2) the **intrapetrosal segment** courses through the petrous portion of the temporal bone; (3) the **intracavernous segment** courses through the cavernous sinus, a venous structure overlying the sphenoid bone (see Figure 4–16); and (4) the **cerebral segment** extends to where the internal carotid artery bifurcates into the anterior and middle cerebral arteries. The intracavernous and cerebral portions form the **carotid siphon,** an important radiological landmark.

Branches emerging directly from the cerebral segment of the internal carotid artery supply deep cerebral and other cranial structures. The major branches of this artery (Figure 4–4B), in caudal to rostral order, are (1) the **ophthalmic artery,** which supplies the optic nerve and the inner portion of the retina, (2) the **posterior communicating artery,** which primarily nourishes diencephalic structures, and (3) the **anterior choroidal artery,** which supplies diencephalic and subcortical telencephalic structures.

The Anterior and Posterior Circulations Supply the Diencephalon and Cerebral Hemispheres

The internal carotid artery divides near the basal surface of the cerebral hemisphere to form the **anterior cerebral** and **middle cerebral arteries** (Figure 4–1).

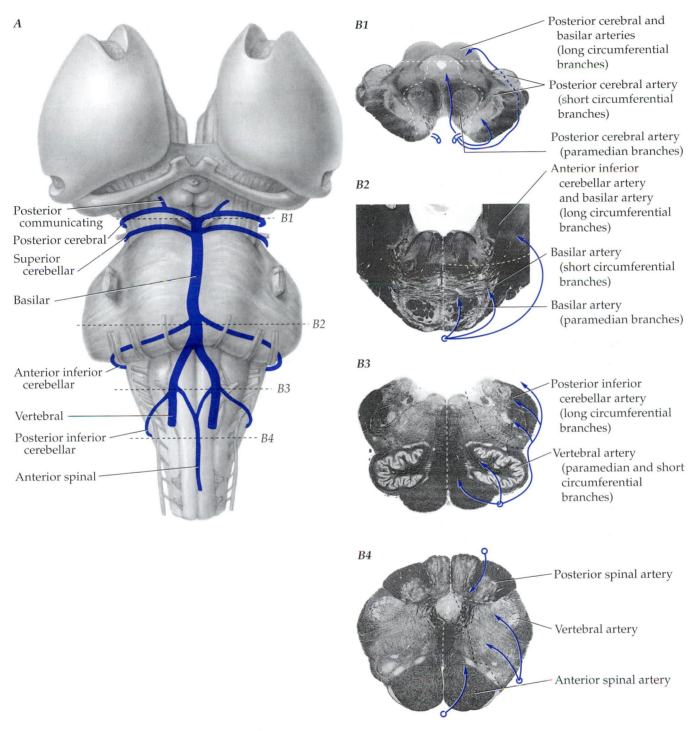

A

Posterior communicating

Posterior cerebral

Superior cerebellar

Basilar

Anterior inferior cerebellar

Vertebral

Posterior inferior cerebellar

Anterior spinal

B1

B2

B3

B4

B1

Posterior cerebral and basilar arteries (long circumferential branches)

Posterior cerebral artery (short circumferential branches)

Posterior cerebral artery (paramedian branches)

B2

Anterior inferior cerebellar artery and basilar artery (long circumferential branches)

Basilar artery (short circumferential branches)

Basilar artery (paramedian branches)

B3

Posterior inferior cerebellar artery (long circumferential branches)

Vertebral artery (paramedian and short circumferential branches)

B4

Posterior spinal artery

Vertebral artery

Anterior spinal artery

Figure 4–3. **A.** Arterial circulation of the brain stem is schematically illustrated on a view of the ventral surface of the brain stem. **B.** Four transverse sections through the brain stem are shown, illustrating the distribution of arterial supply. In the upper medulla (**B3**), pons (**B2**), and midbrain (**B1**), portions of tissue from medial to dorso-lateral are supplied by paramedian, short circumferential, and long circumferential branches. The caudal medulla receives its arterial supply from the vertebral and spinal arteries (**B4**). The dashed lines in **A** indicate the planes of section in **B**.

A

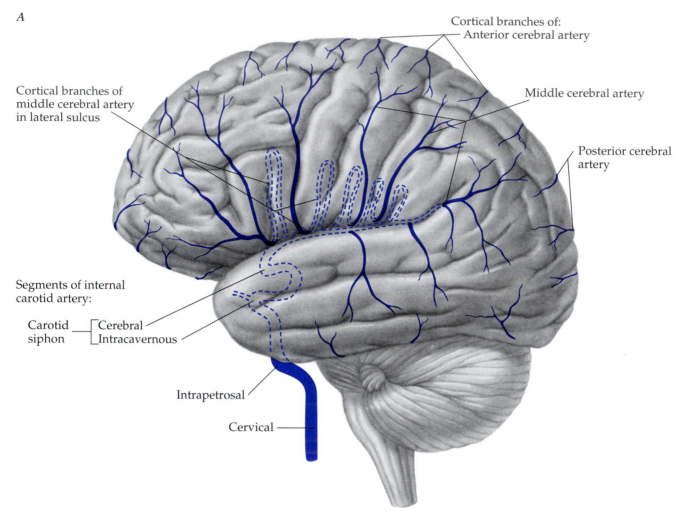

Cortical branches of:
Anterior cerebral artery

Middle cerebral artery

Posterior cerebral artery

Cortical branches of
middle cerebral artery
in lateral sulcus

Segments of internal
carotid artery:

Carotid
siphon

Cerebral

Intracavernous

Intrapetrosal

Cervical

Figure 4–4. The courses of the three cerebral arteries are illustrated in views of the lateral (*A*) and midsagittal (*B*) surfaces of the cerebral hemisphere. Note that the anterior cerebral artery (*B*) courses around the genu of the corpus callosum.

The **posterior cerebral artery** is part of the vertebral-basilar system and originates at the bifurcation of the basilar artery at the midbrain (Figures 4–1 and 4–3A). The posterior cerebral artery develops from the anterior system, thereby receiving blood from the carotid arteries. However, later in development much more blood comes from the basilar artery, making the posterior cerebral artery functionally part of the posterior circulation in maturity.

*The Circle of Willis Is Formed by the
Communicating and Cerebral Arteries*

The anterior and posterior arterial systems connect at several locations. This is clinically important because increased flow in one system can compensate for decreased flow in the other. One site of intercon-

nection is on the ventral brain surface, where the communicating arteries are located. Together the proximal portions of the cerebral arteries and the communicating arteries form the **circle of Willis.** This is an example of a network of interconnected arteries, or an **anastomosis.** The **posterior communicating artery** allows blood to flow between the middle and posterior cerebral arteries, and the **anterior communicating artery** allows blood to flow between the anterior cerebral arteries on both sides of the cerebral hemispheres (Figure 4–1). When either the posterior or the anterior arterial circulation becomes occluded, collateral circulation may occur through the circle of Willis to rescue the region deprived of blood. Many individuals, however, lack one of the components of the circle of Willis. In these individuals, a functional "circle" may not be achieved, resulting in incomplete cerebral perfusion by the surviving system.

B

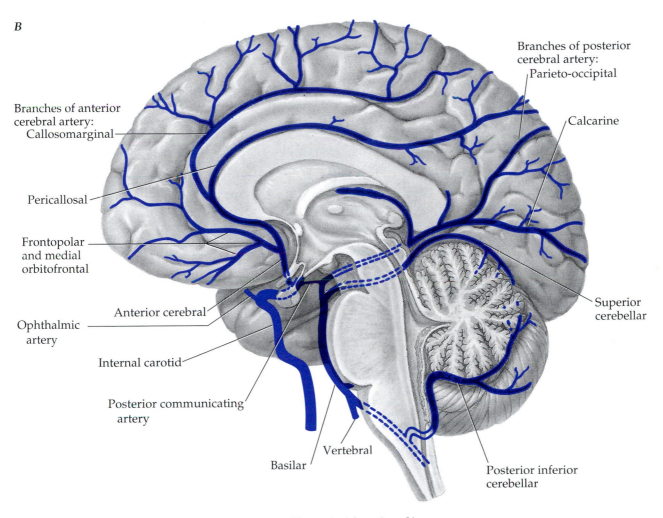

Branches of posterior cerebral artery:
Parieto-occipital

Calcarine

Branches of anterior cerebral artery:
Callosomarginal

Pericallosal

Frontopolar and medial orbitofrontal

Anterior cerebral

Ophthalmic artery

Internal carotid

Posterior communicating artery

Superior cerebellar

Vertebral

Basilar

Posterior inferior cerebellar

Figure 4–4 (continued.)

Deep Branches of the Anterior and Posterior Circulations Supply Subcortical Structures

The arterial supply of the diencephalon, basal ganglia, and internal capsule derives from both the anterior and posterior circulations (Figures 4–5 and 4–6; Table 4–1). This supply is complex, and there are many individual variations. The branches supplying these structures emerge from the proximal portions of the cerebral arteries or directly from the internal carotid artery. The **internal capsule,** the structure through which axons pass to and from the cerebral cortex, contains three separate parts: the **anterior limb,** the **genu,** and the **posterior limb.** Each part contains axons with different functions. Each part of the internal capsule also has a somewhat different arterial supply. The superior halves of the anterior and posterior limbs and the genu are supplied primarily by branches of the middle cerebral artery (Figure 4–6). The inferior half

of the internal capsule is supplied primarily by the anterior cerebral (anterior limb and part of the genu) and anterior choroidal arteries (Figures 4–5 and 4–6). The **basal ganglia** receive their arterial blood supply from the anterior and middle cerebral arteries (the lenticulostriate arteries) and the anterior choroidal artery (Figure 4–5). The **thalamus** is nourished by branches of the posterior cerebral and posterior communicating arteries. The **hypothalamus** is fed by branches of the anterior and posterior cerebral arteries and the two communicating arteries.

Different Functional Areas of the Cerebral Cortex Are Supplied by Different Cerebral Arteries

The cerebral cortex is supplied by the distal branches of the anterior, middle, and posterior cerebral arteries

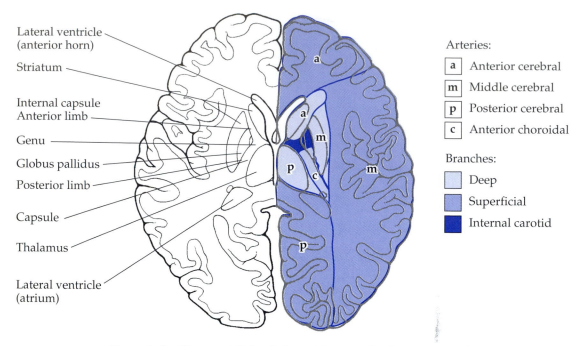

Lateral ventricle (anterior horn)
Striatum
Internal capsule Anterior limb
Genu
Globus pallidus
Posterior limb
Capsule
Thalamus
Lateral ventricle (atrium)

Arteries:
| a | Anterior cerebral
| m | Middle cerebral
| p | Posterior cerebral
| c | Anterior choroidal

Branches:
Deep
Superficial
Internal carotid

Figure 4–5. The arterial circulation of deep cerebral structures is illustrated in schematic horizontal section. (*Adapted from Fisher CM: Modern concepts of cerebrovascular disease. In Meyer JS (editor): The Anatomy and Pathology of the Cerebral Vasculature. Spectrum Publications; 1975:1–41.*)

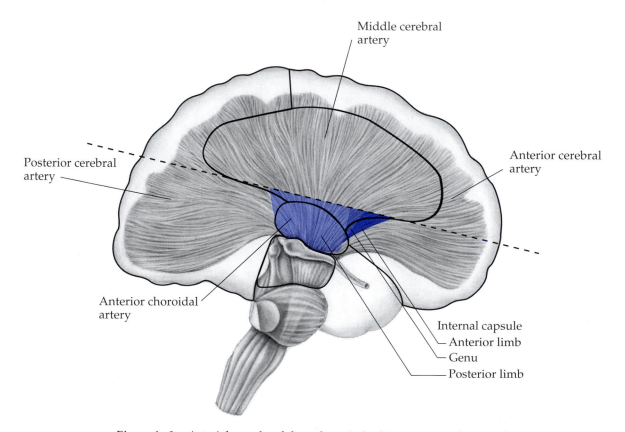

Middle cerebral artery
Posterior cerebral artery
Anterior cerebral artery
Anterior choroidal artery
Internal capsule
Anterior limb
Genu
Posterior limb

Figure 4–6. Arterial supply of the subcortical white matter and internal capsule. Different dorsoventral levels of the internal capsule and limbs receive their arterial supply from different cerebral arteries. The dashed line indicates the plane of the horizontal section in Figure 4–5.

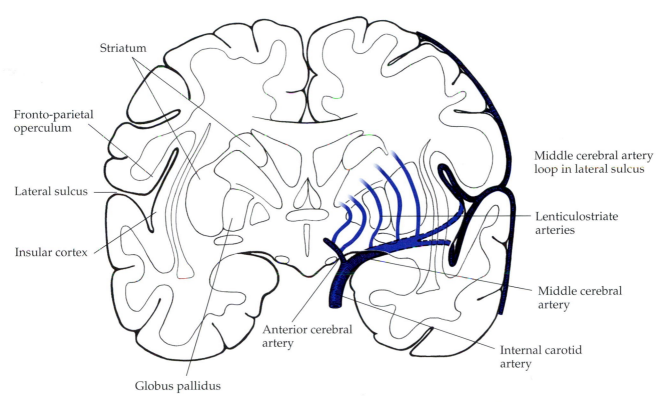

Striatum

Fronto-parietal operculum

Lateral sulcus

Insular cortex

Middle cerebral artery loop in lateral sulcus

Lenticulostriate arteries

Middle cerebral artery

Anterior cerebral artery

Internal carotid artery

Globus pallidus

Figure 4–7. The course of the middle cerebral artery through the lateral sulcus and along the insular and opercular surfaces of the cerebral cortex is shown in a schematic coronal section. *(Adapted from DeArmond SJ, Fusco MM, Dewey MM: Structure of the Human Brain. Oxford University Press, 1976.)*

(Figure 4–7 and 4–8). These branches are often termed cortical branches to differentiate them from the deep branches supplying the diencephalon, basal ganglia, and internal capsule. The **anterior cerebral artery** is c-shaped, like many parts of the cerebral hemispheres (see Figure 3–16). It originates where the internal carotid artery bifurcates and courses within the sagittal fissure and around the rostral end (termed the genu; see Figure 1–9B) of the corpus callosum (Figure 4–4B).

Knowledge of the approximate boundaries of the cortical regions supplied by the different cerebral arteries helps explain the functional disturbances that follow vascular obstruction, or other pathology, of the cerebral vessels. As its gross distribution would suggest (Figure 4–4B), the anterior cerebral artery supplies the dorsal and medial portions of the frontal and parietal lobes (Figure 4–8, medium blue).

The **middle cerebral artery** supplies blood to the lateral convexity of the cortex (Figure 4–8A, light blue). The middle cerebral artery begins at the bifurcation of the internal carotid artery and takes an indirect course through the lateral sulcus (Figure 4–7), along the surface of the **insular cortex**, and over the inner opercular surfaces of the frontal, temporal, and parietal lobes. It finally emerges on the lateral convex-

ity. This complex configuration of the middle cerebral artery can be seen on angiograms (Box 4–1).

The **posterior cerebral artery,** originating where the basilar artery bifurcates (Figures 4–1 and 4–3A), courses around the lateral margin of the midbrain (Figure 4–4B). This artery supplies the occipital lobe and portions of the medial and inferior temporal lobes (Figure 4–8, dark blue).

The terminal ends of the cerebral arteries anastomose on the lateral convexity of the cerebral hemisphere (Figure 4–13). These interconnections or networks occur between branches only when they are located on the cortical surface, not when the artery has penetrated the brain. When a major artery becomes occluded, these anastomoses limit the extent of damage. For example, if a branch of the posterior cerebral artery becomes occluded, tissue with compromised blood supply in the occipital lobe may be rescued by collateral circulation from the middle cerebral artery that connects anastomotically with the blocked vessel.

This collateral circulation can rescue the gray matter of the cerebral cortex. In contrast, little collateral circulation exists between the regions perfused by the cerebral arteries in the white matter. Although collat-

A

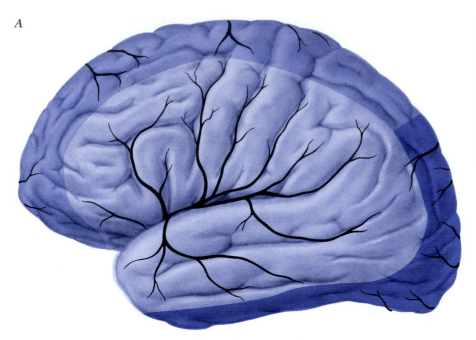

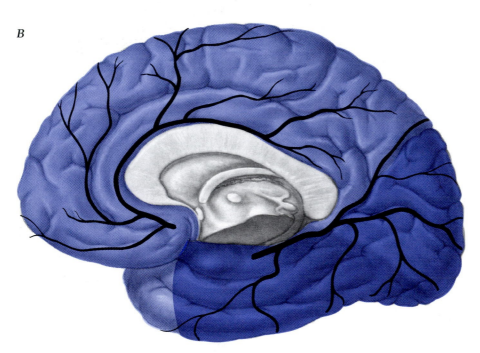

B

Figure 4–8. Cortical territories supplied by the anterior, middle, and posterior cerebral arteries are shown on lateral (*A*) and medial (*B*) views of the cerebral hemispheres. The distribution of the middle cerebral artery is indicated by light blue, the anterior cerebral artery by medium blue, and the posterior cerebral artery by dark blue.

eral circulation provides the cerebral cortex with a margin of safety during arterial occlusion, the anastomotic network that provides such insurance also creates a vulnerability. When systemic blood pressure is reduced, the region served by this network is particularly susceptible to ischemia because such anastomoses occur at the terminal ends of the arteries, regions where perfusion is lowest. The peripheral borders of the territory supplied by major vessels are termed **border zones,** and an infarction occurring in these regions is termed a **border zone infarct.**

Cerebral Veins Drain Into the Dural Sinuses

Venous drainage of the cerebral hemispheres is provided by superficial and deep cerebral veins (Figures 4–14 and 4–15). Superficial veins, arising from the cerebral cortex and underlying white matter, are variable in distribution. Among the more prominent and consistent are the superior anastomotic vein (of Trolard), lying across the parietal lobe, and the inferior anastomotic vein (of Labbé), on the surface of the temporal lobe. The **deep cerebral veins,** such as the in-

Box 4–1.   Radiological Imaging of Cerebral Vasculature

Cerebral vessels can be observed in vivo using **cerebral angiography.** First, radiopaque material is injected into either the anterior or the posterior arterial system. Then a series of skull x-ray films are taken in rapid repetition as the material circulates. Films obtained while the radiopaque material is within cerebral arteries are called **angiograms.** Films obtained later, after the radiopaque substance has reached the cerebral veins or the dural sinuses, are called **venograms.** The entire course of the internal carotid artery is shown in cerebral angiograms in Figure 4–9. Images can be obtained from

different angles with respect to the cranium. Two views are common—from the front (frontal projection, Figure 4–9A) and from the side (lateral projection, Figure 4–9B). The lateral view shows the C-shape of the anterior cerebral artery (and its branches). The medial-to-lateral course of the middle cerebral artery is revealed in the frontal view (Figure 4–9A).

The rostrocaudal course of the middle cerebral artery, from the point at which it enters the lateral sulcus to the point at which it emerges and distributes over the lateral surface of the cerebral cortex, is revealed in the lateral view (Figure 4–9B). The middle cerebral artery

forms loops at the dorsal junction of the insular cortex and the opercular surface of the frontal and parietal lobes (see Figure 4–7). These loops serve as radiological landmarks that aid in estimating the position of the brain in relation to the skull. Figure 4–10 shows the posterior circulation viewed from a lateral perspective. Figure 4–11 shows the two vertebral arteries joining to form the basilar artery and the subsequent bifurcation of the basilar artery into the two posterior cerebral arteries.

Cerebral angiography involves intravascular injection of radiopaque material. The process of injecting this material,

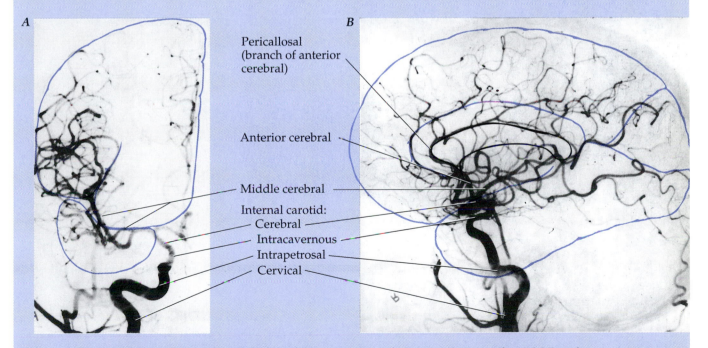

A

B

Pericallosal (branch of anterior cerebral)

Anterior cerebral

Middle cerebral

Internal carotid:
Cerebral
Intracavernous
Intrapetrosal
Cervical

Figure 4–9. Cerebral angiograms of the anterior circulation are shown in frontal (*A*) and lateral (*B*) projections. Overlaying each angiogram is a schematic drawing of the cerebral hemispheres, showing the approximate location of surface landmarks in relation to the arteries. (*Angiograms courtesy of Dr. Neal Rutledge, University of Texas at Austin.*)

(continued)

Box 4–1 (continued.)

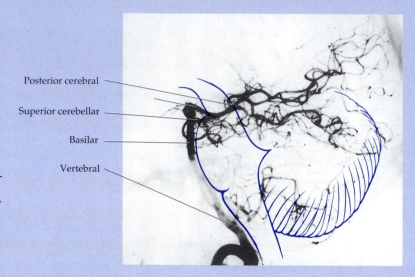

Posterior cerebral

Superior cerebellar

Basilar

Vertebral

Figure 4–10. Cerebral angiogram of the posterior circulation (lateral projection). The overlay drawing is a schematic illustration of the brain stem and cerebellum in relation to the distribution of the posterior circulation. *(Angiogram courtesy of Dr. Neal Rutledge, University of Texas at Austin.)*

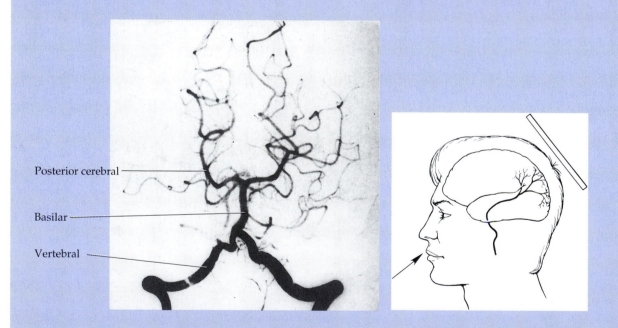

Posterior cerebral

Basilar

Vertebral

Figure 4–11. Cerebral angiogram of the posterior circulation (viewed anteriorly and inferiorly). The inset shows the head and selected cerebral vasculature on the left side (vertebral, basilar, and posterior cerebral arteries) in relation to the direction of transmitted x-rays and the imaging plane. *(Angiogram courtesy of Dr. Neal Rutledge, University of Texas at Austin.)*

Box 4–1 (continued.)

and the material itself, can produce neurological complications; therefore, its use is not without risk. Recently, magnetic resonance imaging has been applied to the study of brain vasculature because it can detect motion of water molecules. This application, termed **magnetic resonance angiography** (MRA), selectively images blood in motion. The MRA scan in Figure 4–12 is a dorsoventral reconstruction (ie, as if looking up from the bottom). The posterior communicating artery is present only on the left side. This patient does not have a complete circle of Willis. The entire cerebral circulation can be reconstructed from the locations of cerebral arteries or veins at multiple levels.

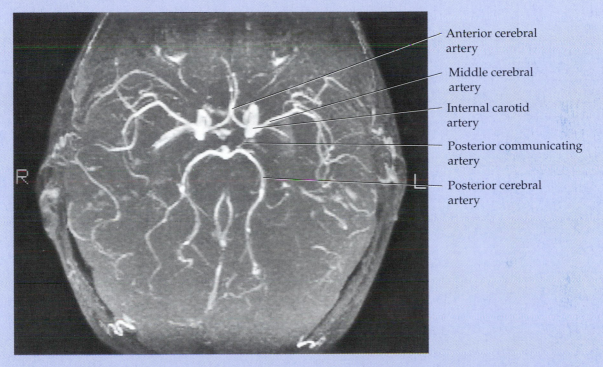

Anterior cerebral artery

Middle cerebral artery

Internal carotid artery

Posterior communicating artery

Posterior cerebral artery

Figure 4–12. Magnetic resonance angiogram. This image is a reconstruction of arteries of the anterior and posterior circulations as if viewed from below. As with conventional angiograms, magnetic resonance angiograms are two-dimensional representations of the three-dimensional arterial system.

ternal cerebral vein (Figure 4–15, inset), drain the more interior portions of the white matter, including the basal ganglia and parts of the diencephalon. Many deep cerebral veins drain into the **great cerebral vein** (of Galen) (Figure 4–15, inset).

Drainage of blood from the central nervous system into the major vessels emptying into the heart—the systemic circulation—is achieved through either a direct or an indirect path. Spinal cord and caudal medullary veins drain directly, through a network of veins and plexuses, into the systemic circulation. By contrast, the rest of the central nervous system drains by an indirect path: The veins first empty into the **dural sinuses** (Figures 4–14 through 4–16; see also Figure 1–12) before returning blood to the systemic circulation. The dural sinuses function as low-pressure channels for venous blood flow back to the systemic circulation. They are located between the periosteal and meningeal layers of the dura (Figure 4–17).

The superficial cerebral veins drain into the superior and inferior sagittal sinuses (Figure 4–15). The **superior sagittal sinus** runs along the midline at

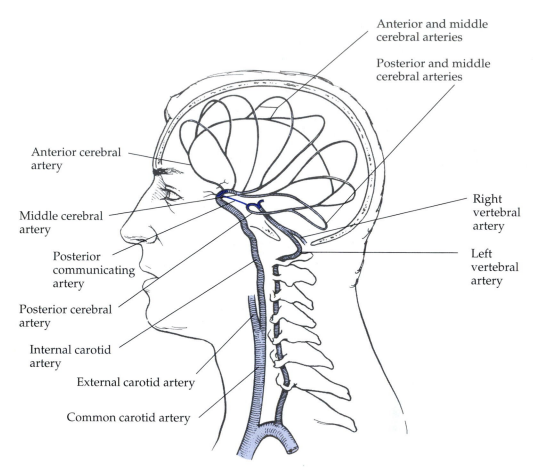

Anterior and middle cerebral arteries

Posterior and middle cerebral arteries

Anterior cerebral artery

Right vertebral artery

Middle cerebral artery

Left vertebral artery

Posterior communicating artery

Posterior cerebral artery

Internal carotid artery

External carotid artery

Common carotid artery

Figure 4–13. Paths for collateral blood supply and the course of the major cerebral arteries over the lateral and medial cortical surfaces. Anastomotic channels between the middle and anterior cerebral arteries—one site for collateral circulation—are depicted. Part of the circle of Willis is shown (dark blue; see Figure 4–1). (*Adapted from Fisher CM: Modern concepts of cerebrovascular disease. In Meyer JS (editor): The Anatomy and Pathology of the Cerebral Vasculature. Spectrum Publications; 1975:1–41.*)

the superior margin of the falx cerebri. The **inferior sagittal sinus** courses along the inferior margin of the falx cerebri just above the corpus callosum. The inferior sagittal sinus, together with the great cerebral vein (of Galen), return venous blood to the **straight** (sometimes called rectus) **sinus** (Figures 4–15 and 4–16). At the occipital pole the superior sagittal sinus and the straight sinus join to form the two **transverse sinuses.** Finally, these sinuses drain into the **sigmoid sinuses,** which return blood to the internal jugular veins. The cavernous sinus, into which drain the ophthalmic and facial veins, is also illustrated in Figure 4–16.

Veins of the midbrain drain into the great cerebral vein, which empties into the straight sinus, whereas the pons and rostral medulla drain into the **superior petrosal sinus** (Figure 4–16). Cerebellar veins drain into the great cerebral vein and the superior petrosal sinus.

The Blood-Brain Barrier Isolates the Chemical Environment of the Central Nervous System From That of the Rest of the Body

The intravascular compartment is isolated from the extracellular compartment of the central nervous system. This feature, the **blood-brain barrier,** was discovered when intravenous dye injection stained most tissues and organs of the body but not the brain. This permeability barrier protects the brain from neuroactive compounds in the blood as well as rapid changes in the ionic constituents of the blood that can affect neuronal excitability.

The blood-brain barrier is thought to result from two characteristics of endothelial cells in the capillaries of the brain and spinal cord. First, in peripheral capillaries, endothelial cells have fenestrations (pores) that allow large molecules to flow into the extracellular space. Moreover, the intercellular spaces between

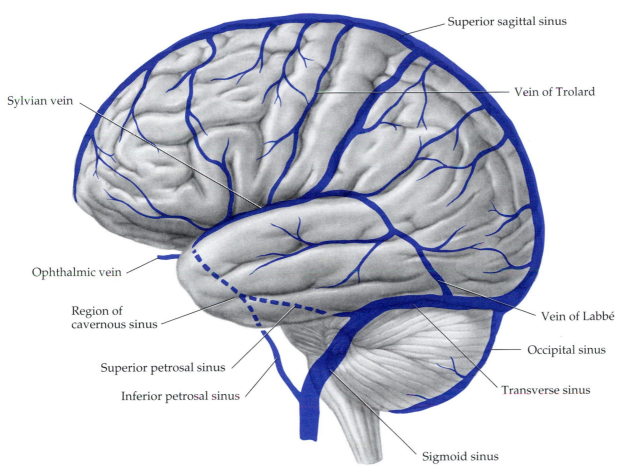

Figure 4–14. Lateral view of the brain, showing major superficial veins and the dural sinuses.

adjacent endothelial cells are leaky. In contrast, in central nervous system capillaries, adjacent endothelial cells are tightly joined, preventing movement of compounds into the extracellular compartment of the central nervous system. Second, there is little transcellular movement of compounds from intravascular to extracellular compartments in the central nervous system because the endothelial cells lack the required transport mechanisms. Moreover, relatively nonselective transport may occur by pinocytosis in peripheral but not central nervous system capillaries.

Although most of the central nervous system is protected by the blood-brain barrier, eight brain structures lack a blood-brain barrier. These structures are close to the midline and, because they are closely associated with the ventricular system, are collectively termed **circumventricular organs** (Figure 4–18). At each of these structures, either neurosecretory products are secreted into the blood or local neurons detect blood-borne compounds as part of a mechanism for regulating the body's internal environment. Regions that lack a blood-brain barrier are not isolated from the rest of the brain. Rather, it has been proposed that

rapid venous drainage from these areas protects surrounding regions.

Cerebrospinal Fluid Serves Many Diverse Functions

Cerebrospinal fluid fills the ventricles. It also fills the subarachnoid space and thus bathes the external brain surface. Together, the ventricles and subarachnoid space contain approximately 140 mL of cerebrospinal fluid, of which 25 mL are in the ventricles and the remaining in the subarachnoid space. Intraventricular pressure is normally around 10–15 mmHg.

Cerebrospinal fluid serves at least three essential functions. First, it provides physical support for the brain, which floats within the fluid. Second, it serves an excretory function and regulates the chemical environment of the central nervous system. Because the brain has no lymphatic system, water-soluble metabolites, which have limited ability to cross the blood-brain barrier, diffuse from the brain into the cerebrospinal fluid. Third, it acts as a channel for chemical communication within the central nervous system.

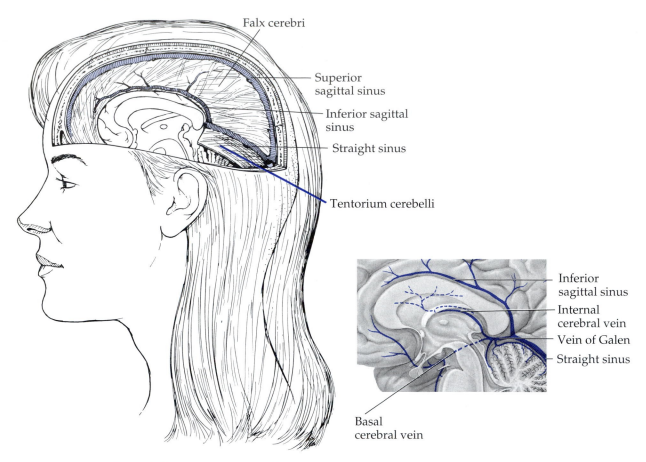

Falx cerebri
Superior sagittal sinus
Inferior sagittal sinus
Straight sinus
Tentorium cerebelli

Inferior sagittal sinus
Internal cerebral vein
Vein of Galen
Straight sinus
Basal cerebral vein

Figure 4–15. Falx cerebri and superior sagittal sinus from a lateral perspective. The inset shows the portion of the medial brain surface that can be seen through the opening in the falx cerebri.

Neurochemicals released by neurons can enter the cerebrospinal fluid and be taken up at sites on the ventricular floor and walls by specialized receptive cells that line the ventricular cavities. Once in the cerebrospinal fluid, these compounds also have relatively free access to neural tissue adjacent to the ventricles because, in contrast to the blood-brain barrier, most of the ventricular lining presents no barrier between the cerebrospinal fluid compartment and the extracellular compartment of the brain.

Most of the Cerebrospinal Fluid Is Produced by the Choroid Plexus

Cerebrospinal fluid is secreted mainly by the **choroid plexus,** which is located in the ventricles (Figure 4–19; see also Figure 3–17). A barrier imposed by the choroidal epithelium prevents the transport of materials from blood into the cerebrospinal fluid. This is the **blood–cerebrospinal fluid barrier,** analogous to the blood-brain barrier. The choroidal epithelium is innervated by autonomic fibers, which serve

a regulatory function. For example, denervation of the sympathetic fibers produces hydrocephalus in animals. A second blood–cerebrospinal fluid barrier exists between the arachnoid and the dural blood vessels.

The rest of the cerebrospinal fluid is secreted by brain capillaries. This extrachoroidal source of cerebrospinal fluid enters the ventricular system through ependymal cells, the ciliated cuboidal epithelial cells that line the ventricles. Total cerebrospinal fluid production by both sources is approximately 500 mL per day. Although the principal function of the choroid plexus is cerebrospinal fluid secretion, the plexus also has a reabsorptive function. The choroid plexus can eliminate from the cerebrospinal fluid a variety of compounds introduced into the ventricles.

Cerebrospinal Fluid Circulates Throughout the Ventricles and Subarachnoid Space

Cerebrospinal fluid produced by the choroid plexus in the lateral ventricles (Figure 4–19) flows through the interventricular foramina and mixes with cerebro-

Figure 4–16. View of the ventral surface of the anterior and middle cranial fossae, and the sinuses on the dorsal surface of the tentorium cerebelli and the ventral cranium.

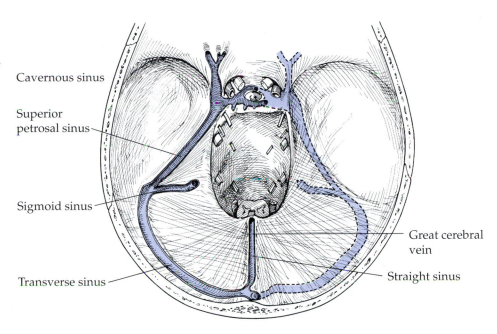

Cavernous sinus

Superior petrosal sinus

Sigmoid sinus

Great cerebral vein

Straight sinus

Transverse sinus

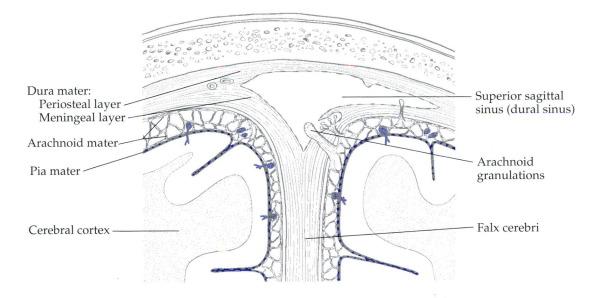

Dura mater:
 Periosteal layer
 Meningeal layer

Arachnoid mater

Pia mater

Cerebral cortex

Superior sagittal sinus (dural sinus)

Arachnoid granulations

Falx cerebri

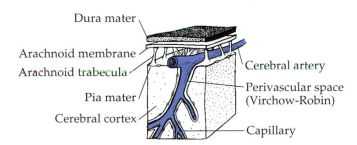

Dura mater

Arachnoid membrane

Arachnoid trabecula

Pia mater

Cerebral cortex

Cerebral artery

Perivascular space (Virchow-Robin)

Capillary

Figure 4–17. A schematic cut through the superior sagittal sinus, illustrating the arachnoid granulations, collections of arachnoid villi containing the unidirectional valves through which cerebrospinal fluid passes to the venous circulation. The inset shows the relationship between cerebral blood vessels and the meningeal layers. *(Adapted from Davson H, Keasley W, Segal MB: Physiology and Pathophysiology of the Cerebrospinal Fluid. Churchill Livingstone, 1987. Inset from Kuffler SW, Nicholls JG: From Neuron to Brain. Sinauer Associates Inc., Publishers, 1976.)*

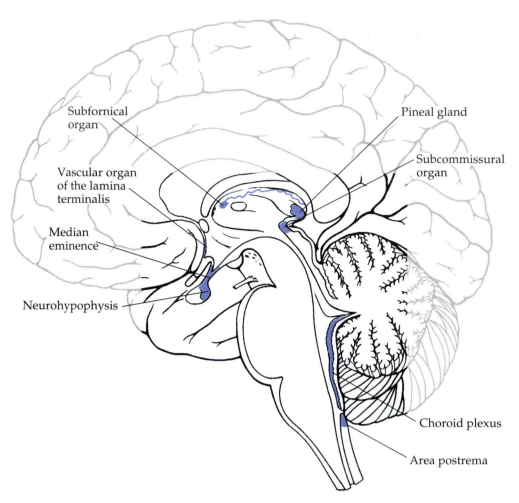

Figure 4–18. Circumventricular organs are brain regions that do not have a blood-brain barrier. The locations of the eight circumventricular organs are shown on a view of the midsagittal brain: neurohypophysis, median eminence, vascular organ of the lamina terminalis, subfornical organ, pineal gland, subcommissural organ, choroid plexus, and area postrema. Note that all of circumventricular organs are located centrally (highlighted region), in close association with the components of the ventricular system.

spinal fluid produced in the third ventricle. From here, it flows through the cerebral aqueduct and into the fourth ventricle, another major site for cerebrospinal fluid production because the choroid plexus is also located there. Three apertures in the roof of the fourth ventricle drain cerebrospinal fluid from the ventricular system into the subarachnoid space: the **foramen of Magendie,** located on the midline, and the two **foramina of Luschka,** located at the lateral margins of the fourth ventricle (Figure 4–19, inset).

The subarachnoid space is dilated in certain locations, termed **cisterns;** cerebrospinal fluid pools here. Five prominent cisterns are located on the midline: (1) the **interpeduncular cistern,** between the basis pedunculi on the ventral midbrain surface, (2) the **quadrigeminal cistern,** dorsal to the superior and inferior colliculi (which are also called the quadrigeminal bodies), (3) the **pontine cistern,** at the ventral por-

tion of the pontomedullary junction, (4) the **cisterna magna,** dorsal to the medulla, and (5) the **lumbar cistern,** in the caudal vertebral canal (Figure 4–19). The subarachnoid space also contains the blood vessels of the central nervous system (Figure 4–17, inset). Blood vessels penetrate the brain together with the pia, creating a perivascular space between the vessels and pia. These spaces, termed the Virchow-Robin spaces, contain cerebrospinal fluid.

The Dural Sinuses Provide the Return Path for Cerebrospinal Fluid

Cerebrospinal fluid passes from the subarachnoid space to the venous blood through small unidirectional valves termed **arachnoid villi.** Arachnoid villi are microscopic evaginations of the arachnoid mater

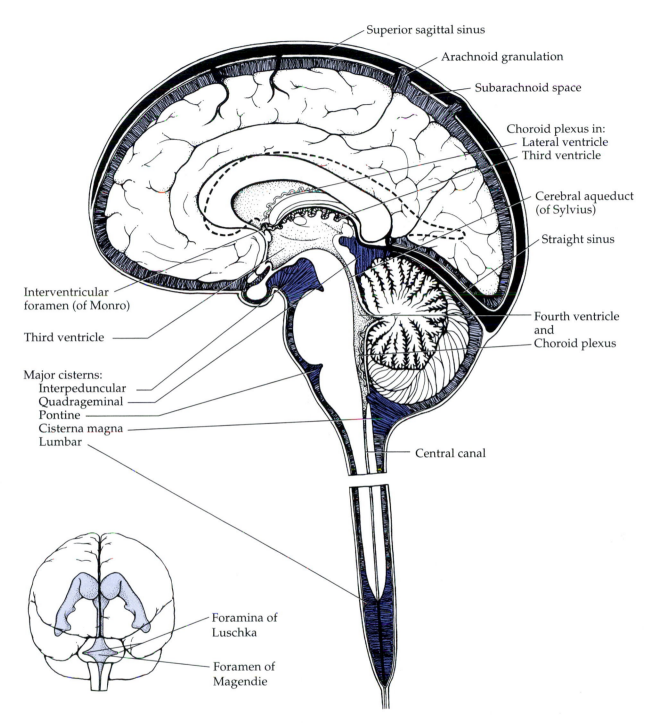

Figure 4–19. The subarachnoid space and ventricular system are shown on a view of the midsagittal surface of the central nervous system. The inset shows the locations of the foramina through which cerebrospinal fluid exits the ventricular system. *(Adapted from Kuffler SW, Nicholls JG: From Neuron to Brain. Sinauer Associates Inc., Publishers, 1976.)*

that protrude into the **dural sinuses** as well as directly into certain veins. The cerebrospinal fluid flows through a system of large vacuoles in the arachnoid cells of the villi and through an extracellular path between cells of the villi. Numerous clusters of arachnoid villi are present over the dorsal (superior) con-

vexity of the cerebral hemispheres in the superior sagittal sinus, where they form a macroscopic structure called the **arachnoid granulations** (Figures 4–17 and 4–19). The arachnoid villi are also present where the spinal nerves exit the spinal dural sac. These villi direct the flow of cerebrospinal fluid into the radicular veins.

Summary

Arterial Supply of the Spinal Cord and Brain Stem

The arterial supply of the spinal cord is provided by the **vertebral** and **radicular arteries** (Figures 4–1 and 4–2). The brain is supplied by the **internal carotid arteries** (the **anterior circulation**) and the **vertebral arteries,** which join at the pontomedullary junction to form the **basilar artery** (collectively termed the **posterior circulation**) (Figure 4–1). The brain stem and cerebellum receive blood only from the posterior system (Figures 4–2 and 4–3A; Table 4–1). The medulla receives blood directly from small branches of the **vertebral arteries** and from the **spinal arteries** and the **posterior inferior cerebellar artery** (PICA) (Figure 4–3). The pons is supplied by **paramedian** and **short circumferential branches** of the **basilar artery.** Two major long circumferential branches are the **anterior inferior cerebellar artery** (AICA) and the **superior cerebellar artery** (Figure 4–3). The midbrain receives its arterial supply primarily from the **posterior cerebral artery** as well as from the basilar artery (Figure 4–3). The PICA supplies the caudal cerebellum, and the AICA and superior cerebellar artery supply the rostral cerebellum.

Arterial Supply of the Diencephalon and Cerebral Hemispheres

The diencephalon and cerebral hemispheres are supplied by the **anterior** and **posterior circulations** (Figures 4–1 and 4–5). The cerebral cortex receives its blood supply from the three cerebral arteries: the **anterior** and **middle cerebral arteries,** which are part of the anterior circulation, and the **posterior cerebral artery,** which is part of the posterior circulation (Figures 4–1 and 4–13). The diencephalon, basal ganglia, and internal capsule receive blood from branches of the **internal carotid artery,** the three **cerebral arteries,** and the **posterior communicating artery** (Figures 4–1, 4–4, 4–5, and 4–13; Table 4–1).

Collateral Circulation

The anterior and posterior systems are interconnected by two networks of arteries: (1) the **circle of Willis**—which is formed by the anterior, middle, and posterior **cerebral arteries;** the **posterior communicating arteries;** and the **anterior communicating artery** (Figure 4–1); and (2) terminal branches of the cerebral arteries, which anastomose on the superior convexity of the cerebral cortex (Figures 4–4 and 4–13).

Venous Drainage

The venous drainage of the spinal cord and caudal medulla is direct to the systemic circulation. By contrast, veins draining the cerebral hemispheres, diencephalon, midbrain, pons, cerebellum, and rostral medulla (Figure 4–13) drain into the **dural sinuses** (Figures 4–14, 4–15, and 4–16). The major dural sinuses are as follows: **superior sagittal, inferior sagittal, straight, transverse, sigmoid, superior,** and **inferior petrosal.**

Blood-Brain Barrier

The internal environment of most of the central nervous system is protected from circulating neuroactive agents in blood by the **blood-brain barrier.** This barrier is formed by a number of specializations in the **capillary endothelium** of the central nervous system. Brain regions without a blood-brain barrier, termed the **circumventricular organs** (Figure 4–18), include the (1) **area postrema** in the medulla, (2) **subcommissural organ,** (3) **subfornical organ,** (4) **vascular organ of the lamina terminalis,** (5) **median eminence,** (6) **neurohypophysis,** (7) **choroid plexus,** and (8) **pineal gland.**

Production and Circulation of Cerebrospinal Fluid

Most of the cerebrospinal fluid is produced by the **choroid plexus,** which is located in the **ventricles** (Figure 4–19). It exits from the ventricular system, through foramina in the fourth ventricle—the two **foramina of Luschka** and the **foramen of Magendie**—directly into the **subarachnoid space.** Cerebrospinal fluid passes into the **dural sinuses** (Figure 4–14) through unidirectional valves termed **arachnoid villi** clustered in the **arachnoid granulations** (Figures 4–17 and 4–19).

Related Sources

Brust JCM: Circulation of the brain. In Kandel ER, Schwartz JH, Jessell TM (editors): Principles of Neural Science, 4th ed. McGraw-Hill; 2000:1302–1316.

Brust JCM: The Practice of Neural Science. McGraw-Hill; 2000. (See ch. 14, cases 49, 50.)

Laterra J, Goldstein GW: Ventricular organization of cerebrospinal fluid: blood brain barrier, brain edema, and hydrocephalus. In Kandel ER, Schwartz JH, Jessell TM (editors): Principles of Neural Science, 4th ed. McGraw-Hill; 2000:1288–1301.

Selected Readings

Davson H, Keasley W, Segal MB: Physiology and Pathophysiology of the Cerebrospinal Fluid. Churchill Livingstone, 1987.

Duvernoy HM: The Superficial Veins of the Human Brain. Springer-Verlag, 1975.

Duvernoy HM: The Human Brain Stem and Cerebellum: Surface, Structure, Vascularization, and Three-dimensional Sectional Anatomy with MRI. Spring-Verlag, 1995.

Duvernoy HM: Human Brain Stem Vessels: Including the Pineal Gland and Information on Brain Stem Infarction. Springer, 1999.

Fisher CM: Modern concepts of cerebrovascular disease. In Meyer JS (editor): The Anatomy and Pathology of the Cerebral Vasculature. Spectrum Publications; 1975:1–41.

Fishman RT: Cerebrospinal Fluid in Diseases of the Nervous System, 2nd ed. Saunders, 1992.

Kistler JP, Ropper AH, Martin JB: Cerebrovascular diseases. In Braunwald E, Isselbacher FJ, Peterdorf RG, et al (editors): Harrison's Principles of Internal Medicine, 11th ed. McGraw-Hill; 1987:1930–1960.

McKinley MJ, Oldfield BJ: Circumventricular organs. In Paxinos G (editor): The Human Nervous System. Academic Press; 1990:415–438.

Sasaki T, Kassell NF: Cerebrovascular system. In Paxinos G (editor): The Human Nervous System. Academic Press; 1990:1135–1149.

Segal MB: The choroid plexuses and the barriers between the blood and the cerebrospinal fluid. Cell Mol Neurobiol 2000;20:183–196.

References

Carpenter MB, Sutin J: Human Neuroanatomy. Williams & Wilkins, 1983.

DeArmond SJ, Fusco MM, Dewey MM: Structure of the Human Brain. Oxford University Press, 1976.

Ferner H, Staubestand J (editors): Sobotta Atlas of Human Anatomy, Vol. 1: Head, Neck, Upper Extremities. Urban & Schwarzenberg, 1983.

Karibe H, Shimizu H, Tominaga T, Koshu K, Yoshimoto T: Diffusion-weighted magnetic resonance imaging in the early evaluation of corticospinal tract injury to predict functional motor outcome in patients with deep intracerebral hemorrhage. J Neurosurg 2000;92:58–63.

Kuffler SW, Nicholls JG: From Neuron to Brain. Sinauer Associates Inc., Publishers, 1976.

Saunders NR, Habgood MD, Dziegielewska KM: Barrier mechanisms in the brain, I. Adult brain. Clin Exp Pharmacol Physiol 1999;26:11–19.

Thompson EJ: Cerebrospinal fluid. J Neurol Neurosurg Psychiatry 1995;59:349–357.

II Sensory Systems

5

Spinal Somatic Sensory Systems

THE SOMATIC SENSORY SYSTEMS mediate touch and limb position senses, as well as pain, itch, and temperature senses. These systems are also criti-cally involved in the maintenance of arousal and in the sensory regulation of limb and trunk movements. To carry out these functions, the somatic sensory systems process stimuli both from the body surface and from within the body—from the muscles, joints, and viscera.

Spinal somatic sensory systems transmit informa-tion from the limbs, neck, and trunk to the brain stem and then to the thalamus and somatic sensory cortex. The trigeminal systems consist of separate pathways that begin in the brain stem and transmit information from the head to the thalamus and then the cortex. The spinal and trigeminal systems remain distinct as they travel to the cortex, contacting separate popu-lations of neurons at each processing stage. However, even though the ascending spinal and trigeminal path-ways are separate, their general organization is remark-ably similar. This chapter considers the spinal somatic sensory pathways; the trigeminal systems are exam-ined in Chapter 6.

The general organization of the spinal sensory systems is discussed first, giving an overview of the functional anatomy of the somatic sensory pathways. Then the regional anatomy is examined at different levels through the nervous system, beginning with the morphology of the somatic sensory receptor neurons and continuing to the cerebral cortex.

FUNCTIONAL ANATOMY OF THE SPINAL SOMATIC SENSORY PATHWAYS

The somatic, or bodily, senses consist of five distinct **modalities:** limb position sense, touch, temperature sense, pain, and itch (Table 5–1). The first two modal-ities comprise the mechanical sensations, whereas the later three comprise the protective sensations. Many of these modalities are engaged during routine activ-ity. For example, in picking up a cup of hot coffee,

Table 5–1. Modalities and submodalities of somatic sensation and afferent fiber groups.

Modality and submodality	Receptor type	Fiber diameter (μm)	Group	Myelination[1]
Touch Texture/superficial Pressure/deep Vibration	Mechanoreceptors Pacinian	6–12	A-β (2)	Myelinated
Position Sense Static Dynamic (kinesthesia)	Mechanoreceptors	13–20 6–12	A-α (1), A-β (2)	Myelinated
Temperature Sense Cold Warmth	Thermoreceptors	1–5 0.2–1.5	A-δ (3), C (4)	Myelinated; unmyelinated
Pain Fast (pricking) Slow (burning)	Nociceptors	1–5 0.2–1.5	A-δ (3) C (4)	Myelinated; unmyelinated Myelinated Unmyelinated
Itch	Histamine	0.2–1.5	C (4)	Unmyelinated

[1]A small number of thinly myelinated and unmyelinated fibers are sensitive to mechanical stimuli. These mechanoreceptors are present in the hairy skin.

you use limb position sense in identifying the shape of your hand as you grasp the handle; contact with the cup is detected by touch. Temperature sense provides information about the temperature of the cup, and if the cup is too hot, you experience pain. Itch is triggered selectively by chemical irritation of the skin, provoking the urge to scratch, thereby tending to remove the offending substance. Each modality can be further subdivided into submodalities, which adds to the richness of somatic sensations. For example, touch consists of several component mechanical sensations including senses of texture and pressure; pain has distinctive pricking and burning sensations.

Somatic sensations are clinically important. Pain typically brings a patient to visit a physician. Somatic sensations also can be important for diagnosing disease. For example, persistent itch can signal liver disease. Vibration sense, a touch submodality (Table 5–1), is routinely used to probe sensory function in humans suspected of having peripheral nerve or central nervous system damage.

The Dorsal Column–Medial Lemniscal System and the Anterolateral System Mediate Different Somatic Sensations

Touch and limb position sense are mediated by the **dorsal column–medial lemniscal system** (Figures 5–1A and 5–2A), named after its two principal components. In contrast, the **anterolateral system** (Figures 5–1B and 5–2B) subserves pain, itch, and temperature senses and, to a much lesser extent, touch. It is named for the location of its spinal axons, which ascend in the anterior portion of the lateral column. Each of these systems consists of a series of neurons from sensory receptor neurons in the periphery to the contralateral cerebral cortex. The dorsal column–medial lemniscal and anterolateral systems are examples of **parallel sensory pathways,** each of which connects the receptive sheet with the cortex but for distinctive functions. The following sections compare the dorsal column–medial lemniscal and anterolateral systems, emphasizing the four key differences in their organization.

The Two Ascending Somatic Sensory Pathways Each Receive Inputs From Different Classes of Sensory Receptor Neurons

The dorsal column–medial lemniscal and anterolateral systems each receive input from different functional classes of dorsal root ganglion neurons, the primary somatic sensory receptor neuron. This is why the two systems have such different functions. Primary sensory receptor neurons sensitive to **mechanical stimulation** of body tissues provide the major sensory input to the dorsal column–medial lemniscal system. In contrast, sensory receptor neurons sensitive to **noxious** (ie, painful), **pruritic** (ie, itch provoking), and **thermal stimuli** provide the major sensory inputs to the anterolateral system.

Although the segregation of the different types of sensory input into the two ascending systems is not absolute, it is sufficiently complete to have important clinical consequences. For example, after a complete lesion of the dorsal column–medial lemniscal system, a crude sense of touch remains, indicating that the anterolateral system receives input from mechanoreceptor neurons but that this information is not organized for fine discriminations. Although simple touch detection thresholds may not be changed, the person's discriminative capabilities are markedly reduced. An individual with such a lesion may not be able to distinguish gradations of rough and smooth (eg, grades of sandpaper), or the difference between two closely spaced mechanical stimuli. Moreover, this individual would have difficulty maintaining balance with his or her eyes closed because of the absence of leg position sense. By contrast, a lesion of the anterolateral system leaves touch and limb position senses unaffected but makes people insensitive or less sensitive to pain.

The Somatic Sensory Pathways Have Different Relay Nuclei in the Spinal Cord and Brain Stem

The first major relay in the dorsal column–medial lemniscal system is in the **dorsal column nuclei,** in the medulla. Here, the first-order neurons in the pathway, the primary sensory neurons, synapse on second-order neurons in the central nervous system (Figure 5–1A). In contrast, the anterolateral system's first relay is in the **dorsal horn** of the spinal cord (Figure 5–1B). Figure 5–2 shows the locations of these structures on schematic myelin-stained sections through key levels of the nervous system.

The Two Ascending Somatic Sensory Pathways Decussate at Different Levels of the Neuraxis

Virtually all sensory and motor pathways have a neuron whose axon decussates, or crosses the midline, somewhere along its course, although the reason for this decussation is unknown. Knowing the level of decussation is clinically important for determining where an injury to the nervous system has occurred (see section below on somatic sensory deficits after spinal cord trauma). The dorsal column–medial lemniscal system decussates in the medulla (Figures 5–1A and 5–2A), whereas the anterolateral system crosses in the spinal cord (Figures 5–1B and 5–2B). Curiously, for both systems, the axon of the second neuron in the circuit decussates.

The Dorsal Column–Medial Lemniscal and Anterolateral Systems Synapse in Different Brain Stem, Diencephalic, and Cortical Regions

Most of the fibers of the dorsal column–medial lemniscal system have similar connections. Axons in the dorsal columns synapse primarily on neurons in the dorsal column nuclei, which transmit information to the **ventral posterior lateral nucleus** of the thalamus and then to the **primary somatic sensory cortex** in the postcentral gyrus (Figure 5–2A). This cortical area is important in localization of mechanical stimuli and in identifying the quality of such stimuli.

Axons of the anterolateral system, in contrast, are distributed within the lateral and ventral spinal columns and contain sets of axons that synapse in separate brain regions: the **spinothalamic tract,** the **spinoreticular tract,** and the **spinomesencephalic tract** (Figures 5–1B and 5–2B). The spinothalamic tract carries information important for pain, itch, and temperature sensations to three major regions of the contralateral thalamus. The first two regions, the **ventral posterior lateral nucleus** and the **ventromedial posterior nucleus,** transmit information to the primary somatic sensory cortex and posterior insular cortex, respectively. These projections, especially the one to the insular cortex, are important in stimulus perception. The third region, the **medial dorsal nucleus** of the thalamus, transmits information to the **anterior cingulate gyrus,** a cortical region important in emotions. The insular and anterior cortical regions are collectively important in behavioral and autonomic responses to pain, temperature, and itch sensations and in the emotions and memories that these stimuli

Figure 5–1. Dorsal view of the brain stem without the cerebellum, illustrating the course of the dorsal column—medial lemniscal system (*A*) and the anterolateral system (*B*). Note that the decussating axons of the anterolateral system (*B*) cross the midline in the ventral commissure. The inset shows the dorsal root ganglion cell and the organization of the primary afferent fiber. The sensory receptor illustrated in the inset is a mechanoreceptor, a pacinian corpuscle.

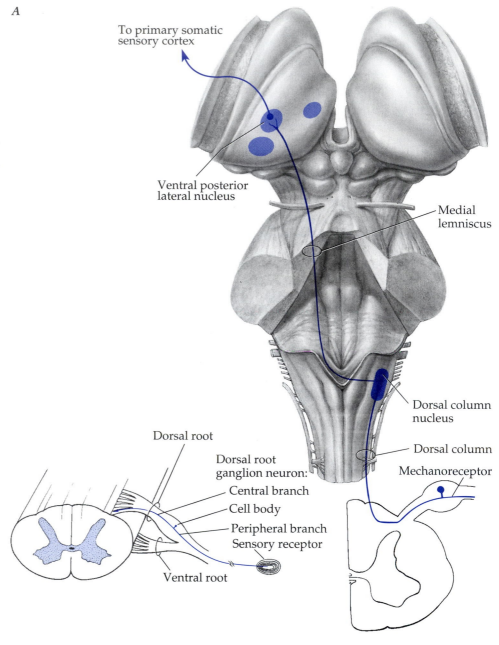

evoke. For example, you may become angry if you are burned when you pick up a hot coffee cup, and your blood pressure and heart rates increase. The salience of the stimulus also helps you to remember not to be so careless the next time!

The spinoreticular tract transmits sensory information to neurons in the reticular formation of the pons and medulla, and many of these neurons project to the intralaminar thalamic nuclei. The reticular formation and intralaminar nuclei are also important in maintaining arousal.

The spinomesencephalic tract terminates in the midbrain tectum and periaqueductal gray matter. The projection to the tectum integrates somatic sensory information with vision and hearing for orienting the head and body to salient stimuli (see Chapter 7). Projections to the **periaqueductal gray matter** play a role in the feedback regulation of pain transmission in the spinal cord. Neurons in the periaqueductal gray matter excite neurons in the **raphe nuclei** and reticular formation (Figure 5–2B), which inhibit pain transmission in the spinal cord.

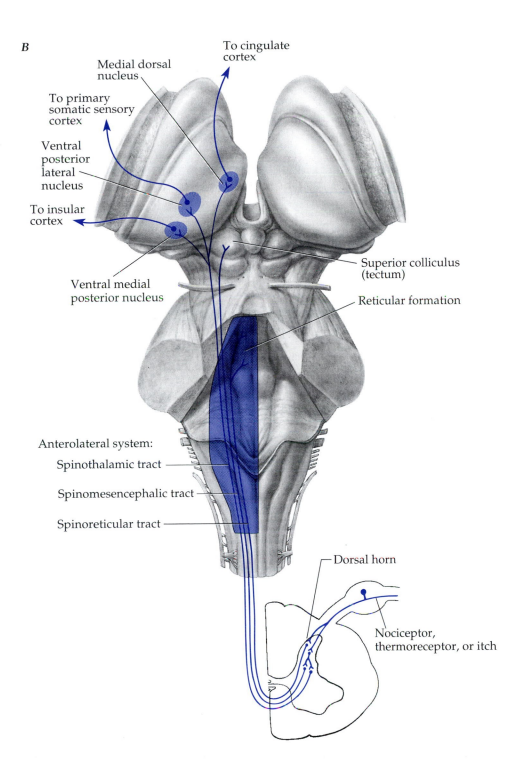

B

To cingulate cortex

Medial dorsal nucleus

To primary somatic sensory cortex

Ventral posterior lateral nucleus

To insular cortex

Ventral medial posterior nucleus

Superior colliculus (tectum)

Reticular formation

Anterolateral system:

Spinothalamic tract

Spinomesencephalic tract

Spinoreticular tract

Dorsal horn

Nociceptor, thermoreceptor, or itch

REGIONAL ANATOMY OF THE SPINAL SOMATIC SENSORY PATHWAYS

The rest of this chapter takes a regional approach to the spinal somatic sensory systems. Progressing in sequence from the periphery to the cerebral cortex, the chapter examines the key components of the dorsal column–medial lemniscal system and the anterolateral system. Knowledge of the regional anatomy is important for understanding how injury to a discrete portion of the central nervous system affects different functional systems indiscriminately.

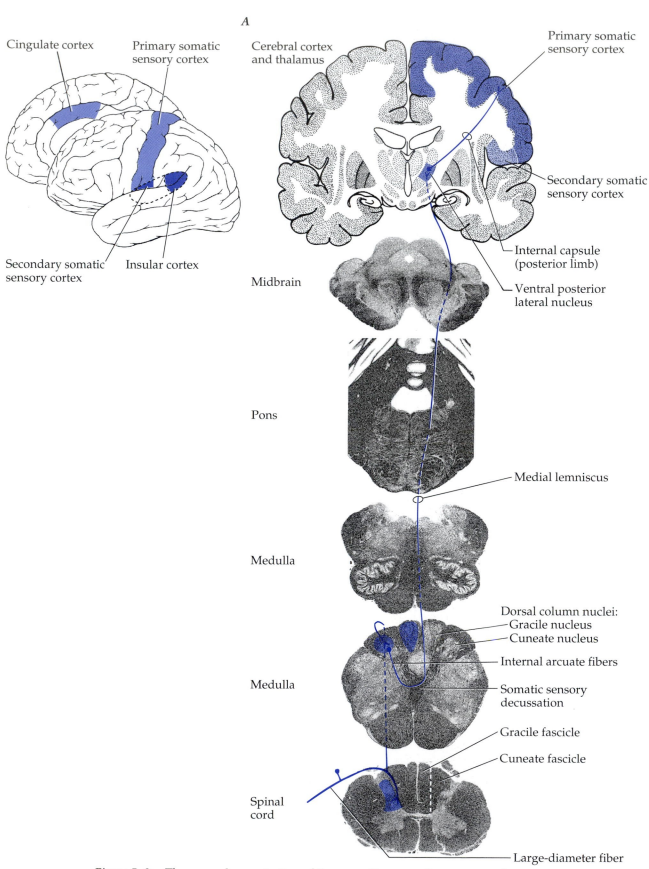

A

Cingulate cortex

Primary somatic sensory cortex

Cerebral cortex and thalamus

Primary somatic sensory cortex

Secondary somatic sensory cortex

Insular cortex

Secondary somatic sensory cortex

Internal capsule (posterior limb)

Midbrain

Ventral posterior lateral nucleus

Pons

Medial lemniscus

Medulla

Dorsal column nuclei:
Gracile nucleus
Cuneate nucleus

Internal arcuate fibers

Medulla

Somatic sensory decussation

Gracile fascicle

Cuneate fascicle

Spinal cord

Large-diameter fiber

Figure 5–2.   The general organization of the ascending somatic sensory pathways. *A.* Dorsal column—medial lemniscal system. *B.* Anterolateral system. The inset shows views of lateral and medial surfaces of the cerebral cortex. Regions that play a key role in somatic sensation are shaded.

B

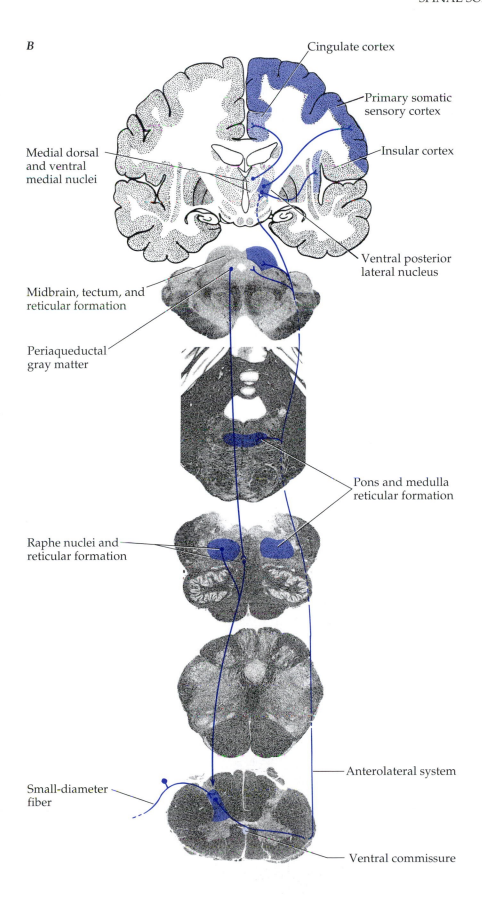

Cingulate cortex

Primary somatic sensory cortex

Medial dorsal and ventral medial nuclei

Insular cortex

Ventral posterior lateral nucleus

Midbrain, tectum, and reticular formation

Periaqueductal gray matter

Pons and medulla reticular formation

Raphe nuclei and reticular formation

Anterolateral system

Small-diameter fiber

Ventral commissure

The Peripheral Axon Terminals of Dorsal Root Ganglion Neurons Contain the Somatic Sensory Receptors

The **dorsal root ganglion neurons** (Figure 5–1, inset), named for the **dorsal root ganglia** in which their cell bodies are located, transduce sensory information into neural signals and transmit these signals to the central nervous system. **Ganglia** are collections of neuronal cell bodies located outside the central nervous system, in contrast to nuclei, which are collections located within the central nervous system. Dorsal root ganglion neurons are **pseudounipolar neurons.** A single axon emerges from the cell body and bifurcates; one axonal branch is directed toward the periphery, where it innervates tissue, and the other, directed centrally, synapses on central nervous system neurons. The peripheral and central axon branches of dorsal root ganglion neurons are often called **primary sensory** (or **afferent**) **fibers.**

The distal axon terminal of the peripheral branch is the receptive portion of the neuron. Here, stimulus energy is **transduced** into neural events by membrane receptor-channel complexes that respond to a particular stimulus energy (eg, thermal, mechanical) or chemical (eg, histamine). **Nociceptors** are sensory receptor neurons that are sensitive to noxious or tissue-damaging stimuli and mediate pain. These receptor neurons respond to chemicals released from traumatized tissue. **Itch-sensitive neurons** respond to histamine. Itch is evoked when histamine is injected intradermally. Receptor neurons sensitive to cold or warmth are termed **thermoreceptors.** The morphology of these three classes of receptor neurons is simple; they are **bare nerve endings** (Figure 5–3A). **Mechanoreceptors** mediate touch and limb position sense (Figure 5–3). Mechanoreceptors are activated when mechanical energy is conducted from the body surface, where stimulation occurs, to the membrane of the receptors, where stretch-activated channels are located. Mechanoreceptors for limb position sense are sensitive to muscle or tendon stretch as well as mechanical changes in the tissues around certain joints. Mechanoreceptors have **encapsulated axon terminals;** however, the capsule does not participate directly in stimulus transduction. Rather, it acts as a filter to shape the mechanoreceptor's response to a stimulus.

Five major types of encapsulated sensory receptor neurons are located in the skin and underlying deep tissue: Meissner's corpuscles, pacinian corpuscles, Ruffini's corpuscles, Merkel's receptors, and hair receptors (Figure 5–3A). These mechanoreceptors mediate touch. Meissner's and pacinian corpuscles are **rapidly adapting.** They respond to a continuous and enduring stimulus by firing a burst of action potentials to mark the beginning and ending of the stimulus. Ruffini's corpuscles and Merkel's receptors are **slowly adapting,** firing action potentials for the duration of the stimulus. Hair receptors may be either slowly or rapidly adapting. Each primary sensory fiber has multiple terminal branches and, therefore, multiple receptive endings.

There are two mechanoreceptors in muscle. The **muscle spindle receptor,** which is located within the muscle belly, measures muscle stretch and serves limb position sense (Figure 5–3B). This structure is innervated by multiple sensory fibers with different properties. The muscle spindle is more complicated than the other encapsulated mechanoreceptors because it also contains tiny muscle fibers, controlled by the central nervous system, that regulate the receptor neuron's sensitivity. The other muscle mechanoreceptor is the **Golgi tendon receptor,** which is entwined within the collagen fibers of tendon and is sensitive to the force generated by contracting muscle. It may have a role in an individual's sense of how much effort it takes to produce a particular motor act. The muscle spindle and Golgi tendon receptors also play key roles in the reflex control of muscle.

The modality sensitivity of a receptor neuron also determines the diameter of its axon and the patterns of connections in the central nervous system. Mechanoreceptors have a **large-diameter axon** covered by a thick myelin sheath. The mechanoreceptors are the fastest conducting sensory receptor neurons in the somatic sensory system. The dorsal column–medial lemniscal system receives sensory input principally from these mechanoreceptors with large-diameter axons. Dorsal root ganglion neurons that are sensitive to noxious stimuli or temperature have **small-diameter axons** that are either myelinated or unmyelinated. Itch-sensitive dorsal root ganglion neurons are unmyelinated. The anterolateral system receives sensory input mostly from receptor neurons with small-diameter axons. The larger the diameter of the axon, the faster it conducts action potentials. Table 5–1 lists the functional categories of primary sensory fibers, including the two fiber nomenclatures based on axonal diameter: A-α (group 1), A-β (group 2), A-δ (group 3), and C (group 4).

The **central branches** of dorsal root ganglion neurons collect into the dorsal roots (Figure 5–1, inset; Figure 5–4, inset). The area of skin innervated by the axons in a single dorsal root is termed a **dermatome.** Dermatomes of adjacent dorsal roots overlap extensively with those of their neighbors (Figure 5–4, inset). This explains the common clinical observation

A

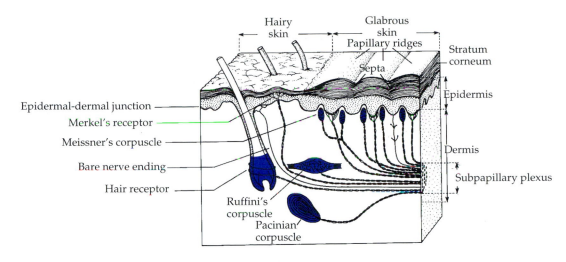

Hairy skin — Glabrous skin
Papillary ridges
Septa
Stratum corneum
Epidermis
Dermis
Subpapillary plexus

Epidermal-dermal junction
Merkel's receptor
Meissner's corpuscle
Bare nerve ending
Hair receptor
Ruffini's corpuscle
Pacinian corpuscle

B

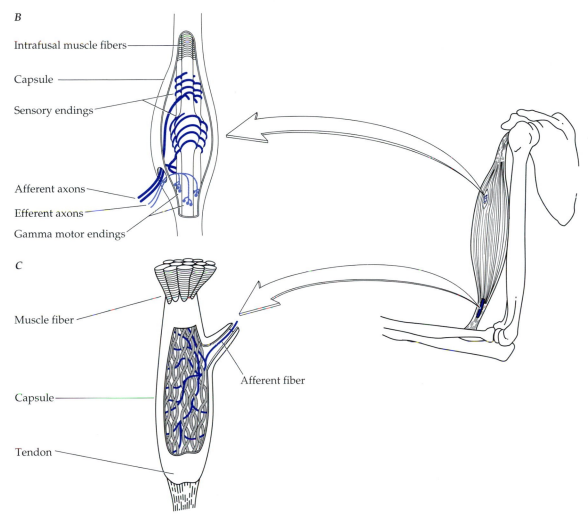

Intrafusal muscle fibers
Capsule
Sensory endings
Afferent axons
Efferent axons
Gamma motor endings

C

Muscle fiber
Afferent fiber
Capsule
Tendon

Figure 5–3. **A.** The morphology of peripheral somatic sensory receptors on hairy skin (*left*) and hairless, or glabrous, skin (*right*). **B.** The muscle spindle organ (***top inset***) is a stretch receptor located within the muscle. It receives an efferent innervation from the spinal cord that maintains receptor sensitivity during muscle contraction. The Golgi tendon organ (***bottom inset***) is most sensitive to active force generated by contracting muscle. (*A, Adapted from Light AR, Perl ER: Peripheral sensory systems. In Dyck PJ, Thomas PK, Lambert EH, Bruge R (editors): Peripheral Neuropathy, 2nd ed. Vol. 1. W. B. Saunders; 1984:210–230. **B**, Adapted from Kandel ER, Schwartz JH, Jessell TM (editors): Principles of Neural Science, 4th edition. McGraw-Hill, 2000.*)

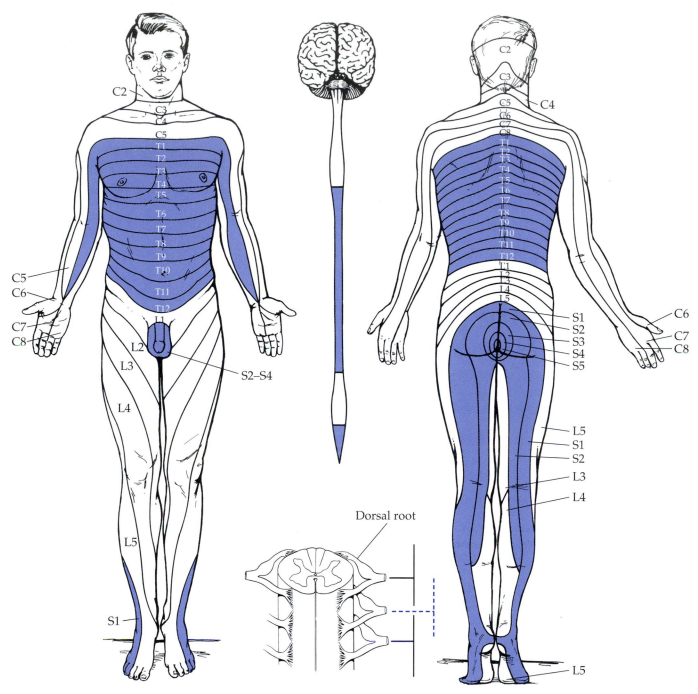

Figure 5–4. The dermatomes of the body have a segmental organization. Note the correspondence between the spinal cord divisions (shown on a ventral view of the central nervous system) and dermatome locations. The inset illustrates dermatomal overlap.

that, when a physician probes sensory capacity after injury to a single dorsal root, typically no anesthetic area is observed, although patients with such damage sometimes experience tingling or even a diminished sensory capacity. Single dorsal root injury commonly produces **radicular pain,** which is localized to the dermatome of the injured root. By comparing the location of radicular pain or other sensory disturbances with a dermatomal map, such as in Figure 5–4, the clinician can localize the site of damage.

Dorsal Root Axons With Different Diameters Terminate in Different Central Nervous System Locations

The central branch of a dorsal root ganglion neuron enters the spinal cord at its dorsolateral margin (Figure 5–5). Even here, axons that serve different sensory functions are segregated. Large-diameter axons, which mediate touch and limb position senses, enter medial to the small-diameter axons, which mediate pain, itch, and temperature senses. Once inside the spinal cord, dorsal root ganglion axons branch extensively. However, the branching patterns of large- and small-diameter sensory fibers are different.

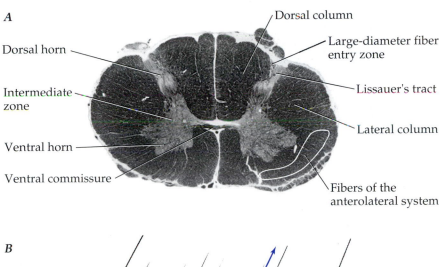

A

Dorsal column

Dorsal horn

Large-diameter fiber entry zone

Intermediate zone

Lissauer's tract

Ventral horn

Lateral column

Ventral commissure

Fibers of the anterolateral system

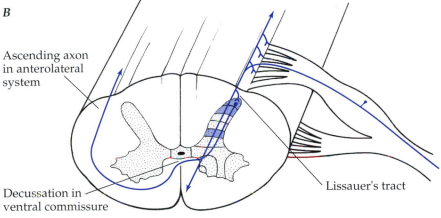

B

Ascending axon in anterolateral system

Decussation in ventral commissure

Lissauer's tract

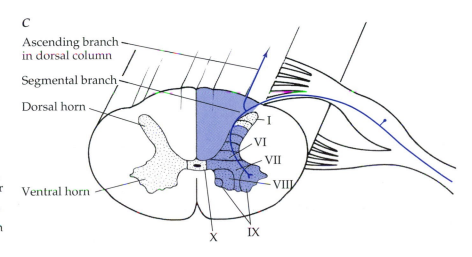

C

Ascending branch in dorsal column

Segmental branch

Dorsal horn

I

VI

VII

VIII

Ventral horn

X   IX

Figure 5–5. **A.** Myelin-stained section through the cervical spinal cord. **B, C.** Schematic drawings based on the section in *A* and illustrating the pattern of termination of small-diameter fibers (*B*) and large-diameter fibers (*C*). Note that small-diameter fibers also terminate in other laminae (see Figure 5–6).

The Spinal Gray Matter Consists of Laminar Sheets of Neurons

The branches of sensory fibers that terminate in the spinal gray matter have specific patterns. To understand these termination patterns, however, the cytoarchitecture of the dorsal and ventral horns (Figure 5–5A) must first be considered briefly. Similar to other areas of the central nervous system, spinal cord neurons are clustered into nuclei. The Swedish neuroanatomist Bror Rexed further recognized that neurons in the dorsal horn are arranged in flattened sheets, termed **Rexed's laminae,** that run parallel to the long axis of the spinal cord (Figure 5–5B,C). He distinguished 10 laminae. The dorsal horn is formed by laminae I through VI:

- **Lamina I,** the outermost, is also termed the **marginal zone.**
- **Lamina II** is also called the **substantia gelatinosa.**
- **Laminae III** and **IV** are also collectively termed the **nucleus proprius.**
- **Laminae V** and **VI** (also termed the base of dorsal horn) of the spinal cord extend rostrally into the base of the spinal trigeminal nucleus.

Laminae VII, VIII, and IX (which contain motor nuclei) comprise the ventral horn; however, these laminae are shaped more like rods or columns than flattened sheets. Lamina X comprises the gray matter surrounding the central canal. Sometimes the dorsal part of lamina VII is termed the intermediate zone, where many interneurons that transmit control signals to motor neurons are located. Because individual laminae contain neurons with distinctive anatomical connections and functions, the laminar nomenclature is more commonly used for describing the spinal gray matter (Figure 5–6, inset).

Small-diameter Sensory Fibers Terminate Primarily in the Superficial Laminae of the Dorsal Horn

Small-diameter axons–which subserve pain, itch, and temperature senses–enter the spinal cord in **Lissauer's tract,** the white matter region that caps the dorsal horn (Figure 5–5A). There they bifurcate and ascend and descend. The dorsal horn terminals derive directly from these ascending and descending branches within the tract. Small-diameter myelinated and unmyelinated axons terminate primarily in laminae I and II (Figure 5–6). These two laminae do not receive input from the large-diameter fibers. Small-diameter fibers also have a small termination within lamina V (Figure 5–6). Although Lissauer's tract is part

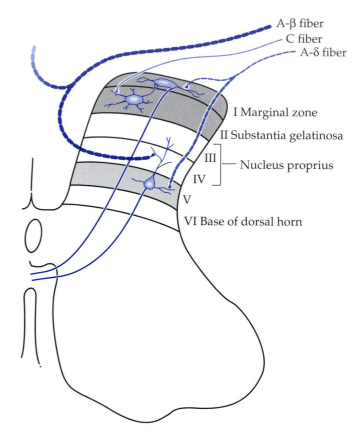

Figure 5–6. Laminar termination patterns of primary sensory axon terminals in the dorsal horn. A-δ and C fibers terminate superficially in the dorsal horn, with a branch of the A-δ fiber also terminating in deeper layers. A-β fibers terminate in the deeper layers of the dorsal horn, as well as in the ventral horn (not shown). However, the major A-β branch ascends in the dorsal column. Projection neurons of the anterolateral system are shown, located in laminae I and V. The axons decussate in the ventral spinal commissure. *(Adapted from Fields HL: Pain. McGraw-Hill, 1987.)*

of the white matter, it stains lightly because its axons either have a thin myelin sheath or are unmyelinated.

Anterolateral System Projection Neurons Are Located in the Dorsal Horn and Decussate in the Ventral Commissure

The laminar organization of the dorsal horn is also important for the projections to the brain stem and thalamus. The pathway to thalamic nuclei important for pain, itch, and temperature sensations originates primarily from neurons in lamina I, which receives direct input from small-diameter sensory fibers (Figure 5–6) and lamina V, which receives both direct and indirect input. Lamina V neurons also receive mechanoreceptive inputs and respond to a range of stimuli from weak mechanical to strong noxious. The spinal cord neurons whose axons project to the intralaminar nuclei and reticular formation of the pons and medulla, involved primarily in arousal, are located more ventrally in the gray matter, in laminae VI through VIII. The projection to the midbrain, important for orienting to salient stimuli and pain suppression, also originates from neurons in laminae I and V, similar to the projection to the ventral posterior lateral nucleus.

Most axons of the anterolateral system decussate in the spinal cord before ascending to the brain stem or thalamus (Figures 5–5B and 5–6). Decussations occur in **commissures,** in this case in the **ventral (anterior) commissure,** ventral to the central canal (Figure 5–5B). During early development this region corresponded to the floor plate (see Figure 3–7), an important site for guiding decussating spinal axons.

Large-diameter Sensory Fibers Terminate in the Dorsal Column Nuclei and the Deeper Laminae of the Dorsal Horn

Large-diameter fibers enter the spinal cord medial to Lissauer's tract, in the **large-diameter fiber entry zone** (in the dorsal column), which is darkly stained because the axons have a thick myelin sheath. The axons skirt over the cap of the gray matter to enter the dorsal column (Figure 5–5C), where they give off an ascending branch into the dorsal column and numerous segmental branches into the gray matter. The ascending branch is the principal one for perception, and it relays information to the dorsal column nuclei. The segmental branches terminate in the deeper layers of the dorsal horn and in the ventral horn (Figures 5–5C and 5–6). The only mechanoreceptors to terminate within the motor nuclei (Figure 5–5B) are the muscle spindle receptors, which mediate the monosynaptic stretch (eg, knee jerk) reflex, and Golgi tendon receptors.

A small number of dorsal horn neurons project their axons into the dorsal columns, comprising approximately 15% of the axons in the path. These neurons receive input from segmental branches of sensory fibers. How their functions differ from those of the primary sensory fibers is not well understood. Many of these neurons respond to mechanical stimulation of the viscera.

The Dorsal Columns Contain Ascending Branches of Mechanoreceptive Sensory Fibers

Each dorsal column transmits sensory information from the ipsilateral side of the body to the ipsilateral medulla. A systematic relationship exists between the position of an axon in the dorsal column and the body location from which it receives input. This organization, termed **somatotopy,** describes how somatic sen-

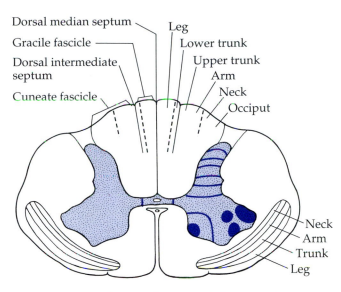

Figure 5–7. The dorsal columns and the ascending axons of the anterolateral system are somatotopically organized.

sory information is represented throughout the central nervous system. Beginning with the sequential ordering of the dorsal roots (Figure 5–4; see also Figure 1–4), somatotopic organization adheres to a simple rule: Adjacent body parts are represented in adjacent sites in the central nervous system. This arrangement ensures that local neighborhood relations in the periphery are preserved in the central nervous system. Similar principles apply to the topographic organization of the peripheral receptive sheet in the visual system (retinotopy) and in the auditory system (tonotopy).

Axons carrying information from the lower limb ascend in the most medial portion of the dorsal column, the **gracile fascicle** (Figure 5–7). Axons from the lower trunk ascend lateral to those from the lower limb, but still within the gracile fascicle. Within the **cuneate fascicle,** axons from the rostral trunk, upper limb, neck, and occiput ascend. The cuneate fascicle begins approximately at the level of the sixth thoracic segment. The gracile and cuneate fascicles are separated by the **dorsal intermediate septum,** and the dorsal columns of the two halves of the spinal cord are separated by the **dorsal median septum** (Figure 5–7).

The Somatotopic Organization of the Dorsal Columns Is Revealed in Human Postmortem Specimens

The somatotopic organization of the dorsal columns can be examined in postmortem tissue from individuals who sustained spinal cord trauma. The sections shown in Figure 5–8A were taken from a patient whose lumbar spinal cord was crushed in a traumatic spinal

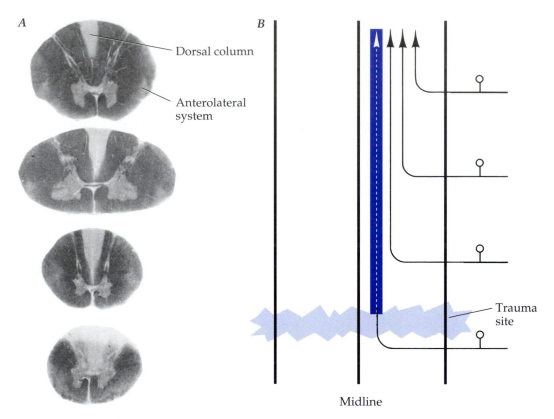

A

Dorsal column

Anterolateral system

B

Trauma site

Midline

Figure 5–8. The somatotopic organization of the dorsal columns can be demonstrated by examining spinal cord sections from a patient who sustained damage to the lumbar spinal cord. *A.* Four levels through the spinal cord, rostrocaudally from top to bottom: a section rostral to the cervical enlargement, a section through the cervical enlargement, and two thoracic sections. *B.* The course taken by the central branches of the dorsal root fibers as they enter the spinal cord and ascend in the dorsal columns. The dashed line depicts the course of a degenerated axon transected by the crush.

injury. The sections are stained for myelin. Axons that have degenerated have lost their myelin sheath and are not stained (see Figure 2–4). In the caudal thoracic spinal cord (Figure 5–8, bottom section), close to the crushed region, nearly all of the axons in both gracile fascicles have degenerated. At more rostral levels the degenerated region becomes confined medially as new contingents of healthy axons continue to enter the spinal cord lateral to the degenerated axons from the lumbar cord. The pattern by which axons enter and ascend in the dorsal columns is shown schematically in Figure 5–8B.

Spinal cord lesions produce particular patterns of somatic sensory loss (Box 5–1). For example, unilateral spinal injury produces ipsilateral loss of mechanical sensations (eg, touch) and contralateral loss of pain, temperature, and itch sensations below the level of the lesion (see Figure 5–9). Spinal damage that interrupts the decussating axons of the anterolateral system (see Figure 5–10) produces bilateral loss of pain, temperature, and itch sensations.

The location of the anterolateral system is revealed by examining the degenerated area in the lateral column in Figure 5–8A. Although the anterolateral system is also somatotopically organized (Figure 5–7), it is not as precise as that for the dorsal columns and only a trend is apparent. Axons transmitting sensory information from more caudal segments are located lateral to those from more rostral segments (Figure 5–7).

The Decussation of the Dorsal Column–Medial Lemniscal System Is in the Caudal Medulla

Dorsal column axons synapse on neurons in the **dorsal column nuclei** (Figure 5–11), the first major relay in the ascending pathway for touch and limb position senses. These and other somatic sensory relay nuclei enhance contrast and spatial resolution so that when adjacent portions of the skin are touched, the person can discern the difference.

Box 5–1. The Patterns of Somatic Sensory Impairments After Spinal Cord Injury

Spinal cord injury results in deficits in somatic sensation and in the control of body musculature at the level of, and caudal to, the lesion. Motor deficits that follow such injury are considered in Chapter 10. Here, somatic sensory deficits are considered. In general, somatic sensory deficits have three major characteristics: (1) the sensory **modality** that is affected, for example, whether pain or touch is impaired, (2) the **laterality,** or side of the body where deficits are observed (ie, ipsilateral versus contralateral), and (3) the **body regions** affected. Damage to one half of the spinal cord, or hemisection, illustrates all three of these characteristic deficits (Figure 5–9). Spinal hemisection can occur, for example, when a tumor encroaches on the cord from one side, or when the cord is injured traumatically. The sensory and motor deficits that follow spinal cord hemisection are collectively termed the **Brown-Séquard syndrome.**

Axons in the dorsal columns are **ipsilateral** in the spinal cord; hence, deficits in touch and limb position sense are present ipsilateral to the spinal

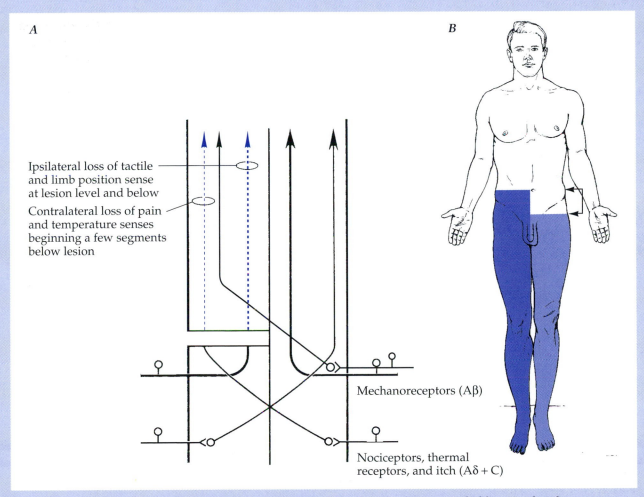

A. Ipsilateral loss of tactile and limb position sense at lesion level and below

Contralateral loss of pain and temperature senses beginning a few segments below lesion

Mechanoreceptors (Aβ)

Nociceptors, thermal receptors, and itch (Aδ + C)

Figure 5–9. ***A.*** The patterns of decussation of the dorsal column—medial lemniscal and anterolateral systems are illustrated in relation to spinal cord hemisection (Brown-Séquard syndrome). ***B.*** Because projection neurons of the anterolateral system ascend as they decussate, spinal hemisection produces a loss of pain, temperature, and itch one to two segments caudal to the lesion. In contrast, loss of mechanical sensations begins at the level of the lesion.

(continued)

Box 5–1   (continued.)

cord lesion (Figure 5–9). In contrast, the axons of the anterolateral system decussate in the spinal cord. Therefore, **pain** and **temperature senses** are impaired on the side of the body that is **contralateral** to the lesion. (Note that itch is not usually tested but presumably also is impaired.)

The spinal cord level at which injury occurs can be determined by comparing the distribution of sensory loss with the sensory innervation patterns of the dorsal roots (ie, the dermatomal maps; Figure 5–4). Because of the differences in the anatomical organization of the two systems mediating somatic sensations, a single level of spinal injury will result in different levels of sensory impairment for touch and pain sensations. For touch sensation the most rostral dermatome in

which sensation is impaired corresponds to the level of injury in the spinal cord. For pain sensation the most rostral dermatome in which sensation is impaired is about two segments lower than the injured spinal cord level. This is because the axons of the anterolateral system decussate over a distance of one to two spinal segments before ascending to the brain stem and diencephalon.

Two pathological processes can selectively impair the function of the dorsal column—medial lemniscal system and the anterolateral system. First, in **tabes dorsalis,** an advanced stage of neurosyphilis, dorsal root ganglion neurons with large-diameter axons are lost. Thus, patients lose touch and limb position sense. Fortunately, tabes dorsalis is rare

today because of antibacterial therapies.

Second, in **syringomyelia,** a cavity (or syrinx) forms in the central portion of the spinal cord (Figure 5–10A), damaging selectively the decussating axons of the anterolateral system. This results in a loss of pain and temperature sense and sparing of mechanical sensations (Figure 5–10B). Syringomyelia interrupts decussating axons from both sides of the body; hence, the sensory loss is usually bilaterally symmetrical. Because the lesion affects the decussating, not the ascending, axons, body regions below the level of injury have normal sensation. By contrast, in spinal cord hemisection, pain and temperature sensations are lost caudal to the lesion because the ascending axons are severed.

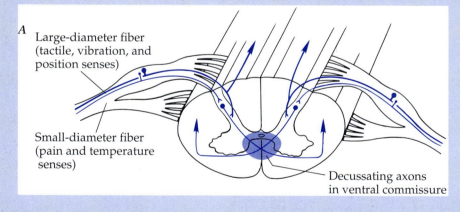

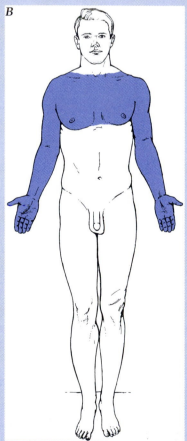

A

Large-diameter fiber (tactile, vibration, and position senses)

Small-diameter fiber (pain and temperature senses)

Decussating axons in ventral commissure

B

Figure 5–10.   Syringomyelia disrupts the decussating fibers of the anterolateral system but usually not the ascending fibers of the dorsal column–medial lemniscal system. **A.** Spinal cord cross section showing the patterns of terminations of small- and large-diameter axons and how the components of the anterolateral system decussate and ascend. The dorsal column–medial lemniscal system ascends ipsilaterally in the spinal cord. The blue-tinted region is affected by the formation of a syrinx (cavity). **B.** Distribution of loss of pain and temperature sense over the body. (*Adapted from Kandel ER, Schwartz JH: Principles of Neural Science. Elsevier, 1985.*)

Figure 5–11. Myelin-stained transverse section through the dorsal column nuclei. Trajectories of internal arcuate fibers from the gracile and cuneate nuclei are shown. Arrow indicates plane of section in Figure 5–12. The inset shows the approximate plane of section.

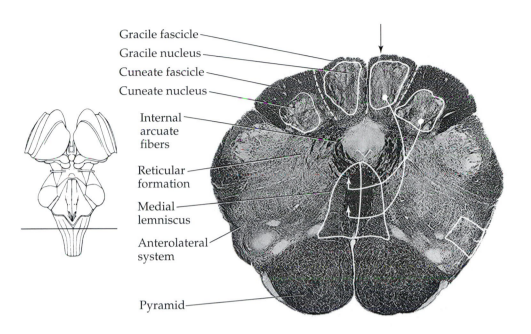

Gracile fascicle
Gracile nucleus
Cuneate fascicle
Cuneate nucleus
Internal arcuate fibers
Reticular formation
Medial lemniscus
Anterolateral system
Pyramid

Axons of the gracile fascicle synapse in the **gracile nucleus,** which is located close to the midline, whereas those from the cuneate fascicle synapse in the **cuneate nucleus.** Figure 5–12 illustrates a parasagittal section close to the midline, through the gracile nucleus (the plane of section is indicated in Figure 5–11). From the dorsal column nuclei, the axons of the second-order neurons sweep ventrally through the medulla, where they are called the **internal arcuate fibers,** and

decussate (Figure 5–11). Immediately after crossing the midline, the fibers ascend to the thalamus in the **medial lemniscus** (Figures 5–11 and 5–13). Axons from the gracile nucleus decussate ventral to axons from the cuneate nucleus and ascend in the ventral part of the medial lemniscus, compared with axons from the cuneate nucleus (Figure 5–11). Because of this pattern, the somatotopic organization of the medial lemniscus in the medulla resembles a person standing upright. In the

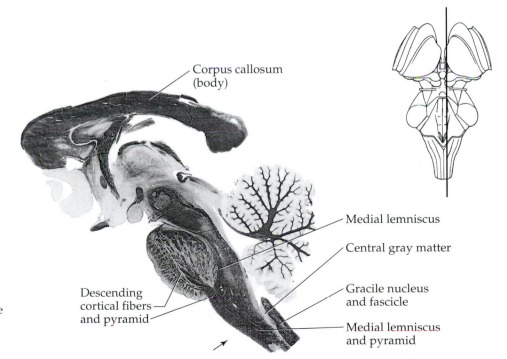

Corpus callosum (body)
Medial lemniscus
Central gray matter
Descending cortical fibers and pyramid
Gracile nucleus and fascicle
Medial lemniscus and pyramid

Figure 5–12. Myelin-stained sagittal section through the brain stem, close to midline. The arrow marks the approximate plane of the section shown in Figure 5–11.

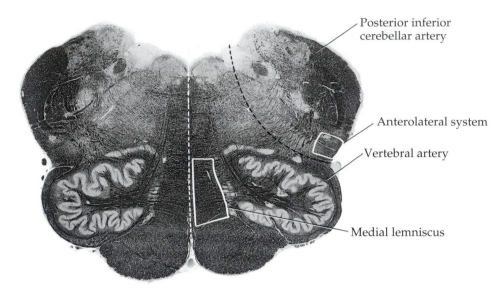

Posterior inferior
cerebellar artery

Anterolateral system

Vertebral artery

Medial lemniscus

Figure 5–13. The pattern of arterial perfusion of the rostral medulla.

pons the medial lemniscus is located more dorsally than in the medulla and is oriented from medial to lateral.

In contrast to the dorsal column–medial lemniscal system, which ascends in the medial medulla, the anterolateral system ascends along its ventrolateral margin (Figures 5–11, 5–13, 5–14). For the spinothalamic and spinomesencephalic tracts the medulla and pons simply serve as a conduit through which axons pass to reach more rostral locations. For the spinoreticular tract the axons terminate in the reticular formation of the pons and medulla (Figure 5–14).

Vascular Lesions of the Medulla Differentially Affect Somatic Sensory Function

The caudal brain stem receives blood from perforating branches of the **vertebral-basilar,** or **posterior, circulation** (see Figure 4–3). The areas served by the **posterior inferior cerebellar artery** (PICA) and smaller branches of the vertebral artery are illustrated in Figure 5–13. Occlusion of the PICA, which supplies the dorsolateral medulla, damages the ascending anterolateral system fibers but not the medial lemniscus. A patient who experiences an infarction of the PICA can have diminished pain sensation on the limbs and trunk but unaffected touch sense. The sensory loss is contralateral to the side of the lesion because the axons of the anterolateral system decussate in the spinal cord (Figure 5–9). (Such sensory loss is one of multiple neurological signs that comprise the **lateral medullary,** or **Wallenberg, syndrome,** which is discussed further in Chapter 6.)

Occlusion of smaller (unnamed) branches of the vertebral artery can damage axons of the medial lemniscus, sparing the anterolateral system. As a consequence, touch and limb position senses, but not pain and temperature senses, are disrupted. Vertebral artery infarction produces mechanosensory deficits on the contralateral side of the body, because the internal arcuate fibers decussate at a more caudal level in the medulla (Figure 5–11). This type of infarction also destroys axons of the corticospinal tract in the pyramid. The motor deficits of vertebral artery infarction are considered in Chapters 10 and 11.

Descending Pain Suppression Pathways Originate From the Brain Stem

For the dorsal column–medial lemniscal system, the midbrain serves as a conduit for the axons of the medial lemniscus, which synapse in the thalamus. The medial lemniscus lies in a horn-shaped collection of myelinated axons adjacent to the red nucleus, which is important for movement control (see Chapter 10) (Figure 5–15). Fibers of the anterolateral system are dorsal and lateral to the medial lemniscus. The **spinothalamic tract,** like the medial lemniscus, courses through the midbrain en route to the thalamus.

One projection of the **spinomesencephalic tract** that is important for orienting to somatic stimuli is to the superior colliculus (Figure 5–15; see Chapter 7). Another projection is to the periaqueductal gray matter, which surrounds the cerebral aqueduct. This midbrain region plays a key role in modulating pain perception. A **descending pain inhibitory system** originates from this region (Figure 5–2B). Pain suppression may be a survival mechanism that allows people to

Figure 5–14. Myelin-stained transverse sections through the medulla (*A*) and pons (*B*). The inset shows the approximate planes of section.

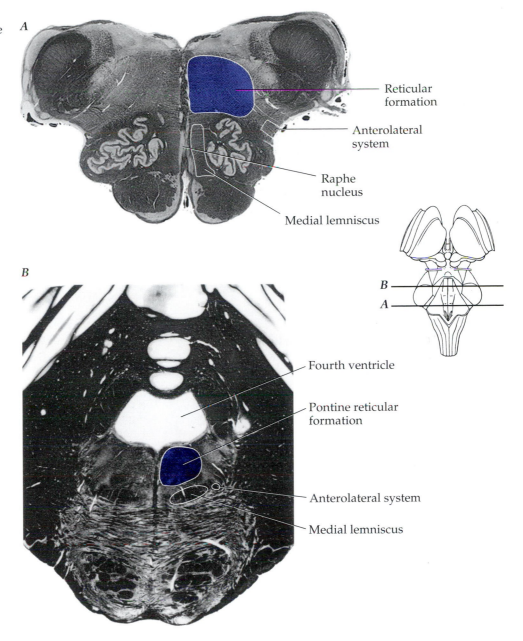

Reticular formation

Anterolateral system

Raphe nucleus

Medial lemniscus

Fourth ventricle

Pontine reticular formation

Anterolateral system

Medial lemniscus

function better despite sudden pain, such as during physical combat or in childbirth. Receiving complex patterns of input from diencephalic and telencephalic structures involved in emotions (see Chapter 16), excitatory neurons of the **periaqueductal gray matter** (Figure 5–15) project to the **raphe nuclei** in the medulla (Figure 5–14A). These raphe neurons, which use **serotonin** as their neurotransmitter, project to the dorsal horn of the spinal cord. Serotonin suppresses pain transmission in the dorsal horn (1) by directly inhibiting ascending projection neurons that transmit information about painful stimuli to the brain and (2) by exciting inhibitory interneurons in the dorsal horn, which use

the neurotransmitter **enkephalin.** Other regions in the brain stem, including the locus ceruleus (see Figure 2–2B2) and the lateral medullary reticular formation (Figure 5–14A), give rise to a descending noradrenergic projection that also suppresses pain transmission.

Three Separate Nuclei in the Thalamus Process Somatic Sensory Information

The **thalamus** (Figure 5–16) is a nodal point for the transmission of sensory information to the cerebral cortex. Indeed, with the exception of olfaction, infor-

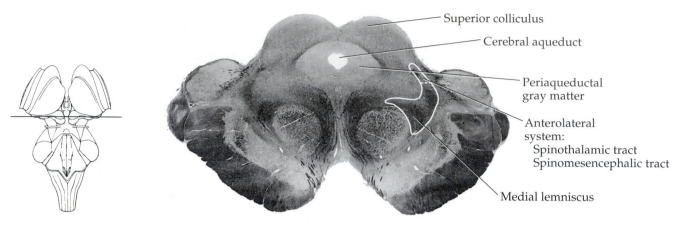

Figure 5–15. Myelin-stained transverse section through the midbrain. The inset shows the approximate plane of section.

mation from all sensory systems is processed in the thalamus and then relayed to the cerebral cortex. The dorsal column–medial lemniscal and anterolateral systems are no exceptions. Three major thalamic regions receive input from these pathways for various aspects of somatic sensation: the ventral posterior nucleus, the ventromedial posterior nucleus, and the medial dorsal nucleus (Figures 5–16 and 5–17).

The **ventral posterior nucleus** has a lateral division, the **ventral posterior lateral nucleus** (Figures 5–16A and 5–17B), which receives input from both the medial lemniscus and the spinothalamic tract and projects to the **primary somatic sensory cortex** (Figure 5–17). Although the spinothalamic tract and the medial lemniscus terminate in the ventral posterior lateral nucleus, their terminal fields hardly overlap, an example of functional localization. The ventral posterior nucleus also has a medial division, the **ventral posterior medial nucleus** (Figures 5–16A and 5–17B), which mediates aspects of somatic sensations from the face and perioral structures. This nucleus is considered in Chapter 6. The ventral posterior nucleus is important in discriminative aspects of the mechanical sensations, such as being able to precisely localize the stimulation site on the body. Its role in pain, temperature senses, and itch is not well understood (see section on cortical pain representations).

The **ventromedial posterior nucleus** (Figure 5–17A) adjoins but is caudal to the ventral posterior nucleus. It projects to the **insular cortex.** This is a major site for processing information from spinothalamic tract neurons in the spinal cord. The **medial dorsal nucleus** (Figure 5–17) also receives spinothalamic input and projects to the **anterior cingulate gyrus.** The ventromedial posterior and medial dorsal

nuclei are thought to play roles in the affective and motivational aspects of pain and in the memory of painful stimuli (see section on cortical pain representations).

Although the **intralaminar nuclei** (such as the central lateral nucleus; Figure 5–17B) also receive spinothalamic input, as well as information from the reticular formation, they are not thought to have a direct sensory function. This is because they also receive inputs from motor and integrative structures of the brain. Moreover, the intralaminar nuclei are diffuse-projecting and may participate in arousal and attention (see Table 2–1).

Several Areas of the Parietal Lobe Process Touch and Proprioceptive Information

Mechanoreceptive sensory information is processed primarily by three cortical areas: (1) the primary somatic sensory cortex, (2) the secondary somatic sensory cortex, and (3) the posterior parietal cortex. (The motor cortical areas also receive mechanoreceptive information, but this information is important in controlling movements.) Located in the postcentral gyrus of the parietal lobe (Figure 5–16B), the primary somatic sensory cortex is the principal region of the parietal lobe to which the ventral posterior lateral nucleus projects. Axons from this nucleus travel to the cerebral cortex through the **posterior limb of the internal capsule** (Figure 5–17B; see also Figure 2–12). The secondary somatic sensory cortex and the posterior parietal cortex receive input from the thalamus and the primary somatic sensory cortex, by cortical association fibers (see below).

A

Leg

Arm

Face

Internal capsule

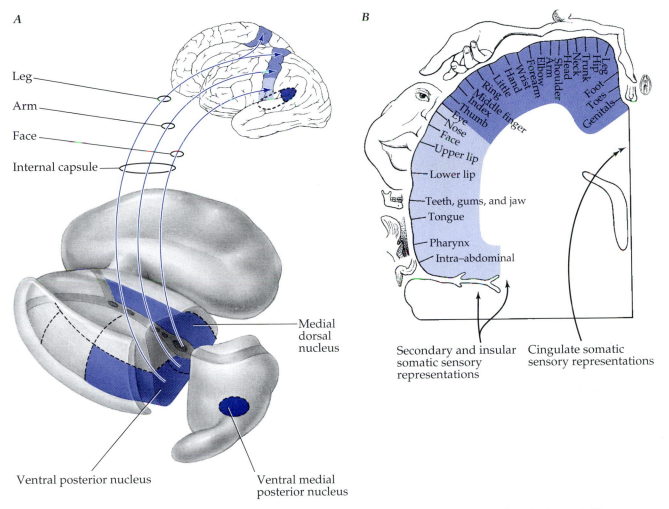

Medial dorsal nucleus

Ventral posterior nucleus

Ventral medial posterior nucleus

B

Leg
Hip
Trunk
Neck
Head
Shoulder
Arm
Elbow
Forearm
Wrist
Hand
Little
Ring
Middle finger
Index
Thumb
Eye
Nose
Face
Upper lip

Lower lip

Teeth, gums, and jaw

Tongue

Pharynx

Intra–abdominal

Foot
Toes
Genitals

Secondary and insular somatic sensory representations

Cingulate somatic sensory representations

Figure 5–16. Organization of the somatic sensory thalamocortical projections. *A.* The ventral posterior nucleus has a somatotopic organization: Neurons receiving input from the leg and arm are located in the lateral division of the nucleus, whereas neurons receiving input from the face are located in the medial division. Axons from the ventral posterior nucleus ascend to the primary somatic sensory cortex in the internal capsule. *B.* A schematic slice through the postcentral gyrus, showing the somatotopic organization of the primary somatic sensory cortex. The relative locations of the cingulate and insular representations are also indicated.

The Primary Somatic Sensory Cortex Has a Somatotopic Organization

The **primary somatic sensory cortex** receives somatotopically organized inputs from the ventral posterior lateral and medial nuclei (Figure 5–16A). This thalamocortical projection imposes a body map on the postcentral gyrus, the **sensory homunculus,** originally described in the human by the Canadian neurosurgeon Wilder Penfield.

The representations of the various body parts on the sensory map do not have the same proportions as the body itself (Figure 5–16B). Rather, the portions of the body used in discriminative touch tasks, such as the fingers, have a disproportionately greater representation on the map than areas that are not as important for touch, such as the leg. It was once thought that these differences were fixed and simply reflected the density of peripheral sensory receptor neurons. We now know that the body map of the brain is not static but is dynamically controlled by the pattern of use of different body parts in touch exploration.

The cerebral cortex is a laminated structure; most regions have at least six cell layers (Figure 5–18). The thalamus projects primarily to layer IV (and the adjoin-

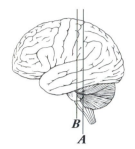

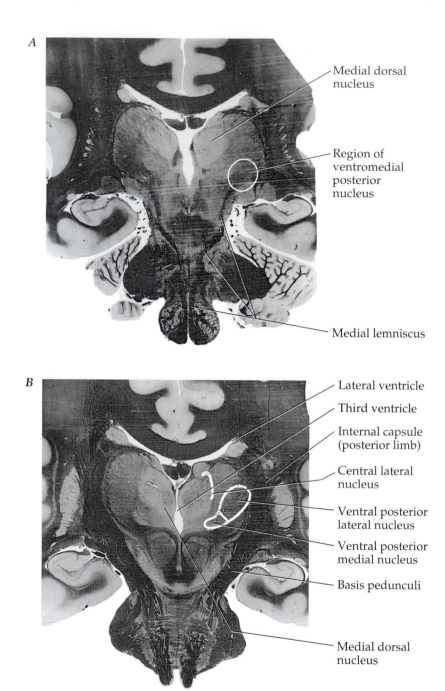

Figure 5–17. Myelin-stained transverse sections through the diencephalon. The section illustrated in *A* is located caudal to the section shown in *B*. The inset shows the approximate planes of section. The central lateral nucleus consists of a thin band of neurons in the internal medullary lamina (*B*).

ing portion of layer III), and this incoming information is distributed to neurons in more superficial and deeper layers. Most of the excitatory connections within a local area of cortex remain somewhat confined to a vertical slice of cortex, termed a **cortical column.** The cortical column constitutes a functional unit. Neurons within a column in the primary somatic sensory cortex, spanning all cortical layers, receive input from the same peripheral location on the body and from the same class of mechanoreceptor. Although originally conceived as cylindrical in shape, the cortical columns have a more irregular configuration.

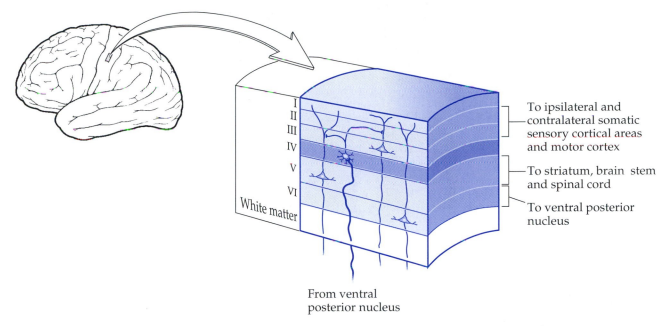

Figure 5–18.   Three-dimensional schematic of a portion of the cerebral cortex. The piece is from the postcentral gyrus (see inset). Within the cortex are six layers in which cells and their processes are located. Neurons whose cell bodies are located in layers II and III project to other cortical areas, those in layer V project their axons to subcortical regions, and those in layer VI project to the thalamus. Neurons in layer IV receive thalamic input and transmit information to neurons in other cortical layers.

The primary somatic sensory cortex consists of four cytoarchitectonic divisions, or **Brodmann's areas** (see Figure 2–17), numbered 1, 2, 3a, and 3b (Figure 5–19). As in other cortical areas, regions of the primary somatic sensory cortex with a different cytoarchitecture have different functions. Areas 3a and 2 process information from mechanoreceptors located in deep structures, such as the muscles and joints, and areas 3b and 1 process information from mechanoreceptors of the skin. Animal experiments have shown that in each

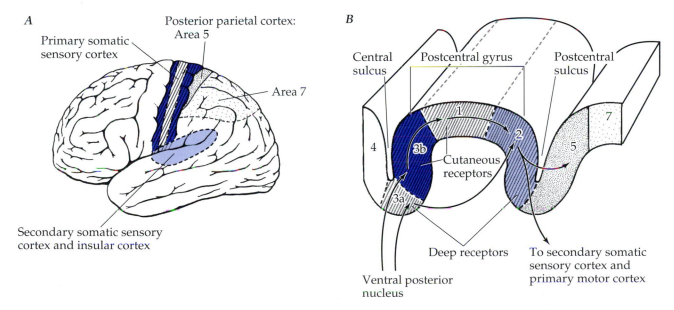

Figure 5–19.   **A.** The locations of the primary and higher order somatic sensory areas are indicated on a lateral view of the cerebral cortex. The light blue region corresponds to the areas beneath the surface, in the insular cortex and the parietal and temporal operculum. **B.** A schematic section cut perpendicular to the mediolateral axis of the postcentral gyrus. *(Adapted from Kandel ER, Schwartz JH: Principles of Neural Science. Elsevier, 1985.)*

of these areas there is a separate representation of the body. In areas 3b and 1 the representations are complete and highly detailed; in areas 3a and 2 the representations appear to be coarser. These differences provide important insights into the functions of the four cytoarchitectonic areas within the primary somatic sensory cortex. Areas 3a and 2 play important roles in limb position sense and shape discrimination of grasped objects; areas 3b and 1 play a major role in superficial touch, including texture discrimination.

Efferent projections arise from the primary somatic sensory cortex (Figure 5–18). **Corticocortical association neurons,** located in layers II and III, project to other cortical areas on the same side, including higher-order somatic sensory cortical areas (see next section) for further processing of sensory information, and the primary motor cortex for movement control. **Callosal neurons,** also located in layers II and III, project their axons to the contralateral somatic sensory cortex through the corpus callosum. One function of these callosal connections may be to join the representations of each half of the body in the primary somatic sensory cortex of each hemisphere. **Descending projection neurons,** located in layers V and VI, send their axons primarily to the thalamus, brain stem, and spinal cord—where somatic sensory information is processed—to act as gatekeepers that regulate the quantity of mechanosensory information that ascends through the central nervous system.

Higher-order Somatic Sensory Cortical Areas Are Located in the Parietal Lobe, Parietal Operculum, and Insular Cortex

Thalamocortical processing of touch and proprioceptive information provides insight into the principles of organization of sensory systems. The main thalamic sensory nucleus for a given modality (eg, ventral posterior nucleus for mechanosensations) projects to the primary sensory cortex. Projections from the primary sensory cortical area distribute the information to multiple cortical regions, although these areas may also receive direct thalamic inputs. These upstream areas are each devoted to processing a specific aspect of the sensory experience. Although sequential pathways from one region to the next can be identified, the primary and higher-order sensory areas are also extensively interconnected and the operations of any one set of connections are dependent on the operations of others. The higher-order sensory areas typically project to cortical regions that receive inputs from the other sensory modalities termed **association areas.**

One such multimodal convergent zone is the large expanse of cortex at the junction of the parietal, temporal, and occipital lobes.

The **secondary somatic sensory cortex** is located on the parietal operculum and insular cortex (Figure 5–19A). Similar to the primary area the secondary somatic sensory cortex is somatotopically organized. This part of the cortex begins a sequence of somatic sensory projections to insular cortical areas and the temporal lobe that are important for object recognition by touch and position sense.

The **posterior parietal cortex** (Figure 5–19A), which includes Brodmann's areas 5 and 7, plays an important role in perception of body image. A lesion of this region in the nondominant hemisphere (typically the right hemisphere) produces a complex sensory syndrome in which the individual neglects the contralateral half of the body. For example, a patient may fail to dress one side of her body or comb half of her hair. Other portions of the posterior parietal cortex receive visual and auditory inputs as well as somatic sensory information. These areas are involved in integrating somatic sensory, visual, and auditory information for perception and attention.

Limbic and Insular Areas Contain the Cortical Representations of Pain, Itch, and Temperature Sensations

Much of what is known of the cortical representation of painful, itch-provoking, and thermal stimuli comes from functional imaging studies conducted in awake human subjects. The primary somatic sensory cortex can become activated with a painful stimulus, but this activation is inconsistent and depends on complex factors, such as the context in which the stimulus is presented or the person's expectation of pain. Moreover, the sites that become active are small and the responses weak. By contrast, the **insular cortex** (Figure 5–20) and **anterior cingulate gyrus** are consistently and intensely activated by a painful stimulus. The insular cortex has direct projections to the limbic system (Chapter 16), which comprises the cortical and subcortical circuitry for emotions. Limbic system structures that receive information about painful stimuli include the amygdaloid complex and limbic association cortex. The anterior cingulate gyrus, which is part of the limbic system, corresponds approximately to Brodmann's area 24 (see Figure 2–16). The insular and anterior cingulate areas are thought to be important in the affective and reactive components of pain.

A

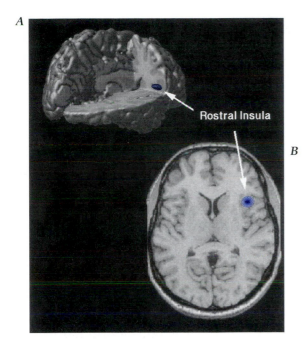

Rostral Insula

B

Figure 5–20. Positron emission tomography using ¹⁵O (see Box 1–1) showing the distribution of selective increase in cerebral blood flow during noxious thermal stimulation. Scans reflect computed differences between activation patterns produced by noxious thermal stimulation and nonnoxious activation. *A.* A three-dimensional view, reconstructed from a series of slices. The highlighted region corresponds to the anterior insular cortex. *B.* A two-dimensional slice through the active region of anterior insular cortex. Darker blue indicates greater ¹⁵O utilization by the tissue. Note that the anterior cingulate gyrus is not shown in this figure. *(Courtesy of Dr. Gary Duncan, University of Montreal and Montreal Neurological Institute; Coghill RC, Talbot JD, Evans AC, et al: Distributed processing of pain and vibration by the human brain. J Neurosci 1994;14:4095–4108.)*

Summary

Somatic Sensory Pathways

There are two major somatic sensory pathways (Figures 5–1 and 5–2; Table 5–1): the **dorsal column–medial lemniscal system,** which mediates **touch** and **limb position sense,** and the **anterolateral system,** which mediates **pain, temperature,** and **itch senses** and crude touch. These systems differ in four major ways: (1) modality sensitivity of input from dorsal root ganglion neurons, (2) location of first relay site, (3) level of decussation, and (4) functional and anatomical homogeneity of the pathway.

Sensory Receptor Neurons

Dorsal root ganglion neurons are **pseudounipolar neurons** (Figure 5–1, inset). They receive somatic sensory information and transmit it from the periphery to the spinal cord. The distal terminal of dorsal root ganglion neurons is the **sensory receptor.** Neurons sensitive to **noxious** and **thermal stimuli** or **histamine** have **bare nerve endings** and **small-diameter axons** (A-δ; C). Those sensitive to **mechanical stimuli** have encapsulated endings and **large-diameter axons** (A-α; A-β). Four major mechanoreceptors innervate glabrous skin and subcutaneous tissue (Figure 5–3): **Meissner's corpuscles, pacinian corpuscles, Merkel's receptors,** and **Ruffini's corpuscles.** The **muscle spindle** is the key receptor for muscle stretch and the Golgi tendon organ, for force. (Figure 5–3B).

Spinal Cord

The axons of dorsal root ganglion neurons enter the spinal cord via the **dorsal root.** A **dermatome** is the area of skin innervated by a single dorsal root (Figure 5–4). The afferent information carried by adjacent dorsal roots overlaps nearly completely on the body surface. Once in the spinal cord, dorsal root ganglion neurons have three major branches: **segmental, ascending,** and **descending.** The principal branching pattern of large-diameter fibers is to ascend to the brain stem in the dorsal columns (Figures 5–5C and 5–6). Whereas small-diameter fibers ascend and descend in **Lissauer's tract,** they eventually terminate in the gray matter of the spinal cord (Figure 5–5B and 5–6).

The ascending somatic sensory pathways course in two locations in the spinal cord. The dorsal column–medial lemniscal system ascends in the **dorsal columns.** The dorsal columns have two fascicles (Figures 5–5, 5–7, and 5–8). The **gracile fascicle** carries axons from the leg and lower trunk, and the **cuneate fascicle** carries axons from the upper trunk, arm, neck, and back of the head. The majority of the axons in the dorsal columns are central branches of dorsal root ganglion neurons. The axons of the anterolateral system derive from dorsal horn neurons and decussate in the **ventral (anterior) commissure** (Figures 5–5B and 5–6). The anterolateral system ascends in the lateral column (Figures 5–6 and 5–7). Spinal cord hemisection has a differential effect on the somatic sensory modalities caudal to the lesion, producing loss of touch and position senses on the side of the lesion and loss of pain and temperature senses on the opposite side (Figures 5–7, 5–9, and 5–10). Central spinal lesions can selectively disrupt the decussating axons of the anterolateral system (Figures 5–9 and 5–10).

Brain Stem

Dorsal column axons terminate in the **dorsal column nuclei** in the caudal medulla (Figures 5–11 and 5–12). Axons of neurons in the dorsal column nuclei decussate and ascend in the **medial lemniscus** (Figures 5–11 through 5–15; and 5–17B) and terminate in the thalamus. Fibers of the anterolateral system terminate in the **reticular formation** (Figures 5–11 and 5–14) (**spinoreticular tract**), **midbrain tectum** and **periaqueductal gray matter** (Figure 5–15) (**spinomesencephalic tract**), and **thalamus** (**spinothalamic tract**) (Figures 5–16 and 5–17).

Thalamus and Cerebral Cortex

The axons of the medial lemniscus synapse in the **ventral posterior lateral nucleus** (Figures 5–16A and 5–17B), which projects to the **primary somatic sensory cortex** (Figures 5–16A and 5–19), via the **posterior limb of the internal capsule**. The **secondary somatic sensory cortex** and **posterior parietal cortex** receive input from the primary somatic sensory cortex. Each of these cortical areas is somatotopically organized. Axons of the spinothalamic tract synapse in the three principal thalamic nuclei. Two of these nuclei— the **ventral posterior lateral nucleus** (Figure 5–17B), which projects to the primary somatic sensory cortex (Figures 5–16A and 5–19), and the **ventromedial posterior nucleus** (Figure 5–17A), which projects to the insular cortex—are important in stimulus perception. The third, the **medial dorsal nucleus** (Figure 5–17), projects to the cingulate cortex for the emotional responses to pain. The insular and anterior cortical regions are also important in the behavioral and autonomic responses to pain, temperature, and itch sensations and the emotions and memories these stimuli evoke.

Inputs from thalamus arrive at layer IV of the cortex (Figure 5–18). Efferent projections from the somatic sensory cortical areas arise from specific cortical layers. **Corticocortical association connections** (with other cortical areas on the same side of the cerebral cortex) are made by neurons in layers II and III. **Callosal connections** (with the other side of the cerebral cortex) are also made by neurons in layers II and III. **Descending projections** to the striatum, brain stem, and spinal cord originate from neurons located in layer V, whereas the projection to the thalamus originates from neurons located in layer VI.

Related Sources

Basbaum AI, Jessell TM: The perception of pain. In Kandel ER, Schwartz JH, Jessell TM (editors): Principles of Neural Science, 4th ed. McGraw-Hill; 2000:472–491.

Brust JCM: The Practice of Neural Science. McGraw-Hill; 2000. (See ch. 5; ch. 8, cases 1–5; ch. 14, cases 43–45, 47; ch. 16, case 68.)

Gardner EP, Kandel ER: Touch. In Kandel ER, Schwartz JH, Jessell TM (editors): Principles of Neural Science, 4th ed. McGraw-Hill; 2000:451–471.

Selected Readings

Brown AG: Organization in the Spinal Cord: The Anatomy and Physiology of Identified Neurons. Springer, 1981.

Brown AG: The terminations of cutaneous nerve fibers in the spinal cord. Trends Neurosci 1981;4:64–67.

Bushnell MC, Duncan GH, Hofbauer RK, Ha B, Chen JI, Carrier B: Pain perception: Is there a role for primary somatosensory cortex? Proc Natl Acad Sci U S A 1999;96: 7705–7709.

Casey KL: Forebrain mechanisms of nociception and pain: Analysis through imaging. Proc Natl Acad Sci USA 1999; 96:7668–7674.

Dubner R: Three decades of pain research and its control. J Dent Res 1997;76:730–733.

Dubner R, Gold M: The neurobiology of pain. Proc Natl Acad Sci U S A 1999;96:7627–7630.

Fields HL: Pain. McGraw-Hill, 1987.

Rustioni A, Weinberg RJ: The somatosensory system. In Bjumörklund A, Hókfelt T, Swanson LW (editors): Handbook of Chemical Neuroanatomy, Vol. 7: Integrated Systems of the CNS, Part II: Central Visual, Auditory, Somatosensory, Gustatory. Elsevier; 1989:219–321.

References

Andrew D, Craig AD: Spinothalamic lamina I neurons selectively sensitive to histamine: A central neural pathway for itch. Nat Neurosci 2001;4:72–77.

Appelberg AE, Leonard RB, Kenshalo DR Jr., et al: Nuclei in which functionally identified spinothalamic tract neurons terminate. J Comp Neurol 1979;188:575–586.

Augustine JR: The insular lobe in primates including humans. Neurol Res 1985;7:2–10.

Blomqvist A, Zhang ET, Craig AD: Cytoarchitectonic and immunohistochemical characterization of a specific pain and temperature relay, the posterior portion of the ventral medial nucleus, in the human thalamus. Brain 2000; 123(part 3):601–619.

Coghill RC, Talbot JD, Evans AC, et al: Distributed processing of pain and vibration by the human brain. J Neurosci 1994;14:4095–4108.

Collins RD: Illustrated Manual of Neurologic Diagnosis. Lippincott, 1962.

Craig AD, Bushnell MC: The thermal grill illusion: Unmasking the burn of cold pain. Science 1994;265:252–255.

Craig AD, Bushnell MC, Zhang ET, Blomqvist A: A thalamic nucleus specific for pain and temperature sensation. Nature 1994;372:770–773.

Friedman DP, Murray EA, O'Neil JB, Mishkin M: Cortical connections of the somatosensory fields of the lateral sulcus of macaques: Evidence for a corticolimbic pathway for touch. J Comp Neurol 1986;252:323–347.

Giesler GJ Jr., Nahin RL, Madsen AM: Postsynaptic dorsal column pathway of the rat. I. Anatomical studies. J Neurophysiol 1984;51:260–275.

Gray D, Gutierrez C, Cusick CG: Neurochemical organization of inferior pulvinar complex in squirrel monkeys and macaques revealed by acetylcholinesterase histochemistry, calbindin and Cat-301 immunostaining, and Wisteria floribunda agglutinin binding. J Comp Neurol 1999;409:452–468.

Gutierrez C, Cola MG, Seltzer B, Cusick C: Neurochemical and connectional organization of the dorsal pulvinar complex in monkeys. J Comp Neurol 2000;419:61–86.

Jones EG: Organization of the thalamocortical complex and its relation to sensory processes. In Darian-Smith I (editor): Handbook of Physiology, Section 1: The Nervous System, Vol. 3: Sensory Processes. American Physiological Society; 1984:149–212.

Jones EG, Friedman DP: Projection pattern of functional components of thalamic ventrobasal complex on monkey somatosensory cortex. J Neurophysiol 1982;48:521–544.

Mesulam MM, Mufson EJ: Insula of the old world monkey. III: Efferent cortical output and comments on function. J Comp Neurol 1982;212:38–52.

Noble R, Riddell JS: Cutaneous excitatory and inhibitory input to neurones of the postsynaptic dorsal column system in the cat. J Physiol 1988;396:497–513.

Rosas-Arellano MP, Solano-Flores LP, Ciriello J: c-Fos induction in spinal cord neurons after renal arterial or venous occlusion. Am J Physiol 1999;276:R120–127.

Talbot JD, Marrett S, Evans AC, et al: Multiple representations of pain in human cerebral cortex. Science 1991;251:1355–1358.

Treede RD, Apkarian AV, Bromm B, Greenspan JD, Lenz FA: Cortical representation of pain: Functional characterization of nociceptive areas near the lateral sulcus. Pain 2000;87:113–119.

Willis WD, Al-Chaer ED, Quast MJ, Westlund KN: A visceral pain pathway in the dorsal column of the spinal cord. Proc Natl Acad Sci USA 1999;96:7675–7679.

Willis WD, Kenshalo DR Jr., Leonard RB: The cells of origin of the primate spinothalamic tract. J Comp Neurol 1979;188:543–574.

6

Cranial Nerves and the Trigeminal and Viscerosensory Systems

IN NEUROANATOMY, *THE STUDY OF SENSATION* and motor control of cranial structures has traditionally been separate from that of the limbs and trunk. This is because cranial nerves innervate the head, and spinal nerves innervate the limbs and trunk. We can see similarities, however, in the functional organization of the cranial and spinal nerves and of the parts of the central nervous system with which they directly connect. For example, sensory axons in cranial nerves synapse in sensory cranial nerve nuclei. Similarly, sensory axons in spinal nerves synapse on neurons of the dorsal horn of the spinal cord and the dorsal column nuclei. The motor cranial nerve nuclei, like the motor nuclei of the ventral horn, contain the motor neurons whose axons project to the periphery.

This chapter examines the general organization of the cranial nerves and the columnar organization of the cranial nerve nuclei, topics introduced in Chapter 3. Knowledge of the columnar organization helps explain the functional organization of the cranial nerves and nuclei because the location of the column provides important information about function. The chapter then examines the trigeminal system, which mediates somatic sensation from the face and head. This system is analogous to the dorsal column–medial lemniscal and anterolateral systems of the spinal cord (see Chapter 5). The chapter also considers the brain stem neural system that processes sensory information from the body's internal organs. This system is closely aligned with the trigeminal system.

■ CRANIAL NERVES AND NUCLEI

Among the 12 pairs of cranial nerves (Figure 6–1 and Table 6–1), the first two—olfactory (I) and optic (II)—are purely sensory. The olfactory nerve, which mediates

135

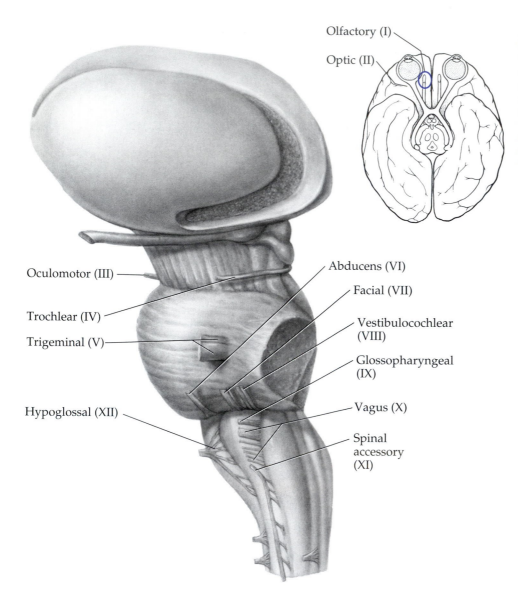

Olfactory (I)

Optic (II)

Oculomotor (III)

Trochlear (IV)

Trigeminal (V)

Hypoglossal (XII)

Abducens (VI)

Facial (VII)

Vestibulocochlear (VIII)

Glossopharyngeal (IX)

Vagus (X)

Spinal accessory (XI)

Figure 6–1. Lateral view of the brain stem, showing the locations of the cranial nerves that enter and exit the brain stem and diencephalon. The inset shows that the olfactory (I) nerve enters the olfactory bulb, which is part of the telencephalon, and that the optic (II) nerve enters the diencephalon via the optic tract.

the sense of smell, directly enters the **telencephalon,** and the optic nerve, for vision, enters the **diencephalon.** The other 10 cranial nerves enter and leave the **brain stem.** The oculomotor (III) and trochlear (IV) nerves, which are motor nerves, exit from the midbrain. They innervate muscles that move the eyes. The trochlear nerve is further distinguished as the only cranial nerve found on the dorsal brain stem surface.

The pons contains four cranial nerves. The trigeminal (V) nerve is located at the middle of the pons. It is termed a **mixed nerve** because it has both sensory and motor functions and it consists of separate sensory and motor roots. This separation is reminiscent of the segregation of function in the dorsal and ventral

spinal roots. The sensory root provides the somatic sensory innervation of the facial skin and mucous membranes of parts of the oral and nasal cavities and the teeth. The motor root contains axons that innervate jaw muscles.

The remaining pontine nerves are found at the pontomedullary junction. The abducens (VI) nerve is a motor nerve that, like the oculomotor and trochlear nerves, innervates eye muscles. The facial (VII) nerve is a mixed nerve and has separate sensory and motor roots. The motor root innervates the facial muscles that determine our expressions, whereas the sensory root primarily innervates taste buds and mediates taste. The facial sensory root is sometimes called the intermediate nerve. (The intermediate nerve also contains axons that innervate various cranial autonomic ganglia [Chapter 11].) The vestibulocochlear (VIII) nerve is a sensory nerve and has two separate components. The vestibular component innervates the semi-circular canals, saccule, and utricle and mediates balance, whereas the cochlear component innervates the organ of Corti and serves hearing.

The medulla has four cranial nerves, each of which contain numerous roots that leave from different rostrocaudal locations. Although the glossopharyngeal (IX) nerve is a mixed nerve, its major function is to provide the sensory innervation of the pharynx and to innervate taste buds of the posterior one third of the tongue. The motor function of the glossopharyngeal nerve is to innervate a single pharyngeal muscle and peripheral autonomic ganglion (see Table 6–1). The vagus (X) nerve, a mixed nerve, has myriad sensory and motor functions that include somatic and visceral sensation, innervation of pharyngeal muscles, and much of the visceral autonomic innervation. The spinal accessory (XI) and hypoglossal (XII) nerves subserve motor function, innervating neck and tongue muscles, respectively (see Table 6–1).

Important Differences Exist Between the Sensory and Motor Innervation of Cranial Structures and That of the Limbs and Trunk

The peripheral organization of sensory (afferent) fibers in cranial nerves is similar to that of spinal nerves. The organization of the primary sensory neurons that innervate the skin and mucous membranes of the head—mediating the somatic senses—is virtually identical to that of the sensory innervation of the limbs and trunk (Figure 6–2). In both cases the distal portion of the axon of **pseudounipolar** primary sensory neurons is sensitive to stimulus energy, and the cell bodies of these primary sensory neurons are located in **peripheral ganglia**. The proximal portion of the axon projects into the central nervous system to synapse on neurons in the medulla and pons. The peripheral sensory ganglia, which contain the cell bodies of the primary sensory neurons of the different cranial nerves, are listed in Table 6–1.

Despite these similarities, three important differences are evident in the anatomical organization of primary sensory neurons in spinal and cranial nerves:

1. For the senses of taste, vision, hearing, and balance, a separate **receptor cell** transduces stimulus energy (Figure 6–2). The receptor activates synaptically the primary sensory neuron, which transmits information—encoded in the form of

action potentials—to the central nervous system. For the spinal and trigeminal somatic sensations, the distal ending of the primary sensory neuron is the sensory receptor. Thus, the primary sensory neuron mediates both stimulus transduction and information transmission.

2. Primary sensory neurons in cranial nerves have either a **pseudounipolar** or a **bipolar morphology** (Figure 6–2). (As is discussed in Chapter 7, a retinal projection neuron is analogous to the primary sensory neurons because it transmits sensory information to the thalamus.)

3. Stretch receptors in jaw muscles, which signal jaw muscle length and thus mediate **jaw proprioception** (or temporal-mandibular joint angle detection), are pseudounipolar primary sensory neurons, but their cell bodies are located within the central nervous system, not in peripheral ganglia. These neurons derive from neural crest cells that do not migrate from the central nervous system to the periphery (see Figure 3–1).

The structures innervated by the motor fibers of cranial nerves, similar to motor fibers in spinal nerves, include striated muscle and autonomic postganglionic neurons. In contrast to striated muscle of the limbs and trunk, which develop from body somites, cranial striated muscle develops from either the cranial **somites** or the **branchial arches**. The extraocular and tongue muscles originate from somites, whereas jaw, facial, laryngeal, palatal, and certain neck muscles are of branchiomeric origin.

There Are Seven Functional Categories of Cranial Nerves

Seven functional categories of cranial nerve enter and exit the brain stem. Four of these categories are similar to those of the spinal nerves (see Table 3–1):

1. **Somatic sensory fibers** subserve touch, pain, itch, and temperature senses and jaw (and limb) proprioception.

2. **Viscerosensory fibers** mediate visceral sensations and chemoreception from body organs and help regulate blood pressure and other bodily functions.

3. **Somatic skeletal motor fibers** are the axons of motor neurons that innervate striated muscle that develops from the somites.

4. **Visceral (autonomic) motor fibers** are the axons of autonomic preganglionic neurons.

Table 6–1. The cranial nerves.

Cranial nerve and root		Function	Cranial formaina	Peripheral sensory ganglia
I	Olfactory	Smell	Cribriform plate	
II	Optic	Vision	Optic	
III	Oculomotor	Somatic skeletal motor	Superior orbital fissure	
		Autonomic		
IV	Trochlear	Somatic skeletal motor	Superior orbital fissure	
V	Trigeminal	Somatic sensory	Superior orbital fissure (Ophthalmic)	Semilunar
			Rotundum (Maxillary)	
		Branchiomeric motor	Ovale (Mandibular)	
VI	Abducens	Somatic skeletal motor	Superior orbital fissure	
VII	Intermediate	Taste	Internal auditory meatus	Geniculate
		Somatic sensory		Geniculate
		Autonomic		
	Facial	Branchiomeric motor	Internal auditory meatus	
VIII	Vestibulocochlear	Hearing	Internal auditory meatus	Spiral
		Balance		Vestibular
IX	Glossopharyngeal	Somatic sensory	Jugular	Superior
		Viscerosensory		Petrosal (inferior)
		Taste		Petrosal
		Autonomic		
		Branchiomeric motor		
X	Vagus	Somatic sensory	Jugular	Jugular (superior)
		Viscerosensory		Nodose (inferior)
		Taste		Nodose (inferior)
		Autonomic		
		Branchiomeric motor		
XI	Spinal accessory	Branchiomeric motor	Jugular	
		Unclassified[1]	Jugular	
XII	Hypoglossal	Somatic skeletal motor	Hypoglossal	

Abbreviation key: CN, cranial nerve.

[1]The accessory nucleus is unclassified because some of the muscles (or compartments of muscles) innervated by this nucleus develop from the occipital somites.

Because cranial nerves are more complex than spinal nerves, innervating highly specialized sensory organs or branchiomeric muscles, there are three additional categories of cranial nerves:

5. Fibers that innervate the retina subserve **vision,** and those that innervate the inner ear mediate **hearing** and **balance.**
6. Fibers that innervate taste buds and the olfactory mucosa mediate **taste** and **smell,** respectively.
7. **Branchiomeric skeletal motor fibers** are the axons of motor neurons that innervate stri-

ated muscle that develops from the branchial arches.

Cranial nerves have historically been classified according to an arcane abbreviated scheme rather than according to their functions. This scheme distinguishes cranial nerves (and their corresponding central nuclei) on the basis of whether the individual component axons provide the **sensory** (afferent) or **motor** (efferent) innervation of the head, whether the innervated structures develop from the **somites** (and therefore are somatic structures) or the **branchial arches** (which are

CNS nucleus	Peripheral autonomic ganglia	Peripheral structure innervated
Olfactory bulb		Olfactory receptors of olfactory epithelium
Lateral geniculate nucleus		Retina (ganglion cells)
Oculomotor		Medial, superior, inferior, rectus, inferior oblique, and levator palpebrae muscles
Edinger-Westphal	Ciliary	Constrictor muscles of iris, ciliary muscle
Trochlear		Superior oblique muscle
Spinal nucleus, main sensory nucleus, mesencephalio nucleus of CN V		Skin and mucous membranes of the head, muscle receptors, meninges
Motor nucleus of CN V		Jaw muscles, tensor tympani, tensor palati, and digastric (anterior belly)
Abducens		Lateral rectus muscle
Solitary nucleus		Taste (anterior two thirds of tongue), palate
Spinal nucleus of CN V		Skin of external ear
Superior salivatory	Pterygopalatine, submandibular	Lacrimal glands, glands of nasal mucosa, salivary glands
Facial		Muscles of facial expression, digastric (posterior belly), and stapedius
Cochlear		Hair cells in organ of Corti
Vestibular		Hair cells in vestibular labyrinth
Spinal nucleus of CN V		Skin of external ear
Solitary nucleus (caudal)		Mucous membranes in pharyngeal region, middle ear, carotid body, and sinus
Solitary nucleus (rostral)		Taste (posterior one third of tongue)
Inferior salivatory nucleus	Otic	Parotid gland
Ambiguus (rostral)		Striated muscle of pharynx
Spinal nucleus of CN V		Skin of external ear, meninges
Solitary nucleus (caudal)		Larynx, trachea, gut, aortic arch receptors
Solitary nucleus (rostral)		Taste buds (posterior oral cavity, larynx)
Dorsal motor nucleus of CN X	Peripheral autonomic	Gut (to splenic flexure of colon), respiratory structures, heart
Ambiguus (middle region)		Striated muscles of palate, pharynx, and larynx
Ambiguus (caudal)		Striated muscles of larynx [Aberrant vague branches] sternocleidomastoid and portion of trapezius muscles
Accesory nucleus, pyramidal decussation to C3–C5		
Hypoglossal		Intrinsic muscles of tongue, hyoglossus, genioglossus, and styloglossus muscles

visceral), and whether the structure innervated has **simple** (general) or **complex** (special) morphology:

- Somatic sensory innervation, as described in Chapter 5, corresponds to general somatic sensory, or GSS.
- Viscerosensory innervation corresponds to general visceral sensory, or GVS.
- Somatic motor innervation, such as the innervation of limb muscles, corresponds to general somatic motor, or GSM.
- Visceral motor, or autonomic, innervation corresponds to general visceral motor, or GVM.

- Vision and hearing corresponds to special somatic sensory, or SSS.
- Taste and smell corresponds to special visceral sensory, or SVS.
- Innervation of branchiomeric muscles corresponds to special visceral motor, or SVM.

The abbreviated nomenclature is fraught with problems and is not intuitive. For example, special visceral motor (or SVM) nerve fibers innervate striated muscles that function just like muscles innervated by the general somatic motor, or GSM, fibers. Vision is described as a special somatic sensory (SSS) modality

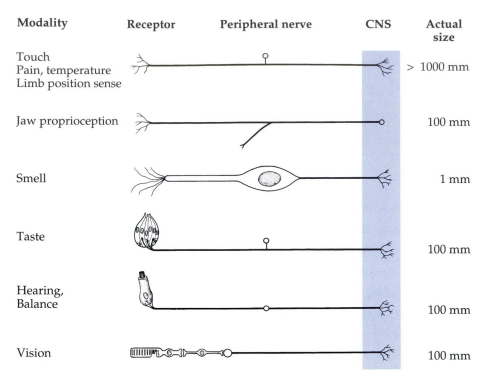

Modality	Receptor	Peripheral nerve	CNS	Actual size
Touch Pain, temperature Limb position sense				> 1000 mm
Jaw proprioception				100 mm
Smell				1 mm
Taste				100 mm
Hearing, Balance				100 mm
Vision				100 mm

Figure 6–2. Schematic illustration of morphology of primary sensory neurons, the location of cell bodies, and the approximate differences in actual sizes. Whereas primary afferent fibers in the spinal cord have a pseudounipolar morphology, in cranial nerves they have either a pseudounipolar or a bipolar morphology. The primary sensory neuron for jaw proprioception is further distinguished because its cell body is located in the central nervous system. For hearing, balance, and taste, separate receptor cells transduce stimulus information, and primary afferent fiber transmits the resulting signals to the central nervous system. The sensory neurons for hearing, balance, and smell are bipolar. For touch, pain, and temperature senses; jaw proprioception; and taste, the primary sensory neurons are pseudounipolar. For vision the retina develops from the central nervous system; thus, none of the neural elements are in the periphery.

and smell, a visceral modality (SVS), but they have little to do with somatic or visceral functions. Because of these inconsistencies and the counterintuitive nature of this system, the cranial nerves and their central nuclei are characterized here on the basis of their functions (see Table 6–1).

Cranial Nerve Nuclei Are Organized Into Rostrocaudal Columns

The primary sensory neurons in cranial nerves that enter the brain stem synapse in **sensory cranial nerve nuclei;** the cell bodies of motor axons in cranial nerves are located in **motor cranial nerve nuclei.** This arrangement is similar to the dorsal roots, which synapse in the dorsal horn and dorsal column nuclei, and the skeletal motor axons of the ventral roots, whose cell bodies are found in the spinal motor nuclei. Each cranial nerve nucleus subserves a single sensory or motor function. This is in contrast to many of the cranial nerves themselves, which contain a mixture of axons that have different functions (see Table 6–1).

Because there are seven functional categories of cranial nerves, there are also seven categories of cranial nerve nuclei. Nuclei of each of these categories form discontinuous columns that extend rostrocaudally through the brain stem (Figures 6–3 and 6–4). The

seven functional categories are distributed through only six discrete columns, however, because two of the sensory categories synapse on neurons in a single column but at separate rostrocaudal locations (see next section).

As discussed in Chapter 3, a systematic relationship exists between the function of each column and its location with respect to the midline (Figures 6–3 and 6–4): The motor columns are located medial to the sensory columns. In the pons and medulla, nuclei on the ventricular floor are separated by the **sulcus limitans.** In the embryonic brain and spinal cord the sulcus limitans separates the developing alar and basal plates (see Chapter 3). The rest of this chapter examines the trigeminal somatic sensory and viscerosensory systems.

■ FUNCTIONAL ANATOMY OF THE TRIGEMINAL AND VISCEROSENSORY SYSTEMS

Somatic sensation of the head, including the oral cavity, is carried by four cranial nerves. The **trigeminal nerve** innervates most of the head and oral cavity and is the most important of the four nerves. The **facial, glossopharyngeal,** and **vagus** nerves innervate small areas of the skin around the external ear and the

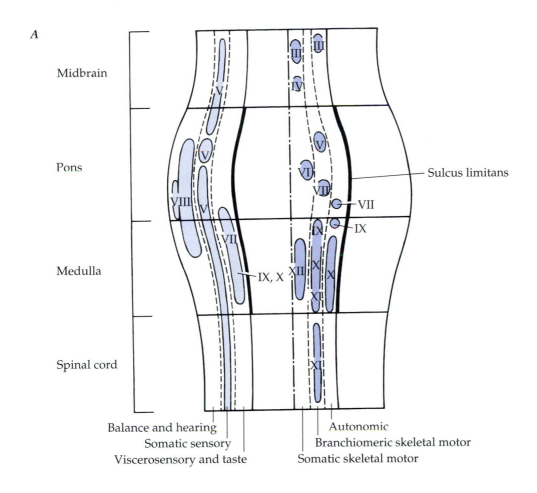

A

Midbrain

Pons

— Sulcus limitans

VII

IX

Medulla

Spinal cord

Balance and hearing
Somatic sensory
Viscerosensory and taste

Autonomic
Branchiomeric skeletal motor
Somatic skeletal motor

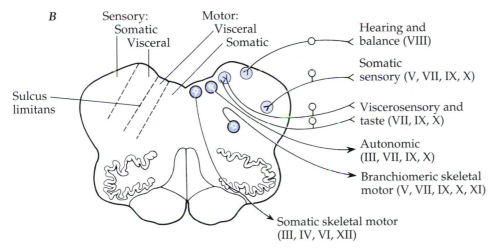

B

Sensory:
Somatic
Visceral

Motor:
Visceral
Somatic

Sulcus
limitans

Hearing and
balance (VIII)

Somatic
sensory (V, VII, IX, X)

Viscerosensory and
taste (VII, IX, X)

Autonomic
(III, VII, IX, X)

Branchiomeric skeletal
motor (V, VII, IX, X, XI)

Somatic skeletal motor
(III, IV, VI, XII)

Figure 6–3. *A.* Schematic dorsal view of brain stem, showing that the cranial nerve nuclei are organized into discontinuous columns. The sulcus limitans separates the afferent and motor nuclei. *B.* Schematic cross section through the medulla, showing the locations of cranial nerve nuclear columns. (*A adapted from Nieuwenhuys R, et al: The Human Central Nervous System: A Synopsis and Atlas, 3rd ed. Springer-Verlag, 1988.*)

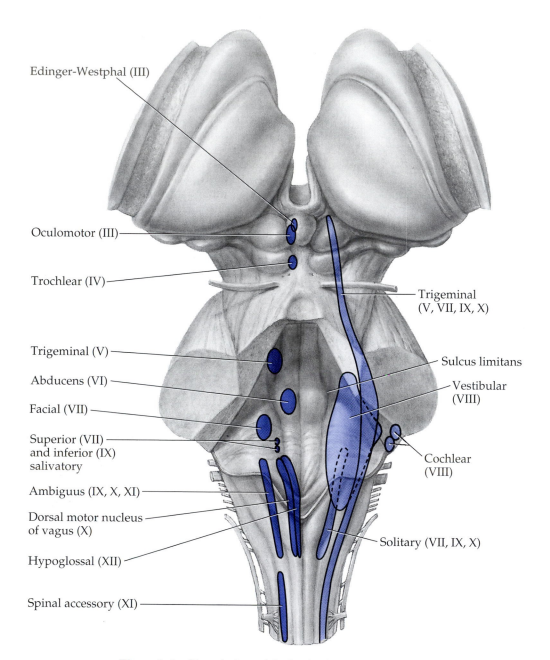

Edinger-Westphal (III)

Oculomotor (III)

Trochlear (IV)

Trigeminal (V)

Abducens (VI)

Facial (VII)

Superior (VII) and inferior (IX) salivatory

Ambiguus (IX, X, XI)

Dorsal motor nucleus of vagus (X)

Hypoglossal (XII)

Spinal accessory (XI)

Trigeminal (V, VII, IX, X)

Sulcus limitans

Vestibular (VIII)

Cochlear (VIII)

Solitary (VII, IX, X)

Figure 6–4. Dorsal view of the brain stem, indicating the locations of cranial nerve nuclei.

mucous membranes and organs of the body. The facial, glossopharyngeal, and vagus nerves also contain sensory fibers that mediate taste (see Chapter 9).

The sensory fibers that innervate surface skin and oral mucosa project into central **trigeminal nuclei,** whereas the sensory fibers that innervate the mucous membranes of the pharynx and larynx and other internal (visceral) structures project to the caudal portion of the **solitary nucleus.** An important exception exists: A small number of sensory fibers that innervate the pharyngeal and laryngeal mucosa project

information to the trigeminal nuclei. Sensory information transmitted to the trigeminal nuclei is thought to contribute to our conscious awareness of cranial sensations. By contrast, information transmitted to the caudal solitary nucleus may not necessarily reach consciousness. Although we become aware of visceral pain, we become conscious of other stimuli only under special circumstances, such as when we become nauseated after eating a certain food or when we feel full after eating a large meal. Some internal stimuli are never perceived. For example, a change in intra-arterial pressure, even a hypertensive episode, can occur unnoticed.

Separate Trigeminal Pathways Mediate Touch and Pain and Temperature Senses

Three trigeminal sensory nuclei serve cranial somatic sensations (eg, from the skin) from the nerves just described. These sensory fibers terminate in two of the trigeminal sensory nuclei, the **main** (or **principal**) **trigeminal sensory nucleus** and the **spinal trigeminal nucleus.** The third sensory nucleus, the **mesencephalic trigeminal nucleus,** is not a site of termination of primary sensory fibers. Rather, it is equivalent to a peripheral sensory ganglion because it contains the cell bodies of certain trigeminal primary sensory fibers (see below).

The sensory axons of the trigeminal nerve enter the ventral pons (Figure 6–1). Sensory axons from the facial, glossopharyngeal, and vagus nerves enter the brain stem more caudally. Just as in spinal nerves, functional differences distinguish individual sensory axons in these nerves. Large-diameter fibers, which mediate mechanical sensations, terminate mostly in the dorsal pons, in the main trigeminal sensory nucleus. Small-diameter fibers—which mediate pain, temperature sensations, and itch—mostly travel in the **spinal trigeminal tract** and terminate in the spinal trigeminal nucleus. (Some large-diameter mechanoreceptive fibers in the spinal trigeminal tract play a role in cranial reflexes; see below.) These differences set the stage for two anatomically and functionally distinct trigeminal ascending sensory systems (Figures 6–5 and 6–6). One system is for cranial touch and dental mechanical senses and is analogous to the dorsal column–medial lemniscal system. The other system is for cranial pain, temperature senses, and itch and is analogous to the anterolateral system.

The Main Trigeminal Sensory Nucleus Mediates Facial Mechanical Sensations

Most neurons in the **main trigeminal sensory nucleus** receive mechanoreceptive information. Projection neurons in this nucleus give rise to axons that decussate in the pons and ascend dorsomedially to fibers from the dorsal column nuclei in the medial lemniscus. The ascending second-order trigeminal fibers—collectively termed the **trigeminal lemniscus**—synapse in the thalamus, in its **ventral posterior medial nucleus** (Figure 6–6A). (Recall that the ventral posterior lateral nucleus is the thalamic spinal somatic sensory relay nucleus.) From here, the axons of thalamic neurons project, via the posterior limb of the internal capsule, to the lateral part of the **primary somatic sensory cortex,** in the **postcentral gyrus.** The **secondary somatic sensory cortex** and the **posterior parietal cortex** also process cranial somatic sensory information (see Chapter 5). These higher-order somatic sensory areas receive their major input from the primary somatic sensory cortex. Because of similarities in connections, the main trigeminal sensory nucleus is anatomically and functionally similar to the dorsal column nuclei (which comprise the gracile and cuneate nuclei).

A smaller pathway also originates from the dorsal portion of the main trigeminal sensory nucleus (Figure 6–6A), sometimes termed the dorsal trigeminothalamic tract. This pathway ascends ipsilaterally to the ventral posterior medial nucleus and processes mechanical stimuli from the teeth and soft tissues of the oral cavity.

The pathway for **jaw proprioception** begins with stretch receptors that encode jaw angle. The cell bodies for these mechanoreceptors are in the **trigeminal mesencephalic nucleus,** and the receptors project to the main trigeminal sensory nucleus and to more rostral portions of the spinal trigeminal nucleus. The projection to the spinal nucleus may be analogous to the small projection of mechanoreceptors to the deep layers of the dorsal horn (see next section). The trigeminal brain stem neurons project to the **ventral posterior medial nucleus** and then to area 3a of the primary somatic sensory cortex. This is the pathway for conscious awareness of temporal-mandibular joint angle. Jaw proprioceptive information also is transmitted to the cerebellum for jaw muscle control (see Chapter 13).

The Spinal Trigeminal Nucleus Mediates Cranial Pain Sensation

The spinal trigeminal nucleus has a rostrocaudal anatomical and functional organization with three components (Figures 6–5 and 6–6B): the **oral nucleus,** the **interpolar nucleus,** and the **caudal nucleus.** The functions of the spinal trigeminal nucleus are similar to those of the dorsal horn of the spinal cord, with which it is continuous. Similar to the dorsal horn, the spinal trigeminal nucleus plays an essential role in facial and dental pain, temperature sensation, and itch and a much lesser role in facial mechanical sensations. In addition, the interpolar and oral nuclei are involved in organizing **trigeminal reflexes** and transmitting sensory information to motor control structures such as the cerebellum and, as described above, also function in jaw proprioception.

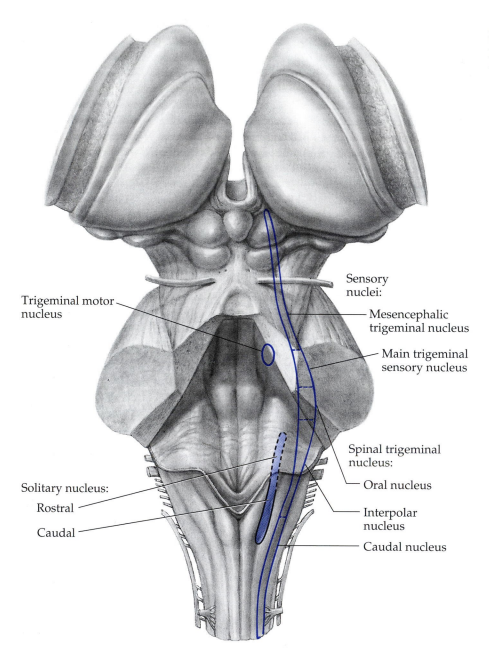

Trigeminal motor nucleus

Solitary nucleus:

Rostral

Caudal

Sensory nuclei:

Mesencephalic trigeminal nucleus

Main trigeminal sensory nucleus

Spinal trigeminal nucleus:

Oral nucleus

Interpolar nucleus

Caudal nucleus

The major ascending trigeminal pathway from the spinal trigeminal nucleus terminates in the contralateral thalamus (Figure 6–6B). The organization of this path, termed the **trigeminothalamic tract,** is similar to that of the **spinothalamic tract,** and it also ascends along with fibers of the **anterolateral system.** Trigeminothalamic axons terminate in three principal locations in the thalamus: the ventral posterior medial nucleus, the ventromedial posterior nucleus, and the medial dorsal nucleus. As discussed in Chapter 5, these thalamic sites have different cortical projections and mediate different aspects of pain and temperature

senses. The **ventral posterior medial nucleus** projects to the primary somatic sensory cortex in the lateral part of the postcentral gyrus, and the **ventromedial posterior nucleus** projects to the insular cortex. These projections, especially from the ventromedial posterior nucleus to the insular cortex, are important in perception of pain, temperature, and itch. The **medial dorsal nucleus** projects to the anterior cingulate gyrus. Both the insular cortex and the anterior cingulate gyrus are thought to participate in the affective and motivational aspects of facial pain, itch, and temperature senses.

The Viscerosensory System Originates from the Caudal Solitary Nucleus

The central branches of glossopharyngeal and vagal axons innervate the pharynx; the larynx; the esophagus; other portions of thoracic and abdominal viscera; and peripheral blood pressure receptive organs. After entering the brain stem the axons collect into the **solitary tract** of the dorsal medulla and terminate in the surrounding **caudal solitary nucleus.** The solitary nucleus is divided into two functionally distinct parts (Figure 6–5): a rostral portion for taste (considered in Chapter 9) and a caudal portion that serves **viscerosensory functions.** The caudal solitary nucleus projects information to various brain structures for a diversity of functions. For conscious awareness of viscerosensory information, such as a sense of fullness or nausea, there is an ascending projection (Figure 6–7), via the parabrachial nucleus of the pons, to the ventral posterior medial nucleus of the thalamus. The viscerosensory thalamic neurons, which are distinct from the ones that process mechanical information, project to the **insular cortex.** Other projections of the caudal solitary and parabrachial nuclei participate in a variety of visceral reflex and autonomic functions (see Chapter 15), such as regulation of blood pressure or gastrointestinal motility.

■ REGIONAL ANATOMY OF THE TRIGEMINAL AND VISCEROSENSORY SYSTEMS

Separate Sensory Roots Innervate Different Parts of the Face and Mucous Membranes of the Head

The trigeminal nerve consists of three sensory roots that innervate the skin and mucous membranes of separate regions of the head: the **ophthalmic division,** the **maxillary division,** and the **mandibular division** (Figure 6–8A). The maxillary and mandibular divisions also innervate the oral cavity. As in the spinal somatic sensory systems, the cell bodies of the trigeminal sensory fibers that mediate cranial touch, pain, temperature, and itch are found in the **semilunar ganglion,** a peripheral sensory ganglion (see Table 6–1). By contrast, the cell bodies of stretch receptors found in jaw muscles are located in the central nervous system, in the **mesencephalic trigeminal nucleus** (Figure 6–5). The trigeminal nerve also innervates stretch receptors in the extraocular muscles, but the cell bodies of these fibers are located in the semilunar ganglion, and their axons course within the ophthalmic division of the trigeminal nerve.

Unlike dorsal roots of adjacent spinal cord segments, where the dermatomes overlap extensively, the trigeminal dermatomes (ie, the area of skin innervated by a single trigeminal sensory nerve division) overlap very little. Thus, a peripheral anesthetic region is more likely to occur after damage to one trigeminal division than after damage to a single dorsal root. Trigeminal neuralgia is an extraordinarily painful neurological condition, often described as a fiery pain that radiates near the border of the ophthalmic and maxillary roots or at the border of the maxillary and mandibular roots.

In addition to the trigeminal nerve, the **intermediate** (a branch of the **facial** nerve), **glossopharyngeal,** and **vagus** nerves innervate portions of the skin of the head. The external ear is innervated by the intermediate and glossopharyngeal nerves, and the external auditory meatus is innervated by the intermediate and vagus nerves (Figure 6–8A). Both the trigeminal and vagus nerves innervate the dura. The cell bodies of the sensory fibers in the facial nerve are located in the **geniculate ganglion,** and those of the glossopharyngeal and vagus nerves are located in the **superior ganglion** of each nerve (see Table 6–1 for nomenclature).

Although the glossopharyngeal and vagus nerves innervate small patches of surface skin, they have a more extensive innervation of the mucous membranes and body organs. The glossopharyngeal nerve innervates the posterior one third of the tongue, the pharynx, portions of the nasal cavity and sinuses, and the eustachian tube. The vagus nerve innervates the hypopharynx, the larynx, the esophagus, and the thoracic and abdominal viscera. The innervation of the pharynx and larynx by the glossopharyngeal and vagus nerves is essential for normal swallowing and for keeping the airway clear of saliva and other liquids during swallowing (see Chapter 11). Branches of the glossopharyngeal and vagus nerves also innervate arterial blood pressure receptors in the **carotid sinus** and **aortic arch,** respectively. These branches are part of the baroreceptor reflex, for blood pressure regulation. For example, they mediate the pressor response to standing. The vagus nerve alone also innervates respiratory structures and the portion of the gut rostral to the splenic flexure. Pelvic visceral organs are innervated by primary sensory fibers that project to the sacral spinal cord. The spinal pathways for pelvic visceral sensation are not well understood but are thought to parallel the organization of the spinal somatic sensory pathways.

After entering the pons the fibers of each nerve division travel into discrete portions of the spinal trigeminal and solitary tracts en route to the trigeminal and solitary nuclei, where they terminate. The

Figure 6–6. General organization of the ascending trigeminal pathways for touch (*A*) and pain and temperature (*B*) senses.

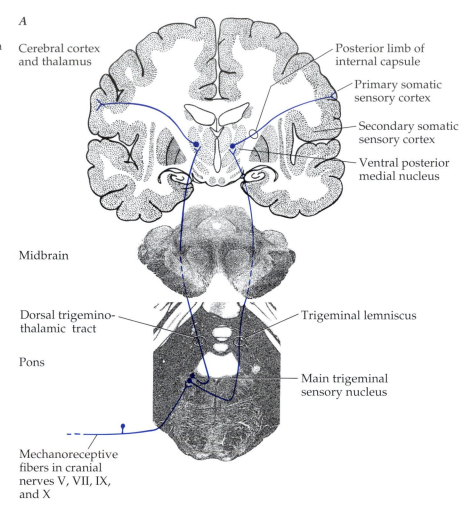

A

Cerebral cortex and thalamus

Posterior limb of internal capsule

Primary somatic sensory cortex

Secondary somatic sensory cortex

Ventral posterior medial nucleus

Midbrain

Dorsal trigemino-thalamic tract

Trigeminal lemniscus

Pons

Main trigeminal sensory nucleus

Mechanoreceptive fibers in cranial nerves V, VII, IX, and X

spinal trigeminal tract (Figure 6–8B) is organized like an inverted face: the roots of the intermediate, glossopharyngeal, and vagus nerves as well as the mandibular division of the trigeminal nerve are located dorsal; the ophthalmic division of the trigeminal nerve is located ventral; and the maxillary division of the trigeminal nerve is in between. Axons in the spinal trigeminal tract, in turn, synapse on neurons in the spinal trigeminal nucleus (Figure 6–8B). The solitary tract is more rostral.

The Key Components of the Trigeminal System Are Present at All Levels of the Brain Stem

The three trigeminal nuclei have distinct sensory functions. The **spinal trigeminal nucleus** is important in facial pain, temperature senses, and itch and is located principally in the medulla and the caudal pons. The **main trigeminal sensory nucleus** mediates

facial touch sense and oral mechanosensation and is located in the pons. The **mesencephalic trigeminal nucleus** contains the cell bodies of stretch receptors that signal jaw muscle length, which is used by the brain for jaw proprioception, and is located in the rostral pons and midbrain.

The Spinal Trigeminal Nucleus Is the Rostral Extension of the Spinal Cord Dorsal Horn

The dorsal horn extends rostrally into the medulla as the spinal trigeminal nucleus. Three nuclear subdivisions comprise the spinal trigeminal nucleus, from caudal to rostral: the caudal nucleus, the interpolar nucleus, and the oral nucleus. The **caudal nucleus** and the dorsal horn of the spinal cord have three key similarities: (1) general morphology and lamination, (2) laminar distribution of sensory fiber terminals, and (3) laminar distribution of projection neurons. In fact,

B

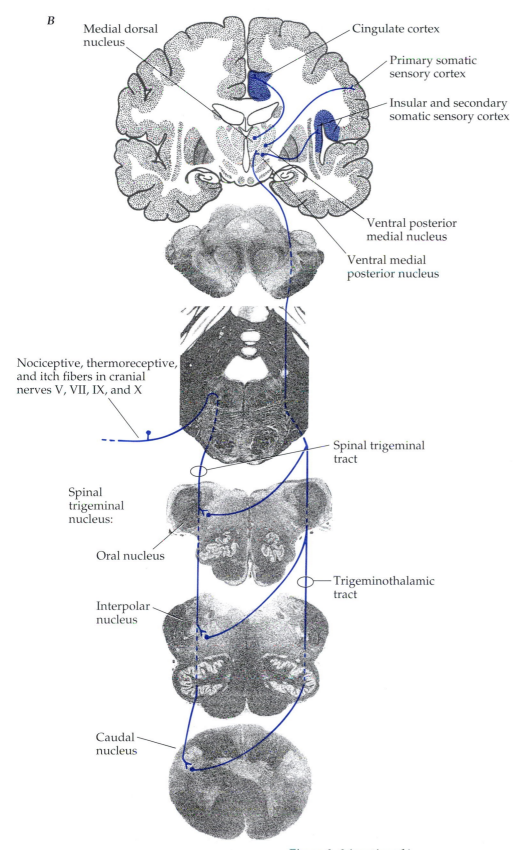

Medial dorsal nucleus

Cingulate cortex

Primary somatic sensory cortex

Insular and secondary somatic sensory cortex

Ventral posterior medial nucleus

Ventral medial posterior nucleus

Nociceptive, thermoreceptive, and itch fibers in cranial nerves V, VII, IX, and X

Spinal trigeminal tract

Spinal trigeminal nucleus:

Oral nucleus

Trigeminothalamic tract

Interpolar nucleus

Caudal nucleus

Figure 6–6 (continued.)

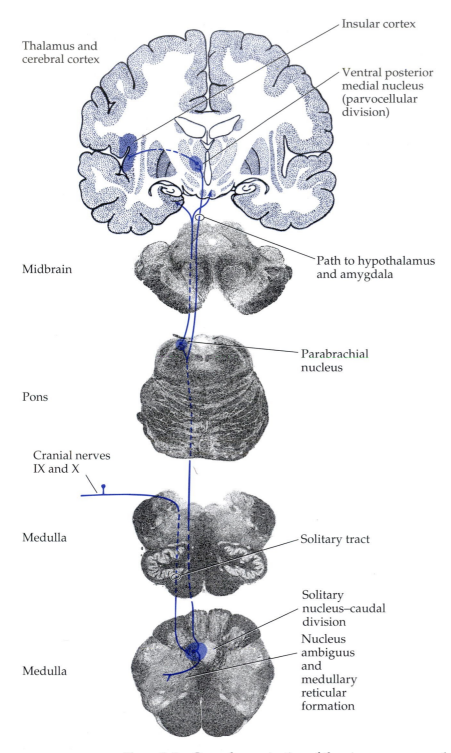

Thalamus and
cerebral cortex

Insular cortex

Ventral posterior
medial nucleus
(parvocellular
division)

Midbrain

Path to hypothalamus
and amygdala

Pons

Parabrachial
nucleus

Cranial nerves
IX and X

Medulla

Solitary tract

Solitary
nucleus–caudal
division

Nucleus
ambiguus
and
medullary
reticular
formation

Medulla

Figure 6–7. General organization of the viscerosensory pathway. Note that neurons in the caudal solitary nucleus contribute to this pathway. Neurons in the rostral solitary nucleus are important in taste (see Chapter 9).

the caudal nucleus is sometimes called the **medullary dorsal horn** because its organization is so similar to that of the spinal cord dorsal horn.

Comparison of sections of the spinal cord and the caudal medulla indicates that the dorsal horn and caudal nucleus have similar morphology and lamination (Figure 6–9):

- **Lamina I,** the outermost, is equivalent to the **marginal zone** of the dorsal horn.

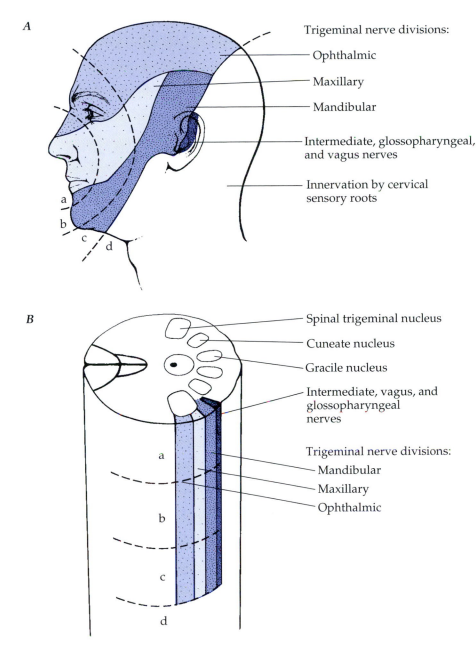

A

Trigeminal nerve divisions:

— Ophthalmic

— Maxillary

— Mandibular

— Intermediate, glossopharyngeal, and vagus nerves

— Innervation by cervical sensory roots

a

b

c / d

B

— Spinal trigeminal nucleus

— Cuneate nucleus

— Gracile nucleus

— Intermediate, vagus, and glossopharyngeal nerves

Trigeminal nerve divisions:

— Mandibular

— Maxillary

— Ophthalmic

a

b

c

d

Figure 6–8. Somatotopic organization of the trigeminal system. *A.* Peripheral innervation territories of the three divisions of the trigeminal nerve and the intermediate and vagus nerves. *B.* The organization of the spinal trigeminal tract for the portion of the medulla that includes the caudal nucleus. The "onion skin" pattern of representation of trigeminal afferents in the caudal nucleus corresponds to **a, b,** and **c; d** corresponds to the rostral spinal cord representation. Regions marked **a** (located rostrally), **b,** and **c** (located caudally) correspond to the concentric zones on the face indicated in *A.* The intraoral representation is located rostral to region **a** in *B;* cervical representation is located caudally (ie, region **d**). *(Adapted from Brodal A: Neurological Anatomy. Oxford University Press, 1981.)*

- **Lamina II** is equivalent to the **substantia gelatinosa.**
- **Laminae III** and **IV** are termed the **magnocellular nucleus** in the trigeminal system and are equivalent to the **nucleus proprius** of the spinal cord.
- **Laminae V** and **VI** (base of dorsal horn) of the spinal cord extend rostrally into the base of the caudal nucleus.

As the nuclear components of the dorsal horn have counterparts in the trigeminal system, so too does the spinal sensory tract. Lissauer's tract extends into the medulla as the **spinal trigeminal tract.** Both Lissauer's tract and the spinal trigeminal tract are lightly stained (Figure 6–9) because they contain thinly myelinated and unmyelinated axons.

An analogy can be made between the organization of other portions of the spinal cord and that of the caudal medulla. Lamina VII of the spinal cord, sometimes termed the intermediate zone, is continuous with the **reticular formation.** Finally, the ventral horn extends rostrally into the medulla to form the cranial nerve motor nuclei.

Important insights into the functions of the spinal trigeminal nucleus and tract have been gained from a neurosurgical procedure to relieve intractable facial pain. This operation transects the spinal trigeminal tract and produces selective disruption of such pain and temperature senses with little effect on touch.

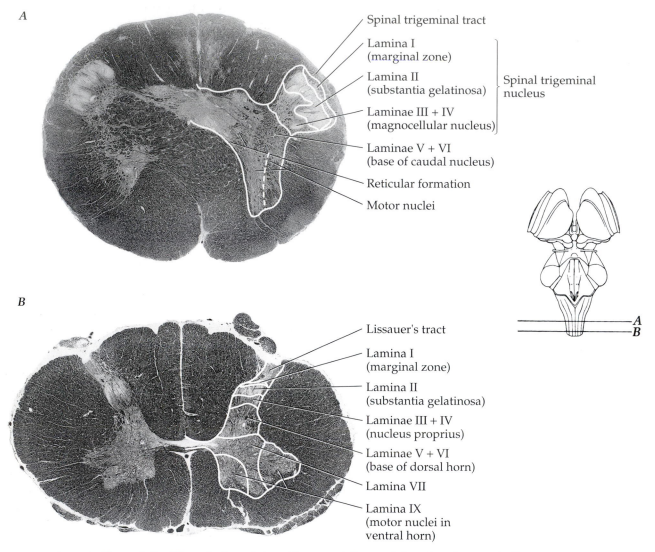

A

Spinal trigeminal tract

Lamina I
(marginal zone)

Lamina II
(substantia gelatinosa)

} Spinal trigeminal
nucleus

Laminae III + IV
(magnocellular nucleus)

Laminae V + VI
(base of caudal nucleus)

Reticular formation

Motor nuclei

B

Lissauer's tract

Lamina I
(marginal zone)

Lamina II
(substantia gelatinosa)

Laminae III + IV
(nucleus proprius)

Laminae V + VI
(base of dorsal horn)

Lamina VII

Lamina IX
(motor nuclei in
ventral horn)

Figure 6–9. The spinal cord dorsal horn and the caudal nucleus have a similar organization. Myelin-stained transverse sections through the caudal nucleus—at the level of pyramidal decussation (*A*)—and the cervical spinal cord (*B*). The inset shows the approximate planes of section.

(Spinal trigeminal tractotomy is rarely done today, however, because analgesic drugs have proved a more effective therapy.) If the tract is transected rostrally, near the border between the caudal and interpolar nuclei, facial pain and temperature senses over the entire face are disrupted. Transection of the tract between its rostral and caudal borders spares pain and temperature senses over the perioral region and nose.

This clinical finding shows that the spinal trigeminal tract has a rostrocaudal somatotopic organization in addition to a mediolateral organization (Figure 6–8B). Trigeminal fibers that innervate the portion of the head adjacent to the cervical spinal cord representation (Figure 6–8A) project more caudally in the spinal trigeminal tract and terminate in more caudal

regions of the caudal nucleus than those that innervate the oral cavity, perioral face, and nose.

Proceeding rostrally from the cervical spinal cord, neurons of the spinal dorsal horn process somatic sensory information (predominantly pain, itch, and temperature senses) from the arm, neck, and occiput (ie, region d in Figure 6–8B). Neurons of the trigeminal caudal nucleus, located near the spinal cord–medulla border, process somatic sensory information from the posterior face and ear (ie, regions b and c in Figure 6–8B). These neurons receive input not only from the mandibular trigeminal division but also from the intermediate, glossopharyngeal, and vagus nerves. Farther rostrally, the neurons process information from the perioral region and nose (ie, region a in Figure 6–8B). Finally, neurons in the most rostral part of the trigeminal caudal nucleus, as well as farther rostrally in the trigeminal spinal nucleus (not shown in Figure 6–8B), process pain and temperature information from the oral cavity, particularly from the **teeth.** This organization is termed "onion skin" because of the concentric ring configuration of the peripheral fields processed at a given level by the medullary dorsal horn.

A second similarity exists between the spinal dorsal horn and the caudal nucleus. As in the dorsal horn of the spinal cord (see Figure 5–6), sensory fibers of different diameters terminate in different laminae of the caudal nucleus. Small-diameter trigeminal sensory fibers mediating pain, itch, and temperature senses terminate primarily in laminae 1 and 2 (the marginal zone and substantial gelatinosa), with only a small termination in lamina V. By contrast, large-diameter fibers mediating aspects of dental and other cranial mechanosensations and reflexes terminate in laminae III through VI (the magnocellular nucleus and deeper).

The third similarity between the spinal dorsal horn and the caudal nucleus is the laminar distribution of ascending projection neurons. The ascending pathway for facial pain is the trigeminothalamic tract, and the ascending projection neurons are located principally in laminae I and V (the marginal zone and base of the caudal nucleus). These neurons project primarily to the contralateral thalamus. Cells that project to other brain stem sites, such as the reticular formation, have a broader distribution. The trigeminal projection to the reticular formation in the rostral medulla, pons, and midbrain—the trigeminoreticular tract—also has a larger ipsilateral component, similar to the spinoreticular tract.

The **caudal nucleus** extends from approximately the first or second cervical segment of the spinal cord to the medullary level (Figures 6–9 and 6–10), at which point the central canal "opens" to form the fourth ventricle. The **interpolar nucleus** extends from the rostral boundary of the caudal nucleus to the rostral medulla (Figure 6–11). Finally, the **oral nucleus** extends from the rostral boundary of the interpolar nucleus to the level at which the trigeminal nerve enters the pons (see Figures 6–5 and AII–9).

Occlusion of the Posterior Inferior Cerebellar Artery Impairs Pain and Temperature Senses on the Same Side of the Face but on the Opposite Side of the Body

The **posterior inferior cerebellar artery** (PICA) provides the arterial supply to the dorsolateral portion of the medulla (Figure 6–11; see Chapter 4). The PICA is an end-artery with little collateral flow from other vessels into the territory it serves. As a consequence, the dorsolateral region of the medulla becomes infarcted when the artery is occluded (Figure 6–11). The major cause of PICA stroke is **vertebral artery** occlusion at the point where the PICA branches off (Figure 6–11, inset). The medial region of the medulla is spared with such an occlusion because of the collateral blood supply to this area from the contralateral vertebral artery and the anterior spinal artery.

Occlusion of the PICA produces a complex set of sensory and motor deficits, termed the **lateral medullary,** or **Wallenberg, syndrome.** This syndrome has a distinctive pattern of somatic sensory signs. First, pain and temperature sensations are lost on the contralateral limbs and trunk due to damage of the ascending axons of the anterolateral system in the **lateral medulla** (see Chapter 5). Sensory loss is on the contralateral side because fibers of the anterolateral system decussate in the spinal cord. Second, there is a loss of pain and temperature sensation on the ipsilateral side of the face. (Presumably itch also is lost, but it is rarely tested.) This is because both the primary sensory fibers in the spinal trigeminal tract and the trigeminal spinal nucleus are destroyed. Because the axons of ascending projection neurons decussate rostral to their cell bodies, similar to the anterolateral

Figure 6–10. Myelin-stained transverse sections through the caudal nucleus.

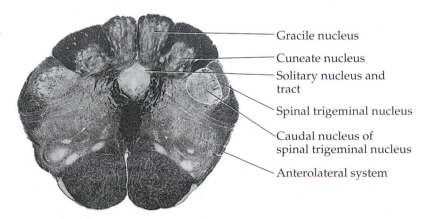

Gracile nucleus

Cuneate nucleus

Solitary nucleus and tract

Spinal trigeminal nucleus

Caudal nucleus of spinal trigeminal nucleus

Anterolateral system

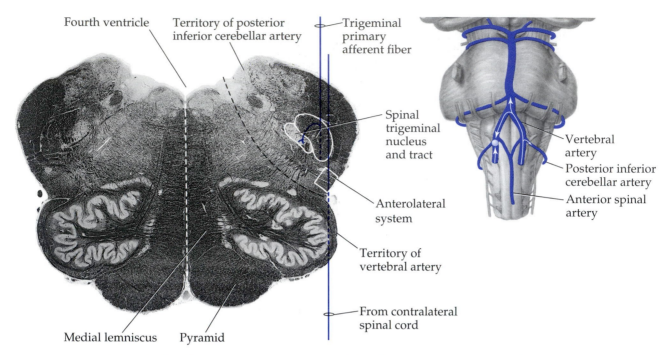

Fourth ventricle   Territory of posterior
                    inferior cerebellar artery

Trigeminal
primary
afferent fiber

Spinal
trigeminal
nucleus
and tract

Vertebral
artery

Posterior inferior
cerebellar artery

Anterior spinal
artery

Anterolateral
system

Territory of
vertebral artery

From contralateral
spinal cord

Medial lemniscus   Pyramid

Figure 6–11.   The arterial supply of the medulla. The inset shows the vasculature on a portion of the ventral brain stem. The large dot on the vertebral artery is the site of occlusion that prevents blood flow into the posterior inferior cerebellar artery. Collateral blood flow from the contralateral vertebral artery supplies the territory of the vertebral artery on the occluded side.

system of the spinal cord (see Figure 5–9), PICA occlusion rarely destroys the axons of decussated trigeminothalamic tract fibers. The anterior inferior cerebellar artery (Figure 4–3) nourishes the lateral brain stem where the decussated trigeminothalamic axons join the anterolateral system. Other sensory and motor deficits are also common neurological signs of the lateral medullary syndrome. These deficits are discussed in Chapters 11, 12, 13, and 15.

The Main Trigeminal Sensory Nucleus Is the Trigeminal Equivalent of the Dorsal Column Nuclei

Rostral to the spinal trigeminal nucleus is the **main trigeminal sensory nucleus** (Figure 6–12). This part of the trigeminal nuclear complex mediates touch sensation of the face and head and mechanosensation from the teeth. Neurons located primarily in the ventral two thirds of this nucleus give rise to axons that decussate and ascend to the **ventral posterior medial nucleus** of the thalamus. Their axons are located in the **trigeminal lemniscus,** dorsomedial to axons of the medial lemniscus. This is another example of seg-

regation of function. The main trigeminal sensory nucleus is the trigeminal equivalent of the dorsal column nuclei because both nuclei project to the contralateral ventral posterior nucleus (but to the medial and lateral subdivisions) and both structures subserve touch sensation (but from different body regions). The trigeminal lemniscus at brain stem levels caudal to the main trigeminal sensory nucleus contains axons from neurons in the spinal trigeminal nucleus. These axons represent a small contingent and may be analogous to the group of dorsal column axons that originate from dorsal horn neurons (see Chapter 5).

The dorsal one third of the main trigeminal sensory nucleus receives mechanoreceptive signals from the soft tissues of the oral cavity and the teeth. Neurons receiving this input give rise to an **ipsilateral pathway** that ascends dorsally in the pons and midbrain and terminates in the ipsilateral ventral posterior medial nucleus of the thalamus. It follows that the ventral posterior medial nucleus receives bilateral inputs from intraoral structures: a contralateral projection from the **trigeminal lemniscus** and an ipsilateral projection from the **dorsal pathway.** This bilateral representation in the thalamus, and presumably also in the somatic sensory cortex, may reflect the function of

Figure 6–12. Myelin-stained sections through the pons at the level of the main sensory nucleus of the trigeminal nerve (*A*) and the parabrachial nucleus (*B*).

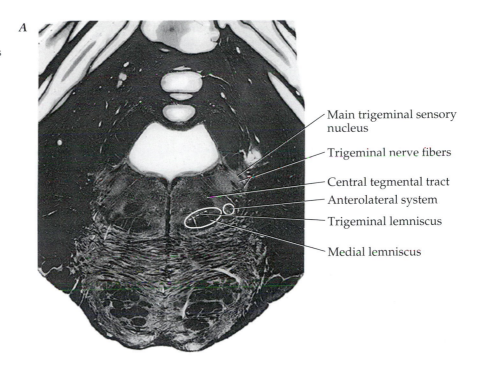

A

Main trigeminal sensory nucleus

Trigeminal nerve fibers

Central tegmental tract

Anterolateral system

Trigeminal lemniscus

Medial lemniscus

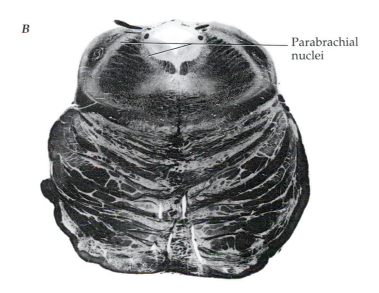

B

Parabrachial nuclei

oral structures on each side, which typically work together during behaviors such as chewing or talking.

The Mesencephalic Trigeminal Nucleus and Tract Contain the Cell Bodies and Axons of Jaw Muscle Stretch Receptors

The mesencephalic trigeminal nucleus, located in the lateral portion of the periventricular and periaqueductal gray matter, contains the cell bodies of

muscle spindle sensory receptors that innervate jaw muscles. Therefore this nucleus is equivalent to a peripheral sensory ganglion. The peripheral branch of the primary sensory neuron (Figure 6–2), carrying sensory information to the central nervous system, ascends to the mesencephalic trigeminal nucleus in the **mesencephalic trigeminal tract** (note its myelinated axons lateral to the nucleus; Figure 6–13). The central branch also projects through the mesencephalic trigeminal tract, to terminate in various brain stem sites important for jaw muscle control and jaw

A

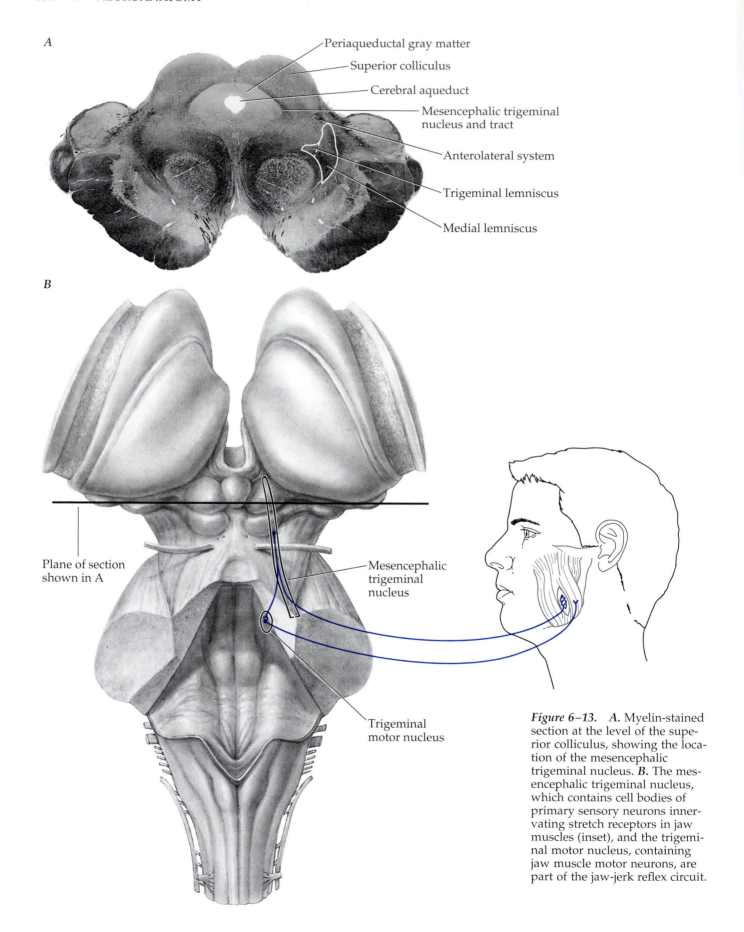

Periaqueductal gray matter

Superior colliculus

Cerebral aqueduct

Mesencephalic trigeminal nucleus and tract

Anterolateral system

Trigeminal lemniscus

Medial lemniscus

B

Plane of section shown in A

Mesencephalic trigeminal nucleus

Trigeminal motor nucleus

Figure 6–13. *A.* Myelin-stained section at the level of the superior colliculus, showing the location of the mesencephalic trigeminal nucleus. *B.* The mesencephalic trigeminal nucleus, which contains cell bodies of primary sensory neurons innervating stretch receptors in jaw muscles (inset), and the trigeminal motor nucleus, containing jaw muscle motor neurons, are part of the jaw-jerk reflex circuit.

proprioception. For example, a monosynaptic projection to the trigeminal motor nucleus mediates the **jaw-jerk** (or **closure**) **reflex** (Figure 6–13B), which is analogous to the knee-jerk reflex. Jaw muscle afferents terminate in the main trigeminal and rostral spinal trigeminal nuclei. Together these regions play a role in jaw proprioception. In the midbrain the medial lemniscus and trigeminal lemniscus have migrated laterally (Figure 6–13A). The trigeminal lemniscus terminates in the **medial division** of the ventral posterior nucleus.

The Caudal Solitary and Parabrachial Nuclei Are Key Brain Stem Viscerosensory Integrative Centers

The **caudal solitary nucleus** (Figure 6–10) receives input from visceral receptors—chemoreceptors (such as receptors sensitive to blood carbon dioxide), mechanoreceptors (such as mechanoreceptors beneath the mucous membrane of the larynx and arterial pressure receptors), vascular pressure receptors (such as baroreceptors in the carotid body), and nociceptors. Neurons in this nucleus have diverse ascending projections. There are also local projections in the medulla and pons that play important roles in controlling blood pressure and respiration rate and in regulating gastrointestinal motility and secretions. Sensory information processed here, especially mechanical and noxious stimuli from the larynx and pharynx, are important for initiating protective reflexes, such as the **laryngeal closure reflex** to prevent fluid aspiration into the lungs. The caudal solitary nucleus has **descending projections** to the spinal cord for directly controlling portions of the autonomic nervous system.

The ascending projections of the caudal solitary nucleus are focused on the **parabrachial nucleus** (Figure 6–12B; see AII–12). This nucleus is located in the pons adjacent to the principal output path of the cerebellum, the superior cerebellar peduncle (see Chapter 13). (Another name for the superior cerebellar peduncle is the brachium conjunctivum; hence, the term *parabrachial.*) One ascending projection of the parabrachial nucleus is to the parvocellular division of the **ventral posterior medial nucleus** of the thalamus, which is the thalamic viscerosensory relay (see next section). (Parvocellular means small celled.) The parabrachial nucleus also transmits viscerosensory information rostrally to the **hypothalamus** and the **amygdala** (see Figure 6–7), two brain structures thought to participate in a variety of autonomic and endocrine functions, for example, feeding and reproductive behaviors (see Chapters 14 and 15). Viscerosensory control of bodily functions is considered in Chapter 14, which covers the hypothalamus and autonomic nervous system.

The Ventral Posterior Nucleus Contains Separate Trigeminal and Spinal Subdivisions and Projects to the Postcentral Gyrus

The ventral posterior nucleus contains several divisions that mediate mechanical sensations, such as touch and pressure. The **ventral posterior lateral division** mediates mechanical sensations from the limbs and trunk and projects to the postcentral gyrus on the superior and medial surfaces. The **ventral posterior medial division** (Figure 6–14) processes mechanosensations from the head and projects to the lateral postcentral gyrus, forming the face and head representations (Figure 6–15). Similar to the over-representation of the hands (see Chapter 5), the representations of the tongue and perioral region in the primary somatic sensory cortex are larger than the cortical representations of other body parts because they are used more extensively during speech and chewing, for example. In many species of rodents and carnivores, the face representation is more extensive than that of the fingers or tongue and perioral regions, because the large whiskers of these species are their principal tactile discriminative and exploratory organs. The primary somatic sensory cortex, in turn, projects to higher-order somatic sensory areas in the posterior cortex for the further elaboration of the sensory message (see Figure 5–19).

Similar to the systems for spinal somatic sensory information processing, cranial somatic sensory information about cranial pain, itch, and temperature is transmitted to the **ventral posterior medial** and **ventromedial posterior nuclei**. These thalamic nuclei project to the postcentral gyrus and the insular cortex, respectively. As discussed in Chapter 5, although both of these cortical regions play a role in perception of pain, itch, and temperature senses, the insular cortex may be more important. In addition, the insular representation is important in memories of painful experiences and the somatic and autonomic behaviors that pain evokes. The **medial dorsal nucleus** receives spinothalamic and trigeminal thalamic pain, temperature, and itch information and projects to the anterior cingulate cortex, which is important in the emotional aspects of pain, itch, and temperature perception.

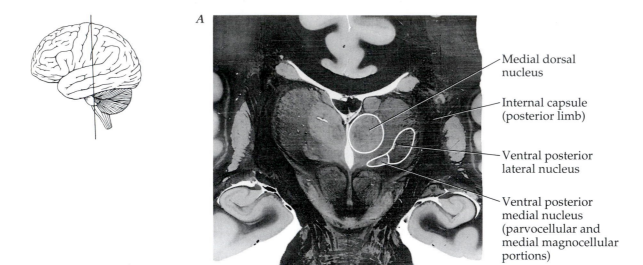

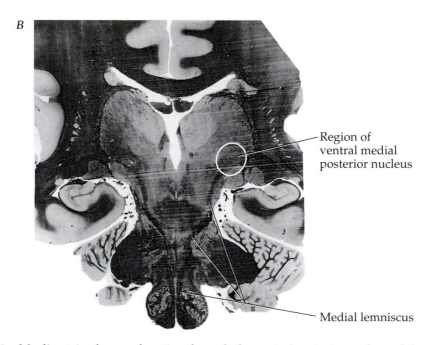

Figure 6–14. Myelin-stained coronal section through the ventral posterior nucleus of the thalamus. The magnocellular and parvocellular portions of the medial division (ventral posterior medial nucleus) are the trigeminal and taste relay nuclei, whereas the lateral division (ventral posterior lateral nucleus) is the relay nucleus for the medial lemniscus (ie, spinal sensory input).

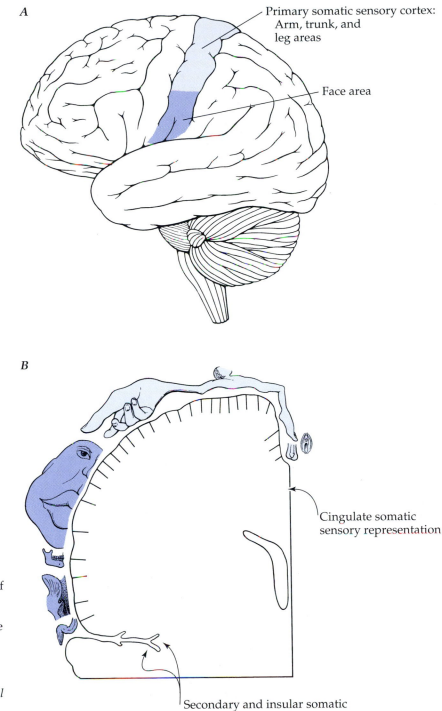

Figure 6–15. *A.* Lateral view of the cerebral hemisphere, with the representation of the limbs, trunk, and face indicated on the postcentral gyrus. *B.* Somatotopic organization of the postcentral gyrus. (*B,* *Adapted from Penfield W, Rasmussen T: The Cerebral Cortex of Man: A Clinical Study of Localization of Function. Macmillan, 1950.*)

The Thalamic Viscerosensory Relay Nucleus Projects to the Insular Cortex

Medial to the trigeminal sensory relay nucleus is the **parvocellular division** of the ventral posterior medial nucleus (Figure 6–14A). This division processes viscerosensory information from the pharynx, larynx, esophagus, and other internal organs and projects within the lateral sulcus, where the viscera are represented (Figure 6–15B). Pelvic visceral organs, which are innervated by primary sensory fibers that project to the sacral spinal cord, are represented more medially in the cortex. The parvocellular ventral posterior medial nucleus also processes taste (see Chapter 9).

Summary

The Cranial Nerves

Of the 12 cranial nerves (Table 6–1 and Figure 6–1), the first two, the **olfactory** (I) and **optic** (II) nerves, are sensory and enter the telencephalon and diencephalon directly. The 3rd through 12th cranial nerves enter and exit from the brain stem directly. Two cranial nerves, the **oculomotor** (III) and the **trochlear** (IV), are motor nerves located in the midbrain. The pons contains the **trigeminal** (V), a mixed nerve; the **abducens** (VI), a motor nerve; the **facial** (VII), a mixed nerve; and the **vestibulocochlear** (VIII), a sensory nerve. The medulla also contains four cranial nerves: the **glossopharyngeal** (IX) and **vagus** (X) are mixed nerves, whereas the **spinal accessory** (XI) and **hypoglossal** (XII) are motor nerves.

Cranial Nerve Nuclei Columns

Separate columns of cranial nerve nuclei course through the brain stem along its rostrocaudal axis (Figures 6–3 and 6–4). Each column has a separate sensory (afferent) or motor function, and the nomenclature conforms to that for the cranial nerves: (1) **skeletal somatic motor,** (2) **branchiomeric skeletal motor,** (3) **visceral (autonomic) motor,** (4) **viscerosensory and taste,** (5) **somatic sensory,** and (6) **hearing and balance** (Table 6–1). Each column has its own mediolateral location (Figures 6–3 and 6–4). The **sulcus limitans** separates the sensory from the motor nuclear columns.

Trigeminal Sensory System

Somatic sensation of cranial structures is mediated predominantly by the trigeminal nerve, which has three sensory divisions (Figure 6–8A): **ophthalmic, maxillary,** and **mandibular.** The cell bodies of the primary sensory neurons that innervate the skin and mucous membranes of the head are located in the **semilunar (or trigeminal) ganglion.** Three other cranial nerves also innervate portions of the head. The **intermediate** (VII) nerve (a branch of the **facial** nerve) innervates the skin of the ear; the **glossopharyngeal** (IX) nerve innervates the posterior tongue and portions of the oral cavity, nasal cavity, pharynx, and middle ear (Figure 6–8A). The **vagus** (X) nerve innervates the skin of the ear and mucous membranes of the larynx. The cell bodies of the primary afferent fibers in the facial nerve are located in the **geniculate ganglion,** and those of the glossopharyngeal and vagus nerves are located in the **superior ganglion** of each nerve. Afferent fibers in these four cranial nerves enter the brain stem and ascend and descend in the **spinal trigeminal tract** (Figures 6–8 and 6–9A). The fibers of the trigeminal nerve, whose cell bodies lie in the semilunar ganglion, terminate in two of the three major components of the trigeminal nuclear complex: the **main (or principal) trigeminal sensory nucleus** (Figure 6–12A) and the **spinal trigeminal nucleus** (Figures 6–1 and 6–9). The spinal trigeminal nucleus has three subdivisions: the **oral nucleus,** the **interpolar nucleus,** and the **caudal nucleus** (Figure 6–5). The afferent fibers of the facial, glossopharyngeal, and vagus nerves terminate in the spinal trigeminal nucleus.

Mechanoreceptive afferent fibers of the trigeminal nerve terminate predominantly in the **main trigeminal sensory nucleus.** The majority of the ascending projection neurons of this nucleus send their axons to the **contralateral ventral posterior medial nucleus** of the thalamus (Figure 6–14). From here, thalamic neurons project, via the posterior limb of the internal capsule, to the face representation of the **primary somatic sensory cortex,** which is located in the lateral portion of the **postcentral gyrus** (Figure 6–15). Projections from the primary cortex engage the secondary somatic sensory cortex and the posterior parietal lobe. A small pathway ascends ipsilaterally to the thalamus and cortex, conveying mechanical information from the mouth, especially the teeth.

Pain, temperature, and **itch** afferents from cranial structures enter and descend in the spinal trigeminal tract. The ascending pathway for pain and temperature sensations originates from the **spinal trigeminal nucleus,** primarily from the **caudal** and **interpolar nuclei** (Figure 6–5). The axons of projection neurons of this nucleus either remain on the ipsilateral side or decussate. The ascending fibers course with the anterolateral system in the lateral medulla and pons en route to the rostral brain stem and thalamus. The thalamic nuclei in which the fibers terminate are the **ventral posterior medial nucleus,** the **ventromedial posterior nucleus,** and the **medial dorsal nucleus** (Figure 6–14).

Afferent fibers carrying proprioceptive information from the jaw muscles form the **mesencephalic trigeminal tract** (Figure 6–13, inset). Their cell bodies are located in the **mesencephalic trigeminal nucleus** and are unique because they are the only primary sensory neurons with cell bodies located in the central nervous system (Figure 6–2). These afferents project to the main and rostral parts of the **spinal trigeminal nucleus,** which give rise to a pathway to the **ventral posterior medial nucleus** and **primary somatic sensory cortex.**

Viscerosensory System

Viscerosensory receptors are innervated by the **glossopharyngeal** (IX) and **vagus** (X) nerves, which project into the caudal solitary nucleus (Figure 6–5). Axons ascend ipsilaterally from the solitary nucleus to the parabrachial nucleus in the rostral pons (Figure 6–12B). The third-order neurons project to the **hypothalamus** and **limbic systems,** structures for regulating behavior and autonomic responses. Other third-order neurons project to the medial part of the **ventral posterior nucleus** and then to the visceral representation in the **insular cortex** (Figures 6–7 and 6–15). Pelvic visceral organs are innervated by primary sensory fibers that project to the sacral spinal cord. The pathways for pelvic visceral sensation are not well understood.

Related Sources

Basbaum AI, Jessell TM: The perception of pain. In Kandel ER, Schwartz JH, Jessell TM (editors): Principles of Neural Science, 4th ed. McGraw-Hill; 2000:472–491.

Brust JCM: The Practice of Neural Science. McGraw-Hill; 2000. (See ch. 3, p. 27; ch. 14, case 54.)

Selected Readings

Brodal A: Neurological Anatomy. Oxford University Press, 1981.

Capra NF: Mechanisms of oral sensation. Dysphagia 1995; 10:235–247.

Dubner R: Three decades of pain research and its control. J Dent Res 1997;76:730–733.

Dubner R, Gold M: The neurobiology of pain. Proc Natl Acad Sci U S A 1999;96:7627–7630.

References

Al-Chaer ED, Feng Y, Willis WD: Comparative study of viscerosomatic input onto postsynaptic dorsal column and spinothalamic tract neurons in the primate. J Neurophysiol 1999;82:1876–1882.

Altschuler SM, Bao XM, Bieger D, Hopkins DA, Miselis RR: Viscerotopic representation of the upper alimentary tract in the rat: Sensory ganglia and nuclei of the solitary and spinal trigeminal tracts. J Comp Neurol 1989;283:248–268.

Altschuler SM, Escardo J, Lynn RB, Miselis RR: The central organization of the vagus nerve innervating the colon of the rat. Gastroenterology 1993;104:502–509.

Arvidsson J, Gobel S: An HRP study of the central projections of primary trigeminal neurons which innervate tooth pulp in the cat. Brain Res 1981;210:1–16.

Arvidsson J, Thomander L: An HRP study of the central course of sensory intermediate and vagal fibers in peripheral facial nerve branches in the cat. J Comp Neurol 1984;223:35–45.

Augustine JR: The insular lobe in primates including humans. Neurol Res 1985;7:2–10.

Barnett EM, Evans GD, Sun N, Perlman S, Cassell MD: Anterograde tracing of trigeminal afferent pathways from the murine tooth pulp to cortex using herpes simplex virus type 1. J Neurosci 1995;15:2972–2984.

Barry MA, Halsell CB, Whitehead MC: Organization of the nucleus of the solitary tract in the hamster: Acetylcholinesterase, NADH dehydrogenase, and cytochrome oxidase histochemistry. Microsc Res Tech 1993;26:231–244.

Beck PD, Kaas JH: Thalamic connections of the dorsomedial visual area in primates. J Comp Neurol 1998;396:381–398.

Blomqvist A, Zhang ET, Craig AD: Cytoarchitectonic and immunohistochemical characterization of a specific pain and temperature relay, the posterior portion of the ventral medial nucleus, in the human thalamus. Brain 2000;123 (part 3):601–619.

Broussard DL, Altschuler SM: Brainstem viscerotopic organization of afferents and efferents involved in the control of swallowing. Am J Med 2000;108(suppl 4a):79S–86S.

Bruggemann J, Shi T, Apkarian AV: Viscero-somatic neurons in the primary somatosensory cortex (SI) of the squirrel monkey. Brain Res 1997;756:297–300.

Burton H, Craig AD Jr.: Distribution of trigeminothalamic projection cells in cat and monkey. Brain Res 1979;161: 515–521.

Capra NF, Ro JY, Wax TD: Physiological identification of jaw-movement-related neurons in the trigeminal nucleus of cats. Somatosens Mot Res 1994;11:77–88.

Chien CH, Shieh JY, Ling EA, Tan CK, Wen CY: The composition and central projections of the internal auricular nerves of the dog. J Anat 1996;189:349–362.

Esaki H, Umezaki T, Takagi S, Shin T: Characteristics of laryngeal receptors analyzed by presynaptic recording from the cat medulla oblongata. Auris Nasus Larynx 1997;24:73–83.

Grelot L, Barillot JC, Bianchi AL: Central distributions of the efferent and afferent components of the pharyngeal branches of the vagus and glossopharyngeal nerves: An HRP study in the cat. Exp Brain Res 1989;78:327–335.

Hanamori T, Smith DV: Gustatory innervation in the rabbit: Central distribution of sensory and motor components of the chorda tympani, glossopharyngeal, and superior laryngeal nerves. J Comp Neurol 1989;282:1–14.

Hayakawa T, Takanaga A, Maeda S, Seki M, Yajima Y: Subnuclear distribution of afferents from the oral, pharyngeal and laryngeal regions in the nucleus tractus solitarii of the rat: A study using transganglionic transport of cholera toxin. Neurosci Res 2001;39:221–232.

Hayashi H, Sumino R, Sessle BJ: Functional organization of trigeminal subnucleus interpolaris: Nociceptive and innocuous afferent inputs, projections to thalamus, cerebellum, and spinal cord, and descending modulation from periaqueductal gray. J Neurophysiol 1984;51:890–905.

Hu JW, Sessle BJ: Comparison of responses of cutaneous nociceptive and nonnociceptive brain stem neurons in trigeminal subnucleus caudalis (medullary dorsal horn) and subnucleus oralis to natural and electrical stimulation of tooth pulp. J Neurophysiol 1984;52:39–53.

Jones EG, Schwark HD, Callahan PA: Extent of the ipsilateral representation in the ventral posterior medial nucleus of the monkey thalamus. Exp Brain Res 1984;63:310–320.

Kruger L: Functional subdivision of the brainstem sensory trigeminal nuclear complex. In Bonica JJ, Liebeskind JC, Albe-Fessard DG (editors): Advances in Pain Research and Therapy, Vol. 3. Raven Press; 1984:197–209.

Kuo DC, de Groat WC: Primary afferent projections of the major splanchnic nerve to the spinal cord and gracile nucleus of the cat. J Comp Neurol 1985;231:421–434.

Kuo DC, Nadelhaft I, Hisamitsu T, de Groat WC: Segmental distribution and central projections of renal afferent fibers in the cat studied by transganglionic transport of horseradish peroxidase. J Comp Neurol 1983;216:162–174.

Lenz FA, Gracely RH, Zirh TA, Leopold DA, Rowland LH, Dougherty PM: Human thalamic nucleus mediating taste and multiple other sensations related to ingestive behavior. J Neurophysiol 1997;77:3406–3409.

Martin GF, Holstege G, Mehler WR: Reticular formation of the pons and medulla. In Paxinos G (editor): The Human Nervous System. Academic Press; 1990:203–220.

Menetrey D, Basbaum AI: Spinal and trigeminal projections to the nucleus of the solitary tract: A possible substrate for somatovisceral and viscerovisceral reflex activation. J Comp Neurol 1987;255:439–450.

Mifflin SW: Laryngeal afferent inputs to the nucleus of the solitary tract. Am J Physiol 1993;265:R269–276.

Nomura S, Mizuno N: Central distribution of primary afferent fibers in the Arnold's nerve (the auricular branch of the vagus nerve): A transganglionic HRP study in the cat. Brain Res 1984;292:199–205.

Paxinos G, Törk I, Halliday G, Mehler WR: Human homologs to brainstem nuclei identified in other animals as revealed by acetylcholinesterase activity. In Paxinos G (editor): The Human Nervous System. Academic Press; 1990:149–202.

Ro JY, Capra NF: Physiological evidence for caudal brainstem projections of jaw muscle spindle afferents. Exp Brain Res 1999;128:425–434.

Satoda T, Takahashi O, Murakami C, Uchida T, Mizuno N: The sites of origin and termination of afferent and efferent components in the lingual and pharyngeal branches of the glossopharyngeal nerve in the Japanese monkey (Macaca fuscata). Neurosci Res 1996;24:385–392.

Shigenaga Y, Chen IC, Suemune S, et al: Oral and facial representation within the medullary and upper cervical dorsal horns in the cat. J Comp Neurol 1986;243:388–408.

Shigenaga Y, Nishimura M, Suemune S, et al: Somatotopic organization of tooth pulp primary afferent neurons in the cat. Brain Res 1989;477:66–89.

Smith RL: Axonal projections and connections of the principal sensory trigeminal nucleus in the monkey. J Comp Neurol 1975;163:347–376.

Sweazey RD, Bradley RM: Central connections of the lingual-tonsillar branch of the glossopharyngeal nerve and the superior laryngeal nerve in lamb. J Comp Neurol 1986;245:471–482.

Sweazey RD, Bradley RM: Response characteristics of lamb pontine neurons to stimulation of the oral cavity and epiglottis with different sensory modalities. J Neurophysiol 1993;70:1168–1180.

Takagi S, Umezaki T, Shin T: Convergence of laryngeal afferents with different natures upon cat NTS neurons. Brain Res Bull 1995;38:261–268.

Takemura M, Nagase Y, Yoshida A, et al: The central projections of the monkey tooth pulp afferent neurons. Somatosens Mot Res 1993;10:217–227.

Treede RD, Apkarian AV, Bromm B, Greenspan JD, Lenz FA: Cortical representation of pain: Functional characterization of nociceptive areas near the lateral sulcus. Pain 2000;87:113–119.

Wild JM, Johnston BM, Gluckman PD: Central projections of the nodose ganglion and the origin of vagal efferents in the lamb. J Anat 1991;175:105–129.

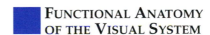

7

The Visual System

I N MANY WAYS THE VISUAL SYSTEM IS ORGANIZED LIKE the systems for touch and pain considered in Chapters 5 and 6. For instance, the topography of connections in the visual system is determined largely by how the receptive sheet is organized. In fact, these connections are so systematized and predictable that clinicians can use a visual sensory defect to pinpoint with remarkable precision the location of central nervous system damage. Another similarity is that all three systems have a **hierarchical and parallel organization.** In a hierarchically organized system, distinct functional levels can be discerned with respect to one another, each with clear anatomical substrates. In vision, as in somatic sensation, multiple hierarchically organized pathways carry information from receptors to structures in the central nervous system. Each pathway processes visual information for a different purpose. For example, separate systems participate in perception of the shape, motion, and color of objects.

Visual perception, like perception for the other senses, is not a passive process; our eyes do not simply receive visual stimulation. Rather, the position of the eyes is precisely controlled to scan the environment and to attend selectively and orient to specific visual stimuli. In addition to the pathways from the retina to the cortex for visual perception, a separate pathway to the brain stem exists for controlling eye movements. This chapter begins with an overview of the visual pathways for perception and eye movement control. It then considers the structure and anatomical connections of the components of these pathways. Finally, the chapter examines how the clinician can, with precision, localize disturbances of brain function by using knowledge of the organization of the visual system.

FUNCTIONAL ANATOMY OF THE VISUAL SYSTEM

Anatomically Separate Visual Pathways Mediate Perception and Ocular Reflex Function

The visual pathway that mediates perception and the pathway that controls eye movement originate in the retina, a thin sheet of neurons and glial cells that adheres to the posterior inner surface of the eyeball (Figure 7–1A). Also located here are the photoreceptors (Figure 7–1A, inset), which synapse on retinal interneurons that, in turn, synapse on ganglion cells. **Ganglion cells** are the retinal projection neurons, which synapse in the thalamus and brain stem. The axons of ganglion cells travel in the **optic nerve** (cranial nerve II), and ganglion cells from each eye contribute axons to the optic nerve on the same side. Some ganglion cell axons decussate in the **optic chiasm** (Figure 7–1A,B) en route to the thalamus and brain stem, whereas other axons remain uncrossed. Together the crossed and uncrossed ganglion cell axons, reordered according to a precise plan (see below), course in the **optic tract** (Figure 7–1B). Each optic tract contains axons from both eyes.

The Pathway to the Primary Visual Cortex Is Important for Perception of the Form, Color, and Motion of Visual Stimuli

The principal thalamic target for ganglion cells is the **lateral geniculate nucleus.** This thalamic relay nucleus is analogous to the ventral posterior nucleus, the somatic sensory relay nucleus. The lateral geniculate nucleus projects to the **primary visual cortex** via a pathway called the **optic radiations.** This projection is important for perception. It comprises several functional pathways, including one for perceiving the form of visual stimuli, another for color, and a third for the location and speed of motion of stimuli.

The primary visual cortex is located in the occipital lobe, along the banks and within the depths of the **calcarine fissure** (Figure 7–1A). The primary visual cortex is also referred to as the **striate cortex** because myelinated axons form a prominent striation. Efferent projections from the primary visual cortex follow one of three principal pathways. One pathway projects to the **secondary** and **higher-order visual cortical areas** in the occipital lobe (see Figure 7–9). Whereas the primary visual cortex is important in visual signal processing that is fundamental to all aspects of visual perception, many of the higher-order cortical areas are each important in different aspects of vision. For example, the primary visual cortex processes information for stimulus form, color, and motion; one of the higher-order areas is important for color vision; and a different area is important for discriminating the direction and speed of a moving stimulus (see Figures 7–1B and 7–16). The axons of the second path from the primary visual cortex decussate in the corpus callosum and terminate in the contralateral primary visual cortex. This projection is also for visual perception. It helps to unify images from the two eyes into a perception of a single visual world. Finally, the third path

from the primary visual cortex descends to the visuomotor centers of the midbrain for eye movement control and for focusing the images on the retina.

The Pathway to the Midbrain Is Important in Voluntary and Reflexive Control of the Eyes

Certain ganglion cells project to the midbrain directly (Figure 7–1A,C), principally to two structures: the **superior colliculus** and the **pretectal nuclei.** The ganglion cell axons traveling to the midbrain skirt the lateral geniculate nucleus and course in the **brachium of superior colliculus** (Figure 7–1B; see also Figure 7–7A). The superior colliculus, found in the **tectum** of the midbrain (see Figure 2–9), is dorsal to the cerebral aqueduct (Figure 7–1C). In lower vertebrates, such as amphibians and birds, the superior colliculus is termed the **optic tectum** and is the principal brain structure for vision, in lieu of a visual cortex. In mammals and especially humans, the superior colliculus has a minimal role in perception but an important role in the control of **saccades.** These rapid eye movements are quick shifts in visual gaze that are used to look from one object to another. The pretectal nuclei are rostral to the tectum, at the midbrain-diencephalic junction (see Figure 7–8C). The pretectal nuclei participate in **pupillary reflexes,** which regulate the amount of light reaching the retina, as well as other visual reflexes (see Chapter 11).

Additional brain stem and diencephalic projections of the optic tract serve other functions. For example, one projection reaches midbrain nuclei that are important in the reflexive control of eye position to stabilize images on the retina when the head is moving. These nuclei comprise the **accessory optic system.** As another example, a retinal projection to the hypothalamus is important for diurnal regulation of hormone secretion (see Chapter 15).

The next section examines the detailed anatomy of each major visual system component, beginning with the optical properties of the eye, which will help explain the functional anatomy of visual system neural connections.

■ REGIONAL ANATOMY OF THE VISUAL SYSTEM

Optical Properties of the Eye Transform Visual Stimuli

When the eyes are fixed straight ahead, the total area seen is called the **visual field** (Figure 7–2A). Although the visual field can be divided into right

A

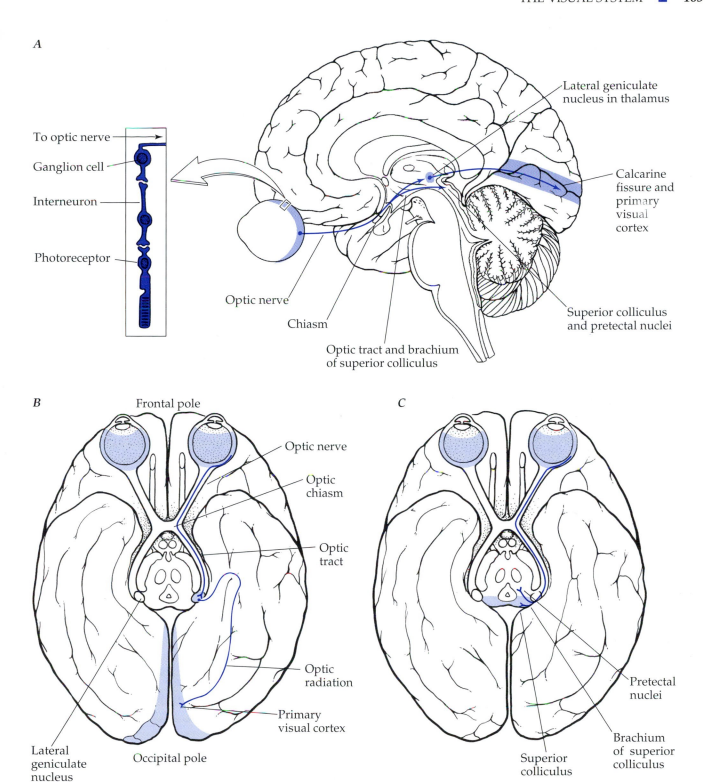

To optic nerve

Ganglion cell

Interneuron

Photoreceptor

Lateral geniculate
nucleus in thalamus

Calcarine
fissure and
primary
visual
cortex

Optic nerve

Chiasm

Superior colliculus
and pretectal nuclei

Optic tract and brachium
of superior colliculus

B

Frontal pole

Optic nerve

Optic
chiasm

Optic
tract

Optic
radiation

Primary
visual cortex

Lateral
geniculate
nucleus

Occipital pole

C

Pretectal
nuclei

Brachium
of superior
colliculus

Superior
colliculus

Figure 7–1. Organization of the two visual pathways, the retinal-geniculate-calcarine
pathway (*A*, *B*) and the pathway to the midbrain (*A*, *C*). The inset on the left shows the
general organization of the retina. The photoreceptor transduces visual stimuli and transmits the sensory information, encoded in the form of nonpropagated potentials, to retinal interneurons. The interneurons transmit the visual information to the ganglion cells.
Ganglion cell axons form the optic nerve once they exit the eyeball. *A.* Midsagittal view
of the brain, showing visual paths to the thalamus and cortex and the path to the midbrain. *B.* Inferior brain view, showing the retinal-geniculate-calcarine pathway. *C.* Inferior brain view, showing the pathway to the midbrain.

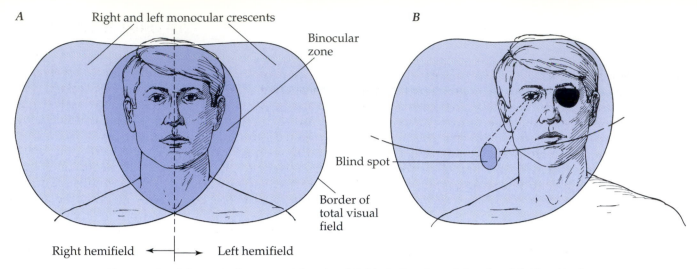

Figure 7–2. Schematic diagram of the visual field. **A.** Overlap of the visual fields of both eyes. **B.** Visual field for the right eye (with a patch over the left eye) with the projection of the blind spot indicated. *(Adapted from Patten H: Neurological Differential Diagnosis. Springer-Verlag, 1977.)*

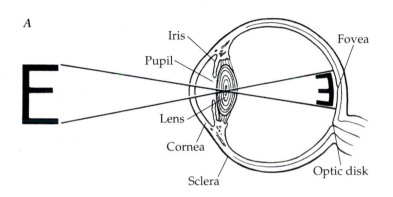

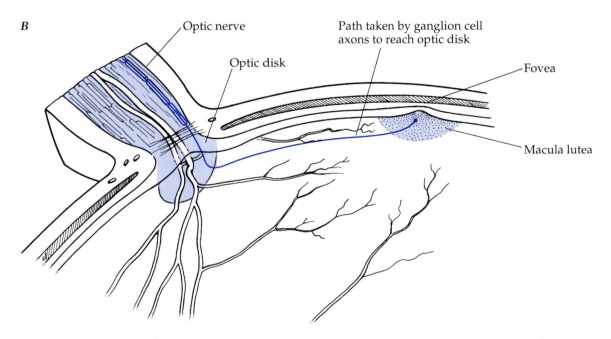

Figure 7–3. **A.** Sagittal view shows the key features of the optical properties of the eye. **B.** Course of ganglion cell axons along the surface of the retina and into the optic nerve at the optic disk. (**B,** *Adapted from Patten H: Neurological Differential Diagnosis. Springer-Verlag, 1977.*)

and left hemifields, the field of view of each eye is not simply one hemifield. Just as when you look through binoculars, the field of view of each eye overlaps extensively. As a result, the visual field includes a central binocular zone (Figure 7–2A, dark blue), where there is stereoscopic vision, and two monocular zones (Figure 7–2A, light blue). Each hemifield is therefore seen by parts of the retina of each eye.

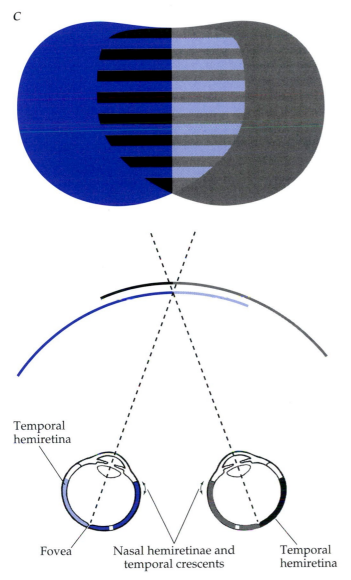

Temporal hemiretina

Fovea   Nasal hemiretinae and temporal crescents   Temporal hemiretina

Figure 7–3 (continued.) **C.** Horizontal view showing the location of the visual fields for each eye and how information projects on the two retinae. The left and right visual fields are shown in blue and gray/black. Information from the dark blue region falls on the left nasal hemiretina, and from the light blue region, on the left temporal hemiretina. Information from the black region falls on the right temporal hemiretina, and from the gray region, on the right nasal hemiretina. The regions of the visual fields in which there is binocular overlap are shown by the stripes.

After light enters the eye through the **cornea,** the transparent avascular portion of the **sclera,** it is focused onto the retinal surface by the **lens** (Figure 7–3A). The lens inverts and reverses the visual image projected on the retina. When you look at an object, you move your eyes so that the object's image falls upon the **fovea,** a specialized high-resolution portion of the retina. The fovea is centered within a morphologically distinct region of the retina called the **macula lutea** (Figure 7–3B). The brain precisely controls the position of the eyes to ensure that the principal portion of an image falls on the fovea of each eye. A vertical line passing through the fovea divides the retina into two halves, a **nasal hemiretina** and a **temporal hemiretina.** Each hemiretina includes half of the fovea and the remaining perifoveal and peripheral portions of the retina. The anterior portions of the nasal hemiretinae correspond to the temporal crescents, which are monocular zones receiving visual information from the temporal parts of the visual fields (Figure 7–3C).

Consider the relationship between an object being viewed and where its image falls on the retina (Figure 7–3C). When you look at someone's face and, for example, fixate on the person's nose, the left side of the face is within the left visual hemifield. The image of the left side falls on the nasal hemiretina of the left eye and the temporal hemiretina of the right eye. Although each eye views the entire face, visual information from the visual hemifield on one side is processed by the visual cortex on the opposite side (see below).

Figure 7–3B also shows the **optic disk,** where retinal axons leave the eyeball and the blood vessels serving a part of the retina enter and leave the eye. This corresponds to the **blind spot** (Figure 7–2B) because the optic disk has no photoreceptors. Interestingly, an individual is not aware of his or her own visual blind spot until it is demonstrated. The fovea and optic disk can be examined clinically using an ophthalmoscope to peer into the back of the eye.

The Retina Contains Five Major Layers

The retina is a laminated structure, as revealed in a section oriented at a right angle to its surface (Figure 7–4A). Other components of the visual system also have a laminar organization. Lamination is one way the nervous system packs together neurons with similar functions and patterns of connections. The spatial reference point for describing the location of the different layers is the **three-dimensional center** of the eye. The **inner,** or proximal, retinal layers are close to the center of the eye; the **outer,** or distal, layers are farther from the center (Figure 7–4A, inset).

A

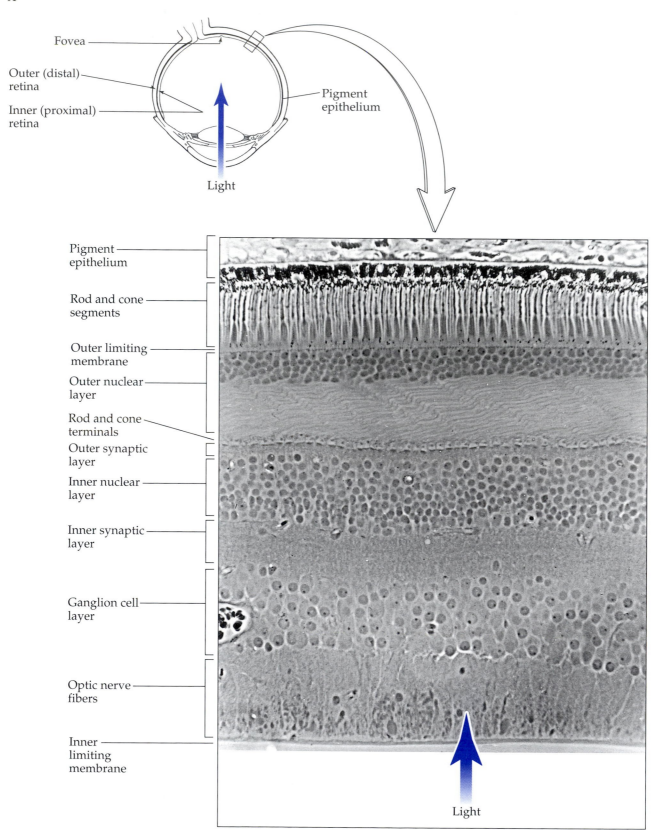

Figure 7–4. *A.* Transverse section of the retina. Inset shows a schematic diagram of the eyeball, indicating the inner and outer portions of the retina.

B

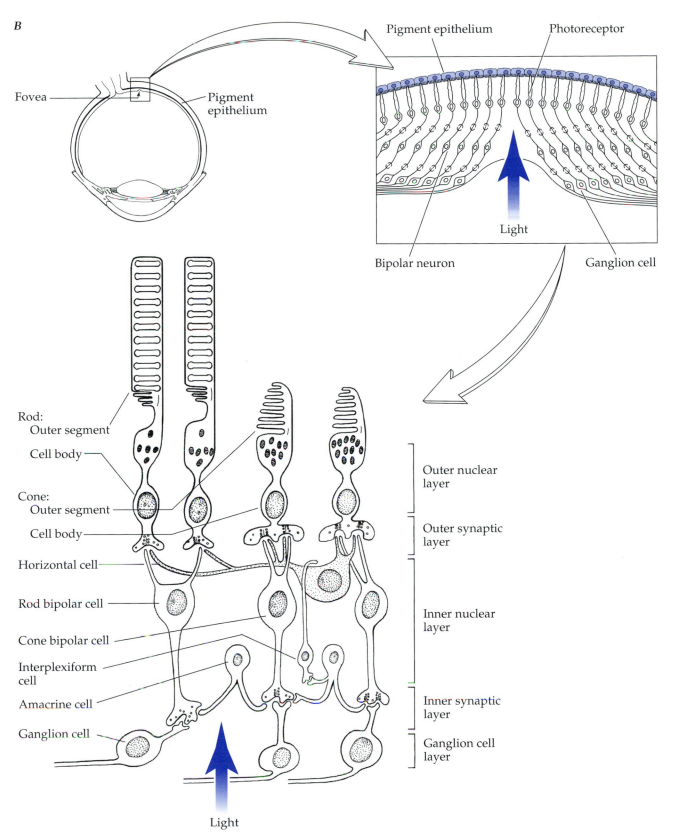

Fovea

Pigment epithelium

Pigment epithelium   Photoreceptor

Light

Bipolar neuron   Ganglion cell

Rod:
  Outer segment
  Cell body

Cone:
  Outer segment
  Cell body

Horizontal cell

Rod bipolar cell

Cone bipolar cell

Interplexiform cell

Amacrine cell

Ganglion cell

Outer nuclear layer

Outer synaptic layer

Inner nuclear layer

Inner synaptic layer

Ganglion cell layer

Light

Figure 7–4 (continued.)   ***B.*** Wiring diagram of the generalized vertebrate retina. The interplexiform cell, identified in numerous species, feeds processed visual information from amacrine cells in the inner retina back to horizontal cells in the outer retina. In the mammalian retina, horizontal cells do not synapse on cones. Boxed inset shows an expanded view of the retina at the fovea. Retinal interneurons are displaced away from the fovea so that the photoreceptors are exposed directly to incoming light. (***A,*** *Courtesy of Dr. John E. Dowling, Harvard University.* ***B,*** *Adapted from Dowling JE, Boycott BB: Organization of the primate retina: Electron microscopy. Proc R Soc Lond B 1966;166:80–111.)*

Although the retina has many layers, there are five principal ones (Figure 7–4B): (1) the outer nuclear layer, (2) the outer synaptic (or plexiform) layer, (3) the inner nuclear layer, (4) the inner synaptic (or plexiform) layer, and (5) the ganglion cell layer. Synapses are present in the two plexiform layers, and cell bodies are located in the other three layers. In addition to the five principal layers, numerous strata contain processes of particular retinal cells.

The **outer nuclear layer** contains the cell bodies of the two classes of photoreceptors: rods, which are for night vision, and **cones,** for daylight and color vision. Cones mediate the most discriminative aspects of visual perception, and they are densest in the fovea, where they number approximately 200,000 per square millimeter. Cone density decreases continuously by about one order of magnitude for every 1 mm from the fovea (Figure 7–5A). This is why visual acuity decreases continuously from the fovea to the peripheral retina. Cones contain the photopigments for color vision and come in three different classes according to their absorption spectra: red, green, or blue.

By contrast, rods are absent in the fovea and are densest along an elliptical ring in the perifoveal region passing through the optic disk (Figure 7–5B). Along

this ring is a site of maximal density of approximately 175,000 per square millimeter. These photoreceptors contain the photopigment **rhodopsin** and are optimally suited for detecting low levels of illumination, such as at dusk or at night. In fact, a single photon can activate a rod cell. The location of maximal rod density, along the parafoveal elliptical ring, corresponds approximately to the location of maximal light sensitivity. This factor helps to explain why, when discerning a faint object at night, we do not look directly at it but rather off to one side.

Connections between photoreceptors and retinal interneurons are made in the **outer synaptic (or plexiform) layer.** The **inner nuclear layer** contains the cell bodies and proximal processes of the retinal interneurons—bipolar, horizontal, and amacrine cells (Figure 7–4B).

Bipolar cells link photoreceptors directly with the ganglion cells. Of the two principal classes of bipolar cells, **cone bipolar cells** and **rod bipolar cells,** the former receive synaptic input from a small number of cone cells to give high visual acuity and color vision. By contrast, rod bipolar cells receive convergent input from many rods for less visual acuity but increased sensitivity to low levels of illumination. The actions of

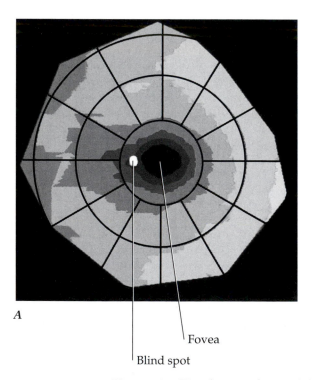

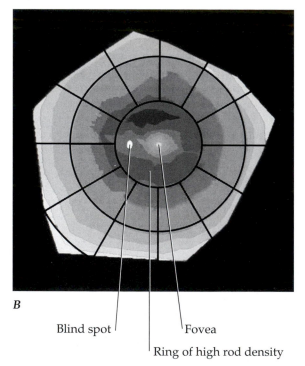

A

B

Fovea

Blind spot

Blind spot   Fovea

Ring of high rod density

Figure 7–5.   Distribution of cones (*A*) and rods (*B*) in the human retina. The density of photoreceptors is indicated by a gray scale: Retinal regions containing a higher density of photoreceptors are shaded darker than regions with a low photoreceptor density. The white spot to the left of center in both *A* and *B* corresponds to the optic disk, where no photoreceptors are located. *(Courtesy of Dr. Christine Curcio; Curcio CA, Sloan KR, Kalina RE, Hendrickson AE: Human photoreceptor topography. J Comp Neurol 1990;292:497–523, Figure 5.)*

horizontal cells and amacrine cells enhance visual contrast through interactions between laterally located photoreceptors and bipolar cells. Horizontal cells are located in the outer part of the inner nuclear layer, whereas amacrine cells are found in the inner portion. Many amacrine cells contain dopamine, which plays a role in adapting retinal synaptic activity to the dark. Synaptic connections between the bipolar cells and the ganglion cells are made in the inner synaptic (or plexiform) layer. The innermost retinal cell layer, the ganglion cell layer, is named after the retinal output cells. Ganglion cell axons collect along the inner retinal surface (Figures 7–3B and 7–4) and leave the eye at the optic disk (Figure 7–3B), where they form the optic nerve.

The cellular organization of the retina might seem unexpected because light must travel through retinal layers that contain axons, projection neurons, and interneurons to reach the photoreceptors. Although this is puzzling, the consequences of this organization on visual acuity are minimized by an anatomical specialization at the fovea. Here the retinal interneurons and ganglion cells are displaced, exposing the photoreceptors directly to visual stimuli and optimizing the optical quality of the image (Figure 7–4B, inset). Moreover, ganglion cell axons are unmyelinated while they are in the retina, which increases the transparency of the retina and facilitates light transmission to the photoreceptor layer in the outer retina. Ganglion cell axons become myelinated once they enter the optic nerve.

Müller cells are the principal retinal neuroglial cells. These cells have important structural and metabolic functions. Their nuclei are located in the inner nuclear layer, and their processes stretch vertically from the outer to the inner limiting membranes (Figure 7–4A). The other nonneural elements associated with the retina are clinically important. The pigment epithelium is external to the photoreceptor layer (Figure 7–4A). It serves a phagocytic role, removing rod outer segment disks that are discarded as part of a normal renewal process. In the retinal disease retinitis pigmentosa, this phagocytic process becomes defective. Because the retina does not tightly adhere to the pigment epithelium, it can become detached following a blow to the head or eye. This results in a partially detached retina and loss of vision in the detached portion.

The circulation of the retina has a dual organization. The arterial supply of the inner retina is provided by branches of the ophthalmic artery, which is a branch of the internal carotid. The outer retina is devoid of blood vessels. Its nourishment derives from arteries in the choroid, the layer of ocular tissue between the inner retina and the outer sclera.

Each Optic Nerve Contains All of the Axons of Ganglion Cells in the Ipsilateral Retina

The optic nerve is cranial nerve II, but it is a central nervous system pathway rather than a peripheral nerve. This is because the retina develops from a displaced portion of the diencephalon (see Figure 3–2), rather than the neural crest, from which the somatic sensory receptors derive.

The optic nerves from both eyes converge at the optic chiasm (Figure 7–6). The axons of ganglion cells of each nasal hemiretina decussate in the optic chiasm and enter the contralateral optic tract, whereas those of each temporal hemiretina remain on the same side and enter the ipsilateral optic tract (Figure 7–6A). Thus, each optic tract contains axons from the contralateral nasal hemiretina and the ipsilateral temporal hemiretina (Figure 7–6B). Despite the incomplete decussation of the optic nerves in the chiasm, there is a complete crossover of visual information: Visual stimuli from one half of the visual field are processed within the contralateral thalamus, cerebral cortex, and midbrain (Figure 7–6A).

The Superior Colliculus Is Important in Oculomotor Control and Orientation

The optic tract splits on the ventral diencephalic surface. The major contingent of axons terminates in the lateral geniculate nucleus and gives rise to the pathway for visual perception (see next section). A smaller contingent skirts the lateral geniculate nucleus and passes over the surface of the medial geniculate nucleus, which is the thalamic auditory nucleus (see Chapter 8). These axons collectively are termed the brachium of superior colliculus (Figure 7–7) because their major site of termination is the superior colliculus.

The superior colliculus is laminated: Incoming visual information is processed by the dorsal layers, whereas somatic sensory, auditory, and other information is processed by neurons in the ventral layers. The spinotectal tract, one component of the anterolateral system (see Chapter 5), brings somatic sensory information to the ventral layers of the superior colliculus.

The superior colliculus helps to orient the eyes and head to salient stimuli in the environment. It does this by combining sensory information from the different modalities in a unique way. The dorsal layers are retinotopically organized, similar to other parts of the visual system. The representations of somatic sensory and auditory information, in deeper collicular layers, are aligned with the visual representation in superficial layers according to a spatial map of the external world.

A

B

From nasal
hemiretina

From temporal
hemiretina

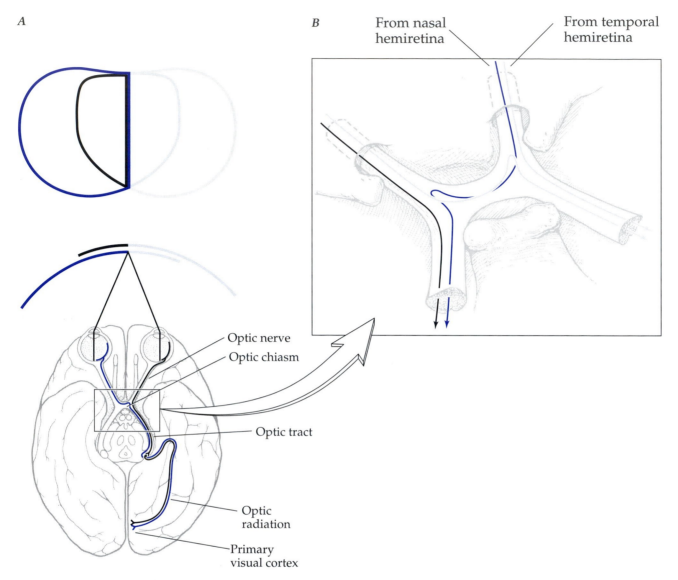

Optic nerve

Optic chiasm

Optic tract

Optic
radiation

Primary
visual cortex

Figure 7–6. **A.** Horizontal view of the visual system, showing the portions of the retina of each eye that receive information from the left visual field. Ganglion neuron axons from the nasal hemiretinae decussate; those from the temporal hemiretinae project to the brain ipsilaterally. **B.** View of the base of the skull showing the regional anatomy of the optic chiasm. Direction of arrows indicates axon trajectory toward lateral geniculate nucleus and midbrain. (**B,** *Adapted from Patten H: Neurological Differential Diagnosis. Springer-Verlag, 1977.*)

Aggregates of neurons in the superior colliculus that are located above one another, but in different layers, all respond to stimuli from the same spatial location. For example, neurons that respond to visual information from the superior visual field are dorsal to neurons that respond to sounds from in front of and above the head and neurons that respond to tactile stimulation of the forehead. For example, such a collection of neurons in the superior colliculus might be important in orienting an individual to a buzzing insect that

lands on his or her forehead. The ventral layers of the superior colliculus contain part of the neural apparatus for eye and neck muscle control (see Chapter 12).

The neural systems for visuomotor function and visual perception appear to converge in the cerebral cortex. Certain superior colliculus neurons have an axon that ascends to the **lateral posterior** and **pulvinar nuclei** of the thalamus (see Figure 2–11). These thalamic nuclei project primarily to **higher-order visual areas** and to the **parietal-temporal-occipital associa-**

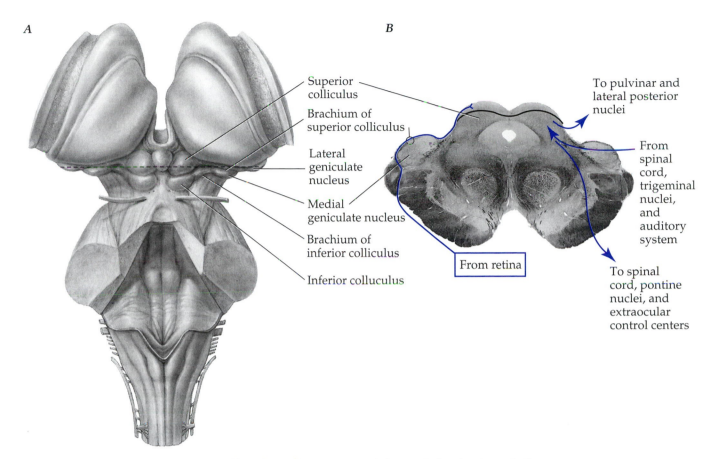

Figure 7–7. **A.** Dorsal surface of brain stem and diencephalon (with cerebellum removed), showing the locations of components of the visual system in the diencephalon and midbrain. **B.** Myelin-stained transverse section through the rostral midbrain (superior colliculus). The path of a ganglion cell axon from the retina to the superior colliculus is shown in blue. The dashed line in *A* shows the plane of section in *B*.

tion areas. One function of this ascending projection from the superior colliculus may be to inform cortical areas important for visual perception about the speed and direction of eye movements. This information is important for distinguishing between movement of a stimulus and movement of the eyes.

The Retinotopic Maps in Each Layer of the Lateral Geniculate Nucleus Are Aligned

The major retinal projection is to the **lateral geniculate nucleus** of the thalamus. This nucleus forms a surface landmark on the ventral diencephalon that is sometimes called the lateral geniculate body (Figure 7–7A). The main contingent of optic tract fibers terminates in the lateral geniculate nucleus (Figure 7–8), where projection neurons send their axons to the primary visual cortex through the **optic radiations** (Figure 7–8A).

The lateral geniculate nucleus contains six major cell layers, stacked on top of one another. Whereas all of these cell layers process input from the **contralateral visual field,** each layer receives projections exclusively from either the **ipsilateral** or the **contralateral retina.** Each layer of the lateral geniculate nucleus contains a complete and orderly representation of the contralateral visual field. Visual representations in the various layers are aligned. In other words, cells oriented along an axis orthogonal to the plane of the layers receive input from the same portion of the contralateral visual field. Neurons in the dorsal and ventral layers have a different morphology and different functions (see below). Neurons located between these cell layers, sometimes called **interlaminar neurons,** receive retinal input and project to the primary visual cortex. The principal function of these neurons is to transmit information about the color of a stimulus to clusters of neurons in the primary visual cortex.

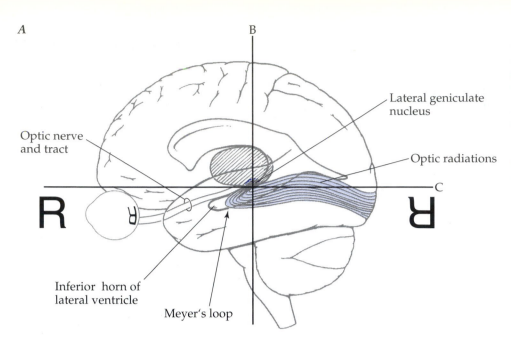

A

Lateral geniculate nucleus

Optic nerve and tract

Optic radiations

Inferior horn of lateral ventricle

Meyer's loop

Figure 7–8. *A.* Course of the axons of the optic radiations from the lateral geniculate nucleus, over the lateral ventricle, to reach the primary visual cortex. *B.* Myelin-stained coronal section through the lateral geniculate nucleus. *C.* Transverse section through the midbrain-diencephalic juncture. (*A, Adapted from Brodal A: Neurological Anatomy. Oxford University Press, 1981.*)

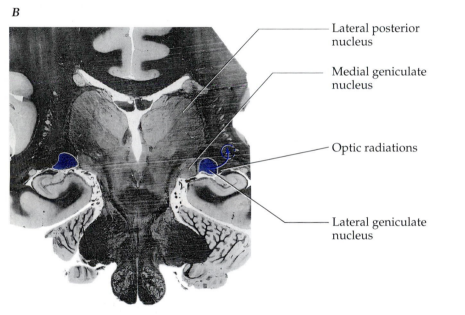

B

Lateral posterior nucleus

Medial geniculate nucleus

Optic radiations

Lateral geniculate nucleus

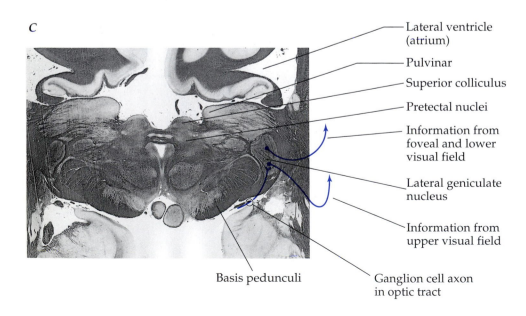

C

Lateral ventricle (atrium)

Pulvinar

Superior colliculus

Pretectal nuclei

Information from foveal and lower visual field

Lateral geniculate nucleus

Information from upper visual field

Basis pedunculi

Ganglion cell axon in optic tract

The Primary Visual Cortex Is the Target of Projections From the Lateral Geniculate Nucleus

Projection neurons in all six layers of the lateral geniculate nucleus send their axons to the primary visual cortex via the optic radiations (Figure 7–8A). The optic radiations take an indirect course around the lateral ventricle to reach their cortical targets. A portion of the optic radiations mediating vision from the superior visual field courses rostrally within the temporal lobe (termed **Meyer's loop**), before heading caudally to the primary visual cortex.

The primary visual cortex, which is located mostly on the medial brain surface, corresponds to Brodmann's cytoarchitectonic **area 17** (Figure 7–9; see also Figure 2–17). It has six principal layers, with layer IV further subdivided into several sublaminae (Figure 7–10). One layer IV sublamina contains the **stripe of Gennari,** a dense plexus of myelinated fibers that are axon collaterals of primary visual cortex neurons. The presence of this stripe gives the primary visual cortex its other name, the **striate cortex.** Similar to the primary somatic sensory cortex, neurons in different layers of the primary visual cortex have different patterns of input and output connections. The higher-order visual areas are located in Brodmann's **areas 18** and **19** (Fig-

ure 7–9), which encircle area 17. The boundary between areas 17 and 18 is distinct because it is where the stripe of Gennari ends (Figure 7–10A).

The Magnocellular and Parvocellular Systems Have Differential Laminar Projections in the Primary Visual Cortex

The different layers of the lateral geniculate nucleus, in addition to receiving input from either the ipsilateral or the contralateral retina, also receive input from a distinct class of retinal ganglion cells, either **magnocellular** (M) cells or **parvocellular** (P) cells (Figure 7–11). The M and P cells give rise to two visual information channels that process distinct features of a visual stimulus.

The **M cell** has a large dendritic arbor, enabling it to integrate visual information from a wide portion of the retina. M cells are thought to play a key role in the analysis of stimulus motion as well as gross spatial features of a stimulus. The ventral two layers of the lateral geniculate nucleus receive input from the M cells. Because the thalamocortical neurons located in these two layers are larger than those in the other layers, they are also called magnocellular layers. The **P cell,** with its small dendritic arbor, processes visual information from a small portion of the retina. These

Figure 7–9. The primary and higher-order visual areas are located on the medial and lateral surfaces of the occipital lobe. *A.* Lateral view of the brain. *B.* Medial view of the brain. Lines correspond to cytoarchitectonic boundaries. V3, V4, and V5 comprise part of cytoarchitectonic area 19. The borders of V1 and V2 are better established, whereas those of V4 and V5 are only approximate. (*Adapted, with permission, from Clarke S, Miklossy J: Occipital cortex in man: Organization of callosal connections, related myelo and cytoarchitecture, and putative boundaries of functional visual areas. J Comp Neurol 1990;298:188–214, and Sereno MI, Dale AM, Reppas JB, et al: Borders of multiple visual areas in humans revealed by functional magnetic resonance imaging. Science 1995;268:889–893.*)

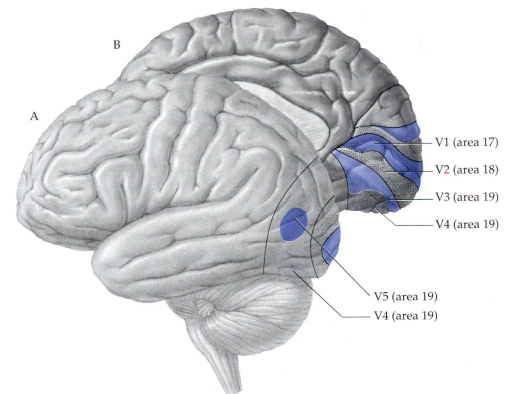

B

A

V1 (area 17)
V2 (area 18)
V3 (area 19)
V4 (area 19)
V5 (area 19)
V4 (area 19)

A

Stripe of Gennari

Calcarine
fissure

Area 17
Area 18

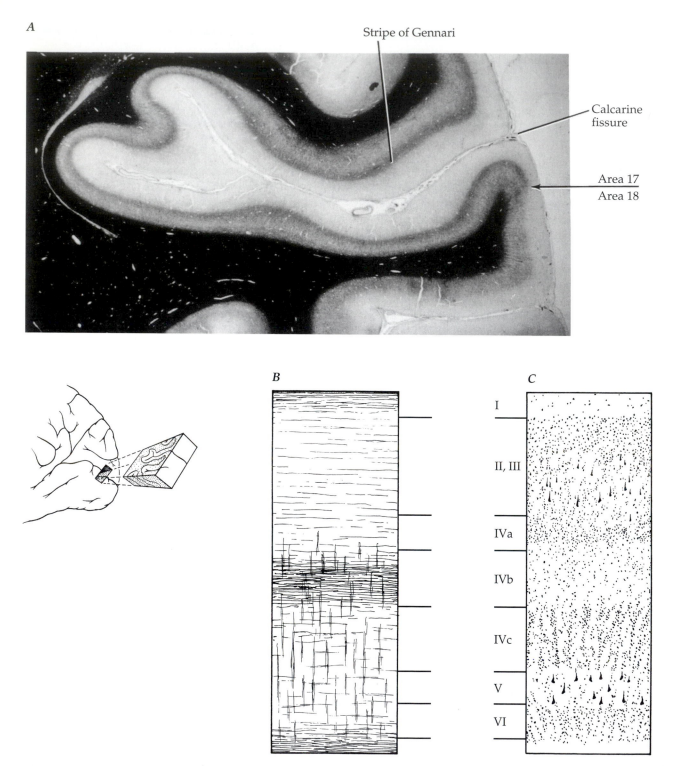

B

C

I

II, III

IVa

IVb

IVc

V

VI

Figure 7–10. **A.** The pattern of lamination in the primary visual cortex is shown in a myelin-stained section. **B.** Schematic drawing of a myelin-stained section through the striate cortex and a Nissl-stained section (**C**), illustrating the cytoarchitecture of the primary visual cortex. The inset shows the orientation of the section in **A.**

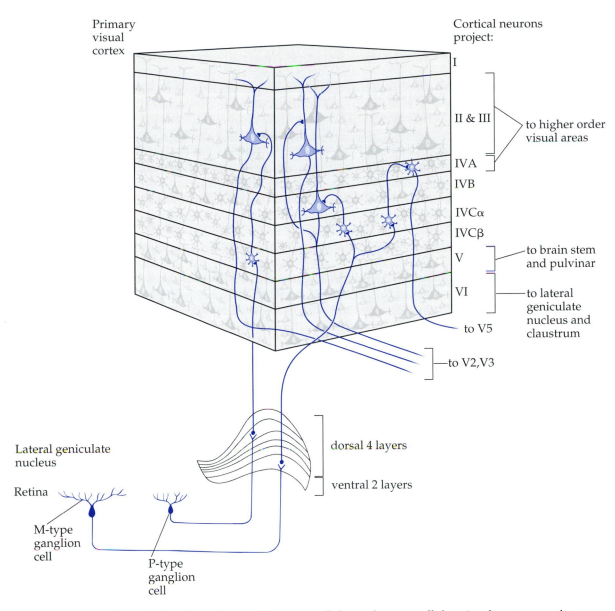

Figure 7–11. Projections of the parvocellular and magnocellular visual systems to the primary visual cortex. The magnocellular projection from the lateral geniculate nucleus terminates primarily in layer IVCα, whereas the parvocellular projection terminates primarily in layers IVA and IVCβ. In addition, both projections terminate in layer VI, which contains neurons that project back to the thalamus. (Only laminae receiving major thalamic projections are tinted blue.)

cells are color sensitive and are important for discriminative aspects of vision, such as distinguishing form and color. The P-type ganglion cells terminate in the dorsal four layers of the lateral geniculate nucleus. Here the thalamocortical neurons are small, hence, the name parvocellular layers.

Whereas neurons in the lateral geniculate nucleus have a light projection to many layers in the primary visual cortex, the densest projections are to **layer IV.** Neurons in the magnocellular and parvocellular layers

project to different sublaminae in layer IV. The magnocellular system projects primarily to layer IVCα, whereas the parvocellular system projects primarily to layers IVA and IVCβ.

Interneurons in the layer IV sublaminae connect with neurons in superficial and deeper cortical layers, which distribute visual information to other cortical and subcortical regions (Figure 7–11). The differential laminar projections of the magnocellular and parvocellular systems set the stage for distinct visual processing channels that distribute information about different aspects of a stimulus to the secondary and higher-order visual cortical areas.

The Primary Visual Cortex Has a Columnar Organization

Different areas of the cerebral cortex share a similar functional organization: The properties of neurons located above and below one another—yet in different layers—have similar properties. This is the **columnar organization** of the cerebral cortex. In the primary somatic sensory cortex, neurons in a cortical column all process sensory information from the same **peripheral location** and the same somatic **submodality** (see Chapter 5; Figure 5–18). The primary visual cortex also has a columnar organization. This organization was first revealed by recording the electrical responses of neurons to simple visual stimuli presented to one or the other eye. Neurons in a cortical column have similar functions because local connections primarily distribute the thalamic input vertically, from layer IV to superficial and deeper layers, rather than horizontally within the same layer. Horizontal connections do exist; however, they mediate other kinds of functions, such as enhancing contrast and binding together visual information from different parts of a scene to form perceptions. These horizontal connections run in the **stria** (or **stripe**) **of Gennari.**

The primary visual cortex has at least three types of columns: **Ocular dominance columns** contain neurons that receive visual input primarily from the ipsilateral or the contralateral eye (Figure 7–12). **Orientation columns** contain neurons that are maximally sensitive to simple visual stimuli with similar spatial orientations (see Figure 7–14). **Color columns,** termed **blobs,** are vertically oriented aggregates of neurons in layers II and III that are sensitive to the color of visual stimuli (see Figure 7–15).

Ocular Dominance Columns Segregate Input From the Two Eyes

The axon terminals of lateral geniculate neurons that receive input from the ipsilateral retina remain segregated from the terminals of neurons that receive their input from the contralateral retina (Figure 7–12). The lateral geniculate terminals carrying input from one eye form bands in layer IV that alternate with terminals transmitting input from the other eye. This means that neurons in layer IV are monocular; they receive visual input from one eye or the other.

Researchers can visualize the projections from one eye to layer IV in the primary visual cortex using transneuronal transport of a tracer substance (Figure 7–12). The tracer was injected into one eye of an anesthetized animal and transported, via the thalamus, to the primary visual cortex. Labeled patches in Figure 7–12A (bright spots) correspond to the projections from the injected eye. Portions of layer IV receiving input from the uninjected eye are unlabeled and alternate with the labeled regions. The labeled patches in layer IV form stripes when viewed in a plane tangential to the cortical surface. This is shown in Figure 7–12B, which presents a photographic montage through layer IV (the inset indicates the plane of section in A and montage sections in B). Remarkably, ocular dominance columns can be shown in human primary visual cortex at autopsy in a person that had one eye removed before death, for example, because of an ocular tumor. When stained for the mitochondrial enzyme cytochrome oxidase, tissue sections show alternating stripes of reduced and normal staining (Figure 7–13A). The stripes with reduced staining correspond to the ocular dominance columns of the removed eye, and normal staining corresponds to the columns of the intact eye. The ocular dominance columns can be analyzed on histological sections and the three-dimensional configuration of the columns drawn on the surface of the primary visual cortex (Figure 7–13B,C).

Mixing of information from both eyes, giving rise to binocular inputs, occurs in neurons located above and below layer IV. These binocular interactions are mediated by cortical interneurons. The binocular neurons receive a stronger synaptic input from the same eye that projected information to the monocular neurons in layer IV, and a weaker input from the other eye. This pattern of lateral geniculate axon terminations in layer IV and blending of connections above and below layer IV forms the anatomical basis of the **ocular dominance columns** (Figure 7–12, inset). A given retinal location in each eye is represented in the cortex by a pair of adjacent ocular dominance columns. Horizontal connections between neurons in adjacent ocular dominance columns are thought to be important for depth perception.

Orientation Columns Are Revealed by Mapping Cortical Functional Organization

Physiological studies have shown that most neurons in the primary visual cortex respond to imple bar-shaped stimuli with a particular orientation. However, unlike ocular dominance, which is an attribute based on anatomical connections from one eye or the other,

A

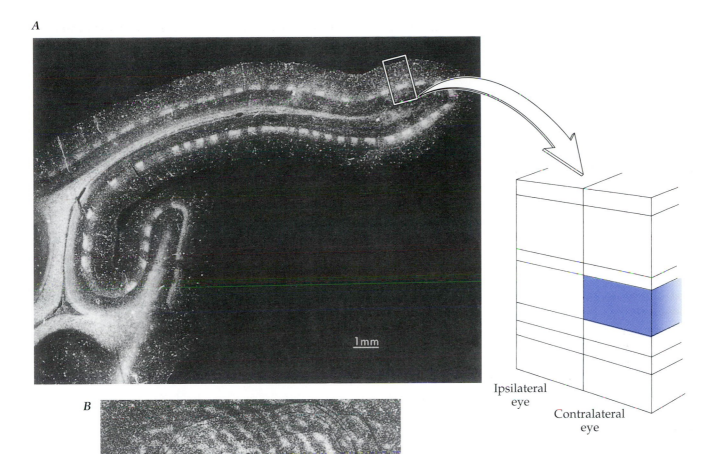

1mm

Ipsilateral eye

Contralateral eye

B

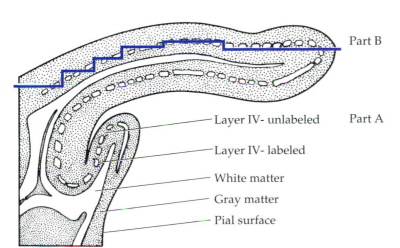

Part B

Part A

Layer IV- unlabeled

Layer IV- labeled

White matter

Gray matter

Pial surface

Figure 7–12. Projections from the retina, through the lateral geniculate nucleus to the primary visual cortex, can be demonstrated using autoradiography. **A.** The section was cut orthogonal to the pial surface. **B.** A montage approximating a plane parallel to the pial surface. The inset is a schematic drawing of the section in **A,** showing the composite plan of the montage in **B.** (**A,** *From Hubel DH, Wiesel TN: Ferrier lecture: Functional architecture of macaque monkey visual cortex. Proc R Soc Lond B 1977;198:1–59.* **B,** *From Hubel DH, Wiesel TN, LeVay S: Plasticity of ocular dominance columns in monkey striate cortex. Philos Trans R Soc Lond B 1977;278:377–409.*)

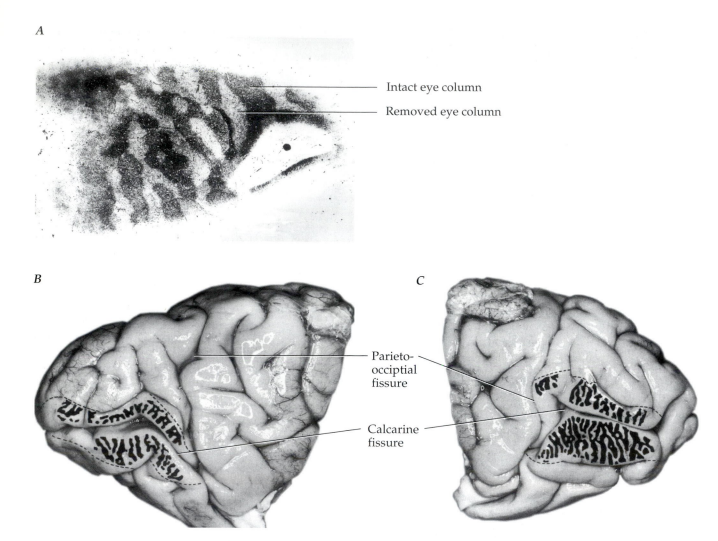

A

Intact eye column

Removed eye column

B

C

Parieto-occiptial fissure

Calcarine fissure

Figure 7–13. Ocular dominance columns in the human brain from a person that had one eye removed 23 years prior to death. *A.* A section cut approximately parallel to the surface of the cortex stained for the presence of the mitochondrial enzyme cytochrome oxidase. The alternating dark and light bands correspond to the locations of the ocular dominance columns for the intact and removed eyes. Enucleation resulted in very low levels of the enzyme in columns for that eye. *B* and *C.* Photographs of the left (*B*) and right (*C*) occipital lobes, with the ocular dominance columns from the intact eye drawn directly on the surface of the cortex. The intervening spaces correspond to the columns for the removed eye. Calibration bar is 1 cm. (*Courtesy of Dr. Jonathan C. Horton. Adapted from Horton JC, Hedley-White ET: Mapping of cytochrome oxidase patches and ocular dominance columns in human visual cortex. Phil Trans R Soc Lond B 1984;304, 255–272.*)

orientation specificity of neurons in a column in the primary visual cortex is a property produced by connections between local cortical neurons (Figure 7–14).

Orientation columns can be revealed in experimental animals using methods that provide an image of neuronal function, such as neuronal activity or local blood flow, which correlates with neural activity. Figure 7–14 is an image of a small portion of the surface of the primary visual cortex of a monkey as it viewed

contours of different orientations. The figure shows the reflectance of a particular wavelength of light, which indicates neural activity. Neurons sensitive to particular stimulus orientations are located within territories of one or another shading. Neurons sensitive to all orientations are present within a local area, but they are distributed in a radial pattern resembling a pinwheel. Cells selective for stimulus orientation (and therefore the orientation columns themselves) are

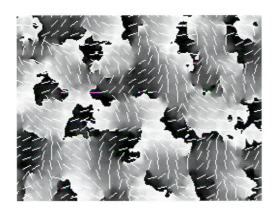

Figure 7–14. Orientation columns in primary visual cortex. This is an image of a portion of the primary visual cortex of the monkey, obtained using an optical imaging technique that measures local changes in tissue reflectance, which indicates neuronal activity. The gray scale shows the orientation sensitivity of neurons, which is also indicated by the short white lines. Note the swirling pattern of orientation sensitivity, sometimes resembling a pinwheel. Neurons sensitive to all orientations are present within a local area. *(Courtesy of Anirrhuda Das, Columbia University.)*

located from layer II to layer VI, and spare a portion of layer IV, which contains neurons that are insensitive to stimulus orientation.

Clusters of Color-sensitive Neurons in Layers II and III Are Distinguished by High Levels of Cytochrome Oxidase Activity

Parvocellular color-sensitive neurons project to layer IVCβ. They also have a small projection, more superficially, to layers II and III. Neurons sensitive to the wavelength of the visual stimulus are clustered within the ocular dominance columns in layers II and III. The locations of these color-sensitive cells correspond to regions of primary visual cortex that have high levels of activity of the mitochondrial metabolic enzyme **cytochrome oxidase** (Figure 7–15A). The regions of increased enzyme activity, which correspond to the clusters of color-sensitive neurons, are termed **blobs** (Figure 7–15A, small dots).

The secondary visual cortex (area 18; V2) shows alternating stripes of increased (thick and thin stripes) or decreased (pale interstripe) cytochrome oxidase

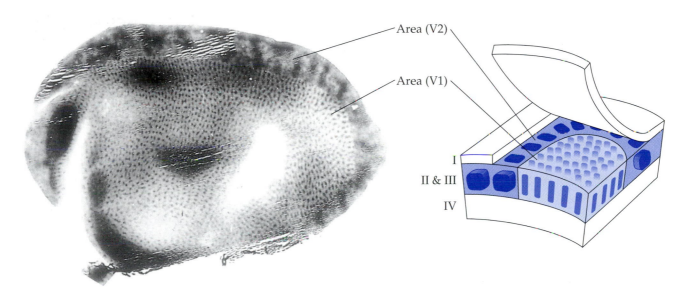

Area (V2)

Area (V1)

I
II & III
IV

Figure 7–15. Clusters of neurons involved in color vision are identified by histochemical localization of cytochrome oxidase. The section was cut parallel to the pial surface and predominantly through layers II and III of the occipital lobe of the visual cortex in a rhesus monkey (inset). Cytochrome oxidase activity is greater in the dark regions than in the light regions. In area 17 (primary visual cortex), regions that have high cytochrome oxidase activity have a spherical shape in cross section and are cylindrical in three dimensions. Cytochrome oxidase staining in area 18 (secondary visual cortex) reveals thick and thin stripes rather than the polka-dot pattern. *(Courtesy of Drs. Margaret Livingstone and David Hubel, Harvard University.)*

activity (Figure 7–15). The next section addresses how neurons in the thick stripe, thin stripe, and pale interstripe are part of distinct visual processing channels.

Higher-Order Visual Cortical Areas Analyze Distinct Aspects of Visual Stimuli

Also located in the occipital lobe are the higher-order visual areas (Figure 7–9). Each area contains a partial or complete representation of the retina. Higher-order visual areas are collectively termed the **extrastriate cortex** because they lie outside area V1, which contains the stripe of Gennari (Figure 7–10). Extrastriate areas receive input directly or indirectly from the primary visual area. Many of the extrastriate areas also receive input from the pulvinar and lateral posterior nuclei. It has been proposed that the **pulvinar nucleus** is important in distinguishing relevant from irrelevant visual stimuli, or **visual salience.** The lateral geniculate nucleus has little projection to the extrastriate areas.

Studies of the extrastriate areas have shown that the intracortical connections between the visual areas are both hierarchical and parallel. For example, V1 projects to V2, which in turn projects to V3. This is a hierarchically organized projection to V3. In contrast, the parallel projection to V3 is a direct one from V1, skipping V2. Although it can be deduced that less information processing occurs in the parallel projection, it is not yet clear how the parallel and hierarchical paths differ functionally.

Research analyzing connections of the monkey visual system suggest that, out of the myriad cortico-cortical projections from the primary and higher-order visual areas, different pathways are involved in perceiving stimulus motion, color, and form (Figure 7–16A):

- The **motion pathway** derives from the M-type ganglion cells. Information passes through the magnocellular layers of the lateral geniculate nucleus, to neurons in layer IVCα of the primary visual cortex (Figure 7–11), and from there to neurons in layer IVB (Figure 7–16A). Neurons in layer IVB project directly to V5 and indirectly via neurons in the thick cytochrome oxidase stripes of V2 (Figure 7–16A, dark blue). There also is a small projection to more superficial layers in V1. The function of this projection is unclear. In the rhesus monkey, V5 corresponds to a region named MT, for middle temporal area. This region is important not only for motion detection but also for regulating slow eye movements (see Chapter 12). The pathway from V1 (and V2) to V3 may be important for analyzing aspects of visual **form in motion.** A region thought to be analogous to V5 in the human can be imaged using positron emission tomography (PET) (Box 7–1).

- The **color pathway** derives from the P-type ganglion cells, which terminate in the parvocellular layers of the lateral geniculate nucleus. From there the thalamocortical projection is, via neurons in layer IVCβ (Figure 7–11), to neurons in the color blobs (layers II and III), then to the thin stripes in V2 (Figure 7–16A, medium blue), and next to V4. The region that may be equivalent to V4 in the human cortex has been described using PET (Box 7–1). The color blobs also receive a direct projection from the interlaminar neurons in the lateral geniculate neurons, which are located in the region between the principal magnocellular and parvocellular cell layers.

- The **form pathway** also derives primarily from the P-type ganglion cells and the parvocellular layers of the lateral geniculate nucleus. In V1, neurons in layer IVCβ (Figure 7–11) project to the interblob regions of layers II and III, and from there to the pale interstripe portion of V2 (Figure 7–16A, light blue). Next, V2 neurons project to V4. Whereas the motion and form systems are thought to contribute to depth perception, the color system does not.

The notion of functionally distinct pathways for different attributes of a visual stimulus helps to explain the remarkable perceptual defects that occur in humans following damage to the temporal and parietal lobes. Damage to the inferior temporal lobe produces a selective defect in **object recognition.** By contrast, damage to the posterior parietal lobe impairs the patient's capacity for **object localization** in the environment but spares the patient's ability to recognize objects. These findings suggest that there are two streams of visual processing in the cortex (Figure 7–16B): The ventral stream carries information about specific features of objects and scenes to the inferior temporal lobe, and the dorsal stream carries spatial information. Thus, the ventral stream is concerned with seeing *what,* as opposed to *where,* which is the function of the dorsal stream. Although extensive interconnections exist, the ventral stream for object recognition may receive a preferential input from the parvocellular, or form and color, system. In contrast, the dorsal stream for localization receives input primarily from the magnocellular system. As is discussed in Chapter 8, there are distinct pathways

Text continued on p. 184

A

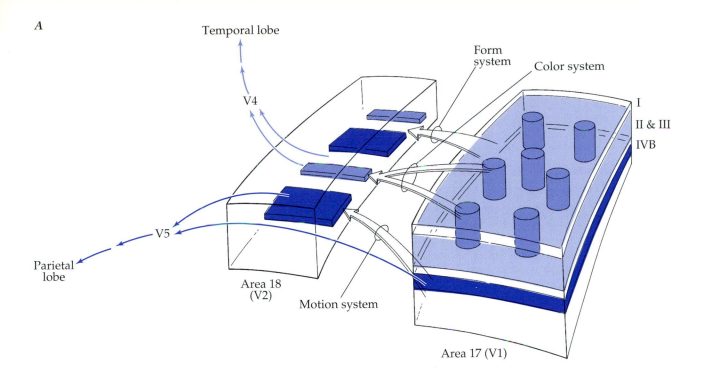

Temporal lobe

Form
system

Color system

V4

I

II & III

IVB

Parietal
lobe

V5

Area 18
(V2)

Motion system

Area 17 (V1)

B

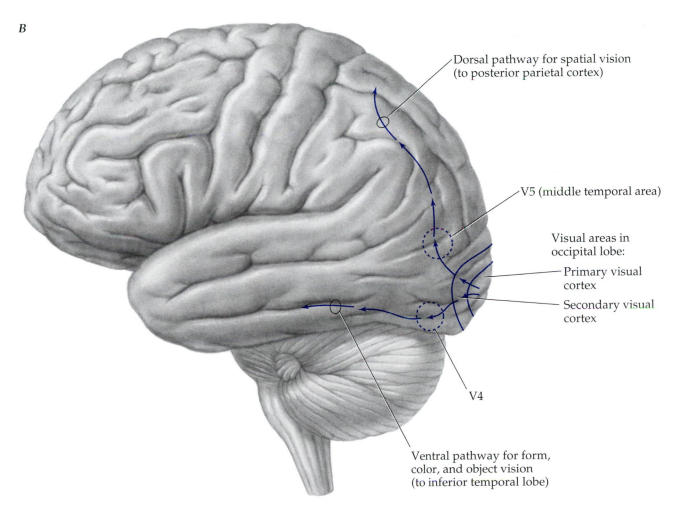

Dorsal pathway for spatial vision
(to posterior parietal cortex)

V5 (middle temporal area)

Visual areas in
occipital lobe:

Primary visual
cortex

Secondary visual
cortex

V4

Ventral pathway for form,
color, and object vision
(to inferior temporal lobe)

Figure 7–16. Projections from the primary visual cortex. *A.* There are separate VI origins
for motion (dark blue), color (medium blue), and form (light blue). The primary visual
cortex (area 17) is shown on the right, and the secondary visual cortex (area 18) is shown
on the left. *B.* Separate pathways into the parietal and temporal lobes are thought to
mediate spatial vision (the analysis of motion and location of visual stimuli) and object
vision (the analysis of form and color of visual stimuli).

Box 7–1. The Functions of the Different Higher-Order Visual Areas Are Revealed by Imaging and Analysis of Deficits Produced by Lesions

The functions of the different higher-order visual areas of the cortex are sufficiently distinct that selective damage to one can impair a remarkably specific aspect of vision. This specificity derives in part from the duality of the parvocellular and magnocellular pathways, as well as the projection from interlaminar lateral geniculate neurons to the color blobs in layers II and III of the primary visual cortex. But, because the different systems do not remain completely separate in the cortex (eg, see Figure 7–11), greater functional specificity appears to be achieved by combining information from the two systems in complex ways.

Functional localization in the visual system can be revealed by imaging techniques such as PET and functional magnetic resonance imaging (fMRI) as well as by considering the deficits in visual perception that occur following localized damage to the different visual cortical areas. Figure 7–17A is an fMRI scan of the first through

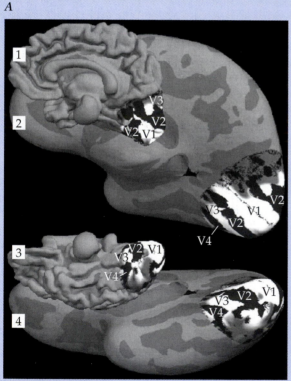

A

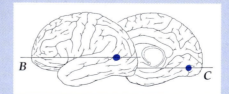

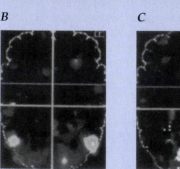

B   C

Figure 7–17. Visual cortical areas imaged in the human brain. **A.** Functional magnetic resonance imaging scans of human brains showing several visual cortical areas in the occipital lobe. **A1** and **A3** are lateral and ventral views of the brain reconstructed from MR images. **A2** and **A4** are data from "smoothed" brains in which data from within sulci are revealed on an unfolded brain surface. These images were obtained while subjects viewed a checkerboard stimulus that was rotated slowly. **B.** Positron emission tomography (PET) scans through the human brain, showing increased cerebral blood flow in a cortical region thought be V5, while the subject views a monochromatic scene in motion. **C.** PET scan showing increased cerebral blood flow in a cortical region thought be V4, while the subject views a stationary color scene. (**A,** *From Sereno MI, Dale AM, Reppas JB, et al: Borders of multiple visual areas in humans revealed by functional magnetic resonance imaging. Science 1995;268:889–893.* **B,** *Courtesy of Professor S. Zeki, Oxford University.*)

Box 7–1 *(continued.)*

fourth visual areas of the human brain. The image was created by taking advantage of the retinotopic organization of the different areas.

Whereas the primary and secondary visual areas become active irrespective of whether an individual views a monochromatic scene in motion or a stationary colorful scene, the higher visual areas are driven by particular stimulation patterns. A parallel situation exists with visual system trauma. Damage to the lower-order visual areas (and subcortical centers) produces **scotomas,** or blind spots, of different configurations (see section on visual field changes). By contrast, damage to the higher-order visual areas produces more subtle defects.

Imaging and Lesion of the "Where" Pathway

An area on the lateral surface of the occipital lobe, close to the juncture of the inferior temporal sulcus and one of the lateral occipital gyri, becomes selectively activated by visual motion (Figure 7–19A). This area closely corresponds to V5. Damage to this region can produce a remarkable visual disorder, motion blindness (hemiakinetopsia), in the contralateral visual field. Patients with this disorder do not report seeing an object move. Rather, objects undergo episodic shifts in location. An approaching form is in the distance at one time and close by the next.

Lesions farther along the "where" pathway, in the posterior parietal association cortex (Figure 7–16B), impair spatial vision and orientation. A lesion here alters complex aspects of perception that involve more than vision, because this region receives convergent inputs from the somatic sensory and auditory cortical areas. Patients can experience deficits in pointing and reaching and in avoiding obstacles. As discussed in Chapter 5, patients also can neglect a portion of their body and a portion of the external world around them. Deficits are most profound when the right hemisphere becomes damaged, a reflection of lateralization of spatial awareness. This pattern of progressively more complex, and more specific, sensory and behavioral impairment illustrates the hierarchical organization of the higher visual pathways.

Posterior Cerebral Artery Infarction Can Produce a Lesion of the "What" Pathway

A region on the medial brain surface, in the caudal portion of the fusiform gyrus, becomes active when a subject views a colorful scene (Figure 7–17B). This may correspond to area V4 in the human brain. A lesion of this portion of the fusiform gyrus can produce cortical color blindness (hemiachromatopsia) in the contralateral visual field. Individuals with such damage may not experience severe loss of form vision, presumably because of the residual capabilities of the intact lower-order visual areas. Whereas color blindness due to the absence of certain photopigments is a common condition, color blindness due to a cortical lesion is rare because it depends on damage to a localized portion of the cortex. Larger lesions, common with infarction of the posterior cerebral artery territory, would more typically produce some form of contralateral blindness because of damage to the primary visual cortex.

Medial to the color territory, in the posterior fusiform gyrus, is a cortical area activated by viewing faces. Patients with a lesion of this posterior and medial portion of the fusiform gyrus can have the bizarre condition termed **prosopagnosia,** in which they lose the ability to recognize faces, even of persons well known to them. Similar to spatial awareness, which is preferentially organized by the right hemisphere, face recognition is also right-side dominant. However, unilateral lesions produce less marked effects. Unfortunately, bilateral vascular lesions can occur because this region is within the territory of the posterior cerebral artery. Recall that the posterior cerebral artery derives its blood supply from the basilar artery, an unpaired artery. Depending on the effectiveness of collateral circulation, basilar artery occlusion can occlude the posterior cerebral arteries bilaterally (see Chapter 4). Lesions that produce prosopagnosia also commonly produce some degree of color blindness (achromatopsia) as well as generalized object recognition impairment (agnosia). This is because vascular lesions are often large enough to encompass several distinct functional regions.

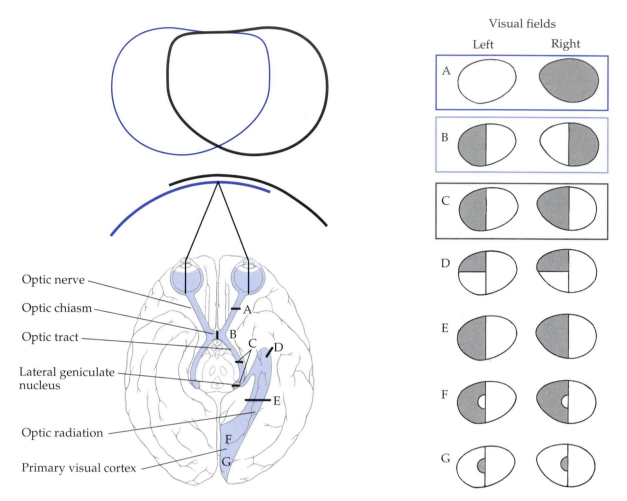

Figure 7–18. Visual field defects. The left portion of the figure illustrates schematically a horizontal view of the visual system, as if viewed from top, showing the right visual field on the right side, and the left, on the left. Visual field defects are shown to the right and are listed in Table 7–1. For each defect, the visual fields of the right and left eyes are separated. All defects are presented schematically. Rarely do such defects present as bilaterally symmetrical. ***A,*** optic nerve; ***B,*** optic chiasm; ***C,*** optic tract (which is similar to lateral geniculate nucleus); ***D,*** Meyer's loop component of optic radiations; ***E,*** main component of optic radiations; ***F*** and ***G,*** primary visual cortex (***F***—infarction producing macular sparing, ***G***—direct trauma to the occipital pole). Insets ***1–3*** show the essential circuit components of the visual pathway that are affected by the injuries shown in parts ***A, B,*** and ***C,*** respectively. ***1.*** With optic nerve damage, the nasal and temporal hemiretinae from the right eye are affected. ***2.*** With an optic chiasm lesion, the nasal hemiretinae from both eyes are affected. ***3.*** With optic tract damage, the nasal hemiretina from the left eye and the temporal hemiretina of the right eye are affected. (*Adapted from Patten H: Neurological Differential Diagnosis. Springer-Verlag, 1977.*)

from the primary auditory cortex for analyzing the spatial characteristics of sounds, such as location, and nonspatial aspects, such as language.

The Visual Field Changes in Characteristic Ways After Damage to the Visual System

The pattern of projection of retinal ganglion cells to the lateral geniculate nucleus and then to the cerebral

cortex is remarkably precise, defined by the retinotopic organization. Damage at specific locations in the visual pathway produces characteristic changes in visual perception. This section examines how clinicians can apply knowledge of the topography of retinal projections in order to localize central nervous system damage.

Functional connections in the visual system can be understood by delineating the visual field. Recall that the **visual field** corresponds to the total field of view

1

2

3

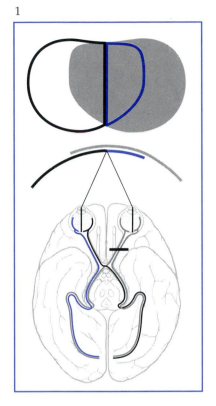

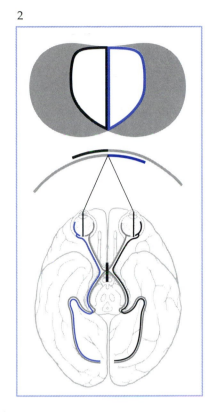

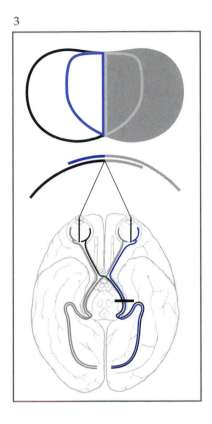

Figure 7–18 (continued.)

of both eyes when their position remains fixed (Figure 7–2). The visual fields of the two eyes overlap extensively. A change in the size and shape of the visual field—a **visual field defect**—often points to specific pathological processes in the central nervous system (Table 7–1). Such defects may reflect damage to any of six key visual system components (Figure 7–18).

Optic Nerve: Complete destruction of the optic nerve produces **blindness** in one eye (Figure 7–18A; Table 7–1); partial damage often produces a **scotoma,** a small blind spot. When a scotoma occurs in the central field of vision, for example, in the fovea, the patient notices reduced visual acuity. Remarkably, a peripheral scotoma is often unnoticed. This emphasizes the importance of foveal vision in our day-to-day activities (see below). Optic nerve damage also produces characteristic changes in the appearance of the optic disk (Figure 7–3B) because the damaged ganglion cell axons degenerate. Tumors and vascular disease commonly cause optic nerve damage.

Optic Chiasm: Ganglion cell axons from the nasal halves of the retina decussate in the optic chiasm (Figure 7–6A). These fibers transmit visual information from the temporal visual fields. A common cause for chiasmal damage is a **pituitary tumor.** The pituitary

gland is located ventral to the optic chiasm. As the tumor grows it expands dorsally, because the bony floor of the cavity in which the pituitary gland is located (the sella) is ventral to the pituitary gland. The mass encroaches on the optic chiasm from its ventral surface. This results in preferential damage of the decussating fibers and produces a **bilateral temporal visual field defect** (bitemporal heteronymous hemianopia) (Figure 7–18B; Table 7–1). Patients may not notice such a defect because it occurs in their peripheral vision. They commonly come to a physician following an accident caused by peripheral visual loss, for example, a traumatic injury incurred from the side, such as being hit by an automobile.

Optic Tract or the Lateral Geniculate Nucleus: Damage to the optic tract or the lateral geniculate nucleus, also due to tumors or a vascular accident, produces a defect in the **contralateral visual field** (homonymous hemianopia) (Figure 7–18C; Table 7–1). If a lesion is due to compression, such as produced by a tumor, the basis pedunculi can become affected (Figure 7–8C), resulting in contralateral limb motor control impairments.

Optic Radiations: Axons of lateral geniculate neurons course around the rostral and lateral surfaces of the

Table 7–1. Visual field defects.[1]

Site of lesion	Location in Figure 7–18	Deficit
Optic nerve	A	Unilateral blindness
Optic chiasm	B	Bitemporal heteronymous hemianopia
Contralateral Defects		
Optic tract	C	Homonymous hemianopia
Lateral geniculate nucleus	C	Homonymous hemianopia
Optic radiations		
Meyer's loop	D	Upper visual quadrant homonymous hemianopia (quadrantanopia)
Main radiations	E	Homonymous hemianopia
Visual cortex		
Rostral	F	Homonymous hemianopia with macular sparing
Caudal	G	Homonymous hemianopia of the macular region

[1]Visual field defects are termed *homonymous* (or congruous) if they affect similar locations for the two eyes and are termed *heteronymous* (or incongruous) if they are different. Hemianopia is loss of half of the visual field in each eye.

lateral ventricle en route to the primary visual cortex at the occipital pole (Figure 7–8A). Neurons in the medial portion of the lateral geniculate nucleus, which mediate vision from the **superior visual fields,** have axons that course rostrally into the **temporal lobe (Meyer's loop)** before they course caudally to the primary visual cortex. Temporal lobe lesions can produce a visual field defect limited to the **contralateral upper quadrant** of each visual field (quadrantanopia) (Figure 7–18D; Table 7–1). This is sometimes referred to as a "pie in the sky" defect because it is often wedge shaped. Neurons in the intermediate and lateral portions of the lateral geniculate nucleus serve the macu-

lar region and the lower visual field, respectively. Their axons have a more direct course around the ventricle and through the white matter underlying the parietal cortex. On rare occasions a lesion of the white matter within the parietal lobe can affect the optic radiations and produce visual field defects (homonymous hemianopia) (Figure 7–18E; Table 7–1).

Primary Visual Cortex: Visual space is precisely represented in the primary visual cortex (Figure 7–19). The representation of the macula lutea region of the retina (commonly termed the macular region) is caudal to the perimacular and peripheral portions. The

Figure 7–19. The primary visual cortex has a retinotopic organization in which the macula is located caudally and the perimacular and peripheral parts of the retina are represented rostrally. The portions of the left visual field (inset) are coded to match the corresponding representations in the right visual cortex.

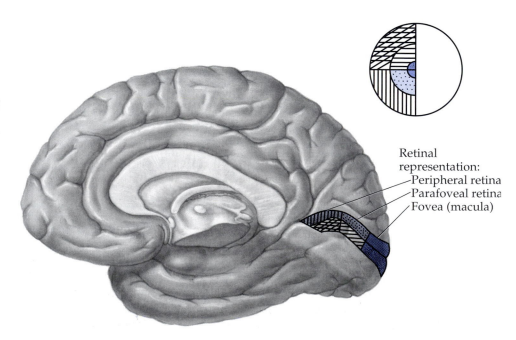

Retinal representation:
Peripheral retina
Parafoveal retina
Fovea (macula)

upper visual field is represented in the inferior bank of the calcarine fissure, and the lower visual field, in the superior bank. Although the macular region is a small portion of the retina, the area of primary visual cortex devoted to it is greatly expanded with respect to the rest of the retina. This organization is similar to the large representation of the fingertips in the primary somatic sensory cortex (see Figure 5–16).

Damage to the primary visual cortex, which commonly occurs after an infarction of the **posterior cerebral artery,** produces a **contralateral visual field** defect that often spares the **macular region** of the visual field (homonymous hemianopia with macular sparing) (Figure 7–18F; Table 7–1). Two factors contribute to **macular sparing.** First, the area of cortex that mediates central vision is so large that a single infarction, or other pathological process, rarely destroys it entirely. Second, in the case of infarctions, the arterial supply to the cortical area that serves the macular region is provided primarily by the **posterior cerebral artery,** with a collateral supply coming from the **middle cerebral artery** (see Figure 4–8). After occlusion of the posterior cerebral artery, the middle cerebral artery can rescue the macular representation. Although rare, a traumatic injury to the occipital pole can produce a defect involving only the macular region (Figure 7–18G; Table 7–1).

Summary

Retina

The retina is the peripheral portion of the visual system (Figures 7–1 and 7–4). Retinal neurons and their synaptic connections are organized into five layers. The cell bodies of photoreceptors are located in the **outer nuclear layer** (1): **Cones** are the photoreceptors for **color vision** and **high-acuity vision; rods** are for **night vision.** Photoreceptors synapse on **bipolar cells** in the **outer synaptic** (or **plexiform**) **layer** (2), but their cell bodies are located in the **inner nuclear layer** (3). Bipolar cells synapse on the **ganglion cells**—the output neurons of the retina—in the **inner synaptic** (or **plexiform**) **layer** (4). Amacrine cells and horizontal cells are the retinal interneurons that mediate lateral interactions among populations of photoreceptors, bipolar cells, and ganglion lls. Ganglion cells are located in the **ganglion cell layer** (5) (Figure 7–3). Light must pass through the ganglion cells and interneurons before reaching the photoreceptors. Müller cells are the principal retinal neuroglia.

Visual Field and Optic Nerves

The retina receives a visual image that is transformed by the optical elements of the eye (Figure 7–3): The image becomes inverted and reversed. Images from one half of the **visual field** (Figure 7–2) are projected on the **ipsilateral nasal hemiretina** and the **contralateral temporal hemiretina** (Figure 7–3). The axons from ganglion cells exit from the eye at the optic disk (Figure 7–6B). Axons from ganglion cells in the temporal hemiretina project into the **ipsilateral optic nerve** and **ipsilateral optic tract** (Figure 7–1B). Ganglion cell axons from the nasal hemiretina project into the ipsilateral optic nerve, decussate in the **optic chiasm,** and course through the **contralateral optic tract** (Figure 7–6A).

Midbrain

Ganglion cell axons destined for the midbrain leave the optic tract and course in the **brachium of superior colliculus** (Figures 7–1C and 7–7). A key midbrain site for the ganglion cell axon terminals is the **superior colliculus,** a laminated structure (Figure 7–7). The **superficial layers** of the superior colliculus mediate **visuomotor and visual reflex function,** and the **deeper layers** subserve **orientation of the eyes and head to salient stimuli.** The **pretectal nuclei,** where interneurons for the pupillary light reflex are located, also receive retinal input (Figure 7–8C; see Chapter 11).

Thalamus

The **lateral geniculate nucleus (dorsal division)** is the thalamic nucleus that receives the principal projection from the retina (Figures 7–7 and 7–8). Like other structures in the visual system, the lateral geniculate nucleus is laminated, and each of the **six layers** receives input from either the **ipsilateral** or **contralateral retina.** Visual information comes from the **contralateral visual hemifield.** The **pulvinar** and **lateral posterior nuclei** receive an ascending projection from the superior colliculus.

Visual Cortical Areas

The lateral geniculate nucleus projects to the **primary visual cortex** (Figures 7–9 and 7–10) via the **optic radiations** (Figure 7–8), which course through the white matter of the temporal, parietal, and occipital lobes. Thalamic input terminates principally in **layer**

IV (Figure 7–11)—in sublaminae A and C (Figure 7–11)—of the primary visual cortex. Input from the ipsilateral and contralateral eyes remains segregated in this layer (Figures 7–12 and 7–13). This is the anatomical substrate of the **ocular dominance columns.** Another type of column is the **orientation column** (Figure 7–14). Vertically oriented aggregates of neurons in layers II and III, centered in the ocular dominance columns, are **color-sensitive columns** (or color blobs) (Figure 7–5), the third column type.

The primary visual cortex is retinotopically organized (Figure 7–19). The primary area projects to the higher-order visual areas of the occipital, parietal, and temporal lobes (Figures 7–9 and 7–16). There are at least three functional pathways from the primary visual cortex to higher-order visual areas: (1) for perception of stimulus **form,** (2) for perception of stimulus **color** (form and color together are important for object recognition), both of which project ventrally into the temporal lobe, and (3) for perception of stimulus **motion,** which projects dorsally into the parietal lobe.

Visual Field Defects

Damage to the visual pathway produces characteristic changes in visual perception (Figure 7–18, Table 7–1): (1) complete transection of the optic nerve, **total blindness in the ipsilateral eye,** (2) optic chiasm, **bitemporal heteronymous hemianopia,** (3) optic tract and lateral geniculate nucleus, **contralateral homonymous hemianopia,** (4) optic radiation in the temporal lobe (Meyer's loop), **contralateral upper quadrant homonymous hemianopia,** (5) optic radiations in parietal and occipital lobes, **contralateral homonymous hemianopia,** and (6) primary visual cortex, **contralateral homonymous hemianopia with macular sparing.**

Related Sources

Brust JCM: The Practice of Neural Science. McGraw-Hill; 2000. (See ch. 3, p. 16; ch. 7, p. 78; ch. 9, cases 6–11; ch. 16, cases 65, 69, 70.)

Kandel ER, Wurtz RH: Constructing the visual image. In Kandel ER, Schwartz JH, Jessell TM (editors): Principles of Neural Science, 4th ed. McGraw-Hill; 2000:492–506.

Lennie P: Color vision. In Kandel ER, Schwartz JH, Jessell TM (editors): Principles of Neural Science, 4th ed. McGraw-Hill; 2000:572–589.

Tessier-Lavigne M: Visual processing in the retina. In Kandel ER, Schwartz JH, Jessell TM (editors): Principles of Neural Science, 4th ed. McGraw-Hill; 2000:507–522.

Wurtz RH, Kandel ER: Central visual pathways. In Kandel ER, Schwartz JH, Jessell TM (editors): Principles of Neural Science, 4th ed. McGraw-Hill; 2000:523–547.

Wurtz RH, Kandel ER: Perception of motion, depth, and form. In Kandel ER, Schwartz JH, Jessell TM (editors): Principles of Neural Science, 4th ed. McGraw-Hill; 2000: 548–571.

Selected Readings

Das A: Orientation in visual cortex: A simple mechanism emerges. Neuron 1996;16:477–480.

Dowling JE: The Retina: An Approachable Part of the Brain. Harvard University Press, 1987.

Merigan WH: Human V4? Curr Biol 1993;3:226–229.

Mishkin M, Ungerleider LG, Macko KA: Object vision: Two cortical pathways. Trends Neurosci 1983;6:414–416.

Patten H: Neurological Differential Diagnosis. 2nd Ed. Springer-Verlag, 1996.

Van Essen DC: Visual areas of the mammalian cerebral cortex. Annu Rev Neurosci 1979;2:227–263.

Van Essen DC, Maunsell JHR: Hierarchical organization and functional streams in the visual cortex. Trends Neurosci 1983;6:370–375.

Zeki S: A Vision of the Brain. Blackwell Scientific Publications, 1993.

References

Adams MM, Hof PR, Gattass R, Webster MJ, Ungerleider LG: Visual cortical projections and chemoarchitecture of macaque monkey pulvinar. J Comp Neurol 2000;419:377–393.

Bachevalier J, Meunier M, Lu MX, Ungerleider LG: Thalamic and temporal cortex input to medial prefrontal cortex in rhesus monkeys. Exp Brain Res 1997;115:430–444.

Baleydier C, Morel A: Segregated thalamocortical pathways to inferior parietal and inferotemporal cortex in macaque monkey. Vis Neurosci 1992;8:391–405.

Beck PD, Kaas JH: Thalamic connections of the dorsomedial visual area in primates. J Comp Neurol 1998;396:381–398.

Berne RM, Levy MN: Physiology. Mosby, 1983.

Clarke S, Miklossy J: Occipital cortex in man: Organization of callosal connections, related myelo and cytoarchitecture, and putative boundaries of functional visual areas. J Comp Neurol 1990;298:188–214.

Curcio CA, Sloan KR, Kalina RE, Hendrickson AE: Human photoreceptor topography. J Comp Neurol 1990;292:497–523.

DeYoe EA, Van Essen DC: Concurrent processing streams in monkey visual cortex. Trends Neurosci 1988;11:219–226.

Dowling JE, Boycott BB: Organization of the primate retina: Electron microscopy. Proc R Soc Lond B 1966;166:80–111.

Fox PT, Miezin FM, Allman JM, et al: Retinotopic organization of human visual cortex mapped with positron emission tomography. J Neurosci 1987;7:913–922.

Gray D, Gutierrez C, Cusick CG: Neurochemical organization of inferior pulvinar complex in squirrel monkeys and macaques revealed by acetylcholinesterase histochemistry, calbindin and Cat-301 immunostaining, and Wisteria floribunda agglutinin binding. J Comp Neurol 1999; 409:452–468.

Gutierrez C, Cola MG, Seltzer B, Cusick C: Neurochemical and connectional organization of the dorsal pulvinar complex in monkeys. J Comp Neurol 2000;419:61–86.

Hendry SH, Reid RC: The koniocellular pathway in primate vision. Annu Rev Neurosci 2000;23:127–153.

Hendry SH, Yoshioka T: A neurochemically distinct third channel in the macaque dorsal lateral geniculate nucleus. Science 1994;264:575–577.

Horton JC, Hedley-Whyte ET: Mapping of cytochrome oxidase patches and ocular dominance columns in human visual cortex. Philos Trans R Soc Lond B 1984;304:255–272.

Horton JC, Hocking DR: Effect of early monocular enucleation upon ocular dominance columns and cytochrome oxidase activity in monkey and human visual cortex. Vis Neurosci 1998;15:289–303.

Horton JC, Hocking DR: Monocular core zones and binocular border strips in primate striate cortex revealed by the contrasting effects of enucleation, eyelid suture, and retinal laser lesions on cytochrome oxidase activity. J Neurosci 1998;18:5433–5455.

Hubel DH, Wiesel TN: Ferrier lecture: Functional architecture of macaque monkey visual cortex. Proc R Soc Lond B 1977;198:1–59.

Huerta MF, Harting JK: Connectional organization of the superior colliculus. Trends Neurosci 1984;7:286–289.

Kosslyn SM, Pascual-Leone A, Felician O, et al: The role of area 17 in visual imagery: Convergent evidence from PET and rTMS. Science 1999;284:167–170.

Levitt JB: Function following form. Science 2001;292:232–233.

Livingston CA, Mustari MJ: The anatomical organization of the macaque pregeniculate complex. Brain Res 2000;876:166–179.

Livingstone MS, Hubel DH: Anatomy and physiology of a color system in the primate visual cortex. J Neurosci 1984;4:309–356.

Markowitsch HJ, Emmans D, Irle E, Streicher M, Preilowski B: Cortical and subcortical afferent connections of the primate's temporal pole: A study of rhesus monkeys, squirrel monkeys, and marmosets. J Comp Neurol 1985;242:425–458.

Merigan WH, Maunsell JHR: How parallel are the primate visual pathways? Annu Rev Neurosci 1993;16:369–402.

Newman E, Reichenbach A: The Müller cell: A functional element of the retina. Trends Neurosci 1996;19:307–312.

Robinson DL, Petersen SE: The pulvinar and visual salience. Trends Neurosci 1992;15:127–132.

Schiller PH: The superior colliculus and visual function. In Darian-Smith I (editor): Handbook of Physiology, Section 1: The Nervous System, Vol. 3. Sensory Processes. American Physiological Society; 1984:457–506.

Sereno MI, Dale AM, Reppas JB, et al: Borders of multiple visual areas in humans revealed by functional magnetic resonance imaging. Science 1995;268:889–893.

Sereno MI, Pitzalis S, Martinez A: Mapping of contralateral space in retinotopic coordinates by a parietal cortical area in humans. Science 2001;294:1350–1354.

Soares JG, Gattass R, Souza AP, Rosa MG, Fiorani M Jr., Brandao BL: Connectional and neurochemical subdivisions of the pulvinar in Cebus monkeys. Vis Neurosci 2001;18:25–41.

Stepniewska I, Qi HX, Kaas JH: Do superior colliculus projection zones in the inferior pulvinar project to MT in primates? Eur J Neurosci 1999;11:469–480.

Stepniewska I, Qi HX, Kaas JH: Projections of the superior colliculus to subdivisions of the inferior pulvinar in New World and Old World monkeys. Vis Neurosci 2000;17:529–549.

Yabuta NH, Sawatari A, Callaway EM: Two functional channels from primary visual cortex to dorsal visual cortical areas. Science 2001;292:297–300.

Yeterian EH, Pandya DN: Corticothalamic connections of extrastriate visual areas in rhesus monkeys. J Comp Neurol 1997;378:562–585.

Yoshioka T, Levitt JB, Lund JS: Independence and merger of thalamocortical channels within macaque monkey primary visual cortex: Anatomy of interlaminar projections. Vis Neurosci 1994;11:467–489.

Zeki S, Watson JDG, Lueck CJ, et al: A direct demonstration of functional specialization in human visual cortex. J Neurosci 1991;11:641–649.

8

The Auditory System

T*HE AUDITORY SYSTEM MEDIATES THE SENSE* of hearing. The sensory experience described as hearing is as broad as the sound spectrum itself. From signals of impending danger, like a car horn, to the pleasing sounds that fill a concert hall, much of our daily behavior is determined by the sounds around us. The auditory system is also our principal communication portal, allowing us to understand speech. This system, like the somatic sensory and visual systems, has a topographic organization determined by the peripheral receptive sheet. And similar to the other systems, the auditory system consists of multiple parallel pathways that engage multiple cortical regions, either directly or via complex corticocortical networks. Each auditory pathway is hierarchically organized and has the connections and properties to mediate different aspects of hearing.

The complexity of the auditory pathways derives from the particular properties of natural sounds, with their diverse frequency characteristics, multiple sources of origin, and large dynamic ranges. However, an added measure of complexity is imposed on the human auditory system by the demands of understanding speech. Although the physical characteristics of a spoken word may not be any more complex than many nonlinguistic sounds, the linguistic quality of the stimulus engages unique cortical areas.

This chapter first considers the general organization of the auditory system. Then it examines key levels through the brain stem, where auditory information is processed. Finally, the connections of the auditory system with the thalamus and cerebral cortex are examined.

FUNCTIONAL ANATOMY OF THE AUDITORY SYSTEM

Parallel Ascending Auditory Pathways May Be Involved in Different Aspects of Hearing

The process of hearing begins on the body surface, as sounds are conducted by the auricle and external auditory meatus to the tympanic membrane. Mechanical displacement of the tympanic membrane, produced by changes in sound pressure waves, is transmitted to the inner ear by tiny bones termed the middle ear ossicles (see Figure 8–2). The inner ear transductive machinery is located within the temporal bone in a coiled structure called the **cochlea.** This is the location of the auditory receptors, termed **hair cells** because they each have a cilia or hair bundle on their apical surface. Each auditory receptor is sensitive to a limited frequency range of sounds. Hair cells in the human cochlea are not mitotically replaced, and their numbers decline throughout life. This reduction results from conditions such as ear infections, exposure to loud sounds or drugs with ototoxic properties, and aging.

A topographic relationship exists between the location of a hair cell in the cochlea and the sound frequency to which the receptor is most sensitive. As discussed below, from the base of the cochlea to the apex, the frequency to which a hair cell is maximally sensitive changes systematically from high frequencies to low frequencies. This differential frequency sensitivity of hair cells along the length of the cochlea is the basis of the **tonotopic organization** of the auditory receptive sheet. Many of the components of the auditory system are tonotopically organized. The topographic relationship between the receptor sheet and the central nervous system is similar to that of the somatic sensory and visual systems, where the subcortical nuclei and cortical areas have a somatotopic or retinotopic organization. In each of these cases, the topographic organization of the central representations is determined by the spatial organization of the peripheral receptive sheet. An important difference exists, however. The receptor sheets of the somatic sensory and visual systems are spatial maps representing stimulus location (eg, hand versus foot, macular versus peripheral). The cochlea represents the frequency of sounds. Sound source localization is computed by central nervous system auditory neurons, on the basis of the timing, loudness, and spectral characteristics of sounds (see below).

Hair cells are innervated by the distal processes of bipolar primary sensory neurons located in the **spiral ganglion.** The central processes of the bipolar neurons form the **cochlear division** of the **vestibulocochlear nerve (cranial nerve VIII).** These axons project to the ipsilateral **cochlear nuclei** (Figure 8–1), which are located in the rostral medulla.

The cochlear nuclei consist of the ventral cochlear nucleus, which has anterior and posterior subdivisions, and the dorsal cochlear nucleus. Neurons in these three components have distinct connections with the rest of the auditory system and give rise to parallel auditory pathways that serve different aspects of hearing. A key function of the anteroventral division of the cochlear nucleus is **horizontal localization of sound.** The posteroventral division contributes to a system of connections that regulate **hair cell sensitivity.** The two divisions of the ventral cochlear nucleus project to the **superior olivary complex,** a cluster of nuclei in the caudal pons. Most neurons in the superior olivary complex project via an ascending pathway called the **lateral lemniscus** to the **inferior colliculus,** located in the midbrain. The projection from the ventral cochlear nucleus to the inferior colliculus is bilateral. The dorsal cochlear nucleus is thought to play a role in identifying **sound source elevation.** It projects directly to the contralateral **inferior colliculus,** also via the lateral lemniscus. The inferior colliculus is the site of convergence of all lower brain stem auditory nuclei. It is tonotopically organized and contains a spatial map of the location of sounds.

In sequence, the next segment of the ascending auditory pathway is the **medial geniculate nucleus,** the thalamic auditory relay nucleus. The medial geniculate nucleus projects to the primary auditory cortex, located within the lateral sulcus (also called the Sylvian fissure) on the superior surface of the temporal lobe. The primary auditory cortex contains multiple tonotopically organized territories, all located on **Heschl's gyri** (Figure 8–1B, inset; see Figure 8–8). The primary cortex forms a central core surrounded by multiple **secondary auditory areas.** Neurons in the primary area are activated by simple tones, whereas those in the secondary areas are better activated by complex sounds. In animals, neurons in these areas are also activated by species-specific calls. The secondary areas are surrounded by several **higher-order auditory areas,** located on the superior and lateral surfaces of the temporal lobe in the **superior temporal gyrus** and **sulcus** (Figure 8–1B). This is where several areas are located that are important for understanding speech (see below).

The auditory pathways contain decussations and commissures—where axons cross the midline—at multiple levels, so that sounds from one ear are processed by both sides of the brain. What is the clinical significance of this bilateral organization of cen-

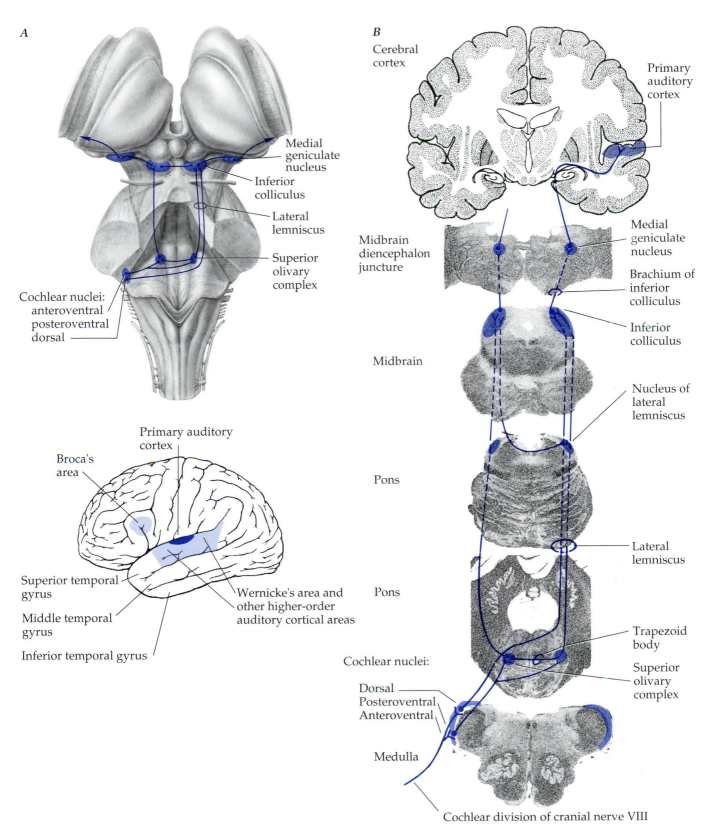

Figure 8–1. *A.* Dorsal view of brain stem, illustrating the organization of major components of the auditory system. *B.* Organization of the auditory system revealed in cross section at different levels through the brain stem and in coronal section through the diencephalon and cerebral hemispheres. The inset shows the auditory and speech-related areas of the cerebral cortex. Wernicke's area, for understanding speech, is located in the superior temporal gyrus. Broca's area, for articulating speech, is located in the inferior frontal gyrus. Heschl's gyri are located within the lateral sulcus and cannot be seen on the surface.

tral auditory connections? Unilateral brain damage does not cause deafness in one ear unless the injury destroys the cochlear nuclei or the entering fascicles of the cochlear nerve. Unilateral deafness is thus a sign of injury to the peripheral auditory organ or the cochlear nerve. In addition to being clinically important, the bilateral representation of sounds has a more general significance in providing a mechanism for sound localization (see below) and enhancing the detection of sounds through summation of converging inputs.

■ REGIONAL ANATOMY OF THE AUDITORY SYSTEM

The Auditory Sensory Organs Are Located Within the Membranous Labyrinth

The membranous labyrinth is a complex sac within the bony labyrinth, cavities in the petrous portion of the temporal bone (Figure 8–2). The membranous labyrinth consists of the auditory sensory organ, the **cochlea,** and five vestibular sensory organs, the three **semicircular canals** and the **saccule** and **utricle** (Figure 8–2A). (Another name for the semicircular canals, utricle, and saccule is the vestibular labyrinth.) The morphological complexity of the auditory and vestibular sensory organs rivals that of the eyeball. Vestibular sensory organs mediate our sense of acceleration, such as during takeoff in a jet, and are important in balance and eye movement control. The vestibular system is considered in Chapter 12.

Much of the membranous labyrinth is filled with **endolymph,** an extracellular fluid resembling intracellular fluid in its ionic constituents. Endolymph has a high potassium concentration and low sodium concentration. In contrast, **perilymph,** a fluid resembling extracellular fluid and cerebrospinal fluid, fills the space between the membranous labyrinth and the temporal bone.

The cochlea is a coiled structure about 30 mm long (Figure 8–2A). The hair cells are located in the **organ of Corti,** a specialized portion of the cochlear duct that rests on the **basilar membrane** (Figure 8–2C). Hair cells of the organ of Corti are covered by the **tectorial membrane** (Figure 8–2C). The basilar membrane, hair cells, and tectorial membrane collectively form the basic auditory transductive apparatus. Two kinds of hair cells are found in the organ of Corti, and their names reflect their position with respect to the axis of the coiled cochlea: **inner** and **outer hair cells.** Inner hair cells are arranged in a single row, whereas outer hair cells are arranged in three or four rows.

Although there are fewer inner than outer hair cells (approximately 3500 versus 12,000), the inner hair cells are responsible for frequency and other fine discriminations in hearing. This is because most of the axons in the cochlear division of cranial nerve XIII innervate the inner hair cells. Each inner hair cell is innervated by as many as ten auditory nerve fibers, and each auditory fiber contacts only a single, or at most a few, inner hair cells. This is a high-resolution system, like that of the innervation of the fingertips and the fovea. By contrast, only a small fraction of auditory nerve fibers innervates the outer hair cell population. Each fiber branches to contact multiple outer hair cells. Research has shown that outer hair cells could be important as **efferent** structures, modulating the sensitivity of the organ of Corti (see the section on the olivocochlear system, below).

The organ of Corti transduces sounds into neural signals. This organ is mechanically coupled to the external environment by the tympanic membrane and the middle ear ossicles (malleus, incus, and stapes) (Figure 8–2A). Pressure changes in the external auditory meatus, resulting from sound waves, cause the **tympanic membrane** to vibrate. The **middle ear ossicles**—the **malleus, incus,** and **stapes**—conduct the external pressure changes from the tympanic membrane to the **scala vestibuli** of the inner ear (Figure 8–2B). These pressure changes are conducted from the scala vestibuli through the fluid to the other compartments of the cochlea, the **scala media** to the **scala tympani** (Figure 8–2B). Pressure changes resulting from sounds set up a traveling wave along the compliant **basilar membrane** (Figure 8–2C), on which the hair cells and their support structures rest. Because the hair cells have hair bundles that are embedded in the less compliant **tectorial membrane,** the traveling wave results in shearing forces between the two membranes. These shearing forces cause the hair bundles to bend, resulting in a membrane conductance change in the hair cells.

Hearing thus depends on movement of the basilar membrane produced by sounds. Outer hair cells can enhance this movement, thereby amplifying the signal generated by the organ of Corti in response to sound. They do so by changing their length in response to sounds (see section on the olivocochlear system, below). This results in a small additional displacement of the basilar membrane that increases the mechanical oscillation produced by changes in sound pressure on the tympanic membrane.

The traveling wave on the basilar membrane, established by changes in sound pressure impinging on the ear resulting from sounds, is extraordinarily complex. High-frequency sounds generate a wave on

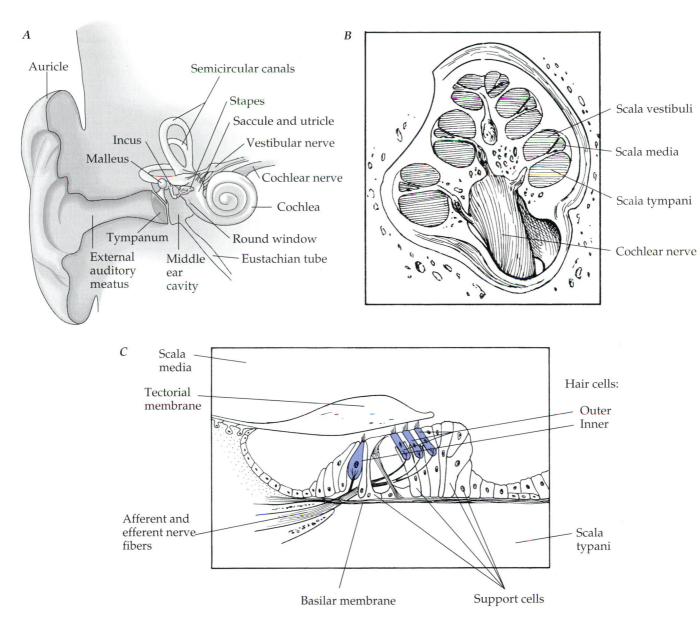

Figure 8–2. Structure of the human ear. ***A.*** The external ear (auricle) focuses sounds into the external auditory meatus. Alternating increasing and decreasing air pressure vibrates the tympanum (ear drum). These vibrations are conducted across the middle ear by the three ear ossicles: malleus, incus, and stapes. Vibration of the stapes stimulates the cochlea. ***B.*** Cut-away view of the cochlea, showing the three coiled channels: scala vestibuli, scala media, and scala tympani. ***C.*** Expanded view of a section through the cochlear duct, illustrating the organ of Corti. (***A,*** *Adapted from Hudspeth AJ: Hearing. In Kandel ER, Schwartz JH, Jessell TM (editors): Principles of Neural Science, 4th ed. McGraw-Hill; 2000:590–613,* ***C,*** *Adapted from Dallos P: Peripheral mechanisms of hearing. In Darian-Smith I (editor): Handbook of Physiology, Section 1: The Nervous System, Vol. 3. Sensory Processes. American Physiological Society; 1984:595–637.)*

the basilar membrane with a peak amplitude close to the base of the cochlea; consequently, these sounds preferentially activate the **basal hair cells.** As the frequency of the sound source decreases, the location of the peak amplitude of the wave on the basilar membrane shifts continuously toward the **cochlear apex.**

This results in the preferential activation of hair cells that are located closer to the cochlear apex. Although the mechanical properties of the basilar membrane are a key determinant of the auditory tuning of hair cells and the tonotopic organization of the organ of Corti, other factors play important roles. For example, the length of the hair bundle varies with position within the cochlea. The bundles act as miniature tuning forks: The shorter bundles are tuned to high frequencies (and are located on hair cells at the cochlear base), whereas the longer bundles are tuned to low frequencies (and are located on hair cells at the apex).

The electrical membrane characteristics of hair cells also contribute to frequency tuning. As is discussed in the next section, the tonotopic organization underlies the topography of connections in the central auditory pathways.

The Topography of Connections Between Brain Stem Auditory Nuclei Provides Insight Into the Functions of Parallel Ascending Auditory Pathways

The brain stem has three major auditory relay nuclei: the **cochlear nuclei,** where the auditory nerve from the ipsilateral ear terminates; the **superior olivary nuclear complex,** which receives auditory information from the cochlear nuclei on both sides of the brain stem; and the **inferior colliculus,** where information from different brain stem auditory nuclei is integrated. Each of these nuclei is located in a different brain stem division: The cochlear nuclei are located in the medulla, the superior olivary nuclei in the pons, and the inferior colliculus in the midbrain. Knowing the connections among auditory relay nuclei is an essential first step toward understanding the anatomical substrates of hearing.

The Cochlear Nuclei Are the First Central Nervous System Relays for Auditory Information

The three divisions of the cochlear nuclei—dorsal, anteroventral, and posteroventral (Figure 8–3C)—each have a tonotopic organization. They also have different patterns of efferent connections and functions, which are discussed further in the next two sections. The anteroventral cochlear nucleus projects bilaterally to the **superior olivary complex,** for horizontal sound localization. The posteroventral cochlear nucleus also projects to the superior olivary complex, where it engages a system for regulating hair cell sensitivity. The dorsal cochlear nucleus, important for vertical sound localization, projects directly to the **inferior colliculus,** bypassing the superior olivary complex.

Most of the axons from each division of the cochlear nucleus decussate and reach the superior olivary complex or the inferior colliculus by a different pathway.

Axons from the dorsal cochlear nucleus course in the dorsal acoustic stria. Axons from the posteroventral cochlear nucleus decussate in both the intermediate acoustic stria and the **trapezoid body** (located most ventral), whereas those from the anteroventral cochlear nucleus cross over only in the trapezoid body. Of the three auditory decussations, only the trapezoid body can be readily discerned. It is present on a myelin-stained section through the caudal pons (Figure 8–3B). The trapezoid body obscures the medial lemniscus at this level.

The cochlear nucleus is the most central site in which a lesion can produce deafness in the **ipsilateral ear.** This is because it receives a projection from only the ipsilateral ear. Lesions of the other central auditory nuclei do not produce deafness, because at each of these sites there is convergence of auditory inputs from both ears. The **anterior inferior cerebellar artery** supplies the cochlear nuclei, and unilateral occlusion can produce deafness in one ear (see Figures 4–1 and 4–3A).

The Superior Olivary Complex Processes Stimuli From Both Ears for Horizontal Localization

The **superior olivary complex** contains three major components (Figure 8–3B): the medial superior olivary nucleus, the lateral superior olivary nucleus, and the nucleus of the trapezoid body. The superior olivary complex should be distinguished from the inferior olivary nucleus (Figure 8–3C), which contains neurons that are important in movement control (see Chapter 13).

The superior olivary complex receives input primarily from the anteroventral cochlear nucleus, and together these structures give rise to the pathway for **horizontal localization of sounds.** To understand how the anatomical connections between the anteroventral cochlear nucleus and the superior olivary complex contribute to this function, consider how sounds in the horizontal plane are localized. A sound is recognized as coming from one side of the head or the other by two means, depending on its frequency. **Low-frequency sounds** activate the two ears at slightly different times, producing a characteristic **interaural time difference.** The farther a sound source is located from the midline, the greater the interaural time difference. For **high-frequency sounds,** the interaural timing difference is an ambiguous cue. However, the head acts as a shield and attenuates these sounds. A high-frequency sound arriving at the distant ear is softer than at the closer ear. This is because

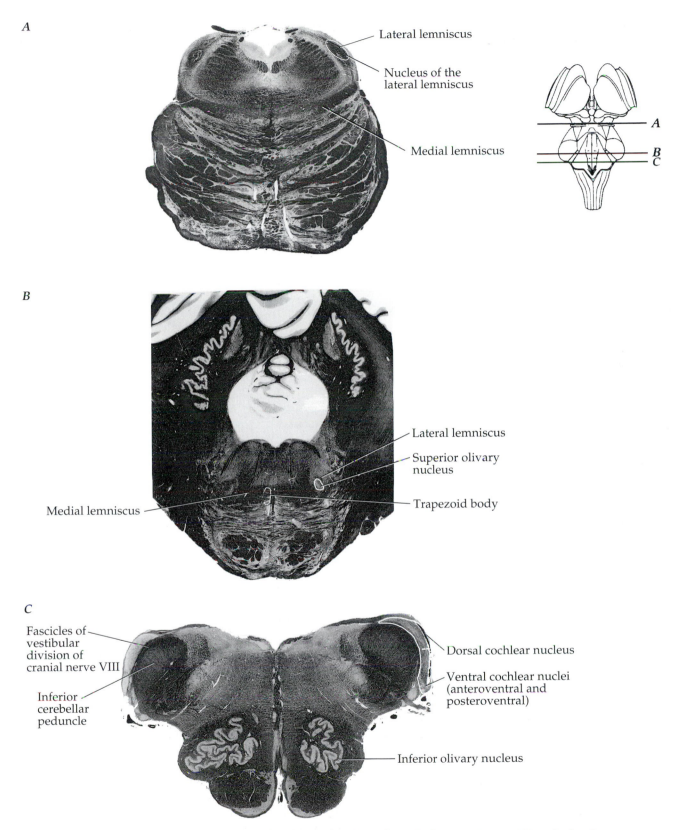

A

Lateral lemniscus

Nucleus of the
lateral lemniscus

Medial lemniscus

A
B
C

B

Lateral lemniscus

Superior olivary
nucleus

Trapezoid body

Medial lemniscus

C

Fascicles of
vestibular
division of
cranial nerve VIII

Inferior
cerebellar
peduncle

Dorsal cochlear nucleus

Ventral cochlear nuclei
(anteroventral and
posteroventral)

Inferior olivary nucleus

Figure 8–3. Myelin-stained transverse sections through the rostral pons (*A*) at the level of the caudal pons (*B*) and cochlear nuclei (*C*). The inset shows the planes of section.

sound energy is absorbed by the head, resulting in an **interaural intensity difference.** This is the duplex theory of sound localization because the mechanisms for low and high frequencies differ.

There are distinct neuroanatomical substrates for the localization of low- and high-frequency sounds. Neurons in the **medial superior olivary nucleus** are sensitive to **interaural time differences,** and in accord with the duplex theory, they respond selectively to low-frequency tones. Individual neurons in the medial superior olive receive monosynaptic connections from the anteroventral cochlear nuclei on both sides, but these inputs are spatially segregated on their medial and lateral dendrites (Figure 8–4). This segregation of inputs is thought to underlie the sensitivity to interaural time differences. In contrast, neurons in the **lateral superior olivary nucleus** are sensitive to **interaural intensity differences,** and they are tuned to high-frequency stimuli. Sensitivity to interaural intensity differences is thought to be determined by convergence of a monosynaptic excitatory input from the ipsilateral anteroventral cochlear nucleus and a disynaptic inhibitory connection from the contralateral anteroventral cochlear nucleus, relayed through the **nucleus of the trapezoid body** (Figure 8–4).

Sounds can also be localized along the vertical axis. Here the structure of the external ear is important. The ridges in the auricle reflect sound pressure in complex ways, creating sound spectra that depend on the direction of the source. Specialized neurons within the dorsal cochlear nucleus appear to use this information to determine the elevation of the sound source. Not surprisingly, the ascending projection of the dorsal cochlear nuclei bypasses the superior olivary complex to reach the inferior colliculus directly.

The Olivocochlear System May Regulate Hair Cell Sensitivity

Some neurons in the superior olivary complex are not directly involved in processing the horizontal location of the source of sounds. These neurons receive auditory information from the posteroventral cochlear nucleus and give rise to axons that project back to the cochlea via the vestibulocochlear nerve. This efferent pathway is called the **olivocochlear bundle.** This **olivocochlear projection** is thought to regulate hair cell sensitivity.

The olivocochlear control system affects the outer and inner hair cells differently. The outer hair cells receive dense synaptic connections directly from the axons of the olivocochlear bundle. In-vitro studies have shown that outer hair cells contract when acetylcholine, a neurotransmitter of the olivocochlear projection, is directly applied to the receptor cell. This mechanical change can modulate cochlea sensitivity and frequency tuning by boosting the basilar membrane traveling wave. Olivocochlear efferents do not synapse on the inner hair cells. Rather, they make inhibitory synapses on auditory nerve fiber terminals that innervate the inner hair cells.

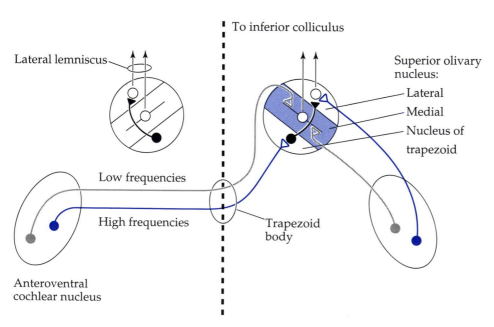

Figure 8–4. Key connections between the cochlear nuclei in the medulla and the superior olivary complex in the pons. Low-frequency tones are conducted over the gray pathway and high-frequency tones, over the blue pathway. Within the superior olivary complex, neurons with open cell bodies and terminals are excitatory, while those with black-filled cell bodies and terminals are inhibitory.

To inferior colliculus

Lateral lemniscus

Superior olivary nucleus:
- Lateral
- Medial
- Nucleus of trapezoid

Low frequencies

High frequencies

Trapezoid body

Anteroventral cochlear nucleus

Auditory Brain Stem Axons Ascend in the Lateral Lemniscus

The **lateral lemniscus** is the ascending brain stem auditory pathway (Figure 8–3A,B). (The lateral lemniscus should be distinguished from the medial lemniscus [Figure 8–3B], which relays somatic sensory information to the thalamus.) The lateral lemniscus carries axons from the contralateral dorsal and posteroventral cochlear nuclei and from the superior olivary complex (medial and lateral nuclei) to the inferior colliculus (Figure 8–5). Many of the axons in the lateral lemniscus, especially those from part of the ventral cochlear nucleus, also send collateral (ie, side) branches into the **nucleus of the lateral lemniscus** (Figure 8–3A). Ventral cochlear neurons that project to the nucleus of the lateral lemniscus process sound characteristics that are important for understanding speech. The nucleus of the lateral lemniscus is another site in the auditory pathway where information crosses the midline.

The Inferior Colliculus Is Located in the Midbrain Tectum

The inferior colliculus is located on the dorsal surface of the midbrain, caudal to the superior colliculus (Figure 8–5A). The inferior colliculus is an auditory relay nucleus where virtually all ascending fibers in the lateral lemniscus synapse. Recall that the superior colliculus is part of the visual system. It is not a relay

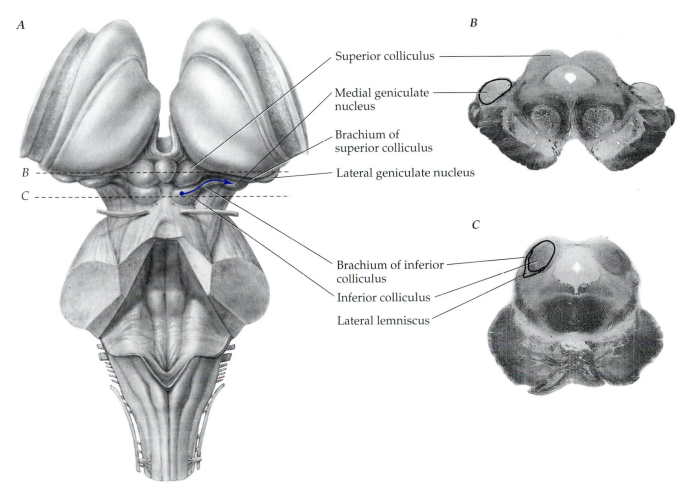

A

B

Superior colliculus

Medial geniculate nucleus

Brachium of superior colliculus

Lateral geniculate nucleus

C

Brachium of inferior colliculus

Inferior colliculus

Lateral lemniscus

Figure 8–5. The inferior colliculi and medial geniculate nuclei are shown on the surface of the brain stem view (*A*) and in myelin-stained transverse sections through the rostral (*B*) and caudal (*C*) midbrain. The dashed lines indicate the planes of section in *B* and *C*.

nucleus but, rather, participates in visuomotor control (see Chapter 12). Although the two colliculi look similar on myelin-stained sections, they can be distinguished by the configuration of structures within the center of the midbrain at the two levels. The superior and inferior colliculi are cut parasagittally in the myelin-stained section in Figure 8–6.

Three component nuclei comprise the inferior colliculus: the central and external nuclei and the dorsal cortex. The **central nucleus** of the inferior colliculus is the principal site of termination of the lateral lemniscus. This nucleus receives convergent input from three sources: (1) pathways originating from the ipsilateral and contralateral **superior olivary nuclei,** (2) the direct pathway from the contralateral **dorsal cochlear nucleus,** and (3) axons from the ipsilateral and contralateral **nucleus of the lateral lemniscus.** The central nucleus receives convergent inputs from the anteroventral and dorsal cochlear nuclei, which participate in horizontal and vertical sound source localization, respectively. Reflecting this convergence, the central nucleus contains a map of auditory space.

The central nucleus is **tonotopically organized** and **laminated** (although not apparent on myelin-stained sections): Neurons in a single lamina are maximally sensitive to **similar tonal frequencies.** Lamination of neurons and the presynaptic terminals of ascending auditory fibers is the structural basis for tonotopy in the central nucleus. As in the somatic sensory and visual systems, lamination is used in the auditory system for packaging neurons with similar functional attributes or connections. The central nucleus gives

rise to a tonotopically organized ascending auditory pathway to the thalamus, which continues to the primary auditory cortex.

The functions of the **external nucleus** are not well understood. Animal studies suggest that it participates in **acousticomotor function,** such as orienting the head and body axis to auditory stimuli. This function of the external nucleus may use somatic sensory information, which is also projected to this nucleus from the spinal cord and medulla, via the spinotectal and trigeminotectal tracts. The functions of the **dorsal cortex** are not known. The external nucleus and dorsal cortex give rise to diffuse ascending thalamocortical pathways.

The tract through which the inferior colliculus projects to the thalamus is located just beneath the dorsal surface of the midbrain, the **brachium of inferior colliculus** (Figure 8–5A). As different as the superior and inferior colliculi are, so too are their brachia. The brachium of superior colliculus brings afferent information to the superior colliculus, whereas that of the inferior colliculus is an efferent pathway carrying axons away from the inferior colliculus to the medial geniculate nucleus (see next section).

The Medial Geniculate Nucleus Contains a Division That Is Tonotopically Organized

The **medial geniculate nucleus** is the thalamic auditory relay nucleus. It is located on the inferior surface of the thalamus, medial to the visual relay, the

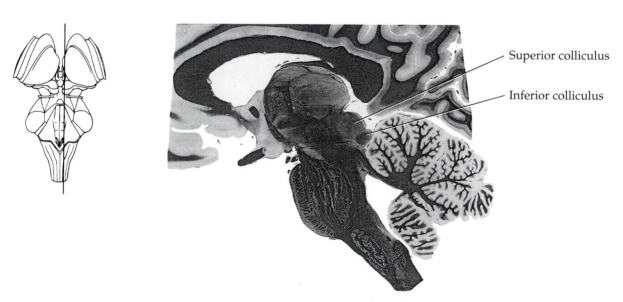

Superior colliculus

Inferior colliculus

Figure 8–6. The superior and inferior colliculi can be identified on this sagittal section through the brain stem.

lateral geniculate nucleus (Figure 8–5A). The medial geniculate nucleus is composed of several divisions, but only the ventral division is the principal auditory relay nucleus (Figure 8–7). This component, referred to simply as the medial geniculate nucleus, is the only portion that is tonotopically organized. It receives the major ascending auditory projection from the central nucleus of the inferior colliculus. Although not observable on the myelin-stained section in Figure 8–7, the ventral division of the medial geniculate nucleus is laminated. Like the central nucleus of the inferior colliculus, individual laminae in the medial geniculate nucleus contain neurons that are maximally sensitive to similar frequencies. The medial geniculate nucleus terminates predominantly in layers III and IV of primary auditory cortex.

The other divisions of the medial geniculate nucleus (dorsal and medial) receive inputs from the three components of the inferior colliculus as well as somatic sensory and visual information. Rather than relay auditory information to the cortex, they seem to serve more integrated functions, such as participating in arousal mechanisms. (The dorsal division is shown in Figure AII–15.)

The Auditory Cortical Areas Are Located on the Superior Surface of the Temporal Lobe

The auditory cortical areas have a concentric and hierarchical organization. The primary cortex is surrounded by the secondary auditory cortex, which is surrounded by the higher-order auditory areas (Figure 8–8). The primary cortex, receiving direct thalamic inputs, processes basic auditory stimulus attributes, such as simple tones, and is the lowest level of the cortical auditory hierarchy (Figure 8–9). The secondary areas, receiving their principal input from the primary areas, and the higher-order areas, receiving input from the secondary areas, process progressively more complex aspects of sounds (Figure 8–9). In animals, neurons in the secondary auditory cortex respond to species-specific calls, and in humans, higher-order auditory areas respond specifically to speech.

The Primary Auditory Cortex Has a Tonotopic Organization

The primary auditory cortex (cytoarchitectonic area 41) is located in the temporal lobe within the lateral sulcus, on **Heschl's gyri** (Figures 8–8 and 8–9). These gyri, which vary in number from one to several depending on the side of the brain and the individual, run obliquely from the lateral surface of the cortex medially to the insular region (Figure 8–9). The orientation of Heschl's gyri is nearly orthogonal to the gyri on the lateral surface of the temporal lobe. The primary auditory cortex is tonotopically organized along the axis of Heschl's gyri, from low frequencies lateral to high frequencies medial (Figure 8–8). Although not yet well characterized in humans, several tonotopically organized subregions are found within this primary sensory area. This organization of multiple rep-

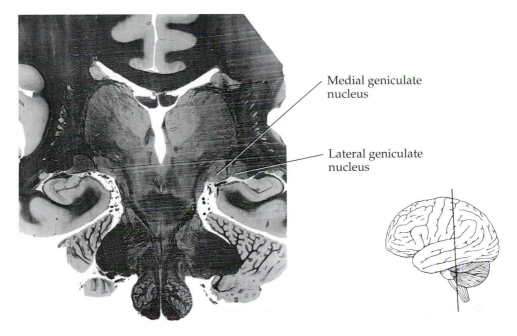

Figure 8–7. Myelin-stained coronal section through the medial geniculate nucleus. The inset shows the plane of section.

Medial geniculate nucleus

Lateral geniculate nucleus

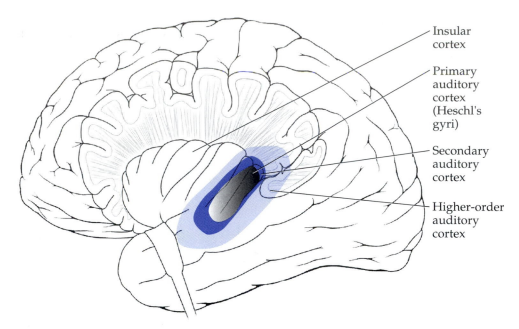

Insular
cortex

Primary
auditory
cortex
(Heschl's
gyri)

Secondary
auditory
cortex

Higher-order
auditory
cortex

Figure 8–8. The auditory areas are indicated. The primary auditory cortex has a tonotopic organization, from high frequencies medially (dark gray) to low frequencies laterally (white). The secondary cortex surrounds the primary cortex; the higher-order auditory areas surround the secondary areas. The auditory areas are located within the lateral sulcus and extend onto the lateral surface.

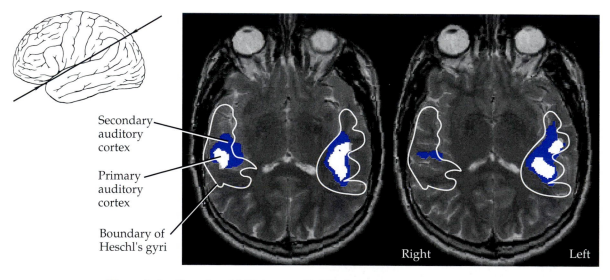

Secondary
auditory
cortex

Primary
auditory
cortex

Boundary of
Heschl's gyri

Right   Left

Figure 8–9. Functional MR images (fMRI) showing activation of the human auditory cortex. The image on the left is slightly more ventral than the one on the right. The white region corresponds approximately to the primary auditory cortex; this area responds to both pure and complex tones (ie, relatively nonselective). The surrounding blue area corresponds to secondary auditory cortex (ie, surrounding belt), which responds preferentially to complex sounds. Small gray areas correspond to sites responding to pure tones only. *(Courtesy of Dr. Josef Rauschecker, Georgetown University; adapted from Wessinger CM, VanMeter J, Tian B, Van Lare J, Pekar J, Rauschecker JP: Hierarchical organization of the human auditory cortex revealed by functional magnetic resonance imaging. J Cogn Neurosci 2001;13:1–7.)*

resentations of the receptor sheet may be similar to the primary somatic sensory cortex, which has multiple somatotopically organized subdivisions (see Figure 5–19). As in other sensory cortical areas, primary auditory cortex has a columnar (or vertical) organization: Neurons sensitive to similar frequencies are arranged across all six layers, from the pial surface to the white matter. Within the primary cortex, neurons represent other features of auditory stimuli, including particular binaural interactions, stimulus timing, and additional tuning characteristics.

Secondary and Higher-order Auditory Areas Give Rise to Projections for Distinguishing the Location and Other Characteristics of Sounds

Although there are myriad cortical auditory areas, up to 15 by some counts, there may be two major streams of auditory information flow. Research in animals, using anatomical tracing techniques, and in humans, using noninvasive functional imaging techniques, has revealed a dual set of cortical networks, strikingly similar to the "what" and "where" visual pathways (see Figure 7–16). The pathway for auditory spatial localization, or "where," originates from the primary cortex and projects to caudal portions the secondary and then higher-order areas (Figure 8–10). This pathway projects to the **posterior parietal lobe** and to the **dorsolateral prefrontal cortex.** The posterior parietal lobe contains a spatial map of extrapersonal space that, together with the prefrontal area, may be used for planning movements to particular targets.

Although the other auditory pathway does not seem to participate in the localization of sounds, its precise function is not well defined. It is thought to be the verbal **"what"** pathway. Also originating from the primary auditory cortex but projecting to rostral portions of the secondary and higher-order areas, this pathway engages more **ventral** and **medial prefrontal cortical areas** (Figure 8–10). These frontal areas are involved in visual object identification, processing of complex sounds, and linguistic functions (see next section). The distinction between spatial and nonspatial streams (ie, where and what) is particularly intriguing for understanding speech mechanisms because the ventral frontal lobe in humans is the location of the motor speech area.

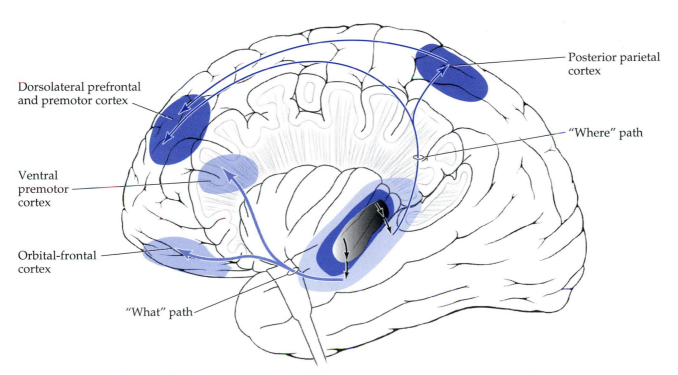

Figure 8–10. Separate "what" and "where" pathways originate from the auditory cortex and project to different regions of the prefrontal cortex and parietal cortex.

Cortical Areas in the Human Selectively Process Speech

Several higher-order auditory cortical areas on the lateral surface of the left temporal lobe in the human brain (cytoarchitectonic areas 42 and 22) comprise important substrates for understanding speech. It is well-known that, in most humans, damage to the left temporal lobe produces an impairment in **understanding speech.** This has been attributed to an interruption in the function of **Wernicke's area** (posterior area 22) (Figures 8–1B, inset; and 8–9). In the right temporal lobe the equivalent cortex is a higher-order auditory area involved in interpreting the emotional content of language—for instance, noting the anger in a person's voice—not speech per se. Whereas Wernicke's area and other linguistic regions in the left temporal lobe are important in the sensory processing underlying speech, **Broca's area** in the left inferior frontal gyrus (including the frontal operculum; corresponding approximately to cytoarchitectonic area 44) is the **motor speech** area (Figure 8–1B, inset).

Consistent with the long-standing finding that in most humans the left cerebral hemisphere is specialized for linguistic function, functional imaging studies have shown that the left temporal lobe becomes activated when people listen to speech or read. In addition to Wernicke's area, more anterior areas also become active when humans listen to speech sounds. One area in the rostral temporal lobe that is specifically activated by speech is located in the superior temporal sulcus, anterior and lateral to the primary auditory cortex. This area may correspond to the region that gives rise to the verbal "what" pathway to the ventral frontal lobe.

Summary

Peripheral Auditory Apparatus

The auditory transductive apparatus, the **organ of Corti,** is located in the **cochlea,** a coiled structure within the temporal bone (Figure 8–2A,B). The **hair cells** (Figure 8–2C) are the auditory receptors. They are organized into a receptive sheet within the cochlea. This sheet has a precise **tonotopic organization:** Receptors sensitive to high frequencies are located near the cochlear base, and those sensitive to low frequencies are located near the apex. The hair cells are innervated by the peripheral processes of **bipolar cells,** whose cell bodies are located in the spiral ganglion. The central processes of the bipolar cells collect into the **cochlear division** of the **vestibulocochlear (VIII) nerve** (Figure 8–1).

Medulla and Pons

The cochlear division of the vestibulocochlear nerve synapses in the **cochlear nuclei.** The cochlear nuclei, which are located in the **rostral medulla,** have three main divisions (Figures 8–1A and 8–3C): the **anteroventral cochlear nucleus,** the **posteroventral cochlear nucleus,** and the **dorsal cochlear nucleus.** Many neurons in the anteroventral cochlear nucleus project to the **superior olivary complex** in the pons (Figures 8–3B and 8–4), on either the ipsilateral or the contralateral side. Neurons in the superior olivary complex project to either the ipsilateral or the contralateral inferior colliculus via the lateral lemniscus. Some of these decussating axons form a discrete commissure, the **trapezoid body** (Figures 8–3B and 8–4). The function of this pathway is in the **horizontal localization of sounds.** The posteroventral nucleus is involved in regulating hair cell sensitivity, together with the olivary cochlear system. Most of the neurons in the dorsal cochlear nucleus give rise to axons that decussate and then ascend in the **lateral lemniscus** (Figure 8–3A,B) to terminate in the **inferior colliculus** (Figures 8–5 and 8–6).

Midbrain and Thalamus

The inferior colliculus contains three main nuclei (Figures 8–5 and 8–6). The **central nucleus,** the principal auditory relay nucleus in the inferior colliculus, has a precise **tonotopic organization.** It projects to the medial geniculate nucleus (Figure 8–7), which in turn projects to the **primary auditory cortex** (cytoarchitectonic area 41) (Figure 8–8). The other two nuclei, the **external nucleus** and the **dorsal cortex** of the inferior colliculus, give rise to diffuse thalamocortical projections, primarily to **higher-order auditory areas** (Figure 8–8).

Cerebral Cortex

The primary auditory cortex is located largely on the superior surface of the temporal lobe, in **Heschl's gyri** (Figure 8–8). It has a tonotopic organization. The higher-order auditory areas, which encircle the primary area (Figures 8–8 and 8–9), receive their principal input from the primary auditory cortex (Figure 8–10).

At least two projections emerge from higher-order areas. One projection, important in sound localization (ie, where), targets the posterior parietal cortex and the dorsolateral prefrontal cortex (Figure 8–10). A second projection—which is thought to be important in processing of complex sounds, including linguistic functions in humans—terminates in the ventral and medial prefrontal cortex. **Wernicke's area** is a part of the higher-order auditory cortex on the left side that is important in interpreting speech (Figure 8–1B, inset).

Related Sources

Brust JCM: The Practice of Neural Science. McGraw-Hill; 2000. (See ch. 3, p. 32; ch. 10, cases 12, 13; ch. 16, cases 63, 64.)

Hudspeth AJ: Hearing. In Kandel ER, Schwartz JH, Jessell TM (editors): Principles of Neural Science, 4th ed. McGraw-Hill; 2000:590–613.

Hudspeth AJ: Sensory transduction in the ear. In Kandel ER, Schwartz JH, Jessell TM (editors): Principles of Neural Science, 4th ed. McGraw-Hill; 2000:614–624.

Selected Readings

Eggermont JJ: Between sound and perception: Reviewing the search for a neural code. Hear Res 2001;157:1–42.

Ehret G: The auditory cortex. J Comp Physiol A 1997;181:547–557.

Kaas JH, Hackett TA: "What" and "where" processing in auditory cortex. Nat Neurosci 1999;2:1045–1047.

Kaas JH, Hackett TA, Tramo MJ: Auditory processing in primate cerebral cortex. Curr Opin Neurobiol 1999;9:164–170.

Laszig R, Aschendorff A: Cochlear implants and electrical brainstem stimulation in sensorineural hearing loss. Curr Opin Neurol 1999;12:41–44.

Rauschecker JP, Tian B: Mechanisms and streams for processing of "what" and "where" in auditory cortex. Proc Natl Acad Sci U S A 2000;97:11800–11806.

References

Augustine JR: The insular lobe in primates including humans. Neurol Res 1985;7:2–10.

Bachevalier J, Meunier M, Lu MX, Ungerleider LG: Thalamic and temporal cortex input to medial prefrontal cortex in rhesus monkeys. Exp Brain Res 1997;115:430–444.

Brugge JF: An overview of central auditory processing. In Popper AN, Fay RR (editors): The Mammalian Auditory Pathway: Neurophysiology. Springer-Verlag; 1994:1–33.

Bushara KO, Weeks RA, Ishii K, et al: Modality-specific frontal and parietal areas for auditory and visual spatial localization in humans. Nat Neurosci 1999;2:759–766.

Galaburda A, Sanides F: Cytoarchitectonic organization of the human auditory cortex. J Comp Neurol 1980;190:597–610.

Galuske RA, Schlote W, Bratzke H, Singer W: Interhemispheric asymmetries of the modular structure in human temporal cortex. Science 2000;289:1946–1949.

Geniec P, Morest DK: The neuronal architecture of the human posterior colliculus. Acta Otolaryngol Suppl 1971;295:1–33.

Geschwind N, Levitsky W: Human brain: Left-right asymmetries in temporal speech region. Science 1968;161:186–187.

Hackett TA, Stepniewska I, Kaas JH: Subdivisions of auditory cortex and ipsilateral cortical connections of the parabelt auditory cortex in macaque monkeys. J Comp Neurol 1998;394:475–495.

Hackett TA, Stepniewska I, Kaas JH: Thalamocortical connections of the parabelt auditory cortex in macaque monkeys. J Comp Neurol 1998;400:271–286.

Hackett TA, Stepniewska I, Kaas JH: Prefrontal connections of the parabelt auditory cortex in macaque monkeys. Brain Res 1999;817:45–58.

Kaas JH, Hackett TA: Subdivisions of auditory cortex and processing streams in primates. Proc Natl Acad Sci U S A 2000;97:11793–11799.

Markowitsch HJ, Emmans D, Irle E, Streicher M, Preilowski B: Cortical and subcortical afferent connections of the primate's temporal pole: A study of rhesus monkeys, squirrel monkeys, and marmosets. J Comp Neurol 1985;242:425–458.

Merzenich MM, Brugge JF: Representation of the cochlear partition on the superior temporal plane of the macaque monkey. Brain Res 1973;50:275–296.

Mesulam MM, Mufson EJ: Insula of the old world monkey. III: Efferent cortical output and comments on function. J Comp Neurol 1982;212:38–52.

Moore JK, Osen KK: The human cochlear nuclei. In Creutzfeldt O, Scheich H, Schreiner C (editors): Hearing Mechanisms and Speech. Springer-Verlag; 1979:36–44.

Oertel D, Bal R, Gardner SM, Smith PH, Joris PX: Detection of synchrony in the activity of auditory nerve fibers by octopus cells of the mammalian cochlear nucleus. Proc Natl Acad Sci U S A 2000;97:11773–11779.

Rauschecker JP: Processing of complex sounds in the auditory cortex of cat, monkey, and man. Acta Otolaryngol Suppl 1997;532:34–38.

Recanzone GH, Schreiner CE, Sutter ML, Beitel RE, Merzenich MM: Functional organization of spectral receptive fields in the primary auditory cortex of the owl monkey. J Comp Neurol 1999;415:460–481.

Romanski LM, Tian B, Fritz J, Mishkin M, Goldman-Rakic PS, Rauschecker JP: Dual streams of auditory afferents target multiple domains in the primate prefrontal cortex. Nat Neurosci 1999;2:1131–1136.

Schreiner CE, Read HL, Sutter ML: Modular organization of frequency integration in primary auditory cortex. Annu Rev Neurosci 2000;23:501–529.

Schwartz IR: The superior olivary complex and lateral lemniscal nuclei. In Webster DB, Popper AN, Fay RR (editors): The Mammalian Auditory Pathway: Neuroanatomy. Springer-Verlag; 1992:117–167.

Scott SK, Blank CC, Rosen S, Wise RJ: Identification of a pathway for intelligible speech in the left temporal lobe. Brain 2000;123(part 12):2400–2406.

Spirou GA, Davis KA, Nelken I, Young ED: Spectral integration by type II interneurons in dorsal cochlear nucleus. J Neurophysiol 1999;82:648–663.

Stone JA, Chakeres DW, Schmalbrock P: High-resolution MR imaging of the auditory pathway. Magn Reson Imaging Clin N Am 1998;6:195–217.

Strominger NL, Nelson LR, Dougherty WJ: Second order auditory pathways in the chimpanzee. J Comp Neurol 1977;172:349–366.

von Economo C, Horn J: Über Windungsrelief, Masse und Rinderarchitektonik der Supratemporalfläche, ihre Individuellen und ihre Seitenunterschiede. Z ges Neurol Psychiat 1930;130:678–757.

Webster DB: An overview of mammalian auditory pathways with an emphasis on humans. In Webster DB, Popper AN, Fay RR (editors): The Mammalian Auditory Pathway: Neuroanatomy. Springer-Verlag; 1992:1–22.

Weeks RA, Aziz-Sultan A, Bushara KO, et al: A PET study of human auditory spatial processing. Neurosci Lett 1999; 262:155–158.

Wessinger CM, VanMeter J, Tian B, Van Lare J, Pekar J, Rauschecker JP: Hierarchical organization of the human auditory cortex revealed by functional magnetic resonance imaging. J Cogn Neurosci 2001;13:1–7.

Yu JJ, Young ED: Linear and nonlinear pathways of spectral information transmission in the cochlear nucleus. Proc Natl Acad Sci U S A 2000;97:11780–11786.

Zatorre RJ, Penhune VB: Spatial localization after excision of human auditory cortex. J Neurosci 2001;21:6321–6328.

9

Chemical Senses: Taste and Smell

TWO DISTINCT NEURAL SYSTEMS ARE USED TO SENSE the molecular environment: the gustatory system, which mediates taste, and the olfactory system, which serves smell. These systems are among the phylogenetically oldest systems of the brain. Compared with those of the other sensory systems, the neural systems for processing chemical stimuli are quite different. For example, both taste and smell have ipsilateral brain projections, whereas those of the other systems are either contralateral or bilateral. Moreover, the primary cortical areas for taste and smell are within the limbic system or in adjoining paralimbic areas. The limbic system mediates emotions and their associated behaviors. This anatomical linkage points to how the physical characteristics of chemical stimuli and their affective qualities are analyzed at the first stage of cortical processing. Information from the other sensory modalities reaches the limbic system only after additional processing stages.

The gustatory and olfactory systems work jointly in perceiving chemicals in the oral and nasal cavities, a more essential collaboration than that which occurs between the other sensory modalities. For example, even though the gustatory system is concerned with the four primary taste sensations—sweet, sour, salty, and bitter—the perception of richer and more complex flavors such as those present in wine is dependent on a properly functioning sense of smell. Chewing and swallowing cause chemicals to be released from food that waft into the nasal cavity, where they stimulate the olfactory system. Damage to the olfactory system, as a result of head trauma, or even the common cold, which impairs conduction of airborne molecules in the nasal passages, can dull the perception of flavor even though the basic taste sensations are preserved.

Although taste and smell work together and share similarities in their neural substrates, the anatomical organization of these systems is sufficiently different to be considered separately.

THE GUSTATORY SYSTEM: TASTE

Taste is mediated by three nerves: **facial** (VII), **glossopharyngeal** (IX), and **vagus** (X). As discussed in Chapter 6, the glossopharyngeal and vagus nerves also provide much of the afferent innervation of the gut, cardiovascular system, and lungs. This visceral afferent innervation provides the central nervous system with information about the internal state of the body.

The Ascending Gustatory Pathway Projects to the Ipsilateral Insular Cortex

Taste receptor cells are clustered in the **taste buds,** located on the tongue and at various intraoral sites. Chemicals from food, termed **tastants,** either bind to surface membrane receptors or pass directly through membrane channels, depending on the particular chemical, to activate taste cells. Taste cells are innervated by the distal branches of the primary afferent fibers in

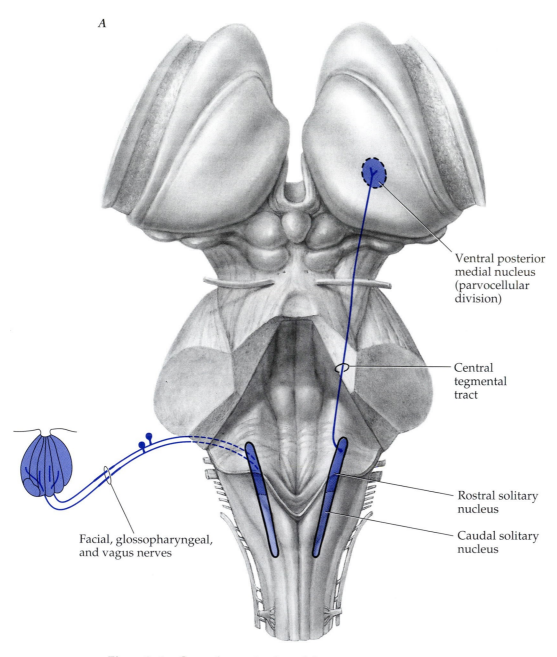

A

Ventral posterior medial nucleus (parvocellular division)

Central tegmental tract

Rostral solitary nucleus

Caudal solitary nucleus

Facial, glossopharyngeal, and vagus nerves

Figure 9–1. General organization of the gustatory system. *A.* Dorsal view of the brain stem, illustrating the location of the solitary nucleus and the projection of the rostral, or gustatory division.

the facial, glossopharyngeal, and vagus nerves (Figure 9–1). These afferent fibers have a pseudounipolar morphology, similar to that of the dorsal root ganglion neurons. In contrast to the nerves of the skin and mucous membranes, where generally the terminal portion of the afferent fiber is sensitive to stimulus energy, taste cells are separate from the primary afferent fibers. For taste, the role of the primary afferent fiber is simply to transmit sensory information to the central nervous system, encoded as a sequence of action potentials. For touch, the role of the primary afferent fiber is both to transduce stimulus energy into action potentials and to transmit this information to the central nervous system.

The central branches of the afferent fibers, after entering the brain stem, collect into the **solitary tract** (Figure 9–1B) of the dorsal medulla and terminate in the rostral portion of the **solitary nucleus** (Figure 9–1A). Recall that the caudal solitary nucleus is a viscerosensory nucleus, critically involved in regulating body functions and transmitting information to the cortex for perception of visceral information.

The axons of second-order neurons in the rostral solitary nucleus ascend **ipsilaterally** in the brain stem, in the **central tegmental tract,** and terminate in the **parvocellular division** of the **ventral posterior medial nucleus** (Figure 9–1A,B). From the thalamus, third-order neurons project to the **insular cortex** and the

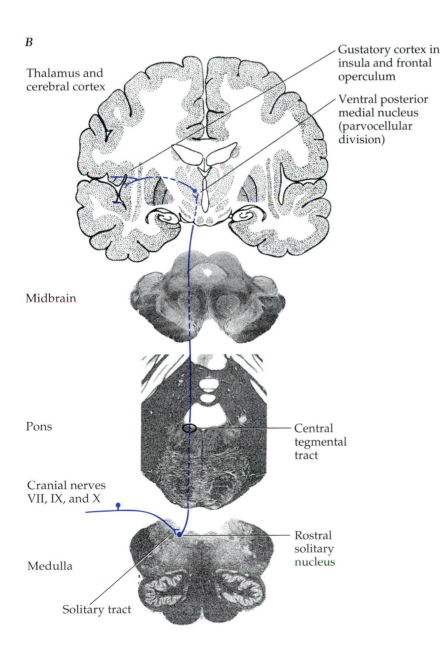

B

Thalamus and cerebral cortex

Gustatory cortex in insula and frontal operculum

Ventral posterior medial nucleus (parvocellular division)

Midbrain

Pons

Central tegmental tract

Cranial nerves VII, IX, and X

Rostral solitary nucleus

Medulla

Solitary tract

Figure 9–1 (continued). **B.** Ascending gustatory pathway.

nearby **operculum,** where the primary gustatory cortical areas are located. This pathway is thought to mediate the discriminative aspects of taste, which enable us to distinguish one quality from another. The insular cortex projects to several brain structures for further processing of taste stimuli. Projections to the **orbitofrontal cortex** are thought to be integrated with olfactory information, for the awareness of flavors. The insular and orbitofrontal cortical areas are considered part of the limbic system, for emotions. In addition to processing stimulus attributes for awareness of tastes, these cortical areas may be important for the behavioral and affective significance of tastes, such as the pleasure experienced with a fine meal or the dissatisfaction after one poorly prepared. A component of the processing of painful stimuli also involves the insular cortex, and pain in humans is not without emotional significance.

Although taste and visceral afferent information (see Chapter 6) are distinct modalities and have separate central pathways, the two modalities interact. In fact, linking information about the taste of a food and its effect on body functions upon ingestion is key to an individual's survival. One of the most robust forms of learning, called **conditioned taste aversion,** associates the taste of spoiled food with the nausea that it causes when eaten. Another name for this learning is bait shyness, referring to a method used by ranchers to discourage predators from attacking their livestock. In this technique, ranchers contaminate livestock meat with an emetic, such as lithium chloride, which causes nausea and vomiting after ingestion. Coyotes, after eating the bait, develop an aversion for the contaminated meat and will not attack the stock. People sometimes experience a phenomenon related to conditioned taste aversion, in which they develop an intense aversion to food they ate before becoming nauseated and vomiting, even if the food was not spoiled and the illness resulted from a viral infection. Experimental studies in rats have shown that such interactions between the gustatory and viscerosensory systems, leading to conditioned taste aversion, may occur in the insular cortex.

■ REGIONAL ANATOMY OF THE GUSTATORY SYSTEM

Branches of the Facial, Glossopharyngeal, and Vagus Nerves Innervate Different Parts of the Oral Cavity

Taste receptor cells are epithelial cells that transduce soluble chemical stimuli within the oral cavity into neural signals. They are present in complex microscopic sensory organs, called **taste buds** (Figure 9–2A).

Taste cells are short lived; they are continuously regenerated. In addition to the taste receptor cells, taste buds contain two additional types of cells: **basal cells,** which are thought to be **stem cells** that differentiate to become receptor cells, and **supporting cells,** which provide structural and possibly trophic support (Figure 9–2A). These cells have a synaptic contact with the distal processes of primary afferent fibers. A single afferent fiber terminal branches many times, both within a single taste bud and between different taste buds, so that it forms synapses with many taste cells.

Taste buds are present on the **tongue, soft palate, epiglottis, pharynx,** and **larynx.** Taste buds on the tongue are clustered on papillae (Figure 9–2B), whereas those at the other sites are located in pseudostratified columnar epithelium or stratified squamous epithelium rather than distinct papillae. Taste receptor cells that are located on the anterior two thirds of the tongue are innervated by the **chorda tympani nerve,** a branch of the facial (VII) nerve. (The facial nerve consists of two separate roots [Figure 9–3], a motor root commonly known as the **facial nerve** and a combined sensory and autonomic root called the **intermediate nerve.**) These anterior taste buds are clustered in the foliate and fungiform papillae (Figure 9–2B).

Taste buds on the posterior third of the tongue, which are located primarily in the circumvallate and foliate papillae (Figure 9–2), are innervated by the **glossopharyngeal (IX) nerve** (Figure 9–3). Taste buds on the palate are innervated by a branch of the intermediate nerve. Taste buds on the epiglottis and larynx are innervated by the vagus (X) nerve, whereas those on the pharynx are innervated by the glossopharyngeal nerve. The familiar taste map of the tongue—showing that sweet and salty are sensed in the front of the tongue, sour laterally, and bitter at the back of the tongue—is wrong. Taste buds in all regions are sensitive to the four basic taste attributes (sweet, sour, salty, and bitter).

The cell bodies of the afferent fibers innervating taste cells are located in peripheral sensory ganglia. The cell bodies of afferent fibers in the intermediate branch of the facial nerve are found in the **geniculate ganglion.** Those of the vagus and glossopharyngeal nerves are located in their respective **inferior ganglia.** As discussed in Chapter 6, the glossopharyngeal and vagus nerves also contain afferent fibers that innervate **cranial skin and mucous membranes;** the cell bodies of these afferent fibers are found in the **superior ganglia.**

The afferent fibers of the intermediate branch of the facial nerve enter the brain stem at the **pontomedullary junction,** immediately lateral to the root that contains somatic motor axons. The taste fibers of the glossopharyngeal and vagus nerves enter the brain stem in the rostral medulla.

A

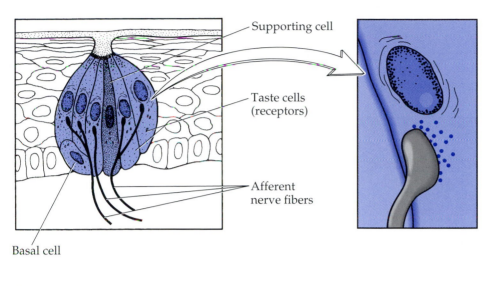

Supporting cell

Taste cells
(receptors)

Afferent
nerve fibers

Basal cell

B

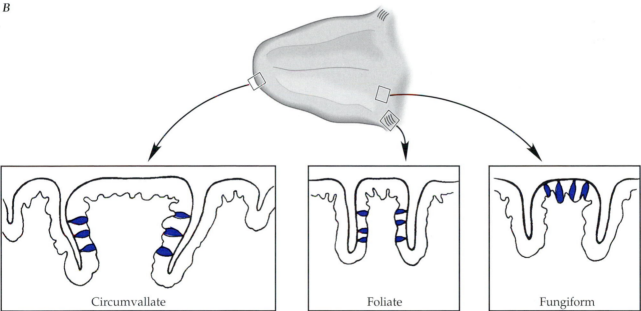

Circumvallate

Foliate

Fungiform

Figure 9–2. Taste buds (*A*) consist of taste receptor cells, supporting cells, and basal cells (not shown). The three types of papillae—circumvallate, foliate, and fungiform—are shown in *B.* Taste buds in papillae are shown in blue. The different classes of taste buds are located in different parts of the tongue.

The Solitary Nucleus Is the First Central Nervous System Relay for Taste

Gustatory fibers innervating the taste buds enter the brain stem and collect in the **solitary tract,** located in the dorsal medulla. The axons of the facial nerve enter the tract rostral to those of the glossopharyngeal and vagus nerves. After entering, however, the fibers send branches that ascend and descend within the tract, similar to the terminals of afferent fibers in Lis-sauer's tract of the spinal cord. The axon terminals leave the tract and synapse on neurons in the surrounding **solitary nucleus.** Second-order neurons in the rostral solitary nucleus (Figures 9–1A and 9–4) send their axons into the ipsilateral **central tegmental tract** (Figure 9–4A) and ascend to the thalamus (see below). The trigeminal and medial lemnisci, which carry the ascending somatic sensory projection from the main trigeminal and dorsal column nuclei, are ventral to the central tegmental tract (Figure 9–4A).

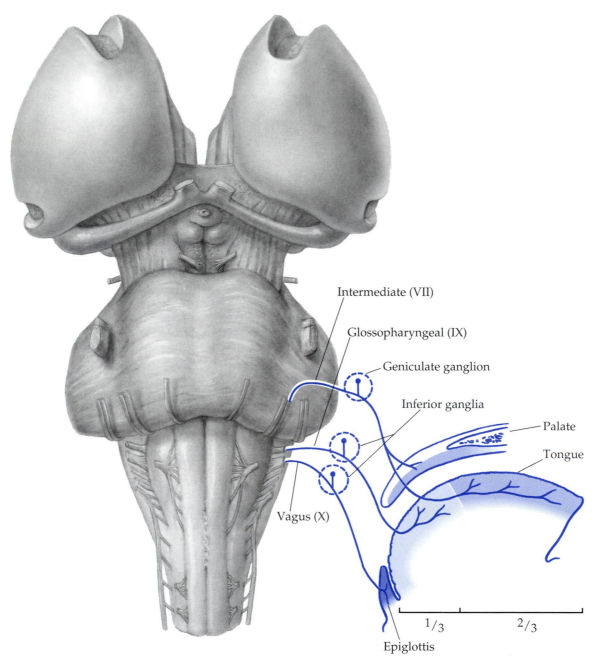

Intermediate (VII)

Glossopharyngeal (IX)

Geniculate ganglion

Inferior ganglia

Palate

Tongue

Vagus (X)

1/3   2/3

Epiglottis

Figure 9–3. Gustatory innervation of the oral cavity by the facial, glossopharyngeal, and vagus nerves. In the periphery the chorda tympani nerve (a branch of cranial nerve VII) supplies taste buds on the anterior two thirds of the tongue, lingual branches of the glossopharyngeal (IX) nerve supply taste buds on the posterior third, and the superior laryngeal (X) nerve supplies taste buds on the epiglottis. The greater petrosal nerve (another branch of cranial nerve VII) supplies taste buds on the palate.

The Parvocellular Portion of the Ventral Posterior Medial Nucleus Relays Gustatory Information to the Insular Cortex and Operculum

Similar to somatic sensations, vision, and hearing, a thalamic relay nucleus receives taste information and projects this information to a circumscribed area of the cerebral cortex. The ascending projection from the rostral solitary nucleus terminates in the **parvocellular division** of the **ventral posterior medial nucleus.** This nucleus has a characteristic pale appearance on myelin-stained sections (Figure 9–5A). The axons of thalamocortical projection neurons in the thalamic gustatory nucleus project into the **posterior limb of the internal capsule** and ascend to the **insular cortex**

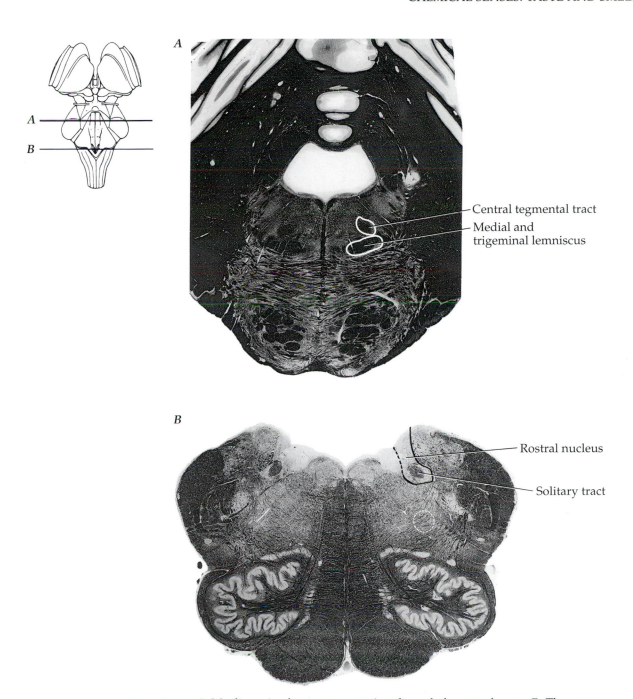

Figure 9–4. ***A.*** Myelin-stained transverse section through the rostral pons. ***B.*** The gustatory component of the solitary nucleus is illustrated in this myelin-stained transverse section through the medulla. The inset shows the planes of section.

and the nearby **operculum** (Figure 9–6). Different nuclei in the ventromedial thalamus receive different inputs and project to different cortical areas (Figure 9–5B). Viscerosensory inputs are processed in adjacent but slightly separated thalamic regions and project to adjoining areas of the insular cortex. Touch and pain also engage different thalamic nuclei and cortical areas.

A schematic coronal section through the cerebral hemisphere reveals the operculum of the frontal lobe

overlying the insular cortex and the approximate locations of the cortical taste areas (Figure 9–6B). Even though the sensory receptors mediating taste and touch on the tongue are intermingled, the cortical areas to which these sensory receptors project their information are relatively distinct. For example, the face area of the primary somatic sensory cortex, where information from mechanoreceptors is relayed, is located on the cortical surface in the postcentral gyrus, whereas the gustatory areas are located deep (Figure 9–6B).

A

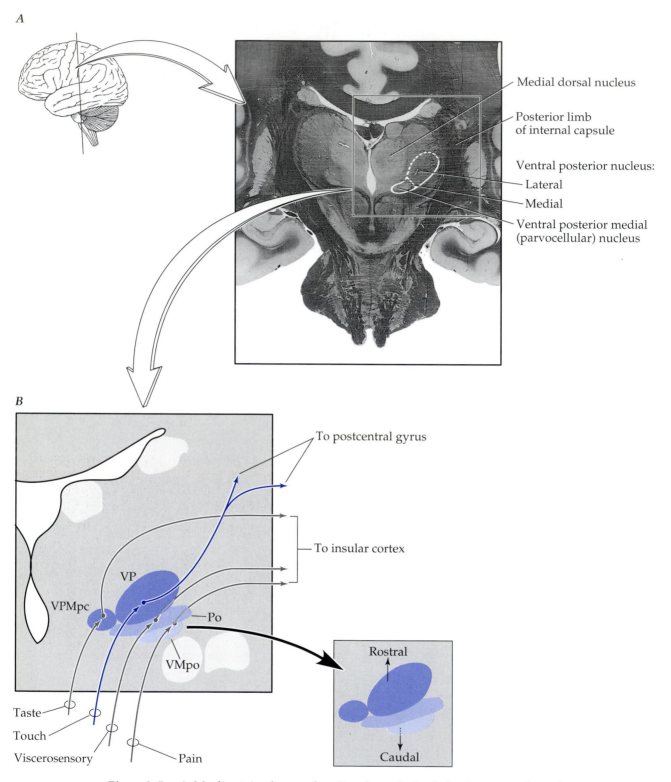

Medial dorsal nucleus

Posterior limb
of internal capsule

Ventral posterior nucleus:
Lateral
Medial

Ventral posterior medial
(parvocellular) nucleus

B

To postcentral gyrus

To insular cortex

VP

VPMpc

Po

VMpo

Taste

Touch

Viscerosensory

Pain

Rostral

Caudal

Figure 9–5. *A.* Myelin-stained coronal section through the thalamic taste nucleus, the
parvocellular portion of the ventral posterior medial nucleus. The medial dorsal nucleus
is also shown on this section; a portion of this nucleus may play a role in olfactory perception. The inset shows the plane of section. *B.* Schematic illustration showing the cortical projections of ventral thalamic somatic sensory, viscerosensory, and taste nuclei.

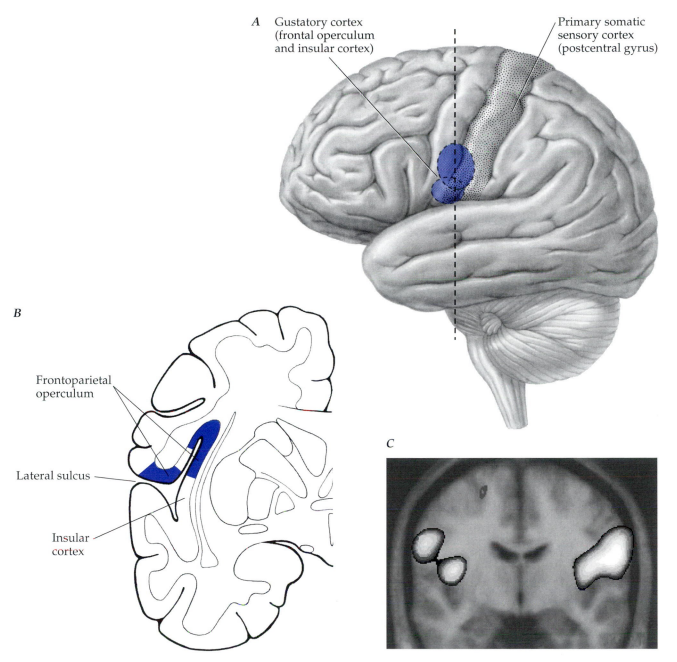

A Gustatory cortex
(frontal operculum
and insular cortex)

Primary somatic
sensory cortex
(postcentral gyrus)

B

Frontoparietal
operculum

Lateral sulcus

Insular
cortex

C

Figure 9–6. Cortical gustatory area. **A.** Lateral view of human cerebral hemisphere; the blue-tinted field corresponds approximately to gustatory areas. These areas, identified in the rhesus monkey, are located entirely beneath the cortical surface on the frontal operculum and the anterior insular cortex. The dotted area corresponds to the primary somatic sensory cortex. **B.** Schematic coronal section through the anterior insular cortex and frontoparietal operculum, showing the approximate locations of the gustatory areas. **C.** $H_2^{15}O$ positron emission tomography scan show bilateral areas of cortical activation in response to tasting a 5% sucrose solution. The gray scale indicates that intensity of activation, measured as cerebral blood flow, which correlates with neural activity. White indicates maximal blood flow (or high neural activity), whereas black indicates low blood flow (or activity). Note that two distinct taste areas are distinguished in the subject's right cortex (left side of image). The single zone on the other side is probably due to blurring of the PET signal. (**C,** *Courtesy of Dr. Stephen Frey, McGill University; Frey S, Petrides M: Re-examination of the human taste region: A positron emission tomography study. Eur J Neurosci 1999;11:2985–2988.*)

Similarly, nociceptive information from the oral cavity (see Chapter 6) is represented posterior to taste in the insular cortex. The presence of separate cortical areas for processing oral tactile, nociceptive, and gustatory stimuli is a reflection of an important principle of cortical organization: Each sensory modality has a separate cortical representation.

THE OLFACTORY SYSTEM: SMELL

The sense of smell is mediated by the **olfactory (I) nerve.** There are two major differences between smell and the other sensory modalities, including taste. First, information about airborne chemicals impinging on the nasal mucosa is relayed to a part of the cerebral cortex without first relaying in the thalamus. The thalamic nucleus that processes olfactory information receives input from the cortical olfactory areas. Second, the cortical olfactory areas are phylogenetically older (allocortex) than the primary cortical regions (neocortex) that process other stimuli (see Chapter 2).

The Olfactory Projection to the Cerebral Cortex Does Not Relay in the Thalamus

Primary olfactory neurons are found in the olfactory epithelium, a portion of the nasal cavity (Figure 9–7A). The primary olfactory neurons have a bipolar morphology (see Figure 6–2). The peripheral portion of the primary olfactory neuron is **chemosensitive,** and the central process is an **unmyelinated axon** that projects to the central nervous system. Recall that taste receptor cells, which transduce chemical stimuli on the tongue, and the primary taste fibers, which transmit information to the brain stem, are separate cells. Primary olfactory neurons are sensitive to airborne chemicals—or **odorants**—because they have transmembrane olfactory receptors on their chemosensitive membranes. Although most odorant molecules are carried into the olfactory epithelium with inhaled air, some travel from the oral cavity during chewing and swallowing. Each primary olfactory neuron has one type of olfactory receptor, which determines the spectrum of odorants to which the neuron is sensitive.

The unmyelinated axons of the primary olfactory neurons collect into numerous small fascicles, which together form the **olfactory nerve.** Olfactory nerve fascicles pass through foramina in a portion of the **ethmoid bone** termed the **cribriform plate** (Figure 9–7A) and synapse on second-order neurons in the **olfactory bulb** (Figures 9–7 and 9–8). Head trauma can shear off these delicate fascicles as they traverse the bone, resulting in **anosmia,** the inability to perceive odors.

But because olfactory neurons regenerate, the sense of smell can return.

Neurons that have a particular olfactory receptor are scattered randomly within a portion of the olfactory epithelium. The axons of these olfactory neurons all converge onto a **glomerulus,** which contains projection neurons and interneurons. The glomerulus is the basic processing unit of the olfactory bulb.

The next link in the olfactory pathway is the projection of second-order neurons in the olfactory bulb through the **olfactory tract,** directly to the primitive allocortex on the ventral surface of the cerebral hemispheres. Five separate areas of the cerebral hemisphere receive a direct projection from the olfactory bulb (Figure 9–8B): (1) the **anterior olfactory nucleus,** which modulates information processing in the olfactory bulb, (2) the **amygdala** and (3) the **olfactory tubercle,** which together are thought to be important in the emotional, endocrine, and visceral consequences of odors, (4) the adjacent **piriform and peri-amygdaloid cortical areas,** which may be important for olfactory perception, and (5) the **rostral entorhinal cortex,** which is thought to be important in olfactory memories.

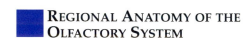

REGIONAL ANATOMY OF THE OLFACTORY SYSTEM

The Primary Olfactory Neurons Are Located in the Nasal Mucosa

Most of the lining of the nasal cavity is part of the respiratory epithelium, which warms and humidifies inspired air. The **olfactory epithelium** is a specialized portion of the nasal epithelial surface that contains the primary olfactory neurons. It is located on the superior nasal concha on each side as well as the midline septum and roof. Primary olfactory neurons, of which there are approximately several million, are short lived, similar to taste cells. These bipolar sensory neurons have an apical portion with hairlike structures (olfactory cilia) that contain the molecular machinery for receiving chemical stimuli (Figure 9–7, inset). In addition to the olfactory neurons, the olfactory epithelium contains two other cell types: (1) glial-like **supporting cells** and (2) **basal cells,** which are stem cells that differentiate into primary olfactory neurons as the sensory neurons die.

The initial step in olfactory perception is the interaction of an odorant molecule with an **olfactory receptor,** a complex transmembrane protein located in the apical membrane of primary olfactory neurons. A series of recent discoveries using molecular tech-

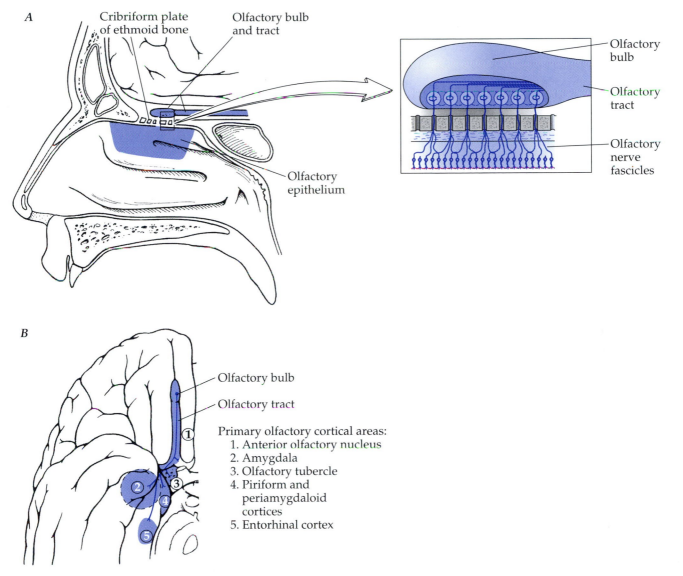

Figure 9–7. Olfactory pathway. *A.* Olfactory epithelium (blue) on the superior nasal concha. The nasal septum is not shown. The inset shows a cutaway view of the olfactory epithelium and olfactory bulb. *B.* Schematic of inferior surface of cerebral hemisphere, illustrating the five main termination sites of olfactory tract fibers.

niques has shown that there are approximately 1000 different types of olfactory receptors and that individual primary olfactory sensory neurons each contain only one olfactory receptor type or a small number of different receptor types. Olfactory receptors bind multiple odorants, indicating that individual primary olfactory neurons are sensitive to multiple odorants. Different odorants therefore appear to be initially processed by sensory neurons that are distributed widely throughout the olfactory epithelium. The scattering of olfactory receptor types within the olfactory epithelium is similar to the distribution of taste cells in the oral cavity.

A second component of the olfactory system, the **vomeronasal organ,** comprises a portion of the olfactory epithelium separate from the main olfactory epithelium. In animals the vomeronasal organ is important in detecting **pheromones** that have important effects on the individual animal's social and sexual behavior. Rather than project to the olfactory bulb, virtually all the neurons of the vomeronasal organ project to a different structure, the accessory olfactory bulb, which projects only to the amygdala. Social and sexual behavior in humans does not depend on pheromonal cues, and humans do not appear to have a vomeronasal organ.

A

Olfactory bulb

Cribriform plate

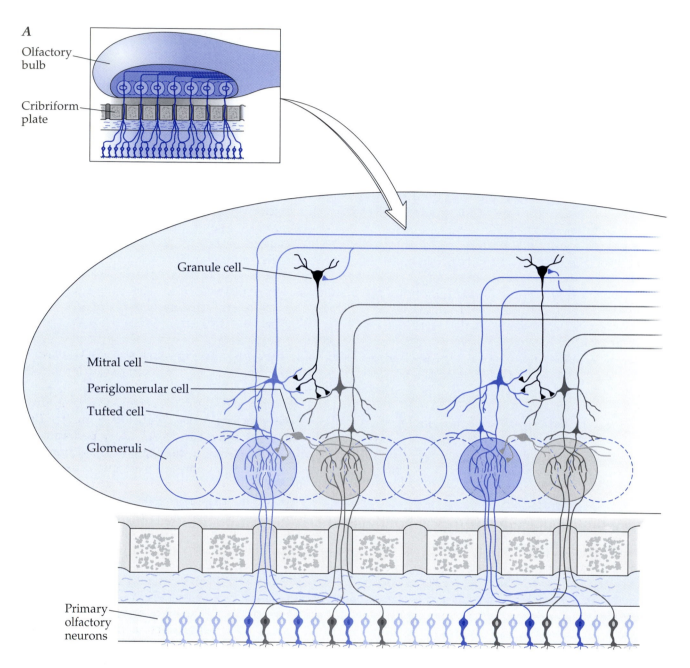

Granule cell

Mitral cell

Periglomerular cell

Tufted cell

Glomeruli

Primary olfactory neurons

B

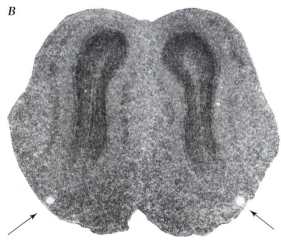

Figure 9–8. Projection of primary olfactory sensory neurons to the olfactory bulb. ***A.*** The axons of bipolar cells synapse on the projection neurons of the olfactory bulb, the mitral cells, and the tufted cells, as well as the periglomerular cells, a type of inhibitory interneuron. ***B.*** In situ hybridization of olfactory receptor mRNA in the axon terminals of primary olfactory sensory neurons in a single glomerulus in the olfactory bulb of the rat. The two bright spots on the ventral surface of the bulb (arrows) correspond to the two labeled glomeruli. (***A,*** *Adapted from Mori K, Nagao H, Yoshihara Y: The olfactory bulb: Coding and processing of odor molecule information. Science 1999;286:712; and Mori K, von Campenhause H, Yoshihara Y: Zonal organization of the mammalian main and accessory olfactory systems. Philos Trans R Soc Lond B Biol Sci 2000;355:1803. **B,** Courtesy of Dr. Robert Vassar, Columbia University; Vassar R, Chao SK, Sticheran R, Nuñez JM, Vosshall LB, Axel R: Topographic organization of sensory projections to the olfactory bulb. Cell 1994;79:981–991.)*

The Olfactory Bulb Is the First Central Nervous System Relay for Olfactory Input

Primary olfactory neurons synapse on neurons in the **olfactory bulb** (Figures 9–7 and 9–8), which is a portion of the cerebral hemispheres. (The olfactory bulb develops as a small outpouching on the ventral surface of the telencephalon [see Figure 3–16].) Compared with rodents and carnivores, the olfactory bulb is reduced in size in monkeys, apes, and humans. Similar to most other components of the cerebral hemisphere, neurons in the olfactory bulb are organized into discrete laminae.

The central processes of olfactory receptor cells synapse on three types of neurons in the olfactory bulb (Figure 9–8A): on **mitral cells** and **tufted cells**, which are the two projection neurons of the olfactory bulb, and on interneurons called **periglomerular cells.** The terminals of the olfactory receptor cells and the dendrites of mitral, tufted, and periglomerular cells form a morphological unit called the **glomerulus** (Figure 9–8). Within a glomerulus, certain presynaptic and postsynaptic elements are ensheathed by **glial cells.** This sheath ensures specificity of action, limiting the spread of neurotransmitter released by the presynaptic terminal. Whereas structures called glomeruli are located in other central nervous system locations, including the cerebellar cortex (see Chapter 13), those in the olfactory bulb are among the largest and most distinct.

Mitral and **tufted cells** are the projection neurons of the olfactory bulb. Their axons project from the olfactory bulb through the **olfactory tract** to the primary olfactory cortical areas (Figure 9–9). The **granule cell** (Figure 9–10A) is an inhibitory interneuron that receives excitatory synaptic input from mitral cells to which it feeds back inhibition. Another inhibitory interneuron in the olfactory bulb is the **periglomerular cell,** which receives a direct input from the primary olfactory neurons. This neuron inhibits mitral cells in the same and adjacent glomeruli. One function of these inhibitory interneurons is to make the neural responses to different odorants more distinct, thereby facilitating discrimination.

A remarkable specificity exists in the projections of olfactory sensory neurons to the glomeruli. Even though primary olfactory neurons that contain a particular type of olfactory receptor are widely distributed throughout part of the olfactory epithelium, they project to one or a small number of glomeruli in the olfactory bulb (Figure 9–8B). Because there are about 1000 different olfactory receptor genes and about 1000 to 3000 glomeruli, researchers have suggested that each glomerulus may receive projections from olfactory sensory neurons that have a particular type of receptor. This finding suggests that the neuronal processes within the glomerulus—the dendrites of mitral, tufted, and periglomerular cells—comprise a **functional unit** for processing a particular set of odorants.

The Olfactory Bulb Projects to Structures on the Ventral Brain Surface Through the Olfactory Tract

The olfactory bulb and tract lie in the **olfactory sulcus** on the ventral surface of the frontal lobe (Figure 9–9). The **gyrus rectus** (or straight gyrus) is located medial to the olfactory bulb and tract. As the olfactory tract approaches the region where it fuses with the cerebral hemispheres, it bifurcates into a prominent **lateral olfactory stria** (Figures 9–9 and 9–10A) and a small **medial olfactory stria** (Figure 9–9). The lateral olfactory stria contains the axons from the olfactory bulb, whereas the medial olfactory stria contains axons from other brain regions that are projecting to the olfactory bulb.

The **anterior perforated substance** is located caudal to the olfactory striae (Figure 9–9, inset). Tiny branches of the anterior cerebral artery perforate the ventral brain surface in this region. These branches provide the arterial supply for parts of the basal ganglia and internal capsule. The anterior perforated substance is gray matter (see below), whereas the olfactory striae are pathways on the brain surface. The **olfactory tubercle,** one of the gray matter regions to which the olfactory bulb projects, is located in the anterior perforated substance (Figures 9–9, inset; and 9–10A). This tubercle and other parts of the anterior perforated substance are part of the **basal forebrain.** One nucleus of the basal forebrain is the basal nucleus of Meynert, which comprises neurons containing acetylcholine that project diffusely throughout the cortex and regulate cortical excitability (see Chapter 2; Figure 2–2A).

The Primary Olfactory Cortex Receives a Direct Input From the Olfactory Bulb

The projection neurons of the olfactory bulb (tufted and mitral cells) send their axons directly to five spatially disparate regions on the ventral and medial surfaces of the cerebral hemispheres. These areas are collectively termed the **primary olfactory cortex:** (1) anterior olfactory nucleus, (2) amygdala, (3) olfactory tubercle, (4) piriform and periamygdaloid cortical areas, and (5) rostral entorhinal cortex.

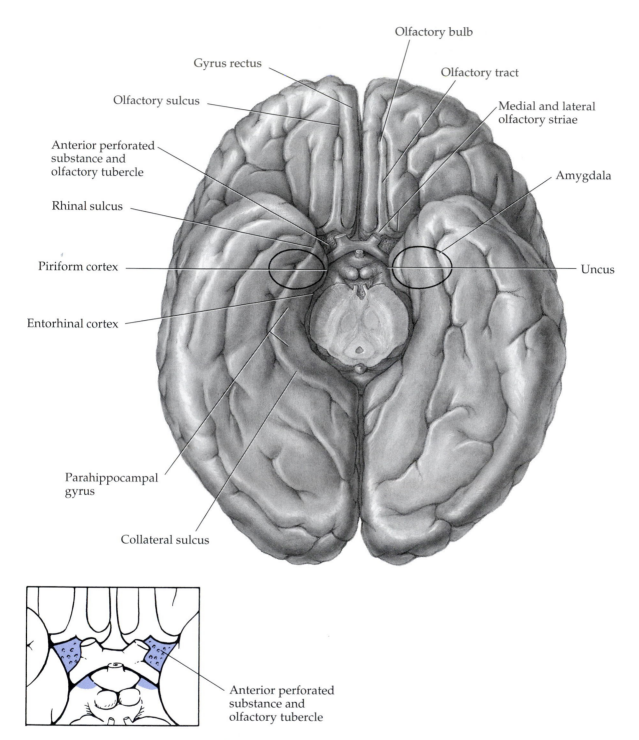

Olfactory bulb

Gyrus rectus

Olfactory tract

Olfactory sulcus

Medial and lateral
olfactory striae

Anterior perforated
substance and
olfactory tubercle

Amygdala

Rhinal sulcus

Piriform cortex

Uncus

Entorhinal cortex

Parahippocampal
gyrus

Collateral sulcus

Anterior perforated
substance and
olfactory tubercle

Figure 9–9. Ventral surface of the cerebral hemisphere. The parahippocampal gyrus contains numerous anatomical and functional divisions, two of which are the entorhinal cortex and piriform cortex. Allocortex is located medial to the collateral sulcus and rhinal fissure. The approximate location of the amygdala is indicated. The inset shows the location of the olfactory tubercle within the region of the anterior perforated substance (blue).

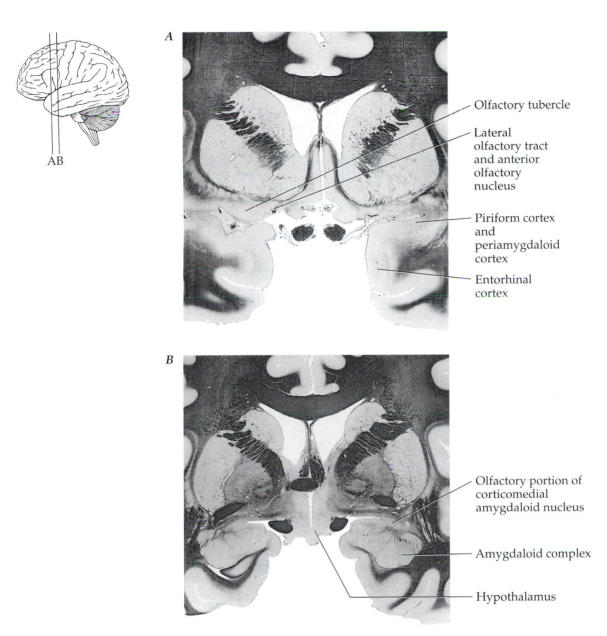

Figure 9–10. Myelin-stained coronal section through the region of the anterior perforated substance (*A*) and amygdala (*B*). The inset shows the planes of section.

Most of the primary olfactory areas on the ventral and medial surfaces of the cerebral hemispheres (Figure 9–9) have a cytoarchitecture that is characteristically different from the nonolfactory cortical regions located lateral to them. Recall that most of the cerebral cortex is **neocortex,** with at least six cell layers (see Chapter 2). Somatic sensory, visual, auditory, and gustatory cortical areas are all part of the neocortex. In contrast, the olfactory cortex has fewer than six layers, termed **allocortex.** With fewer layers, allocortex is more limited than neocortex in its processing capabil-

ities. Allocortex also receives little direct input from the thalamus. There are two major kinds of allocortex: archicortex and paleocortex. **Archicortex** is located primarily in the hippocampal formation (see Chapter 16). **Paleocortex** is located on the basal surface of the cerebral hemispheres, in part of the insular cortex, and caudally along the parahippocampal gyrus and retrosplenial cortex (the area of cortex located caudal to the splenium of the corpus callosum; see Figure AI–4). In addition to archicortex and paleocortex, there are various forms of transitional cortex with characteristics of both neocortex and allocortex. On the ventral brain surface, allocortex and transitional cortex remain medial to the **rhinal sulcus** and its caudal extension, the **collateral sulcus** (Figure 9–9). The paleocortical olfactory areas each have three morphologically distinct layers. Axons of the olfactory tract course in the most superficial layer before synapsing on neurons in the deeper layers.

Neurons in the Anterior Olfactory Nucleus Modulate Information Transmission in the Olfactory Bulb Bilaterally

The anterior olfactory nucleus is located caudal to the olfactory bulb on either side of the olfactory tract, where it fuses with the cerebral hemispheres (Figure 9–10A). Neurons of the anterior olfactory nucleus are also scattered along the olfactory tract. Neurons in this nucleus project their axons back to the olfactory bulb, both ipsilaterally and contralaterally. In Alzheimer disease, a progressive neurological degenerative disease in which individuals become severely demented, the anterior olfactory nucleus undergoes characteristic structural changes. Damage of the anterior olfactory nucleus may underlie the impaired sense of smell in Alzheimer patients.

Projections of the Olfactory Bulb to the Amygdala and Olfactory Tubercle Play a Role in Olfactory Regulation of Behavior

A major projection of the olfactory bulb is to the **amygdala,** a heterogeneous structure located in the anterior temporal lobe (Figures 9–9 and 9–10B). The amygdala has three major nuclear divisions: the corticomedial nuclear group, the basolateral nuclear group, and the central nucleus. The olfactory bulb projects to a portion of the **corticomedial** nuclear group (Figure 9–10B). This olfactory projection is thought to be important in behavior regulation rather than in odor perception and discrimination. For example, neurons in the corticomedial nuclear group are part of a circuit transmitting olfactory information to the hypothalamus (Figure 9–10B), for the regulation of food intake. Also, in certain animals the corticomedial nuclear group plays an essential role in the olfactory regulation of **reproductive behaviors.** The organization of the amygdala is considered in detail in Chapter 16.

The **olfactory tubercle** is a part of the basal forebrain located medial to the olfactory tract (Figure 9–10A). Compared with the amygdala, which receives a major olfactory projection in most animal species, the olfactory projections to the olfactory tubercle are fewer in number in primates. Neurons in the olfactory tubercle receive input from and project their axons to brain regions that play a role in **emotions** (see Chapter 16).

The Olfactory Areas of the Temporal and Frontal Lobes May Be Important in Olfactory Perceptions and Discriminations

The olfactory bulb also projects directly to the caudolateral frontal lobe and the rostromedial temporal lobe. These areas consist of the rostral entorhinal cortex, the piriform cortex, and the periamygdaloid cortex, which overlies the amygdala (Figures 9–10 and 9–11).

The piriform cortex, named for its appearance in certain mammals, where the rostral temporal lobe is shaped like a pear (*pirum* is Latin for "pear"), may be important in the initial processing of odors leading to perception. This connection has been deduced because the piriform cortex projects directly, and indirectly via the **medial dorsal nucleus** (Figure 9–6), to neocortical areas of the **orbitofrontal cortex** that are implicated in olfactory perception (Figure 9–11). Lesions of the orbitofrontal olfactory area in monkeys impair **olfactory discrimination.** The orbitofrontal cortex also receives information from the insular taste cortex. As a site of convergence of olfactory and gustatory information, the orbitofrontal cortex may be important in integrating these two modalities for perception of flavors.

The **rostral entorhinal cortex** is located on the parahippocampal gyrus. This area is thought to be important in allowing a particular smell to evoke memories of a place or event. This cortex projects to the hippocampal formation, which has been shown to be essential for consolidation of short-term memories into long-term memories (see Chapter 16).

Projections From the Olfactory Bulb to the Cortex Have a Parallel Organization

For many years little was known of the pattern of projections from the olfactory bulb to the cortex, apart

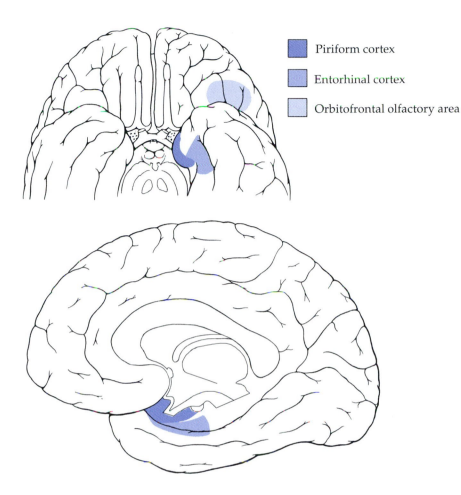

Piriform cortex

Entorhinal cortex

Orbitofrontal olfactory area

Figure 9–11. Olfactory cortical areas that may play a role in perception. Primary olfactory regions of the temporal lobe and the medial orbital surfaces of the frontal lobe (blue). The orbitofrontal cortex receives a projection from the primary olfactory areas (as well as the medial dorsal nucleus of the thalamus).

from the presence of terminations in the five areas described above. What was known suggested that there was little specificity in the connections, quite unlike the somatotopic or retinotopic organizations for touch and vision. Recent experiments using molecular genetics to analyze the topography of the projections from the olfactory bulb to the various olfactory cortical areas have revealed the logic of the anatomy of the cortical inputs connections. In these experiments, mice were genetically modified to express a tracer protein only if they had a particular olfactory receptor gene. Although the tracer was expressed only in the primary sensory neurons with the particular olfactory receptor gene, it was transneuronally transported to the postsynaptic target neurons in the olfactory bulb and the olfactory cortex. The mechanism for this form of transport is not well understood, but the tracer is thought to be released along with neurotransmitters and other compounds at the synaptic cleft in the olfactory bulb. The tracer is picked up by postsyn-

aptic neurons and transported to their terminations in the cortex. From there, tracer is picked up by the cortical neurons that receive synaptic input from the labeled bulb neurons. In this way, entire circuits containing neurons with the genetically identified primary sensory neurons were marked.

Primary olfactory neurons that contain a particular olfactory receptor project, via one or just a few glomeruli (Figures 9–8 and 9–12), to discrete clusters of neurons in multiple olfactory cortical areas (Figure 9–12). When researchers examined the cortical locations receiving input from neurons with one or another olfactory receptor, they found a complex overlapping pattern. In this way, information from different receptors—about different sets of odorants—is integrated by olfactory primary cortical neurons before being distributed to the orbitofrontal and other neocortical areas, for perception and discrimination, and to other limbic system structures, for influencing behavior and emotions.

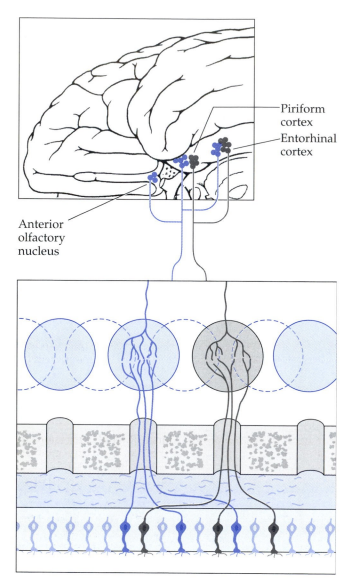

Figure 9–12. Sets of primary olfactory neurons that express a particular olfactory receptor project (i.e., gray or black) to one or a few glomeruli. Projection neurons in the glomeruli project to several olfactory cortical areas. Three areas are shown in the boxed schematic of the olfactory cortical areas: the piriform and entorhinal cortical areas, as well as the anterior olfactory nucleus. (*Adapted from Zou Z, et al: Genetic tracing reveals a stereotyped sensory map in the Olfactory Cortex. Nature 2001;414:173–179.*)

Summary

The Gustatory System

Sensory Receptors and Peripheral Nerves

Gustatory receptors are clustered in **taste buds** (Figure 9–2), which are located on the tongue, palate,

pharynx, larynx, and epiglottis (Figure 9–3). The **facial (VII) nerve** innervates taste buds on the anterior two thirds of the tongue and the **palate;** the **glossopharyngeal (IX) nerve** innervates taste buds on the posterior one third of the tongue and pharynx; and the **vagus (X) nerve** innervates taste buds on the epiglottis and larynx (Figure 9–3).

Brain Stem, Thalamus, and Cerebral Cortex

Afferent fibers of the three cranial nerves serving taste enter the solitary tract and terminate principally in the rostral portion of the **solitary nucleus** (Figures 9–1 and 9–4). Projection neurons from the solitary nucleus ascend ipsilaterally, in the **central tegmental tract** (Figure 9–4), to the parvocellular portion of the **ventral posterior medial nucleus** (Figure 9–5). The cortical areas to which the thalamic neurons project are located in the **insular cortex** and nearby **operculum** (Figure 9–6). These areas are separate from the representation of tactile sensation on the tongue.

The Olfactory System

Receptors and Olfactory Nerve

Primary olfactory neurons, located in the **olfactory epithelium,** are **bipolar neurons** (Figures 9–7 and 9–8). The distal process is sensitive to chemical stimuli, and the central process projects to the olfactory bulb (Figures 9–7 and 9–8) as the **olfactory (I) nerve.** The olfactory nerve is formed by multiple small fascicles of axons of primary olfactory neurons that pass through foramina in a portion of the **ethmoid bone** termed the **cribriform plate** (Figure 9–7). There are about 1000 olfactory receptors, but an individual olfactory neuron contains one type of receptor. The olfactory receptor type determines the odorants to which the neuron is sensitive.

Cerebral Cortex

Olfactory nerve fibers synapse on neurons in the glomeruli of the olfactory bulb (Figure 9–8). Primary olfactory neurons with a particular olfactory receptor send their axons to one or just a few glomeruli (Figure 9–8). Projection neurons in glomeruli send their axons, via the **olfactory tract,** to five regions of the cerebral hemisphere (Figure 9–8B): (1) the **anterior olfactory nucleus** (Figure 9–10A), (2) the **olfactory** tubercle (a portion of the **anterior perforated substance**) (Figure 9–10A), (3) the **amygdala** (Figure 9–10), (4) the **piriform** and **periamygdaloid cortical areas** (Figures 9–10 and 9–11), and (5) the **rostral entorhinal cortex** (Figure 9–11). The piriform cortex projects, via the **medial dorsal nucleus,** to the **orbitofrontal cortex,** which is thought to be important in olfactory discrimination.

Related Sources

Brust JCM: The Practice of Neural Science. McGraw-Hill; 2000. (See ch. 3, pp. 15, 29, 36; ch. 11, cases 15, 16.)

Buck LB: Smell and taste: The chemical senses. In Kandel ER, Schwartz JH, Jessell TM (editors): Principles of Neural Science, 4th ed. McGraw-Hill; 2000:625–647.

Selected Readings

Buck LB: The molecular architecture of odor and pheromone sensing in mammals. Cell 2000;100:611–618.

Cavada C, Company T, Tejedor J, Cruz-Rizzolo RJ, Reinoso-Suarez F: The anatomical connections of the macaque monkey orbitofrontal cortex. A review. Cereb Cortex 2000;10:220–242.

Doty RL: Olfaction. Annu Rev Psychol 2001;52:423–452.

Dulac C: How does the brain smell? Neuron 1997;19:477–480.

Dulac C: The physiology of taste, vintage 2000. Cell 2000;100:607–610.

Finger TE: Gustatory nuclei and pathways in the central nervous system. In Finger TE, Silver WL (editors): Neurobiology of Taste and Smell. John Wiley and Sons; 1987:331–353.

Haberly LB: Olfactory cortex. In Shepherd GM (editor): The Synaptic Organization of the Brain. Oxford University Press; 1990:317–345.

Herness MS, Gilbertson TA: Cellular mechanisms of taste transduction. Annu Rev Physiol 1999;61:873–900.

Meredith M: Human vomeronasal organ function: A critical review of best and worst cases. Chem Senses 2001; 26:433–445.

Norgren R: Gustatory system. In Paxinos G (editor): The Human Nervous System. Academic Press; 1990:845–860.

Price JL: Olfactory system. In Paxinos G (editor): The Human Nervous System. Academic Press; 1990:979–998.

References

Beckstead RM, Morse JR, Norgren R: The nucleus of the solitary tract in the monkey: Projections to the thalamus and brain stem nuclei. J Comp Neurol 1980;190:259–282.

Braak H: Architectonics of the Human Telencephalic Cortex. Springer-Verlag; 1980:147.

Buck LB, Axel R: A novel multigene family may encode odorant receptors: A molecular basis for odor recognition. Cell 1991;65:175–187.

Carmichael ST, Price JL: Limbic connections of the orbital and medial prefrontal cortex in macaque monkeys. J Comp Neurol 1995;363:615–641.

Cechetto DF, Saper CB: Evidence for a viscerotopic sensory representation in the cortex and thalamus in the rat. J Comp Neurol 1987;262:27–45.

Chiavaras MM, Petrides M: Orbitofrontal sulci of the human and macaque monkey brain. J Comp Neurol 2000; 422:35–54.

Frey S, Petrides M: Re-examination of the human taste region: A positron emission tomography study. Eur J Neurosci 1999;11:2985–2988.

Horowitz LF, Montmayeur JP, Echelard Y, Buck LB: A genetic approach to trace neural circuits. Proc Natl Acad Sci U S A 1999;96:3194–3199.

Lenz FA, Gracely RH, Zirh TA, Leopold DA, Rowland LH, Dougherty PM: Human thalamic nucleus mediating taste and multiple other sensations related to ingestive behavior. J Neurophysiol 1997;77:3406–3409.

Markowitsch HJ, Emmans D, Irle E, Streicher M, Preilowski B: Cortical and subcortical afferent connections of the primate's temporal pole: A study of rhesus monkeys, squirrel monkeys, and marmosets. J Comp Neurol 1985;242:425–458.

Mori K, Nagao H, Yoshihara Y: The olfactory bulb: Coding and processing of odor molecule information. Science 1999;286:711–715.

Mori K, von Campenhause H, Yoshihara Y: Zonal organization of the mammalian main and accessory olfactory systems. Philos Trans R Soc Lond B Biol Sci 2000;355:1801–1812.

Pritchard TC, Hamilton RB, Morse JR, et al: Projections of thalamic gustatory and lingual areas in the monkey, *Macaca fascicularis.* J Comp Neurol 1986;244:213–228.

Qureshy A, Kawashima R, Imran MB, et al: Functional mapping of human brain in olfactory processing: A PET study. J Neurophysiol 2000;84:1656–1666.

Reilly S: The role of the gustatory thalamus in taste-guided behavior. Neurosci Biobehav Rev 1998;22:883–901.

Ressler KJ, Sullivan SL, Buck LB: A molecular dissection of spatial patterning in the olfactory system. Curr Opin Neurobiol 1994;4:588–596.

Ressler KJ, Sullivan SL, Buck LB: Information coding in the olfactory system: Evidence for a stereotyped and highly organized epitope map in the olfactory bulb. Cell 1994; 79:1245–1255.

Rolls ET: The orbitofrontal cortex. Philos Trans R Soc Lond B Biol Sci 1996;351:1433–1443; discussion 1443–1434.

Scott TR, Plata-Salaman CR: Taste in the monkey cortex. Physiol Behav 1999;67:489–511.

Shepherd GM, Greer CA: Olfactory bulb. In Shepherd GM (editor): The Synaptic Organization of the Brain. Oxford University Press; 1990:133–169.

Shikama Y, Kato T, Nagaoka U, et al: Localization of the gustatory pathway in the human midbrain. Neurosci Lett 1996;218:198–200.

Small DM, Zatorre RJ, Dagher A, Evans AC, Jones-Gotman M: Changes in brain activity related to eating chocolate: From pleasure to aversion. Brain 2001;124:1720–1733.

Smith DV, Margolskee RF: Making sense of taste. Sci Am 2001;284:32–39.

Steward WB, Kauer JS, Shepherd GM: Functional organization of rat olfactory bulb, analyzed by the 2-deoxyglucose method. J Comp Neurol 1979;185:715–734.

Sweazey RD, Bradley RM: Response characteristics of lamb pontine neurons to stimulation of the oral cavity and epiglottis with different sensory modalities. J Neurophysiol 1993;70:1168–1180.

Uesaka Y, Nose H, Ida M, Takagi A: The pathway of gustatory fibers of the human ascends ipsilaterally in the pons. Neurology 1998;50:827–828.

Vassar R, Chao SK, Sticheran R, Nuñez JM, Vosshall LB, Axel R: Topographic organization of sensory projections to the olfactory bulb. Cell 1994;79:981–991.

Vassar R, Ngai J, Axel R: Spatial organization of odorant receptor expression in the mammalian olfactory epithelium. Cell 1993;74:309–318.

Vogt BA, Pandya DN, Rosene DL: Cingulate cortex of the rhesus monkey: I. Cytoarchitecture and thalamic afferents. J Comp Neurol 1987;262:256–270.

Zou Z, Horowitz LF, Montmayeur JP, Snapper S, Buck LB: Genetic tracing reveals a stereotyped sensory map in the olfactory cortex. Nature 2001;414:173–179.

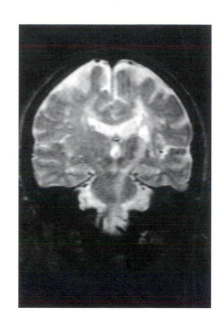

III

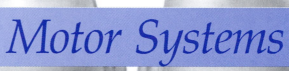

Motor Systems

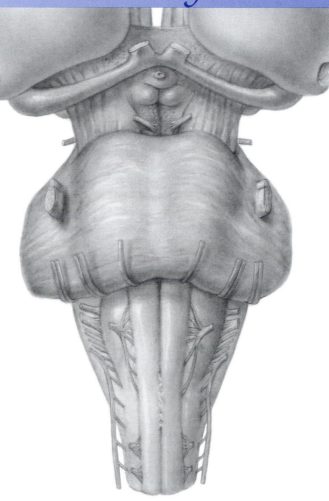

10

Descending Motor Pathways and the Motor Function of the Spinal Cord

THE MOTOR SYSTEMS OF THE BRAIN AND SPINAL CORD work together to control body movements. These systems must fulfill diverse tasks because the functions of the muscles of the body differ markedly. Consider, for instance, the fine control required of skeletal muscles in the hand in grasping a china cup in contrast to the gross strength required of back and leg muscles in lifting a box full of books. The muscles that move the eyes have an entirely different set of tasks, such as positioning the eyes to capture information from the visual world. The principal function of facial muscles is not movement but rather creating facial expressions as well as assisting in speech articulation. These jobs are so varied that it is not surprising that the motor systems have specific components devoted to their control.

The first three chapters covering the motor system examine the components of the brain and spinal cord that are essential for contracting muscle. Damage to these components can produce muscle weakness. This chapter focuses on the neuroanatomy of limb control and posture, first with an overview and then with an examination of the descending spinal motor pathways and the spinal cord motor nuclei to which they project. The pathways that control facial and other head muscles are discussed in Chapter 11. Because eye movement and balance share many neural circuits, and a strong interrelationship with the vestibular system, these topics are covered jointly in Chapter 12.

FUNCTIONAL ANATOMY OF THE MOTOR SYSTEMS AND THE DESCENDING MOTOR PATHWAYS

Diverse Central Nervous System Structures Comprise the Motor Systems

Four separate components of the central nervous system comprise the systems for controlling skeletal muscles that steer movements of the limbs and trunk (Figure 10–1A): (1) descending motor pathways, together with their associated cortical areas and sub-cortical nuclei, (2) motor neurons and interneurons, (3) basal ganglia, and (4) the cerebellum.

The regions of the cerebral cortex and brain stem that contribute to the **descending motor pathways** are organized much like the ascending sensory pathways but in reverse: from the cerebral cortex toward the periphery. The brain stem motor pathways engage in relatively automatic control, such as rapid postural adjustments and correction of misdirected movements. By contrast, the cortical motor pathways participate in more refined and adaptive control, such as reaching to objects and grasping. The motor pathways synapse directly on motor neurons as well as on interneurons that in turn synapse on motor neurons.

These **motor neurons** and **interneurons** comprise the second component of the motor systems. For muscles of the limbs and trunk, motor neurons and most interneurons are found in the **ventral horn** and **intermediate zone** of the spinal cord. (The intermediate zone corresponds primarily to the spinal gray matter lateral to the central canal. It is sometimes included within the ventral horn.) For muscles of the head, including facial muscles, the motor neurons and interneurons are located in the **cranial nerve motor nuclei** and the **reticular formation,** respectively (see Chapter 11).

The third and fourth components of the motor systems, the **cerebellum** and the **basal ganglia** (see Chap-

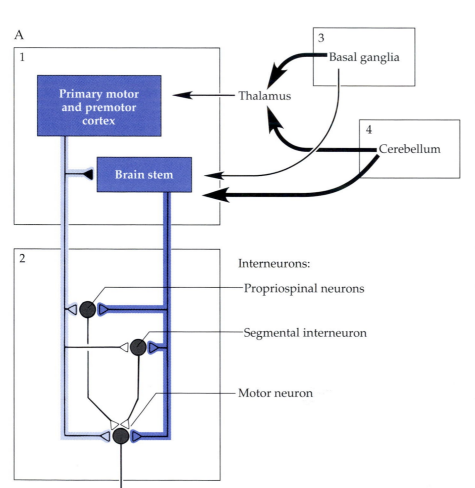

Figure 10–1. *A.* General organization of the motor systems. There are four major components to the motor systems (each enclosed by a box): descending pathways, motor neurons and interneurons, basal ganglia, and cerebellum. This figure also illustrates the parallel and hierarchical organization of the motor systems. In this example there are two parallel pathways: one from the primary motor cortex and the other from the brain stem to motor neurons. Three hierarchical pathways originate in the cortex but contact three different sets of neurons: descending projection neurons in the brain stem, propriospinal neurons, and segmental interneurons.

B

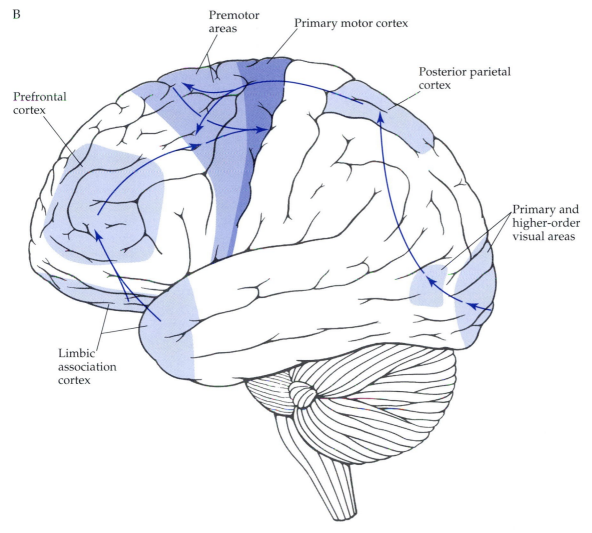

Figure 10–1 (continued). **B.** Key cortical regions for controlling movement. The limbic and prefrontal association areas are involved in the initial decision to move, in relation to motivational and emotional factors. In reaching to grasp an object, the visual areas process information about the location and shape of the object. This information is transmitted, via the posterior parietal lobe, to the premotor areas, which are important in movement planning. From there, information is transmitted to the primary motor cortex, from which descending control signals are sent to the motor neurons.

ters 13 and 14), do not contain neurons that project directly to motor neurons. Nevertheless, these structures have a powerful regulatory influence over motor behavior. They act indirectly in controlling motor behavior through their effects on the descending brain stem pathways and, via the thalamus, cortical pathways (Figure 10–1A).

Many Cortical Regions Are Recruited Into Action During Visually Guided Movements

Other areas of the brain provide the motor systems with information essential for accurate movement control (Figure 10–1B). For example, during visually guided behaviors—such as reaching to grasp a cup—the process of translating thoughts and sensations into action begins with the initial decision to move. This process is dependent on the **limbic** and **prefrontal association areas** (Figure 10–1B), which are involved in emotions, motivation, and cognition.

The **magnocellular visual system** processes visual information for guiding movements. As discussed in Chapter 7, the magnocellular visual system projects to the **posterior parietal lobe** (the "where" path; see Figure 7–16), a cortical area important for identifying the location of salient objects in the environment and for attention (Figure 10–1B). Visual information next is distributed to **premotor areas** of the frontal lobe, where the plan of action to reach to the cup is formed. This plan specifies the path the hand takes to reach the target and prepares the hand for grasping or manipulation once contact with the object occurs. Planning requires determining which muscles to contract, and when. Whereas the decision to move is a conscious experience, much of the planning of a movement is not.

The next step in translating into action the decision to reach is directing the muscles to contract. This step involves the cortical motor areas and the corticospinal tract. The **primary motor cortex** is the most important area because it has the largest projection to the spinal cord. The **corticospinal tract** transmits control signals to motor neurons and to interneurons. As discussed below, most of the premotor areas also contribute axons to the corticospinal tract. The cortical motor pathways also recruit brain stem pathways (Figure 10–1A) for coordinating voluntary movements with postural adjustments, such as maintaining balance when lifting a heavy object.

The specific contributions of the cerebellum and basal ganglia to movement control are surprisingly elusive. The cerebellum is part of a set of neural circuits that compare intention to move with the actual movement that took place. When a disparity between intent and action is detected, the cerebellum can generate an error-correcting control signal. This signal is then transmitted to the cortical and brain stem motor pathways (Figure 10–1A). However, this description only captures a small part of cerebellar function (see Chapter 13). Even less is known about basal ganglia function. The specific contribution of the basal ganglia to motor action plan formulation is unknown, but movements become disordered when the basal ganglia are damaged. For example, in patients with Parkinson disease, a neurodegenerative disease that primarily affects the basal ganglia, movements are slow or fail to be initiated and patients have significant tremors.

There Are Three Functional Classes of Descending Pathways

Descending pathways can be classified as (1) motor control pathways, (2) pathways that regulate somatic sensory processing, and (3) pathways that regulate the functions of the autonomic nervous system. **Motor control pathways** mediate the voluntary and involuntary (or automatic) control of movement. As described earlier, they originate in the cerebral cortex and brain stem and synapse on motor neurons and interneurons.

The descending pathways that regulate **somatic sensory processing** also originate in the cerebral cortex and brain stem but terminate primarily on **dorsal horn neurons** and in brain stem **somatic sensory relay nuclei.** These pathways are important for controlling the flow of somatic sensory information into the central nervous system, which has an important effect on perception. For example, the raphespinal pathway suppresses pain transmission (see Chapter 5).

The descending pathways that regulate the **autonomic nervous system** originate from the cerebral cortex, amygdala, hypothalamus, and brain stem. The neurons comprising these pathways synapse on preganglionic autonomic neurons in the brain stem and spinal cord. The autonomic pathways, together with the autonomic nervous system itself, are examined along with the hypothalamus in Chapter 15.

Multiple Parallel Motor Control Pathways Originate From the Cortex and Brain Stem

Seven major descending motor control pathways terminate in the brain stem and spinal cord (Table 10–1). Three of these pathways originate in layer V of the cerebral cortex, primarily in the frontal lobe: (1) the **lateral corticospinal tract,** (2) the **ventral (or anterior) corticospinal tract,** and (3) the **corticobulbar tract.** The corticobulbar tract terminates primarily in cranial motor nuclei in the pons and medulla and is the cranial equivalent of the corticospinal tracts. It is considered in detail in Chapter 11. The remaining four pathways originate from brain stem nuclei: (4) the **rubrospinal tract,** (5) the **reticulospinal tracts,** (6) the **tectospinal tract,** and (7) the **vestibulospinal tracts.** Similar to the ascending somatic sensory pathways (see Chapter 5), the various parallel motor control pathways serve separate but overlapping functions, which are discussed below. In addition to these seven descending motor pathways, neurotransmitter-specific systems—including the raphe nuclei, locus ceruleus, and midbrain dopaminergic neurons—have diffuse projections to the spinal cord intermediate zone and ventral horn. Other than pain regulation, the functions of these descending pathways are not well understood (see Chapter 2).

Motor Pathways of the Spinal Cord Have a Hierarchical Organization

Each of the descending motor pathways influences skeletal muscle via **monosynaptic, disynaptic,** and **polysynaptic connections** between descending projection neurons and **motor neurons** (Figure 10–1A). Typi-

Table 10–1. Descending pathways for controlling movement.

Tract	Site of origin	Decussation	Spinal cord column	Site of termination	Function
Cerebral Cortex					
Corticospinal					
Lateral	Areas 6, 4, 1, 2, 3, 5, 7, 23	Crossed—pyramidal decussation	Lateral	Dorsal horn, lateral intermediate zone, ventral horn	Sensory control, voluntary movement (limb muscles)
Ventral	Areas 6, 4	Uncrossed[3]	Ventral	Medial intermediate zone, ventral horn	Voluntary movement (axial muscles)
Corticobulbar	Areas 6, 4, 1, 2, 3, 5, 7, 23	Crossed and uncrossed[2]	Brain stem only	Cranial nerve sensory and motor nuclei, reticular formation	Sensory control, voluntary movement (cranial muscles)
Brain Stem					
Rubrospinal	Red nucleus (magnocellular)	Ventral tegmentum	Lateral	Lateral intermediate zone, ventral horn	Voluntary movement, limb muscles
Vestibulospinal					
Lateral	Lateral vestibular nucleus	Ipsilateral[1]	Ventral	Medial intermediate zone, ventral horn	Balance
Medial	Medial vestibular nucleus	Bilateral	Ventral	Medial intermediate zone, ventral horn	Head position/ neck muscles
Reticulospinal					
Pontine	Pontine reticular formation	Ipsilateral[1]	Ventral	Medial intermediate horn, ventral horn	Autonomic movement, axial and limb muscles
Medullary	Medullary reticular formation	Ipsilateral[1]	Ventrolateral	Medial intermediate zone, ventral horn	Autonomic movement, axial and limb muscles
Tectospinal	Deep superior colliculus	Dorsal tegmentum	Ventral	Medial intermediate zone, ventral horn	Coordinates neck with eye movements

[1]Whereas these tracts descend ipsilaterally, they terminate on interneurons whose axons decussate in the ventral commissure and thus influence axial musculature bilaterally.
[2]Most of the projections to the cranial nerve motor nuclei are bilateral; those to the part of the facial nucleus that innervates upper facial muscles are bilateral, and those to the lower facial muscles are contralateral (see Chapter 11).

cally the axon of a descending projection neuron makes all types of connections with motor neurons. Whether disynaptic or polysynaptic, the connections are mediated by two kinds of spinal cord interneurons: segmental interneurons and propriospinal neurons. **Segmental interneurons** (sometimes termed **intrasegmental neurons**) have a short axon that distributes branches within a single spinal cord segment to synapse on motor neurons. In addition to receiving input from the descending motor pathways, segmental interneurons receive convergent input from different classes of somatic sensory receptors for the reflex control of movement. For example, particular inter-

neurons receive input from nociceptors and mediate limb withdrawal reflexes in response to painful stimuli, such as when you jerk your hand away from a hot stove. Segmental interneurons are located primarily in the intermediate zone and the ventral horn on the same side (ipsilateral) as the motor neurons on which they synapse. **Propriospinal neurons** (sometimes termed **intersegmental neurons**) have an axon that projects for multiple spinal segments before synapsing on motor neurons (Figure 10–1A).

The **hierarchical organization** of the motor pathways reflects the fact that there are monosynaptic and polysynaptic pathways to the motor neurons. Three basic hierarchical motor pathways exist: (1) mono-synaptic corticospinal projections to motor neurons, (2) disynaptic corticospinal projections to motor neurons, via segmental and propriospinal interneurons, and (3) polysynaptic pathways to complex spinal interneuronal circuits (not shown in Figure 10–1A).

In addition to the direct corticospinal pathways to the spinal cord, there are **indirect cortical pathways** that route through the brain stem, such as the **cortico-reticulo-spinal pathway.** The first leg of this type of pathway consists of a cortical projection to the brain stem; the second leg is simply the brain stem motor pathway, such as the reticulospinal tract. Considering all combinations of pathways, the projection neurons of the cerebral cortex constitute the highest level in the hierarchy, the brain stem projection neurons comprise the next lower level, and spinal interneurons and the motor neurons are the two lowest levels. Can brain stem motor pathways work independent of the cortical pathways? The answer is probably yes, based on laboratory animal studies. Both the cerebellum and basal ganglia have direct brain stem projections (Figure 10–1A), which could influence brain stem motor pathway function without cortical pathway involvement.

The Functional Organization of the Descending Pathways Parallels the Somatotopic Organization of the Motor Nuclei in the Ventral Horn

The motor neurons innervating **limb muscles,** and the interneurons from which they receive input, are located in the **lateral ventral horn** and **intermediate zone.** In contrast, motor neurons innervating **axial** and **girdle muscles** (ie, neck and shoulder muscles), and their associated interneurons, are located in the **medial ventral horn** and **intermediate zone.** The mediolateral somatotopic organization of the intermediate zone and ventral horn is easy to remember because it mimics the form of the body (Figure 10–2). This mediolateral somatotopic organization also applies to the descending motor pathways in the spinal cord white matter. The pathways that descend in the lateral portion of the spinal cord white matter control limb muscles. In contrast, the pathways that descend in the medial portion of the white matter control axial and girdle muscles.

The Laterally Descending Pathways Control Limb Muscles and Regulate Voluntary Movement

There are two laterally descending pathways: the lateral corticospinal tract, which originates in the cerebral cortex, and the rubrospinal tract, which descends from the midbrain (Table 10–1). The neurons that give rise to these pathways have a **somatotopic** organization. Moreover, the lateral corticospinal and rubrospinal tracts control muscles on the **contralateral** side of the body. The **lateral corticospinal tract** is the principal motor control pathway in humans. A lesion of this pathway anywhere along its path to the motor neuron produces devastating and persistent limb use impairments. One such impairment is the loss of the ability to **fractionate movements,** that is, to move one finger independent of the others. Manual dexterity depends on fractionation, without which hand movements are clumsy and imprecise.

The major site of origin of the lateral corticospinal tract is the primary motor cortex (Figure 10–3A); axons also originate from the premotor cortical regions and the somatic sensory cortical areas. Descending axons in the tract that originate in the primary motor cortex course within the cerebral hemisphere in the **posterior limb of the internal capsule** and, in the mid-

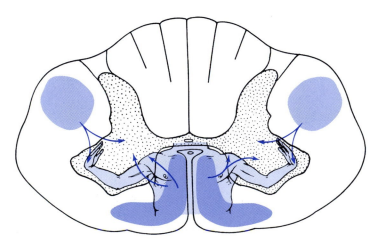

Figure 10–2. Schematic diagram of the spinal cord, showing the somatotopic organization of the ventral horn and indicating the general locations of motor neurons innervating limb and axial muscles and flexor and extensor muscles. A partial homunculus is superimposed on the ventral horns. (*Adapted from Crosby EC, Humphrey T, Lauer EW: Correlative Anatomy of the Nervous System. Macmillan, 1962.*)

brain, in the **basis pedunculi** (Figure 10–3A). Next on its descending course, the tract disappears beneath the ventral surface of the pons only to reappear on the ventral surface of the medulla as the **pyramid.** At the junction of the spinal cord and medulla, the axons **decussate** (pyramidal decussation) and descend in the dorsolateral portion of the lateral column of the spinal cord white matter; hence the name lateral corticospinal tract (see Figure 10–5). This pathway terminates primarily in the lateral portions of the intermediate zone and ventral horn of the cervical and lumbosacral cord, the locations of neurons that control distal limb muscles of the hand and foot.

The **rubrospinal tract** (Figure 10–3B), which has fewer axons than the corticospinal tract, originates from neurons in the **red nucleus,** primarily from the caudal part. This portion is termed the **magnocellular division** because many rubrospinal tract neurons are large. The rubrospinal tract decussates in the midbrain and descends in the dorsolateral portion of the brain stem. Similar to the lateral corticospinal tract, the rubrospinal tract is found in the dorsal portion of the lateral column (see Figure 10–5) and terminates primarily in the lateral portions of the intermediate zone and ventral horn of the cervical cord. In humans, the rubrospinal tract does not descend into the lumbosacral cord, suggesting that it functions in arm but not leg control.

The Medially Descending Pathways
Control Axial and Girdle Muscles
and Regulate Posture

Axial and girdle muscles are controlled primarily by the four medially descending pathways: the ventral corticospinal tract, the reticulospinal tracts, the tectospinal tract, and the vestibulospinal tracts (Table 10–1). (The vestibulospinal tracts are considered in Chapter 12, along with eye and head movement control.) The medial descending pathways exert **bilateral control** over axial and girdle muscles. Even though individual pathways may project unilaterally (either ipsilaterally or contralaterally), they synapse on interneurons whose axons decussate in the **ventral spinal commissure** (see Figure 10–17C). Bilateral control provides a measure of redundancy: Unilateral lesion of a bilateral pathway typically does not have a profound behavioral effect.

The **ventral corticospinal tract** originates predominantly from the **primary motor cortex** and the **premotor cortex** and descends to the medulla along with the lateral corticospinal tract (Figure 10–4A). However, the ventral corticospinal tract remains uncrossed and descends in the **ipsilateral ventral column** of the

spinal cord (Figure 10–5; see Figure 10–19). Many ventral corticospinal tract axons have branches that decussate in the spinal cord. This tract terminates in the medial gray matter, synapsing on motor neurons in the medial ventral horn and on interneurons in the medial intermediate zone. The ventral corticospinal tract projects only to the cervical and upper thoracic spinal cord; thus, it is preferentially involved in the control of the neck, shoulder, and upper trunk muscles.

The **reticulospinal tracts** (Figure 10–4B) originate from different regions of the **pontine and medullary reticular formation**. The pontine reticulospinal tract descends in the ventral column of the spinal cord, whereas the medullary reticulospinal tract descends in the ventrolateral quadrant of the lateral column (Figure 10–5). The reticulospinal tracts descend predominantly in the ipsilateral spinal cord but exert bilateral motor control effects. Laboratory animal studies show that the reticulospinal tracts control relatively automatic movements, such as maintaining posture or walking over even terrain.

The **tectospinal tract** (Figure 10–4B) originates primarily from neurons located in the deeper layers of the superior colliculus, which is also termed the **tectum,** the portion of the midbrain dorsal to the cerebral aqueduct (see Figure 10–11A). The tectospinal tract also has a limited rostrocaudal distribution, projecting only to the cervical spinal segments. It therefore participates primarily in the control of neck, shoulder, and upper trunk muscles. Because the superior colliculus also plays a key role in controlling eye movements (see Chapter 12), it is likely that the tectospinal tract is important for coordinating head movements with eye movements.

The various descending pathways in the spinal cord are illustrated on the right side of Figure 10–5; the ascending somatic sensory pathways (see Chapter 5) are illustrated on the left side. The two spinocerebellar pathways, which transmit sensory information to the cerebellum for controlling movement (see Chapter 13), also are illustrated.

REGIONAL ANATOMY OF THE MOTOR SYSTEMS AND THE DESCENDING MOTOR PATHWAYS

The rest of this chapter examines the brain and spinal cord with the aim of understanding the motor pathways and their spinal terminations. This discussion begins with the cerebral cortex—the highest level of the movement control hierarchy—and proceeds caudally to the spinal cord, following the natural flow of information processing in the motor systems.

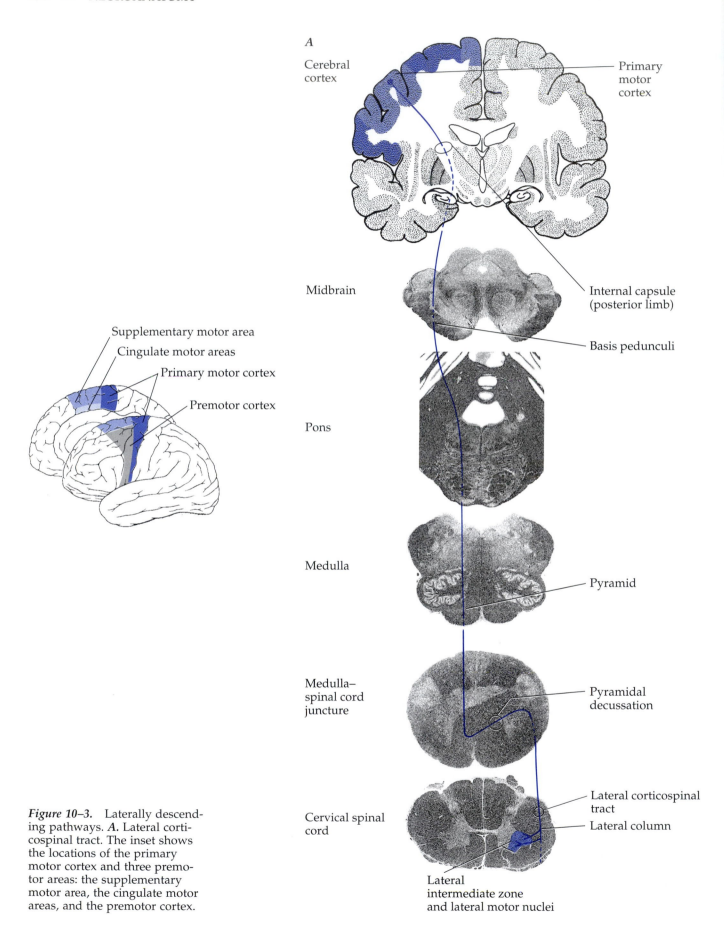

A

Cerebral cortex

Primary motor cortex

Internal capsule (posterior limb)

Midbrain

Basis pedunculi

Pons

Medulla

Pyramid

Medulla–spinal cord juncture

Pyramidal decussation

Lateral corticospinal tract

Lateral column

Cervical spinal cord

Lateral intermediate zone and lateral motor nuclei

Supplementary motor area

Cingulate motor areas

Primary motor cortex

Premotor cortex

Figure 10–3. Laterally descending pathways. *A.* Lateral corticospinal tract. The inset shows the locations of the primary motor cortex and three premotor areas: the supplementary motor area, the cingulate motor areas, and the premotor cortex.

B

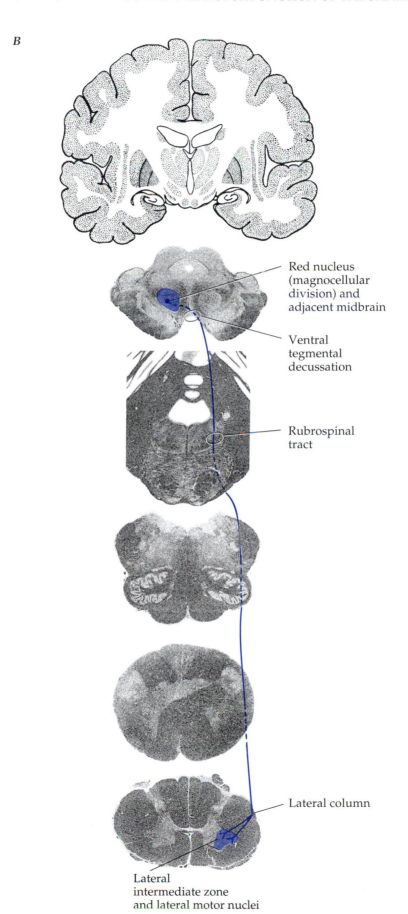

Red nucleus
(magnocellular
division) and
adjacent midbrain

Ventral
tegmental
decussation

Rubrospinal
tract

Lateral column

Lateral
intermediate zone
and lateral motor nuclei

Figure 10–3 (continued).
B. Rubrospinal tract. The lateral corticospinal tract also originates from neurons located in area 6 and the parietal lobe.

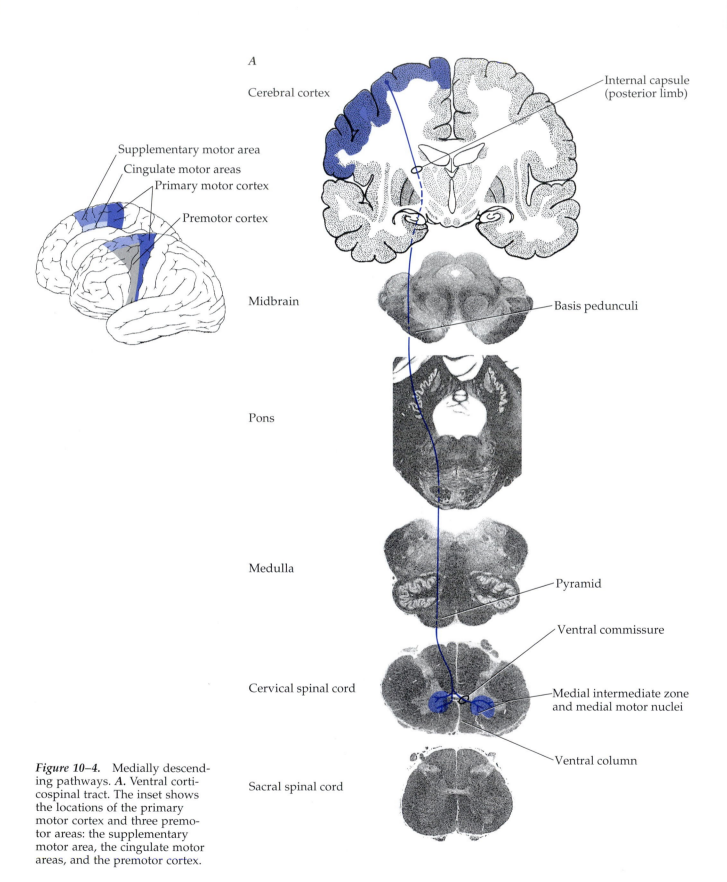

A

Cerebral cortex

Supplementary motor area
Cingulate motor areas
Primary motor cortex
Premotor cortex

Internal capsule (posterior limb)

Midbrain

Basis pedunculi

Pons

Medulla

Pyramid

Ventral commissure

Cervical spinal cord

Medial intermediate zone and medial motor nuclei

Ventral column

Sacral spinal cord

Figure 10–4. Medially descending pathways. *A.* Ventral corticospinal tract. The inset shows the locations of the primary motor cortex and three premotor areas: the supplementary motor area, the cingulate motor areas, and the premotor cortex.

B

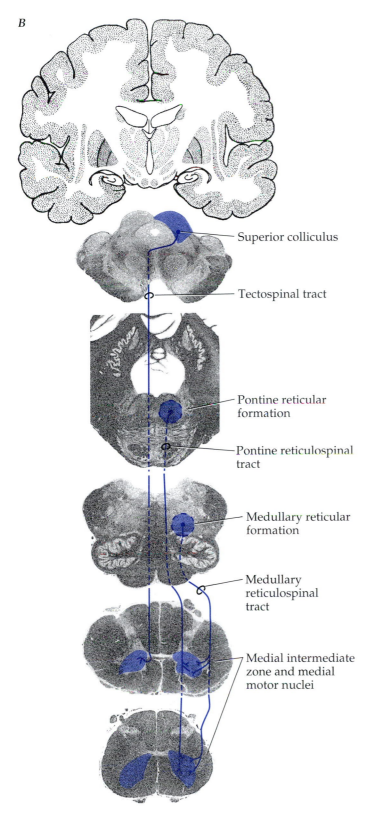

— Superior colliculus

— Tectospinal tract

— Pontine reticular formation

— Pontine reticulospinal tract

— Medullary reticular formation

— Medullary reticulospinal tract

— Medial intermediate zone and medial motor nuclei

Figure 10–4 (continued). **B.** Tectospinal tract and pontine and medullary reticulospinal tracts.

The Cortical Motor Areas Are Located in the Frontal Lobe

Similar to each sensory modality, multiple cortical sites serve motor control functions (Figure 10–6). Four separate motor areas have been identified in the frontal lobe: the primary motor cortex, the supplementary motor area, the premotor cortex, and the cingulate motor area. Many of these areas have distinct subregions.

The **primary motor cortex** (Figure 10–6) gives rise to most of the fibers in the corticospinal tracts and has a complete and somatotopically organized body representation (see below). It plays a key role in the execution of skilled movement. The primary motor cortex is found in the caudal part of the **precentral gyrus,** extending from the lateral sulcus to the medial surface of the cerebral hemisphere. The **premotor cortical regions** are rostral to the primary motor cortex and consist of the **supplementary motor area,** the **premotor cortex,** and the **cingulate motor areas** (Figure 10–6). Collectively the premotor cortical regions receive information from the association cortex—the prefrontal cortex, posterior parietal cortex, and limbic cortex—and participate in movement planning. They have dense projections to the primary motor cortex. They also may participate in movement execution because many premotor cortical regions have direct spinal projections, via the **corticospinal tract.**

The Premotor Cortical Regions Integrate Information From Diverse Sources

The **supplementary motor area** is located primarily on the medial surface of the cerebral hemisphere, in area 6 (Figure 10–6). Its major subcortical input arises from the **ventral anterior nucleus** of the thalamus (see Figure 10–10A), which is a relay nucleus for the **basal ganglia.** One key cortical input is from the prefrontal cortex, which is important in high-level planning of motor behavior. Imaging and lesion studies in humans suggest that the supplementary motor area plays a role in planning voluntary movements that are internally generated—or willed—rather than movements provoked by a stimulus.

The **premotor cortex** is located laterally in area 6 (Figure 10–6A). In contrast to the supplementary motor area, which gets its input from the basal ganglia, the premotor cortex receives its major input from the **cerebellum,** relayed by the **ventrolateral nucleus** of the thalamus (see Figure 10–10A). The premotor cortex has at least two distinct motor fields with separate sets of

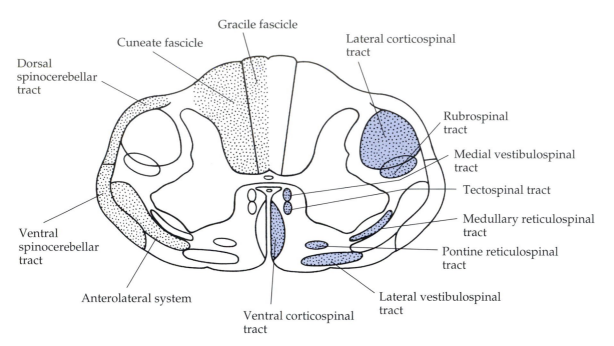

Dorsal spinocerebellar tract

Cuneate fascicle

Gracile fascicle

Lateral corticospinal tract

Rubrospinal tract

Medial vestibulospinal tract

Tectospinal tract

Medullary reticulospinal tract

Pontine reticulospinal tract

Ventral spinocerebellar tract

Anterolateral system

Ventral corticospinal tract

Lateral vestibulospinal tract

Figure 10–5. Schematic diagram of the spinal cord, indicating the locations of the ascending (*left*) and descending (*right*) pathways.

connections: the dorsal and ventral premotor cortices. Parts of the premotor cortex have a major descending projection to the **reticular formation.** This pathway may be important for controlling the actions of girdle muscles by a projection to neurons that give rise to the **reticulospinal tracts.** The premotor cortex plays a role in voluntary movements guided by stimuli, especially vision. Studies in laboratory animals suggest that the dorsal premotor cortex participates in the control of reaching and that the ventral premotor cortex participates in grasping.

The **cingulate motor area** is found on the medial surface of the cerebral hemisphere, in cytoarchitectonic areas 6, 23, and 24, deep within the cingulate sulcus (Figure 10–6B). Curiously this motor area, which in the monkey comprises three separate subfields, is located in a cortical region that is considered part of the **limbic system,** which is important for emotions. This motor area may play a role in motor behaviors that occur in response to emotions and drives.

The Primary Motor Cortex Gives Rise to Most of the Fibers of the Corticospinal Tract

The primary motor cortex, which corresponds to **cytoarchitectonic area 4,** receives input from three

major sources: the premotor cortical regions, the somatic sensory areas (in the parietal lobe), and the thalamus. These input pathways transmit neural control signals that motor cortical neurons integrate to produce accurately directed voluntary movements. As discussed earlier, premotor cortical regions receive input from diverse cortical and subcortical sources. The somatic sensory cortical areas (primary, secondary, and higher-order areas) have privileged access to the primary motor cortex, whereas other sensory cortical areas do not. This may be because somatic sensory information from the limbs and trunk is essential for coordinating all movements. Thalamic input to the primary motor cortex comes primarily from the **ventrolateral nucleus** (see Figure 10–10A), the principal thalamic relay nucleus for the **cerebellum.** The primary motor cortex also receives a smaller input from the basal ganglia, relayed by the **ventral anterior nucleus** (see Figure 10–10A). Thus, the cerebellum and basal ganglia can influence the primary motor cortex by two separate routes: through direct thalamic projections to the primary motor cortex and through corticocortical projections from the premotor cortex and the supplementary motor areas, respectively.

The cytoarchitecture of the primary motor cortex is different from that of sensory areas in the parietal, temporal, and occipital lobes (see Figure 2–17). Whereas the sensory areas have a thick layer IV and a thin

Figure 10–6. Lateral (*A*) and medial (*B*) views of the human brain, indicating the locations of the primary motor cortex, premotor cortex, supplementary motor area, and cingulate motor area. The primary somatic sensory cortex is also shown.

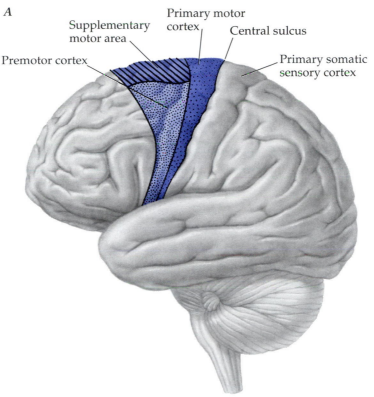

A

Premotor cortex

Supplementary motor area

Primary motor cortex

Central sulcus

Primary somatic sensory cortex

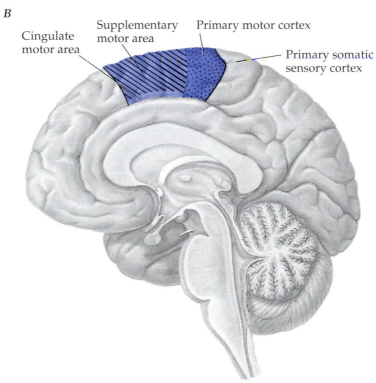

B

Cingulate motor area

Supplementary motor area

Primary motor cortex

Primary somatic sensory cortex

layer V, the primary motor cortex has a **thin layer IV** and a **thick layer V.** Recall that layer IV is the principal input layer of the cerebral cortex, where most of the axons from the thalamic relay nuclei terminate, and that layer V is the layer from which descending projections originate (see Figure 2–16). In the motor areas, thalamic terminations have a wider laminar distribution than sensory areas.

The primary motor cortex, like the somatic sensory cortex (see Chapter 5), is somatotopically organized (Figure 10–7). In the primary motor cortex, somatotopy can be revealed by electrical stimulation of the cortical surface, a procedure often used during neurosurgery or by functional imaging, such as functional magnetic resonance imaging (fMRI) (see Chapter 2). Regions controlling facial muscles (through projections to the cranial nerve motor nuclei; see Chapter 11) are located in the lateral portion of the precentral gyrus, close to the lateral sulcus. Regions controlling other body parts are—from the lateral side of the cerebral cortex to the medial side—neck, arm, and trunk areas. The leg and foot areas are found on and close to the medial surface of the brain. Figure 10–8 shows an example of two fMRI scans of the primary motor cortex while the person made simple movements of the arm and leg. Arm movement activated the lateral part of the primary motor cortex, whereas leg movement activated the medial part. The motor representation in the precentral gyrus forms the **motor homunculus;** it is distorted in a similar way as the **sensory homunculus** of the postcentral gyrus (see Figure 5–16B).

Within the representations of the individual major body parts in the primary motor cortex—face, arm, trunk, and leg—the somatotopic organization does not seem to be as precise as that in the primary somatic sensory cortex. Functional imaging in humans, as well as studies in laboratory animals, suggest that although the primary motor cortex has an overall somatotopic organization—with distinct face, arm, trunk, and leg zones—within a given zone the organization is more complex. For example, muscles of a body part that act together to produce a particular motor behavior, such as reaching, appear to be represented together within a somatotopic zone.

Somatotopic organization means that different mediolateral regions of the primary motor cortex contribute differently to the three descending corticospinal pathways (Figure 10–7). As described above, limb muscles are preferentially controlled by the **lateral corticospinal tract,** and girdle and axial muscles are controlled by the **ventral corticospinal tract.** It follows that arm and leg areas contribute preferentially to the lateral corticospinal tract, and neck, shoulder, and trunk regions to the ventral corticospinal tract. The face area of the primary motor cortex projects to the cranial nerve motor nuclei and thus contributes axons to the **corticobulbar projection** (see Chapter 11).

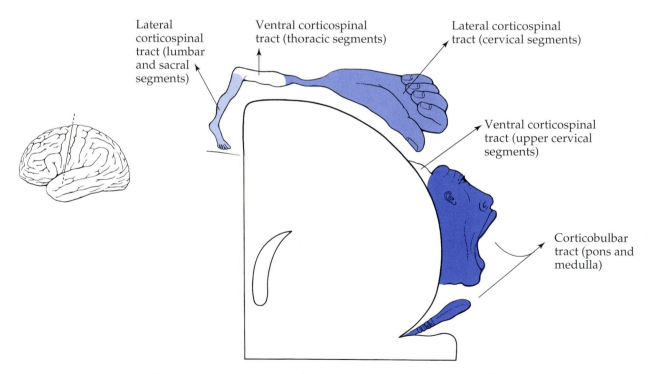

Lateral corticospinal tract (lumbar and sacral segments)

Ventral corticospinal tract (thoracic segments)

Lateral corticospinal tract (cervical segments)

Ventral corticospinal tract (upper cervical segments)

Corticobulbar tract (pons and medulla)

Figure 10–7. Somatotopic organization of the primary motor cortex. The descending pathways by which these areas of primary motor cortex influence motor neurons are indicated. The inset shows the plane of schematic section. (*Adapted from Penfield W, Rasmussen T: The Cerebral Cortex of Man: A Clinical Study of Localization. Macmillan, 1950.*)

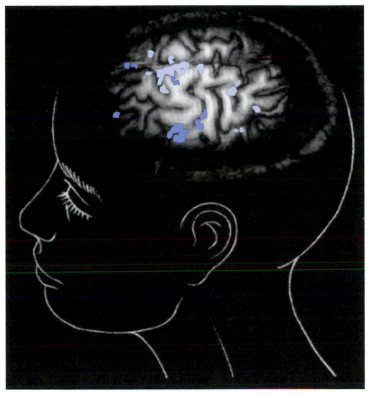

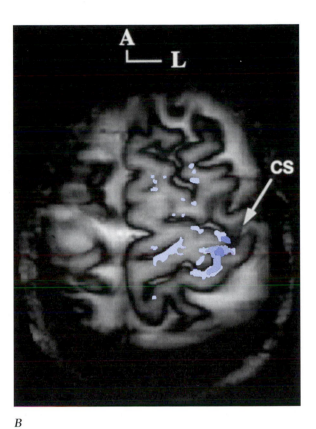

A   B

Figure 10–8. Functional imaging of human primary motor cortex. **A.** Horizontal slice through the cerebral hemispheres while the person made alternating hand and foot movements. Increased neural activity, as monitored by changes in deoxyhemoglobin detected by the magnetic resonance imaging scan, occurred laterally (dark blue)—corresponding to the hand area—and medially, within the interhemispheric fissure (light blue)—corresponding to the foot area. **B.** Horizontal slice obtained while the person made oppositional movements of the thumb with the remaining digits. This task activated only the lateral motor cortex. The strength of activation is indicated by the depth of blue: light blue, weak activation; dark blue, strong activation. (Abbreviations: A, anterior; L, lateral; CS, central sulcus.) (*A, Courtesy of Drs. SG Kim, J Ashe, AP Georgopoulos, and K Ugurbil. B, Courtesy of Drs. SG Kim, J Ashe, AP Georgopoulos, et al: Functional imaging of human motor cortex at high magnetic field. J Neurophysiol 1993; 69:297–302.*)

The Projection From Cortical Motor Regions Passes Through the Internal Capsule En Route to the Brain Stem and Spinal Cord

The **corona radiata** is the portion of the subcortical white matter that contains descending cortical axons and ascending thalamocortical axons (Figure 10–9). The corona radiata is superficial to the **internal capsule,** which contains approximately the same set of axons but is flanked by the deep nuclei of the basal ganglia and thalamus (see Figure 2–12). The internal capsule is shaped like a curved fan (Figure 10–9), with three main parts: (1) the rostral component, termed the **anterior limb,** (2) the caudal component, termed the **posterior limb,** and (3) the **genu** (Latin for "knee"),

which joins the two limbs (Figures 10–9A). The anterior limb is rostral to the thalamus, and the posterior limb is lateral to the thalamus.

Each cortical motor area sends its axons into a different part of the corona radiata and internal capsule. The descending motor projection from the primary motor cortex to the spinal cord courses in the posterior part of the posterior limb. The location of this projection is revealed in an MRI scan from a patient with a small lesion confined to the posterior limb of the internal capsule (Figure 10–9B). The pathway can be seen in this scan because degenerating axons produce a different magnetic resonance signal from that of normal axons. Retrograde degeneration can be followed back toward the cortex, and anterograde degeneration

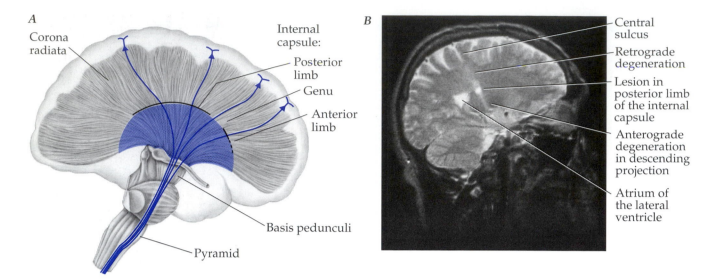

Figure 10–9. *A.* Three-dimensional view of fibers in the white matter of the cerebral cortex. The regions corresponding to the internal capsule, basis pedunculi, and pyramid are indicated. The corona radiata is the portion of the white matter beneath the gray matter of the cerebral cortex. *B.* MRI from a patient with a stroke in the posterior limb of the internal capsule. Degeneration can be followed back (or retrograde) toward the precentral gyrus and forward (or anterograde) toward the brain stem. *(Courtesy of Dr. Adrian Danek, Ludwig Maximilians University, Munich, Germany; Danek A, Bauer M, Fries W: Tracing of neuronal connections in the human brain by magnetic resonance imaging in vivo. Eur J Neurosci 1990;2:112–115.)*

can be followed toward the brain stem. The approximate location of the corticospinal projection in the posterior limb is shown in Figure 10–10A (labeled A, T, and L, for projections controlling muscles of the arm, trunk, and leg). The projection to the caudal brain stem, via the corticobulbar tract, descends rostrally to the corticospinal fibers, in the genu (labeled F for face in Figure 10–10A), as well as to part of the posterior limb of the internal capsule. Most of the path of the descending motor projection within the brain can be followed in a coronal section through the cerebral hemispheres, diencephalon, and brain stem (Figure 10–10B), and in an MRI from another patient who had a stroke in the posterior limb of the internal capsule (Figure 10–10C).

The descending projections from the premotor areas also course within the internal capsule but rostral to those from the primary motor cortex. This separation of the projections from primary and premotor cortical areas is clinically significant. Patients with a small posterior limb stroke can exhibit severe signs because of the high density of corticospinal axons. Typically, however, they can recover some function, such as strength. This recovery is mediated in part by the spinal projections from the premotor cortical regions that are ros-

tral to the injury. Small strokes tend to damage one or the other contingent of descending axons because of the particular vascular distributions in the region of the internal capsule (see Figure 4–6). The **anterior choroidal artery** supplies the posterior limb, where the projections from the primary motor cortex are located. Branches from the **anterior cerebral artery** or the **lenticulostriate branches** (anterior and middle cerebral artery) supply the anterior limb and genu.

The internal capsule also contains ascending axons as well as other descending axons. The **thalamic radiations** are the ascending thalamocortical projections located in the internal capsule (Figure 10–10A). The projections from the ventral anterior and ventrolateral nuclei of the thalamus course here. Corticopontine axons, which carry information to the cerebellum for controlling movements, and corticoreticular axons, which affect the reticular formation and reticulospinal tracts, are also located in the internal capsule. The entire internal capsule appears to condense to form the **basis pedunculi** of the midbrain (Figures 10–9 and 10–11A). The basis pedunculi contains only descending fibers and therefore appears more compact than the internal capsule, which contains both ascending thalamocortical fibers and descending cortical fibers.

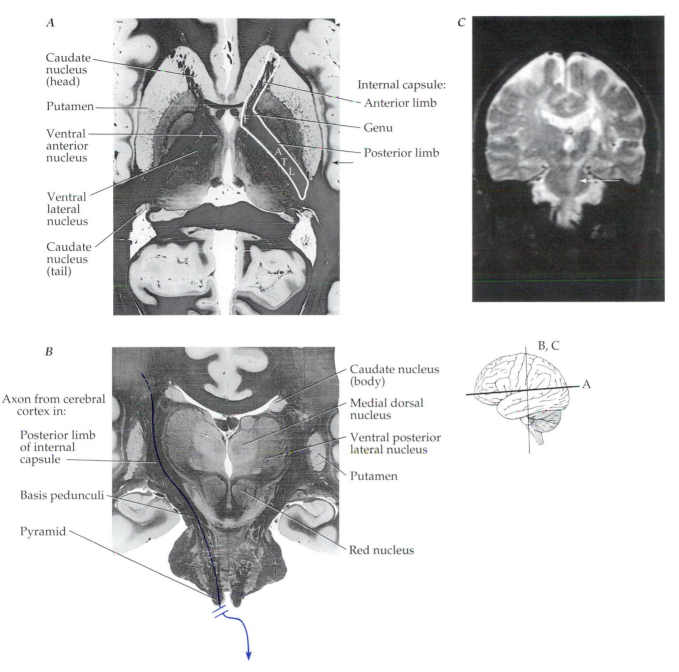

Figure 10–10. ***A.*** Myelin-stained horizontal section through the internal capsule. Note that the thalamus extends rostrally as far as the genu. The head of the caudate nucleus and the putamen are separated by the anterior limb of the internal capsule. The fiber constituents and somatotopic organization of the internal capsule are indicated. The arrow indicates the plane of section shown in ***B.*** (Abbreviations: F, face; A, arm; T, trunk; L, leg.) ***B.*** Myelin-stained coronal section through the posterior limb of the internal capsule. Note that the component of the internal capsule is identified as the posterior limb in this section because the thalamus is medial to the internal capsule. ***C.*** Magnetic resonance imaging scan from a patient with an internal capsule lesion. Coronal slice through the posterior limb of the internal capsule showing bright vertically oriented band extending from the lesion caudally into the pons. This band corresponds to degenerated axons in the internal capsule, basis pedunculi, and pons. (***C,*** *Courtesy of Dr. Jesús Pujol; from Pujol J, Martí-Vilalta JL, Junqué C, Vendrell P, Fernández J, Capdevila A: Wallerian degeneration of the pyramidal tract in capsular infarction studied by magnetic resonance imaging. Stroke 1990;21:404–409.)*

A

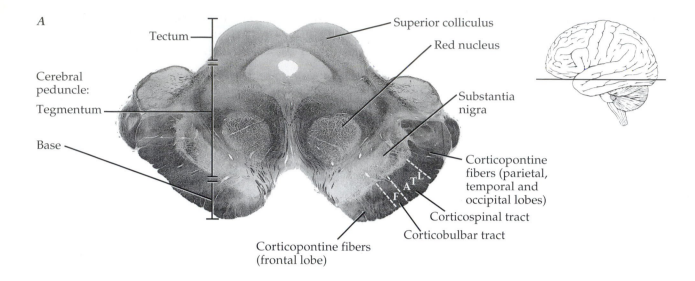

Tectum

Cerebral peduncle:

Tegmentum

Base

Superior colliculus

Red nucleus

Substantia nigra

Corticopontine fibers (parietal, temporal and occipital lobes)

Corticospinal tract

Corticobulbar tract

Corticopontine fibers (frontal lobe)

B

C

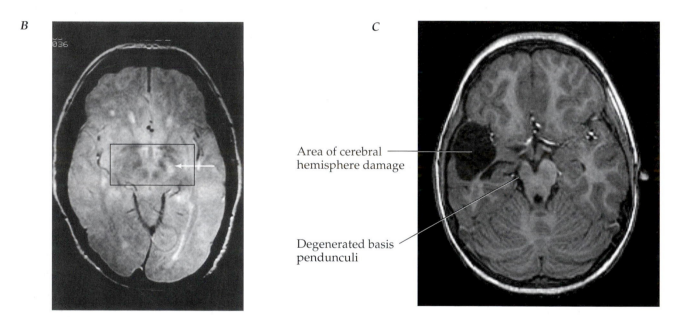

Area of cerebral hemisphere damage

Degenerated basis pedunculi

Figure 10–11. ***A.*** Myelin-stained transverse section through the rostral midbrain. The composition of axons in the basis pedunculi and the somatotopic organization of the corticospinal fibers are shown on the right. ***B.*** Transverse slice through the midbrain (horizontal slice through central hemispheres) showing site of degeneration. ***C.*** Transverse magnetic resonance imaging (MRI) scan through the midbrain of an 8-year-old child with cerebral palsy, produced by a perinatal lesion of the cerebral hemisphere. The MRI scan shows damage to the right cerebral cortex and underlying white matter and degeneration of the basis pedunculi. The area of the degenerated basis pedunculi in this patient was about half that of the other side. She had severe motor impairments of the right arm, especially for highly skilled hand movements. (***B,*** *Courtesy of Dr. Jesús Pujol; from Pujol J, Martí-Vilalta JL, Junqué C, Vendrell P, Fernández J, Capdevila A: Wallerian degeneration of the pyramidal tract in capsular infarction studied by magnetic resonance imaging. Stroke 1990;21:404–409.* ***C,*** *Courtesy of Dr. Etienne Olivier, University of Louvain; Duqué J, et al: Correlation between impaired dexterity and corticospinal tract dysgenesis in congenital hemiplegia. Brain 126:1–16, 2003.*)

The Corticospinal Tract Courses in the Base of the Midbrain

Each division of the brain stem contains three regions from its dorsal to ventral surfaces: **tectum**, **tegmentum**, and **base** (Figure 10–11A). In the rostral midbrain, the tectum consists of the **superior colliculus**. The midbrain base is termed the **basis pedunculi**. Together, the tegmentum and basis pedunculi constitute the **cerebral peduncle**.

Corticospinal tract axons course within the middle of the basis pedunculi, flanked medially and laterally by corticopontine axons (see Chapter 13) and other descending cortical axons (Figure 10–10B). The location of these axons can be seen on an MRI scan from a patient with a lesion of the posterior limb of the internal capsule (Figure 10–11B). Figure 10–11C shows atrophy in the cerebral peduncle on the side in which the patient, an 8-year-old child, had sustained damage to the motor cortex and the underlying white matter during early childhood.

The rostral midbrain is a key level in the motor system because three nuclei that subserve motor function are located here: the superior colliculus, the red nucleus, and the substantia nigra. Neurons from the deeper layers of the **superior colliculus** (Figure 10–11) give rise to the **tectospinal tract**, one of the medial descending pathways. The **red nucleus** (Figures 10–10B and 10–11A) is the origin of the **rubrospinal tract**, a lateral descending pathway that begins primarily in the **magnocellular division** of this nucleus. The other major component of the red nucleus, the **parvocellular** (or **small-celled**) **division**, is part of a multisynaptic pathway from the cerebral cortex to the cerebellum (see Chapter 13). The tectospinal and rubrospinal tracts decussate in the midbrain. The **substantia nigra** is a part of the basal ganglia (see Chapter 14). Substantia nigra neurons that contain the neurotransmitter dopamine degenerate in patients with Parkinson disease.

Descending Cortical Fibers Separate Into Small Fascicles in the Ventral Pons

In the pons the descending cortical fibers no longer occupy the ventral brain stem surface but rather are located deep within the base (Figure 10–12A, B). The pontine nuclei receive their principal input from the cerebral cortex via the **corticopontine pathway**. The corticopontine pathway is an important route by which information from all cerebral cortex lobes influences the cerebellum (see Chapter 13).

The Pontine and Medullary Reticular Formation Gives Rise to the Reticulospinal Tracts

The **reticular formation** is located in the central brain stem (see Figures 2–6 and 2–8). Neurons in the

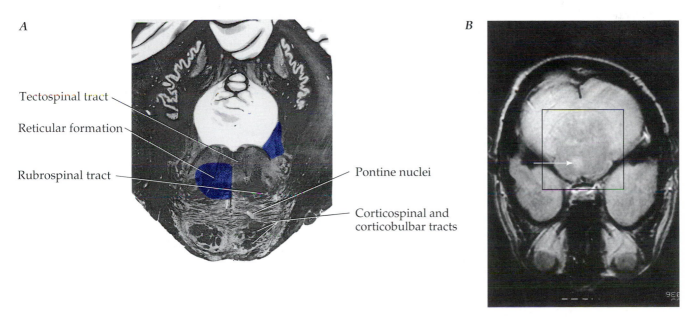

A. Myelin-stained section through the pons, showing the locations of the motor pathways.

Tectospinal tract

Reticular formation

Rubrospinal tract

Pontine nuclei

Corticospinal and corticobulbar tracts

Figure 10–12. **A.** Myelin-stained section through the pons, showing the locations of the motor pathways. **B.** Transverse slice through the pons and cerebellum (horizontal slice through central hemispheres) showing site of degeneration. (**B,** *Courtesy of Dr. Jesús Pujol; from Pujol J, Martí-Vilalta JL, Junqué C, Vendrell P, Fernández J, Capdevila A: Wallerian degeneration of the pyramidal tract in capsular infarction studied by magnetic resonance imaging. Stroke 1990;21:404–409.*)

pontine and medullary reticular formation (Figures 10–12A and 10–13A,B) give rise to the **reticulospinal tracts.** (Few reticulospinal neurons originate from the midbrain.) Experiments in laboratory animals suggest that the reticulospinal tracts control relatively automatic motor responses, such as simple postural adjustments, stepping when walking, and rapid corrections of movement errors. When these automatic responses must occur during voluntary movements, such as maintaining an upright posture when reaching to lift something heavy, the cortico-reticulo-spinal pathway is engaged.

Many reticulospinal neurons have a widespread projection pattern that often includes an axon with ascending and descending branches. The significance of this morphological pattern is that individual neurons can distribute information both to lower levels of the motor systems that are directly involved in executing movements and to higher levels thought to be involved in adapting and correcting ongoing movements.

The Lateral Corticospinal Tract Decussates in the Caudal Medulla

The path of the descending cortical fibers into the medulla can be followed in the sagittal section shown in Figure 10–14. The numerous fascicles of the caudal pons collect on the ventral surface of the medulla to form the **pyramids** (Figures 10–13 and 10–14). The axons of the lateral and ventral corticospinal tracts, which originate primarily from the **ipsilateral frontal lobe,** are located in each pyramid. This is why the terms **corticospinal tract** and **pyramidal tract** are often—but inaccurately—used interchangeably. These terms are *not* synonymous because the pyramids also contain **corticobulbar** and **corticoreticular fibers** that terminate in the medulla. Damage to the corticospinal system produces a characteristic set of motor control and muscle impairments (see section below on brain stem and spinal lesions) that are sometimes called **pyramidal signs.**

The axons descend in the pyramid and decussate in fascicles. One fascicle of decussating axons is cut in the section shown in Figure 10–13C (solid line). Another group from the other side (located just rostrally or caudally) would likely decussate along the path shown by the dotted line. The rubrospinal tract, which had crossed in the midbrain, maintains its dorsolateral position. Here, at the medulla–spinal cord junction, the crossed lateral corticospinal tract axons join the rubrospinal axons and descend in the lateral column (Figures 10–5 and 10–13C). These are the two lateral motor pathways. The reticulospinal and tectospinal

tracts remain medially located and assume a more ventral position as they descend in the spinal cord.

The Intermediate Zone and Ventral Horn of the Spinal Cord Receive Input From the Descending Pathways

The motor pathways descend in the ventral and lateral columns of the spinal cord (Figure 10–5). The lateral corticospinal tract is located in the lateral column, revealed by the zone of degeneration in the lumbar cord from an individual who had a lesion of the internal capsule prior to death (Figure 10–15). (Note that the ventral corticospinal tract descends only as far as the cervical spinal cord. Thus, there are no degenerating fibers in the ventral column.)

As discussed in Chapter 5, the dorsal horn corresponds to Rexed's laminae I through VI, the intermediate zone to lamina VII, and the ventral horn to laminae XIII and IX (Figure 10–16A). The motor nuclei are located in lamina IX. Lamina X surrounds the spinal cord central canal. The premotor, primary motor, and primary somatic sensory cortical regions all have spinal projections, but their target laminae differ. The somatic sensory cortex projects dorsally in the gray matter—preferentially to the dorsal horn—and could regulate sensory processing. Axons from the premotor and primary motor cortical regions synapse on motor neurons in the ventral horn and on interneurons in the intermediate zone, which synapse on motor neurons (Figure 10–16A). Brain stem motor pathways terminate throughout the spinal gray matter.

The Lateral and Medial Motor Nuclei Have Different Rostrocaudal Distributions

The motor neurons that innervate a particular muscle are located within a column-shaped nucleus that runs rostrocaudally over several spinal segments. These column-shaped nuclei of motor neurons collectively form lamina IX (Figure 10–16A). Nuclei innervating distal limb muscles are located laterally in the gray matter, whereas those innervating proximal limb and axial muscles are located medially (Figure 10–2). The medial motor nuclei are present at all spinal levels (illustrated schematically as a continuous column of nuclei in Figure 10–17), whereas the lateral nuclei are present only in the cervical enlargement (C5-T1) and the lumbosacral enlargement (L1-S2).

In the spinal cord, autonomic preganglionic motor neurons are also arranged in a column (see Chapter 15) and, together with the motor nuclei, have a

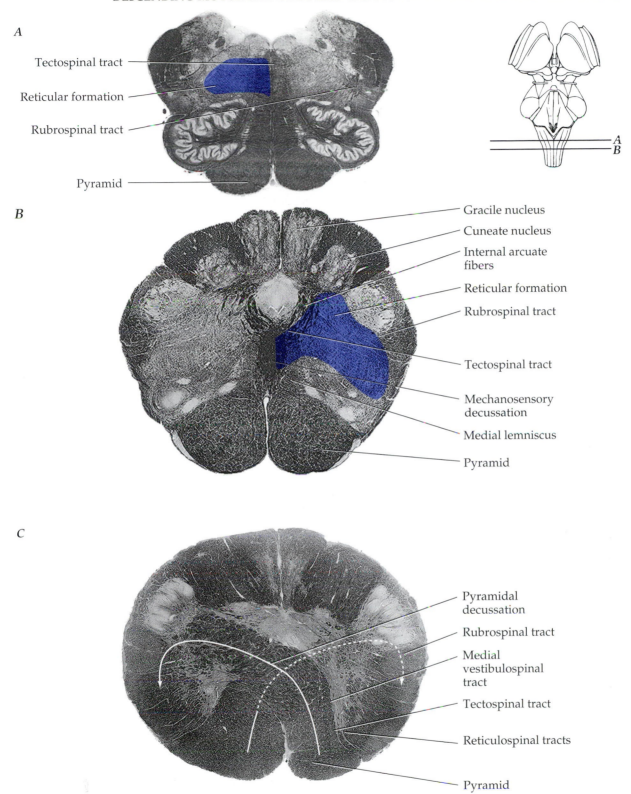

Figure 10–13. *A.* Myelin-stained section through the medulla, showing the locations of the motor pathways. *B* and *C.* Myelin-stained transverse sections through the decussation of the internal arcuate fibers, or mechanosensory decussation (*B*), and the pyramidal, or motor, decussation (*C*). Arrows in *C* indicate the pattern of decussating corticospinal fibers. The solid arrow indicates an axon coursing within the portion of the tract shown in the section. The dashed arrow corresponds to a decussating axon a bit rostral or caudal to this level.

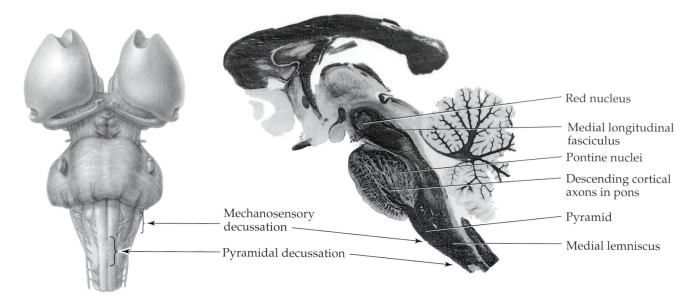

Red nucleus
Medial longitudinal fasciculus
Pontine nuclei
Descending cortical axons in pons
Pyramid
Medial lemniscus

Mechanosensory decussation
Pyramidal decussation

Figure 10–14. Myelin-stained sagittal section (close to the midline) through the brain stem. Brackets show the rostrocaudal levels of the somatic sensory and motor decussations.

three-dimensional organization similar to that of the brain stem cranial nerve nuclei columns (see Chapters 3 and 11). The longitudinal organization of the somatic and autonomic motor nuclei and the cranial nerve nuclei underscores the common architecture of the spinal cord and brain stem (see Chapter 3, section on spinal cord and brain stem development).

Degenerating axons of the lateral corticospinal tract

Figure 10–15. Myelin-stained section through the lumbar spinal cord from an individual who had an internal capsule stroke before death. Region showing degeneration in the lateral column (lightly stained) corresponds to the location of the lateral corticospinal tract. Note that the ventral corticospinal is not present at this level.

Lesions of the Descending Cortical Pathway in the Brain and Spinal Cord Produce Flaccid Paralysis Followed by Spasticity

Lesions involving the posterior limb of the internal capsule, ventral brain stem, and spinal cord isolate motor neurons from their normal voluntary control, producing a common set of motor signs. Initially these signs include **flaccid paralysis** and **reduced muscle reflexes** (eg, knee-jerk reflex). Clinical examination also reveals **decreased muscle tone,** signaled by the marked reduction in resistance felt by the examiner to passive movement of the limb. These signs are attributable largely to interruption of the corticospinal fibers even though the corticoreticular and corticopontine fibers are damaged. The laterality of the signs depends on whether the lesion occurs in the brain or the spinal cord (see below). Spinal cord injury is particularly devastating because all muscles of the body caudal to the level of injury can become affected (Box 10–1).

A few weeks after the occurrence of the lesion, a similar examination reveals **increased muscle tone** and **exaggerated muscle stretch (or myotatic) reflexes.** The increased muscle tone is due to increased reflex activity when the examiner passively stretches the limb. This sign is termed **spasticity,** and it is thought to result primarily from changes that occur after damage to the **indirect cortical pathways** to the spinal cord, for example, the cortico-reticulo-spinal pathway. The indirect pathways can have inhibitory influences on muscle tone, especially the tone of limb extensor muscles. Damage would produce a reduction in this

Figure 10–16. *A.* Schematic drawing of the general organization of the spinal cord gray matter and white matter. *B.* Drawing of a single spinal segment, showing columns of motor nuclei, running rostrocaudally within the ventral horn.

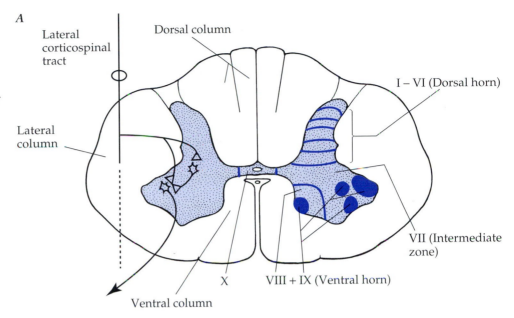

A

Lateral corticospinal tract

Dorsal column

I – VI (Dorsal horn)

Lateral column

VII (Intermediate zone)

X

VIII + IX (Ventral horn)

Ventral column

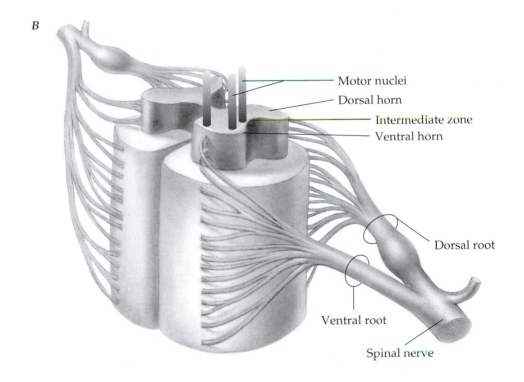

B

Motor nuclei

Dorsal horn

Intermediate zone

Ventral horn

Dorsal root

Ventral root

Spinal nerve

inhibition, thereby elevating tone (ie, disinhibition). Long-term synaptic plasticity appears to play an important role in the delayed time-course of this effect. By contrast, experiments in laboratory animals—in which there is selective damage of corticospinal axons in the pyramid in the caudal medulla—produce decreased, not increased, muscle tone.

In addition to producing spasticity, lesions of the descending cortical projection pathway result in the emergence of abnormal reflexes, the most notable of which is **Babinski's sign.** This sign involves extension (also termed dorsiflexion) of the big toe in response to scratching the lateral margin and then the ball of the foot (but not the toes). Babinski's sign is thought to be a withdrawal reflex. Normally such withdrawal of the big toe is produced by scratching the toe's ventral surface. After damage to the descending cortical fibers, the reflex can be evoked from a much larger area than

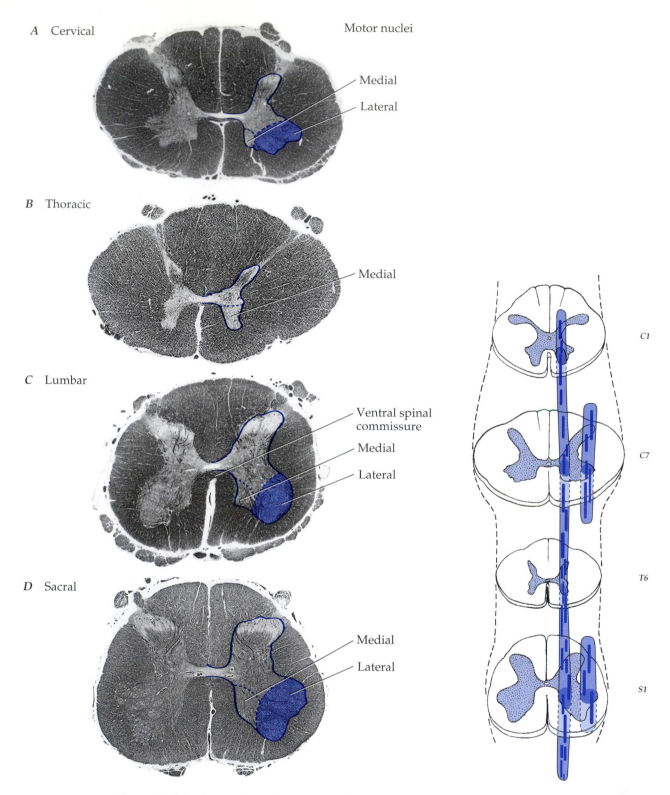

A Cervical

Motor nuclei

— Medial

— Lateral

B Thoracic

— Medial

C Lumbar

Ventral spinal commissure

— Medial

— Lateral

D Sacral

— Medial

— Lateral

C1

C7

T6

S1

Figure 10–17. Approximate locations of the medial and lateral motor nuclei are shown at four spinal cord levels: cervical (**A**), thoracic (**B**), lumbar (**C**), and sacral (**D**). The inset shows the columnar organization of the medial and lateral motor nuclei. The medial column, which contains motor neurons that innervate proximal and axial muscles, runs throughout the entire spinal cord. Motor nuclei that contain the motor neurons that innervate individual muscles also have a columnar shape but are narrower and course for a shorter rostrocaudal distance. The lateral column contains motor neurons that innervate lateral (distal) muscles. This column is present in the cervical and lumbosacral enlargements only. As for the medial column, motor neurons that innervate individual muscles form narrower and shorter columns.

normal. **Hoffmann's sign,** which is thumb adduction in response to flexion of the distal phalanx of the third digit, is an example of an abnormal upper limb reflex caused by damage to the descending cortical fibers.

Damage to different portions of the descending motor pathways can produce similar effects on muscle tone and limb control, but the laterality of effects differs. Vascular lesions of the **internal capsule** are more common than lesions of the ventral brain stem and spinal cord. The arterial supply of the internal capsule is provided primarily by the **anterior choroidal artery** and, at more superior levels, deep branches of the **middle cerebral artery** (see Figure 4–6). Small branches of these arteries commonly occlude and produce focal (ie, lacunar) infarctions. Corticospinal damage at this level produces limb motor control impairments (initially decreased tone and then later spasticity) on the **contralateral side** (Figure 10–19, see arrow and follow boldface line). The laterality of this effect occurs because the pathway crosses the midline in the medulla, in the pyramidal decussation (Figure 10–19). Following a small capsular infarction, the arm and leg can both become affected. Both limbs are affected because the axons that descend from the arm and leg areas of the primary motor cortex converge within a small space in the posterior limb of the internal capsule, even though their cells of origin are widely separated in the cortex (Figure 10–9). Why do only limb motor signs and not axial motor signs occur? This is because the medial descending pathways, including the ventral corticospinal tract, have a bilateral organization. A unilateral lesion does not deprive axial motor neurons of their control because medial pathways from the other side can supply control signals to the motor neurons.

Spinal Cord Hemisection Produces Ipsilateral Limb Motor Signs

Ipsilateral motor deficits are a key feature of spinal cord hemisection (Figure 10–19). The laterality of the motor defects results because the lateral corticospinal

---

Box 10–1. Motor Pathways Can Regenerate When Axonal Growth Inhibition Is Blocked

Descending motor pathways travel long distances from the cerebral cortex or brain stem nuclei to their targets in the spinal cord. Whereas the axons of these pathways are well protected within the skull, they become vulnerable to mechanical damage once they course into the spinal cord. For example, during an automobile accident, excessive relative motion of the vertebrae can cause spinal contusions that kill spinal neurons and sever the axons of spinal pathways, both ascending and descending. When the axon of a descending projection neuron is severed, communication between its cell body in the brain and its terminals in the spinal cord is interrupted. The portion of the axon distal to the injury, now isolated from its cell body, degenerates. This is because the axon's support, including most protein synthesis, derives from the cell body.

Spinal cord injury is almost always seriously debilitating, because it can produce paralysis of the parts of the body located below the level of injury. What makes spinal injury even more devastating is that the axons of neurons in the central nervous system, once severed, rarely regenerate. Researchers are beginning to understand why. Although multiple factors are thought to be important, components of central nervous system myelin itself are strong inhibitors of axonal growth. Among the various proteins associated with myelin, three are now known to be potent axon growth inhibitors: myelin-associated glycoprotein (MAG), a protein named nogo, and oligodendrocyte myelin glycoprotein (OMgp). It is likely that there are more. Researchers have shown that by blocking the actions of myelin growth inhibitory proteins, central nervous system axons gain some capacity to regenerate. One way to block these proteins is by using antibodies. When the antibody binds to the appropriate myelin antigen, it neutralizes its axonal growth inhibitory actions.

In rats treated with an antibody to nogo, severed corticospinal axons are capable of some regeneration, sometimes up to many millimeters beyond the site of damage.

(continued)

tract has already decussated: The damaged axons terminate on the same side as the injury. Initially, **flaccid paralysis** and **reduced myotatic reflexes** occur in the limb innervated by motor neurons caudal to the lesion.

But after a variable period of a few weeks, **spastic paralysis** develops and abnormal reflexes emerge. Because the medial descending pathways terminate bilaterally, axial motor function may not be affected as

---

Box 10–1 (continued).

Another provocative approach to promoting central nervous system axonal regeneration is to induce active immunity against the growth inhibitory proteins, much like development of immunity to measles or polio. Animals can be "vaccinated" with myelin so that they produce antibodies that block the growth-inhibiting actions of myelin. Although a condition similar to multiple sclerosis can occur if immunity to myelin is too strong, researchers developed a milder immune response that permits some corticospinal axonal regeneration in animals (Figure 10–18B), without the untoward side effects. These approaches promote central nervous system pathway regeneration in animals and may form the basis of future therapeutic approaches in humans who have experienced spinal injury.

Descending corticospinal axons   Regenerating corticospinal axons

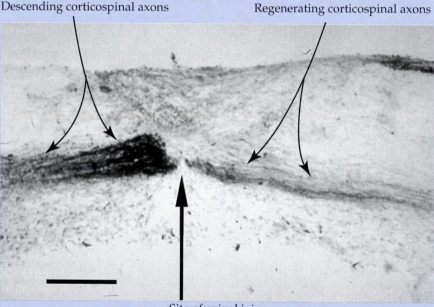

Site of spinal injury

Figure 10–18. Blockade of axon growth inhibitors permits corticospinal axon regeneration after damage. Axonal regeneration occurs in mice immunized against myelin proteins. This is shown in the micrograph of a sagittal section through the mouse spinal cord. The animal was immunized using a special vaccine that resulted in generation of antibodies against myelin inhibitory growth proteins, which neutralized the actions of these proteins but did not cause a large-scale inflammatory reaction, which could result in demyelination. The arrow indicates the site of transection of corticospinal axons. In the rodent, the principal corticospinal axons course in the base of the dorsal columns. Labeled axons appear black. There are many axons to the left of the arrow; they are still attached to their cell bodies in the motor cortex. Labeled axons to the right of the arrow have regenerated and grown through the site of injury. While there are far fewer regenerating axons than the intact group, without immuno-blockade virtually no corticospinal axons regenerated. *(Courtesy of Dr. Sam David; Huang DW et al: A therapeutic vaccine approach to stimulate axon regeneration in the adult mammalian spinal cord. Neuron 1999;24:639–647.)*

Figure 10–19. Brown-Séquard syndrome. Spinal cord hemisection produces motor and somatic sensory signs. This figure shows the cortical pathways producing motor signs; see Figure 5–9A for the effect of such a lesion on touch, position sense, vibration sense, pain, and temperature senses. The lateral descending pathways, which target distal limb muscle motor neurons, decussate in the medulla. In contrast, the medial descending pathways, which target proximal limb motor neurons, typically descend ipsilaterally and terminate bilaterally in the spinal cord. As a consequence of this pattern, spinal cord hemisection affects distal muscles on the ipsilateral limb and, to a much lesser extent, proximal and axial musculature.

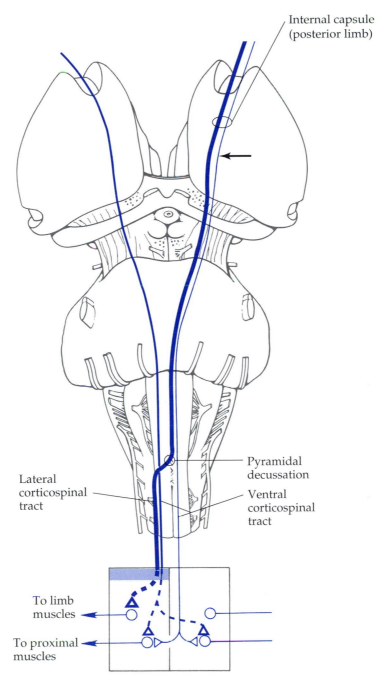

Internal capsule (posterior limb)

Lateral corticospinal tract

Pyramidal decussation

Ventral corticospinal tract

To limb muscles

To proximal muscles

seriously as limb function. However, for the affected body parts, a spinal injury is typically more devastating than a supraspinal injury because all motor pathways can be affected. These are the motor signs of the **Brown-Séquard syndrome.** As discussed in Chapter 5, spinal cord hemisection produces characteristic somatic sensory deficits below the level of the lesion: a loss of **tactile sense, vibration sense,** and **limb position sense** on the **ipsilateral side** and loss of **pain and temperature senses** on the **contralateral side** (see Figure 5–9).

Summary

Descending Pathways

Seven descending motor pathways course in the white matter of the brain stem and spinal cord (Figures 10–3 through 10–5; Table 10–1): the **lateral corticospinal tract,** the **rubrospinal tract,** the **ventral corticospinal tract,** the **reticulospinal tract** (which is further subdivided into separate medullary and pontine components), the **vestibulospinal tract** (which is subdivided into separate medial and lateral components), and the **tectospinal tract.** These pathways project directly on spinal motor neurons through monosynaptic connections and indirectly by synapsing first on segmental interneurons and propriospinal neurons. The corticobulbar tract projects only to the brain stem (see Chapter 11).

Lateral Descending Pathways

The locations of the descending axons in the spinal cord provide insight into their functions (Figure 10–2). Those that control **limb muscles** descend in the **lateral column** of the spinal cord and terminate in the **lateral intermediate zone** and **lateral ventral horn** (Figures 10–2, 10–3, and 10–5). The **lateral corticospinal tract** and the **rubrospinal tract** are the two laterally descending pathways. In humans, the lateral corticospinal tract has more axons than the rubrospinal tract. The **primary motor cortex** (area 4), located on the precentral gyrus (Figures 10–6 and 10–7), contributes most of the fibers of the lateral corticospinal tract. (The other major contributors to the lateral corticospinal tract are the premotor cortical regions located rostral to the primary motor cortex, mainly in cytoarchitectonic **areas 6 and 24** and in the parietal lobe.) The descending projection neurons of the cortex are located in **layer V,** and their axons course through the **posterior limb of the internal capsule** (Figures 10–9 and 10–10A) and then along the ventral brain stem surface (Figures 10–11A through 10–13). The lateral corticospinal tract decussates in the ventral medulla in the **pyramidal decussation,** at the junction of the medulla and the spinal cord (Figures 10–13C; 10–14, inset; and 10–19). In the spinal cord, the lateral corticospinal tract courses in the dorsal portion of the **lateral column** (Figures 10–5 and 10–15) and terminates in cervical and lumbosacral segments. The other laterally descending pathway, the **rubrospinal tract,** originates from the **magnocellular division** of the **red nucleus** (Figures 10–11 and 10–14). The axons decussate in the midbrain, descend in the dorsolateral portion of the brain stem and spinal cord (Figures 10–3B and 10–5), and terminate in the cervical cord. The other division of the red nucleus, the **parvocellular division,** is part of a circuit that involves the cerebellum.

Medial Descending Pathways

The remaining four pathways course in the medial portion of the spinal cord white matter, the **ventral column,** and influence axial and girdle muscles. These medially descending pathways terminate in the medial ventral horn—where axial and girdle motor neurons are located—and the medial intermediate zone (Figure 10–2). These pathways influence motor neurons bilaterally: After descending into the cord, either the axon of the projection neuron decussates in the ventral commissure or its terminals synapse on interneurons and propriospinal neurons whose axons decussate. The **ventral corticospinal tract,** which originates mostly in the primary motor cortex and area 6, descends in the brain stem along with the lateral corticospinal tract but does not decussate in the medulla and courses in the ventral column of the spinal cord (Figure 10–4A and 10–19). The **reticulospinal tracts** (pontine and medullary; Figure 10–4B) originate in the **reticular formation** (Figures 10–12 and 10–13B) and descend ipsilaterally for the entire length of the spinal cord and function in posture and automatic responses, such as locomotion. The **tectospinal tract** (Figure 10–4B) originates from the deeper layers of the **superior colliculus** (Figure 10–11), decussates in the midbrain, and descends medially in the caudal brain stem and spinal cord. This pathway descends only to the cervical spinal cord and plays a role in coordination of head and eye movements. (See Chapter 12 for the vestibulospinal tracts.)

Related Sources

Brust JCM: The Practice of Neural Science. McGraw-Hill; 2000. (See ch. 4; ch. 6; ch 12, cases 22, 26–28, 30–32; ch. 14, cases 45, 46, 51.)

Ghez C, Krakhauer J: The organization of movement. In Kandel ER, Schwartz JH, Jessell TM (editors): Principles of Neural Science, 4th ed. McGraw-Hill; 2000:653–673.

Krakhauer J, Ghez C: Voluntary movement. In Kandel ER, Schwartz JH, Jessell TM (editors): Principles of Neural Science, 4th ed. McGraw-Hill; 2000:756–781.

Loeb GE, Ghez C: The motor unit and muscle action. In Kandel ER, Schwartz JH, Jessell TM (editors): Principles of Neural Science, 4th ed. McGraw-Hill; 2000:674–694.

Melvill Jones G: Posture. In Kandel ER, Schwartz JH, Jessell TM (editors): Principles of Neural Science, 4th ed. McGraw-Hill; 2000:816–831.

Pearson K, Gordon J: Locomotion. In Kandel ER, Schwartz JH, Jessell TM (editors): Principles of Neural Science, 4th ed. McGraw-Hill; 2000:737–755.

Pearson K, Gordon J: Spinal reflexes. In Kandel ER, Schwartz JH, Jessell TM (editors): Principles of Neural Science, 4th ed. McGraw-Hill; 2000:713–736.

Selected Readings

Dum RP, Strick PL: Medial wall motor areas and skeletomotor control. Curr Opin Neurobiol 1992;2:836–839.

Jackson SR, Husain M: Visuomotor functions of the lateral pre-motor cortex. Curr Opin Neurobiol 1996;6:788–795.

Jankowska E, Lundberg A: Interneurons in the spinal cord. Trends Neurosci 1981;4:230–233.

Luppino G, Rizzolatti G: The organization of the frontal motor cortex. News in Physiological Sciences 2000;15:219–224.

Picard N, Strick PL: Imaging the premotor areas. Curr Opin Neurobiol 2001;11:663–672.

Roland PE, Zilles K: Functions and structures of the motor cortices in humans. Curr Opin Neurobiol 1996;6:773–781.

Tanji J: New concepts of the supplementary motor area. Curr Opin Neurobiol 1996;6:782–787.

References

Asanuma H: The pyramidal tract. In Brooks VB (editor): Handbook of Physiology, Section 1: The Nervous System, Vol. 2, Motor Control. American Physiological Society; 1981:703–733.

Brösamle C, Huber AB, Fiedler M, Skerra A, Schwab ME: Regeneration of lesioned corticospinal tract fibers in the adult rat induced by a recombinant, humanized IN-1 antibody fragment. J Neurosci 2000;20:8061–8068.

Burman K, Darian-Smith C, Darian-Smith I: Geometry of rubrospinal, rubroolivary, and local circuit neurons in the macaque red nucleus. J Comp Neurol 2000;423:197–219.

Burman K, Darian-Smith C, Darian-Smith I: Macaque red nucleus: Origins of spinal and olivary projections and terminations of cortical inputs. J Comp Neurol 2000;423:179–196.

Chung CS, Caplan LR, Yamamoto Y, et al: Striatocapsular haemorrhage. Brain 2000;123:1850–1862.

Crosby EC, Humphrey T, Lauer EW: Correlative Anatomy of the Nervous System. Macmillan, 1962.

Danek A, Bauer M, Fries W: Tracing of neuronal connections in the human brain by magnetic resonance imaging in vivo. Eur J Neurosci 1990;2:112–115.

Dum RP, Strick PL: The origin of corticospinal projections from the premotor areas in the frontal lobe. J Neurosci 1991;11:667–689.

Fries W, Danek A, Scheidtmann K, Hamburger C: Motor recovery following capsular stroke. Role of descending pathways from multiple motor areas. Brain 1993;116:369–382.

Fries W, Danek A, Witt TN: Motor responses after transcranial electrical stimulation of cerebral hemispheres with a degenerated pyramidal tract. Ann Neurol 1991;29:646–650.

Huang DW, McKerracher L, Braun PE, David S: A therapeutic vaccine approach to stimulate axon regeneration in the adult mammalian spinal cord. Neuron 1999;24:639–647.

Jenny AB, Saper CB: Organization of the facial nucleus and corticofacial projection in the monkey: A reconsideration of the upper motor neuron facial palsy. Neurology 1987;37:930–939.

Kim SG, Ashe J, Georgopoulos AP, et al: Functional imaging of human motor cortex at high magnetic field. J Neurophysiol 1993;69:297–302.

Kuypers HGJM: Anatomy of the descending pathways. In Brooks VB (editor): Handbook of Physiology, Section 1: The Nervous System, Vol. 2, Motor Control. American Physiological Society; 1981:597–666.

Kuypers HGJM, Brinkman J: Precentral projections to different parts of the spinal intermediate zone in the rhesus monkey. Brain Res 1970;24:151–188.

Lu M-T, Presont JB, Strick PL: Interconnections between the prefrontal cortex and the premotor areas in the frontal lobe. J Comp Neurol 1994;341:375–392.

Martin JH: Differential spinal projections from the forelimb areas of rostral and caudal subregions of primary motor cortex in the cat. Exp Brain Res 1996;108:191–205.

Matsuyama K, Drew T: Organization of the projections from the pericruciate cortex to the pontomedullary brain stem of the cat: A study using the anterograde tracer Phaseolous vulgaris leucoagglutinin. J Comp Neurol 1997;389:617–641.

Molenaar I, Kuypers HGJM: Cells of origin of propriospinal fibers and of fibers ascending to supraspinal levels. An HRP study in cat and rhesus monkey. Brain Res 1978;152:429–450.

Morecraft RJ, Herrick JL, Stilwell-Morecraft KS, et al: Localization of arm representation in the corona radiata and internal capsule in the non-human primate. Brain 2002;125:176–198.

Morecraft RJ, Louie JL, Herrick JL, Stilwell-Morecraft KS: Cortical innervation of the facial nucleus in the non-human primate: A new interpretation of the effects of stroke and related subtotal brain trauma on the muscles of facial expression. Brain 2001;124:176–208.

Murray EA, Coulter JD: Organization of corticospinal neurons in the monkey. J Comp Neurol 1981;195:339–365.

Nathan PW, Smith MC: The rubrospinal and central tegmental tracts in man. Brain 1982;105:223–269.

Penfield W, Rasmussen T: The Cerebral Cortex of Man: A Clinical Study of Localization of Function. Macmillan, 1950.

Pujol J, Martí-Vilalta JL, Junqué C, Vendrell P, Fernández J, Capdevila A: Wallerian degeneration of the pyramidal tract in capsular infarction studied by magnetic resonance imaging. Stroke 1990;21:404–409.

Ross ED: Localization of the pyramidal tract in the internal capsule by whole brain dissection. Neurology 1980;30:59–64.

Schell GR, Strick PL: The origin of thalamic inputs to the arcuate premotor and supplementary motor areas. J Neurosci 1984;4:539–560.

Sterling P, Kuypers HGJM: Anatomical organization of the brachial spinal cord of the cat. III. The propriospinal connections. Brain Res 1967;4:419–443.

Vogt BA, Pandya DN, Rosene DL: Cingulate cortex of the rhesus monkey: I. Cytoarchitecture and thalamic afferents. J Comp Neurol 1987;262:256–270.

Wiesendanger M: Organization of secondary motor areas of cerebral cortex. In Brooks VB (editor): Handbook of Physiology, Section 1: The Nervous System, Vol. 2, Motor Control. American Physiological Society; 1981:1121–1147.

11

Cranial Nerve Motor Nuclei and Brain Stem Motor Functions

A S DISCUSSED EARLIER, STRIKING PARALLELS exist between the functional and anatomical organization of the spinal and cranial somatic sensory systems. In fact, the principles governing the organization of one are nearly identical to those of the other. A similar comparison can be made between motor control of cranial structures and that of the limbs and trunk: Cranial muscles are innervated by motor neurons found in the cranial nerve motor nuclei, whereas limb and axial muscles are innervated by motor neurons in the motor nuclei of the ventral horn. A similar parallel exists with the control of body organs. Control of the glands and smooth muscle of the head, as well as the pupil, is mediated by parasympathetic preganglionic neurons located in cranial nerve autonomic nuclei. Abdominal visceral organs are controlled by parasympathetic neurons in the sacral cord.

This chapter examines in detail the cranial nerve motor nuclei innervating facial, jaw, and tongue muscles, as well as muscles for swallowing. It also examines the control of these nuclei, which is accomplished by the corticobulbar tract. This pathway is the cranial equivalent of the corticospinal tract, and the two pathways share numerous organizational principles. Knowing the patterns of corticobulbar connections with the cranial motor nuclei has important diagnostic value because it helps clinicians to understand the cranial motor signs produced by brain stem damage. This knowledge also helps clinicians to plan the proper therapy for the patient to avert potentially life-threatening sequelae. The autonomic motor nuclei of the brain stem are also examined to achieve greater knowledge of regional anatomy. Such knowledge is essential for localizing central nervous system damage after trauma.

ORGANIZATION AND FUNCTIONAL ANATOMY OF CRANIAL MOTOR NUCLEI

There Are Three Columns of Cranial Nerve Motor Nuclei

Cranial nerve motor nuclei are organized into three columns that run rostrocaudally throughout the brain stem (Figure 11–1): somatic skeletal, branchiomeric, and autonomic. Nuclei in the **somatic skeletal motor column** contain motor neurons that innervate striated muscle of somatic origin (ie, from the occipital somites): the extraocular and tongue muscles. This column is close to the midline. Nuclei of the **branchiomeric motor column** contain motor neurons innervating striated muscle of branchiomeric (visceral) origin: facial, jaw, palatal, pharyngeal, and laryngeal muscles. This column is lateral to the somatic skeletal motor column (Figure 11–1) and is displaced ventrally from the ventricular floor (Figure 11–1, bottom inset). Nuclei of the **autonomic motor column** contain the parasympathetic preganglionic neurons that regulate the functions of cranial exocrine glands, smooth muscle, and many body organs. The autonomic motor column is lateral to the somatic skeletal motor column (Figure 11–1). Sometimes these three columns are termed general somatic motor, special visceral motor, and general visceral motor columns, respectively.

The Cranial Motor Nuclei Are Controlled by the Cerebral Cortex and Diencephalon

Nuclei within the somatic skeletal and branchiomeric motor columns that innervate facial, tongue, jaw, laryngeal, and pharyngeal muscles are controlled by the cortical motor areas: the primary motor cortex, the supplementary motor area, the premotor cortex, and the cingulate motor areas. These are the same cortical regions that control limb and trunk muscles (see Chapter 10). However, the cranial motor representations project to the various brain stem motor nuclei through the **corticobulbar tract.** Nuclei that innervate extraocular muscles are controlled by different cortical areas and not by the corticobulbar tract (see Chapter 12).

Of all the cortical motor areas, the **primary motor cortex** contributes the greatest number of axons to the corticobulbar tract. The cell bodies of these primary motor cortex axons are located within layer V of the cranial representation, which is the lateral precentral gyrus close to the **lateral sulcus** (see Figure 10–7). Their descending axons course within the internal capsule, along with but rostral to the corticospinal fibers. Corticobulbar neurons project to the pons and medulla.

Their axons terminate either bilaterally or contralaterally, depending on the particular nucleus (see below). Muscles innervated by motor nuclei that receive a **bilateral projection** from the corticobulbar tract do not become weak after a unilateral lesion of the motor cortex, the internal capsule, or some other portion of its descending pathway. The projection from the intact side is sufficient for normal (or near-normal) control of force production. This is not the case, however, for muscles receiving only a **contralateral projection.** In these instances, weakness reveals the unilateral damage. This relationship between the laterality of cortical control and the laterality of motor signs after unilateral damage is similar to that of the corticospinal system.

The nuclei comprising the autonomic motor column, which control cranial exocrine glands, smooth muscle, and body organs, are also influenced by projections from higher levels of the nervous system, in particular the **hypothalamus.** This diencephalic structure receives inputs from diverse regions of the cerebral hemispheres, especially the limbic association cortex. The autonomic nervous system and hypothalamus are considered in Chapter 15. This chapter considers the locations and peripheral innervation patterns of the cranial autonomic nuclei.

Neurons in the Somatic Skeletal Motor Column Innervate the Tongue and Extraocular Muscles

Four nuclei comprise the somatic skeletal motor column, which contains motor neurons that innervate striated muscles derived from the **occipital somites** (Figure 11–1; see Figure 3–4). Three of these nuclei contain motor neurons that innervate the extraocular muscles: the **oculomotor nucleus,** the **trochlear nucleus,** and the **abducens nucleus.** The fourth is the **hypoglossal nucleus,** which innervates tongue muscles.

The oculomotor nucleus is located in the rostral midbrain and innervates the **medial rectus, inferior rectus, superior rectus,** and **inferior oblique muscles,** which move the eyes (see Figure 12–3), as well as the **levator palpebrae superioris muscle,** an eyelid elevator. The motor axons course within the **oculomotor (III) nerve.** Motor neurons in the trochlear nucleus course in the **trochlear (IV) nerve** and innervate the **superior oblique muscle.** The **abducens nucleus** contains the motor neurons that project their axons to the periphery through the **abducens (VI) nerve** and innervate the **lateral rectus muscle.**

The **hypoglossal nucleus** is the fourth member of the somatic skeletal motor column (Figures 11–1 and 11–2). The axons of motor neurons in the hypoglossal nucleus course in the **hypoglossal (XII) nerve** and

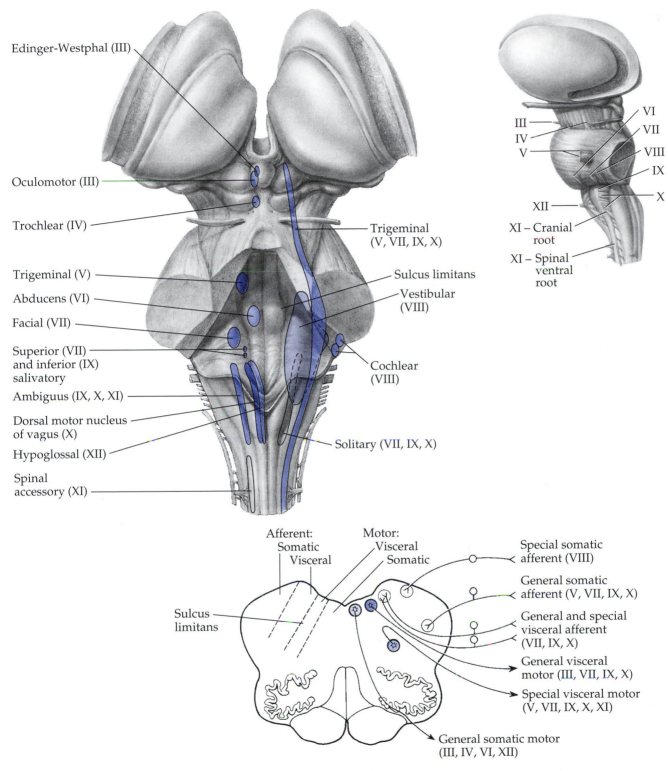

Edinger-Westphal (III)

Oculomotor (III)

Trochlear (IV)

Trigeminal (V)

Abducens (VI)

Facial (VII)

Superior (VII)
and inferior (IX)
salivatory

Ambiguus (IX, X, XI)

Dorsal motor nucleus
of vagus (X)

Hypoglossal (XII)

Spinal
accessory (XI)

Trigeminal
(V, VII, IX, X)

Sulcus limitans

Vestibular
(VIII)

Cochlear
(VIII)

Solitary (VII, IX, X)

III
IV
V

VI
VII

VIII

IX

X

XII

XI – Cranial
root

XI – Spinal
ventral
root

Afferent:
Somatic
Visceral

Motor:
Visceral
Somatic

Sulcus
limitans

Special somatic
afferent (VIII)

General somatic
afferent (V, VII, IX, X)

General and special
visceral afferent
(VII, IX, X)

General visceral
motor (III, VII, IX, X)

Special visceral motor
(V, VII, IX, X, XI)

General somatic motor
(III, IV, VI, XII)

Figure 11–1. Dorsal view of the brain stem (without the cerebellum), showing the locations of cranial nerve nuclei. The top inset, which is a lateral view diencephalon, and basal ganglia, shows the various cranial nerves, the spinal accessory nerve, and a ventral root. The bottom inset is a schematic cross section through the medulla, showing the location of cranial nerve nuclear columns. (*Adapted from Nieuwenhuys R, Voogd J, van Huijzen C: The Human Central Nervous System: A Synopsis and Atlas, 3rd ed. Springer-Verlag, 1988.*)

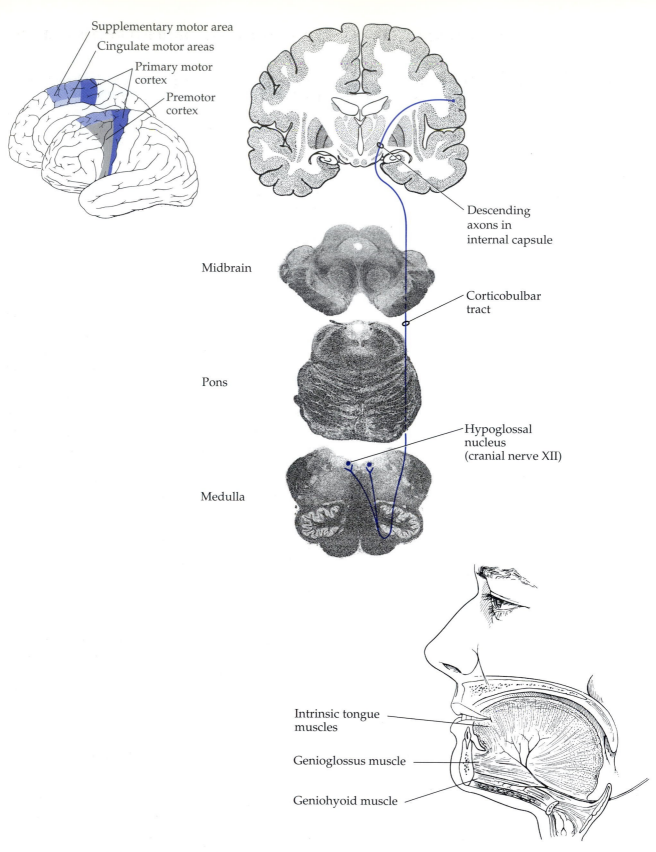

Supplementary motor area

Cingulate motor areas

Primary motor cortex

Premotor cortex

Descending axons in internal capsule

Midbrain

Corticobulbar tract

Pons

Hypoglossal nucleus (cranial nerve XII)

Medulla

Intrinsic tongue muscles

Genioglossus muscle

Geniohyoid muscle

Figure 11–2. Cortical control of the hypoglossal nucleus. The descending cortical projection to the hypoglossal nucleus originates from the lateral motor cortex, which is the location of the cranial nerve motor representation. In most people the hypoglossal nucleus on one side is contacted by motor cortex neurons on both sides. A unilateral corticobulbar tract lesion typically does not produce unilateral weakness. Note that the geniohyoid muscle is innervated by cervical spinal cord motor neurons, whose axons course, for a portion, with the hypoglossal nerve. The top inset shows the locations of the primary motor cortex and the three premotor areas: the supplementary motor area, the cingulate motor areas, and the premotor cortex.

innervate intrinsic tongue muscles, including the genioglossus, hypoglossus, and styloglossus. Similar to the control of limb muscles, the primary motor cortex and other cortical motor areas project to the hypoglossal nucleus via the **corticobulbar tract.**

The corticobulbar projection from the primary motor cortex to the hypoglossal nucleus is most commonly a bilateral one. Unilateral lesion of this projection, for example in the internal capsule, does not produce weakness of tongue muscles in the majority of people. In some individuals, however, contralateral tongue weakness does occur, suggesting a crossed (ie, unilateral) corticobulbar projection to the hypoglossal nucleus in these individuals. By contrast, a lesion of the hypoglossal nucleus or nerve consistently produces ipsilateral tongue paralysis. When such patients are asked to protrude their tongue, it deviates to the side of the lesion.

The Branchiomeric Motor Column Innervates Skeletal Muscles That Develop From the Branchial Arches

The nuclei that comprise the branchiomeric motor column contain motor neurons that innervate striated muscles derived from the **branchial arches.** Three cranial nerve nuclei constitute this nuclear column: the **facial motor nucleus,** the **trigeminal motor nucleus,** and the **nucleus ambiguus.** The branchiomeric motor nuclei in the brain stem each receive a projection from the primary motor cortex via the corticobulbar tract.

The Topography of Cortical Projections to the Facial Motor Nucleus Is Complex

The facial motor nucleus contains the motor neurons that innervate the muscles of **facial expression.** These axons course in the **facial (VII) nerve.** Whereas a facial nerve or nucleus lesion produces facial muscle paralysis over the entire **ipsilateral face,** a unilateral lesion of the primary motor cortex, the internal capsule, or the descending cortical fibers produces differential effects on the voluntary control of upper and lower facial muscles. After the lesion, upper facial muscles retain voluntary control. A patient with such a lesion can furrow his or her brow symmetrically. In contrast, lower facial muscles contralateral to the side of the lesion become weak. A patient with such damage would smile asymmetrically when asked to smile by his or her physician. Surprisingly, if the patient were provoked to smile, for example by hearing a humorous joke, he or she could do so symmetrically, implying no facial weakness.

Knowledge of the origin of corticobulbar neurons and the pattern of their terminations helps to explain these peculiar effects. The primary motor cortex has dense contralateral projections to lower facial muscle motor neurons and sparse bilateral projections to upper facial motor neurons (Figure 11–3). Thus a lesion would be expected to weaken only the contralateral lower facial muscles. Several factors may account for sparing of upper facial muscle control. First, connections to these muscles are less lateralized, with more ipsilateral terminations providing redundancy in control. Second, although the primary motor cortex only weakly drives the upper facial muscles, several premotor areas—especially the premotor cortex and cingulate motor region—have stronger projections, and these are bilateral. Moreover, the descending axons of these premotor regions are separated from those of the primary motor cortex; they are located more rostrally in the corona radiata and internal capsule. They are typically spared with local cortical or internal capsule injury because they receive a different arterial supply (see Figure 4–6). As for the patient who is able to smile symmetrically after hearing a funny joke, that observation also is thought to be related to the intact premotor connections, especially those from the cingulate motor areas, which receive their major inputs from brain regions regulating emotions.

The Trigeminal Motor Nucleus and the Nucleus Ambiguus Receive a Bilateral Projection From the Primary Motor Cortex

The axons of motor neurons of the trigeminal motor nucleus course in the **trigeminal (V) nerve** and innervate principally the muscles of **mastication:** masseter, temporalis, and external and internal pterygoid muscles (see Table 6–1). Because the primary motor cortex projects bilaterally to the trigeminal motor nuclei (Figure 11–4), unilateral cortical or descending pathway lesions do not produce weakness of the target muscles. Bilateral control by the primary motor cortex may reflect the fact that jaw muscles on both sides of the mouth are typically activated in tandem during most motor acts, for example, chewing or talking. This is similar to the bilateral control of axial muscles, for maintaining posture, by the medial descending spinal cord pathways (see Chapter 10).

The nucleus ambiguus contains motor neurons that innervate striated muscles of the **pharynx** and **larynx.** This nucleus and its efferent projections through cranial nerves are organized rostrocaudally. A small number of motor neurons in the most rostral portion

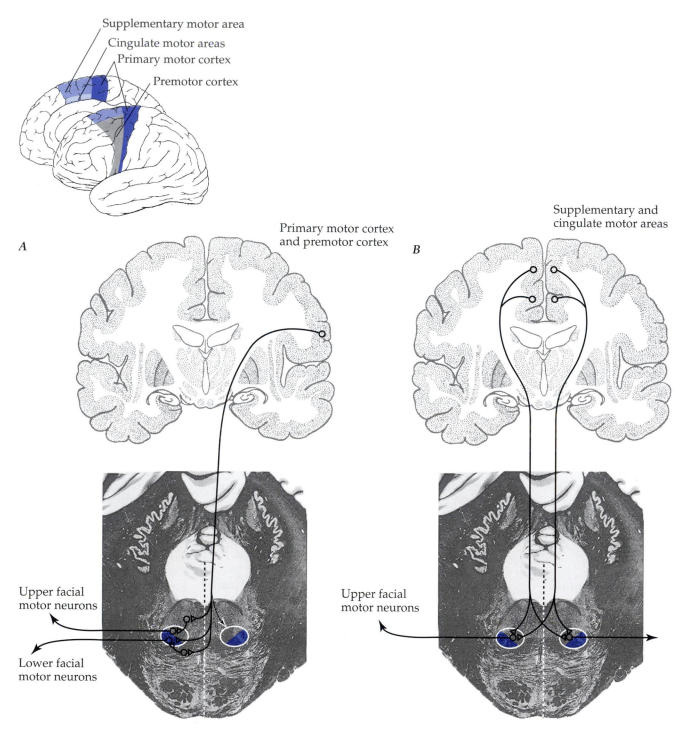

Figure 11–3. Pathways for control of facial motor neurons. **A.** Pathway from the primary motor and premotor cortical areas, which are both located on the lateral surface of the cortex. **B.** Pathway from the supplementary (*top*) and cingulate (*bottom*) motor areas, which are both located on the medial surface. The inset shows the locations of the primary motor cortex and the three premotor areas: the supplementary motor area, the cingulate motor areas, and the premotor cortex.

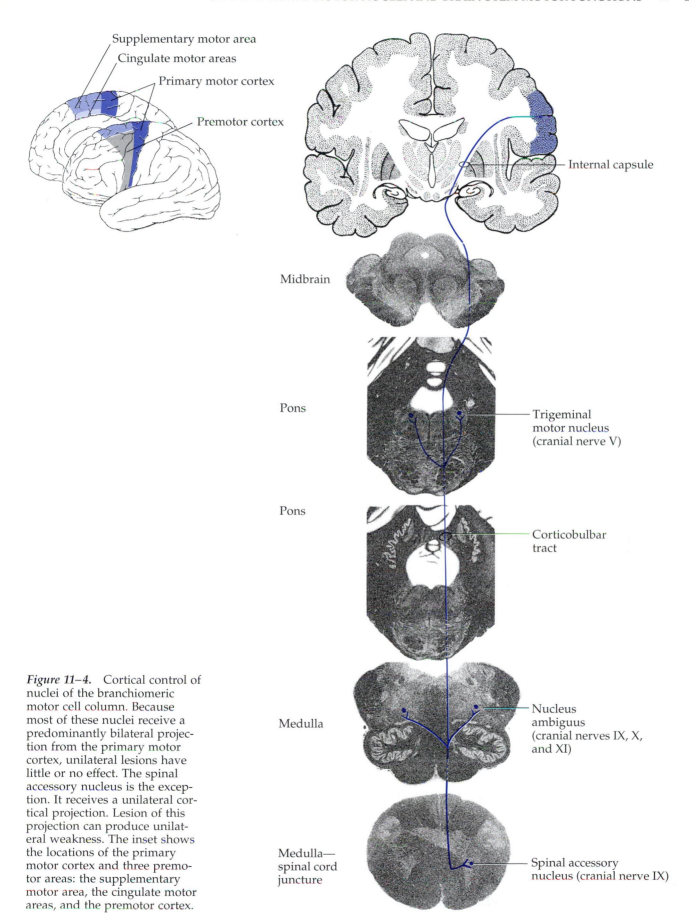

Supplementary motor area
Cingulate motor areas
Primary motor cortex
Premotor cortex

Internal capsule

Midbrain

Pons

Trigeminal
motor nucleus
(cranial nerve V)

Pons

Corticobulbar
tract

Medulla

Nucleus
ambiguus
(cranial nerves IX, X,
and XI)

Medulla—
spinal cord
juncture

Spinal accessory
nucleus (cranial nerve IX)

Figure 11–4. Cortical control of nuclei of the branchiomeric motor cell column. Because most of these nuclei receive a predominantly bilateral projection from the primary motor cortex, unilateral lesions have little or no effect. The spinal accessory nucleus is the exception. It receives a unilateral cortical projection. Lesion of this projection can produce unilateral weakness. The inset shows the locations of the primary motor cortex and three premotor areas: the supplementary motor area, the cingulate motor areas, and the premotor cortex.

of the nucleus ambiguus course in the **glossopharyngeal (IX) nerve** and innervate one pharyngeal muscle, the stylopharyngeus. Because this muscle is located deep within the pharynx, its function cannot be tested noninvasively. Most motor neurons in the nucleus send their axons through the **vagus (X) nerve** to innervate the pharynx and larynx. Because the pharyngeal muscles are innervated by the vagus nerve, a lesion of the nucleus ambiguus produces difficulty in swallowing. The vagus nerve carries the fibers of the efferent limb of the **gag reflex.** In this reflex, mechanical stimulation of the pharynx, using a cotton swab for example, produces a reflex contraction of the pharyngeal muscles. The **glossopharyngeal nerve** contains the afferent fibers that innervate mechanoreceptors of the pharynx that comprise the afferent limb of the gag reflex (see Chapter 6).

The most caudal portion of the nucleus ambiguus contains laryngeal motor neurons whose axons course in a portion of the **spinal accessory (XI) nerve.** This cranial nerve consists of distinct **cranial and spinal roots,** and only axons in the cranial root have their cell bodies in the **nucleus ambiguus.** These axons are probably **displaced vagal fibers** that join the vagus nerve as they exit from the cranium and then innervate the same structures as the vagus.

The motor cortex exerts bilateral control of motor neurons in the nucleus ambiguus (Figure 11–4), leading to the redundancy in their control, as discussed above. Whereas a unilateral lesion of the corticobulbar tract may not produce laryngeal and pharyngeal signs (Box 11–1), brain stem lesions that damage the nucleus ambiguus and surrounding regions produce ipsilateral paralysis of pharyngeal and laryngeal muscles. Such damage results in hoarseness and swallowing impairments and also impairs the airway protective reflex, the automatic closure of the larynx during swallowing to prevent food and fluids from entering the trachea.

Cells bodies of axons in the spinal root of the spinal accessory nerve are located in the **spinal accessory nucleus** (Figure 11–1). This nucleus is a part of the ventral horn of the upper cervical spinal cord—from the pyramidal decussation to about the fourth or fifth cervical segments—not the branchiomeric motor column. Axons in the spinal root of the spinal accessory nerve innervate the **sternocleidomastoid muscle** and the upper part of the **trapezius muscle,** which develop from the somites and not the branchial arches. Unlike the nucleus ambiguus, which is under bilateral cortical control, the spinal accessory nucleus receives a predominantly ipsilateral cortical projection. This ipsilateral projection targets primarily the motor neurons of the sternocleidomastoid muscle, which turns the head to the opposite side. Thus, the cortical projection is ipsilateral, but the motor actions of the muscle produce a movement directed to the contralateral side.

The Autonomic Motor Column Contains Parasympathetic Preganglionic Neurons

The autonomic motor column contains neurons that regulate the function of various body organs, smooth muscles, and exocrine glands. These neurons are part of the **parasympathetic nervous system,** a division of the **autonomic nervous system** (see Chapters 1 and 15). In contrast to the innervation of skeletal muscle, which is mediated by a single motor neuron (Figure 11–4), the innervation of smooth muscle and glands is accomplished by two separate neurons: preganglionic and postganglionic neurons (Figure 11–6). Parasympathetic preganglionic neurons are located in the various nuclei that comprise the autonomic motor column; these neurons also are found in the sacral spinal cord (see Chapter 15). Parasympathetic postganglionic neurons are located in **peripheral autonomic ganglia.**

The autonomic motor column, which is lateral to the somatic skeletal motor column (Figure 11–1), contains four nuclei, from the rostral brain stem to the medulla: the **Edinger-Westphal nucleus,** the **superior salivatory nucleus,** the **inferior salivatory nucleus,** and the **dorsal motor nucleus of the vagus.** (Whereas most of the cranial parasympathetic preganglionic neurons are located in these nuclei, additional preganglionic neurons are found in and around the nucleus ambiguus. The axons of these neurons course in the vagus nerve.) The autonomic motor column is analogous to the **intermediolateral nucleus,** a column of sympathetic preganglionic neurons in the spinal cord.

The **Edinger-Westphal nucleus** is located in the midbrain and in the pretectal region, dorsal to the oculomotor nucleus (Figure 11–6). It participates in pupillary constriction and lens accommodation. The parasympathetic neurons in the nucleus send their axons into the **oculomotor (III) nerve** to synapse on postganglionic neurons in the **ciliary ganglion.** These neurons innervate the **ciliary muscle** and the **constrictor muscles of the iris.**

Parasympathetic preganglionic neurons are also located in nuclei of the caudal pons and medulla (Figure 11–6). Neurons of the **superior** and **inferior salivatory nuclei** are located in the pons and medulla. They are somewhat dispersed, not forming a discrete cell column. The **dorsal motor nucleus of the vagus** forms a column of neurons beneath the floor of the **fourth ventricle** in the medulla.

The axons of neurons of the superior salivatory nucleus course in the **intermediate nerve** (Figure 11–6). They synapse in two peripheral ganglia: (1) the **pterygopalatine** ganglion, where postganglionic neurons innervate the lacrimal glands and glands of the nasal mucosa, and (2) the **submandibular** ganglion, from which postganglionic parasympathetic neurons innervate the submandibular and sublingual salivary

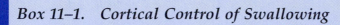

Box 11–1. *Cortical Control of Swallowing*

Swallowing is a coordinated motor response that transports food and fluids from the mouth to the stomach. A swallow comprises multiple phases, beginning with the oral phase when the food is formed into a bolus and leading into the pharyngeal phase when the food bolus is transported into the esophagus. The final, or esophageal phase, carries the food into the stomach. The cerebral cortex plays an important role in initiating swallowing, especially during the oral phase. Brain stem centers organize the patterns of pharyngeal and esophageal muscle contraction for swallowing, much like spinal circuits organize limb muscle patterns for limb reflexes.

There are two key brain stem regions for swallowing (Figure 11–5). The first is the **solitary nucleus** (Figure 11–12B), which is important in **viscerosensory** functions (see Chapter 6) and taste (see Chapter 9). It receives sensory information directly from the nerves innervating the mucous membranes of the pharynx and larynx, especially the superficial laryngeal nerve of the vagus nerve. The solitary nucleus projects to the second key region, comprising the **nucleus ambiguus** and the adjoining **reticular formation** (Figure 11–12B), which contain motor neurons and interneurons responsible for producing the muscle contractions for swallowing. These brain stem centers are also important for organizing the **airway protective reflex,** for closing the larynx during swallowing to prevent aspiration of food and fluids into the lungs.

The frontal lobe motor areas are essential for initiating swallowing and for adapting the patterns of muscle contractions to different foods and fluids. The lateral precentral gyrus, containing the head representations of the primary motor and lateral premotor cortical areas, becomes active during swallowing (Figure 11–5A; transverse image). This activation occurs not only with voluntary swallowing but also during an autonomic and largely subconscious form of swallowing as saliva accumulates in the mouth. These cortical areas are activated bilaterally, reflecting the bilateral organization of the cortical projections to the nucleus ambiguus and the solitary nucleus.

Up to one third of patients who have strokes affecting cortical motor function experience **dysphagia,** a swallowing impairment, such as choking when starting to swallow. **Pulmonary aspiration** and malnutrition are two serious consequences of dysphagia. Why do some stroke victims have swallowing impairments if redundancy exists in the corticobulbar projection?

Researchers suggest that the cortical representation of swallowing is asymmetrical, with dominant and nondominant hemispheres. In many people, functional imaging shows an asymmetry in cortical activation during swallowing, suggesting that the side with the larger response is dominant for swallowing. Consistent with this idea, when the side with the larger response is stimulated noninvasively using transcranial magnetic stimulation, normal subjects show stronger contractions of pharyngeal and esophageal muscles from that side than the other. It is somewhat more common for the right hemisphere to be dominant (Figure 11–5B). (The side does not seem to depend on handedness.) It has been suggested that stroke patients who develop dysphagia sustained a lesion to their dominant hemisphere and that they recover effective swallowing because the nondominant intact hemisphere becomes dominant. The bilateral organization of the corticobulbar projections to the nucleus ambiguus might therefore provide an important anatomical substrate for recovery. Another mechanism for recovery of swallowing function is for other cortical regions, such as the cingulate motor area, to play a more important role after damage.

(continued)

Box 11–1 (continued).

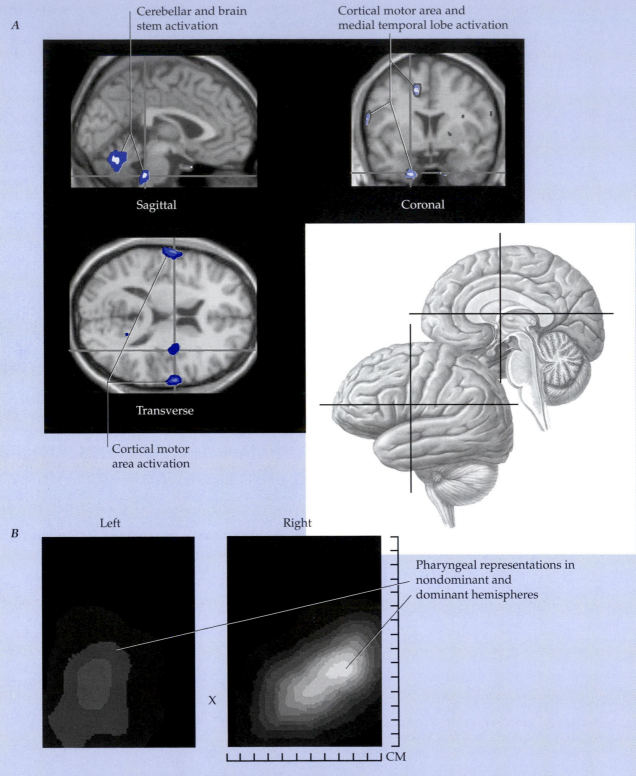

A

Cerebellar and brain stem activation

Cortical motor area and medial temporal lobe activation

Sagittal

Coronal

Transverse

Cortical motor area activation

B

Left

Right

Pharyngeal representations in nondominant and dominant hemispheres

X

CM

Figure 11–5. Cortical control of swallowing. *A.* Functional magnetic resonance imaging scans. The inset shows the planes of section. The transverse slice shows that there is bilateral motor cortical activation. There also is activation of subcortical structures, the cerebellum, and the brain stem. *B.* Functional maps of the primary motor cortex areas where transcranial magnetic stimulation evokes contraction of pharyngeal and esophageal muscles. *(Courtesy of Dr. Shaheen Hamdy, University of Manchester and the Medical Research Council; Hamdy S, Rothwell JC, Brooks DJ, Bailey D, Aziz Q, Thompson DG: Identification of the cerebral loci processing human swallowing with H$_2$^{15}O PET activation. J Neurophysiol 1999;81:1917–1926.)*

A

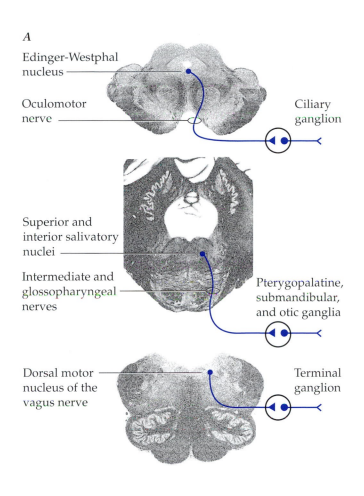

Edinger-Westphal nucleus

Oculomotor nerve

Ciliary ganglion

Superior and interior salivatory nuclei

Intermediate and glossopharyngeal nerves

Pterygopalatine, submandibular, and otic ganglia

Dorsal motor nucleus of the vagus nerve

Terminal ganglion

B

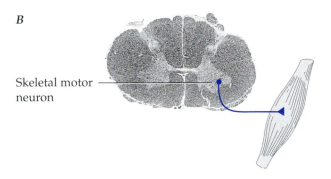

Skeletal motor neuron

Figure 11–6. **A.** Parasympathetic preganglionic neurons are located in nuclei within the central nervous system, whereas postganglionic neurons are located in peripheral ganglia. **B.** Somatic motor neurons project directly to their peripheral targets, which are striated muscles.

glands. The intermediate nerve is sometimes considered to be the sensory branch of the **facial nerve** because it contains afferent fibers, which are the axons of pseudounipolar neurons of the geniculate ganglion (see Chapters 6 and 9).

The inferior salivatory nucleus contains parasympathetic preganglionic neurons whose axons course in the **glossopharyngeal nerve** and synapse on postganglionic neurons in the **otic ganglion** (Figure 11–6). Parasympathetic postganglionic neurons in the otic ganglion innervate the **parotid gland,** which secretes saliva.

The parasympathetic preganglionic neurons in the dorsal motor nucleus of the vagus nerve synapse in extracranial parasympathetic ganglia, called **terminal ganglia** (Figure 11–6). These ganglia are located in the viscera of the thoracic and abdominal cavities, including the gastrointestinal tract proximal to the splenic flexure of the colon. The functions of the vagal parasympathetic neurons include regulating heart rate (ie, slowing), gastric motility (ie, increasing), and bronchial muscle control (ie, contracting to constrict airway). (The colon distal to the flexure is innervated by parasympathetic preganglionic neurons of the sacral spinal cord [see Chapter 15].)

■ REGIONAL ANATOMY OF CRANIAL MOTOR NUCLEI

The rest of this chapter focuses on the spatial relations between the cranial nerve nuclei, cortical motor pathways, and other important brain stem structures. In addition to describing the locations and connections of the cranial nerve motor nuclei, this chapter further explains the three-dimensional organization of the brain stem.

Lesion of the Genu of the Internal Capsule Interrupts the Corticobulbar Tract

Similar to the corticospinal projection, neurons that form the corticobulbar tract originate from multiple cortical sites: the primary motor cortex, the supplementary motor area, the premotor cortex, and the cingulate motor areas. The corticobulbar projection descends in the genu and the posterior limb of the internal capsule, rostral to the corticospinal projection (Figure 11–7). The corticobulbar axons terminate in the cranial motor nuclei innervating muscles of the jaw, face, pharynx, and larynx.

The various parts of the internal capsule are supplied by different cerebral artery branches (see Figure 4–6). The superficial portion is supplied by deep branches of the **middle cerebral artery.** The inferior part of the posterior limb is supplied by the **anterior choroidal artery,** and the inferior parts of the genu and anterior limbs are supplied primarily by deep branches of the **anterior cerebral artery.**

A Posterior limb
(corticospinal tract)

Genu
(corticobulbar tract)

Anterior limb

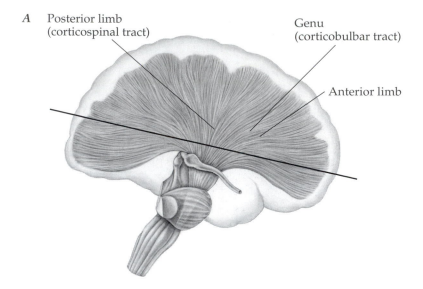

Figure 11–7. *A.* Three-dimensional view of fibers within the white matter of the cerebral cortex. The components of the internal capsule are indicated. The horizontal line indicates the plane of section in part *B.*
B. Horizontal myelin-stained section through the diencephalon and cerebral hemispheres. Note that the thalamus extends rostrally as far as the genu. The head of the caudate nucleus and the putamen are separated by the anterior limb of the internal capsule. The fiber constituents and somatotopic organization of the internal capsule are indicated. (*A,* *Adapted from Carpenter MB, Sutin J: Human Neuroanatomy. Williams & Wilkins, 1983.*)

B

Caudate
nucleus
(head)

Putamen

Ventral
anterior
nucleus

Ventral
lateral
nucleus

Caudate
nucleus
(tail)

Internal capsule:

Anterior limb

Genu
(corticobulbar tract)

Posterior limb
(corticospinal tract)

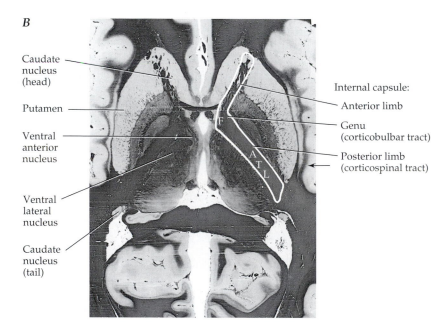

Parasympathetic Neurons in the Midbrain Regulate Pupil Size

The **oculomotor nucleus,** which innervates extraocular muscles, and the **Edinger-Westphal nucleus,** which contains parasympathetic preganglionic neurons, are located at the level of the superior colliculus (Figure 11–8B). Axons from these nuclei course through the red nucleus in their path to the periphery. The oculomotor nerve exits from the medial surface of the cerebral peduncle into the **interpeduncular fossa.** Most of the neurons in the Edinger-Westphal nucleus synapse in the **ciliary ganglion,** which contains the parasympathetic postganglionic neurons. However,

other neurons within and in the vicinity of the nucleus project axons to the spinal cord. These descending projection neurons may coordinate the functions of the parasympathetic and sympathetic divisions of the autonomic nervous system.

The Edinger-Westphal nucleus (Figure 11–8) mediates lens accommodation and pupillary constriction in response to light. It does this through a projection to parasympathetic postganglionic neurons in the ciliary ganglion. Pupillary reflexes are an important component of assessing brain stem function during clinical examination.

The **pupillary light reflex** is the constriction of the pupil that occurs when light hits the retina. Visual

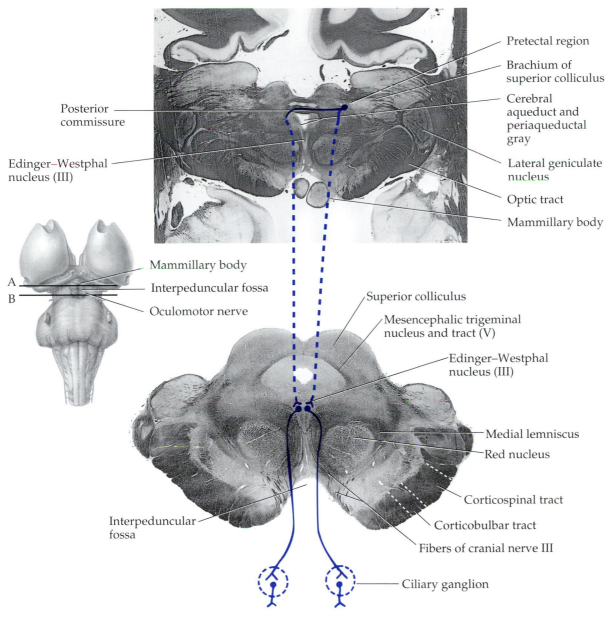

Figure 11–8. Myelin-stained sections through the midbrain-diencephalic junction (**A**) and rostral midbrain (**B**). The circuit for the pupillary light reflex is shown across both sections. The inset shows planes of section in **A** and **B**.

input from the retina passes directly to the **pretectal nuclei** via the **brachium of superior colliculus** (Figure 11–8; see Chapter 7). The pretectal nuclei project bilaterally to the parasympathetic preganglionic neurons in the Edinger-Westphal nucleus. The axons cross to the contralateral side in the **posterior commissure.**

Parasympathetic preganglionic neurons project to the ciliary ganglion through the **oculomotor nerve,** and from there, postganglionic neurons innervate the constrictor muscles of the iris. The bilateral projection of pretectal neurons to the parasympathetic pregan-

glionic neurons in the Edinger-Westphal nucleus ensures that illumination of one eye causes constriction of the pupil on the ipsilateral side (direct response) as well as on the contralateral side (consensual response). **Pupillary dilation** is mediated either by inhibition of the circuit for pupillary constriction or by the separate control of the iris by the sympathetic component of the autonomic nervous system (see Chapter 15).

Parasympathetic preganglionic neurons of the midbrain participate in a second visual reflex, the **accommodation reflex,** which is the increase in lens curvature that occurs during near vision. This reflex is usually part of the **accommodation-convergence reaction,** a complex response that prepares the eyes for near vision by increasing lens curvature, constricting the pupils, and coordinating convergence of the eyes. These responses involve the integrated actions of the visual areas of the occipital lobe, along with motor neurons in the oculomotor nucleus that innervate the extraocular muscles and parasympathetic preganglionic neurons. Central nervous system pathology

can distinguish different components of the visual reflexes. For example, in neurosyphilis the accommodation reaction is preserved but the light reflex is impaired. Patients with this condition have a classic neurological sign, the **Argyll Robertson pupils:** Their pupils are small and unreactive to light but get smaller when the patient accommodates. Distinct portions of the midbrain are supplied by paramedian, short circumferential, and long circumferential branches of the posterior cerebral artery (see Figure 4–3B1).

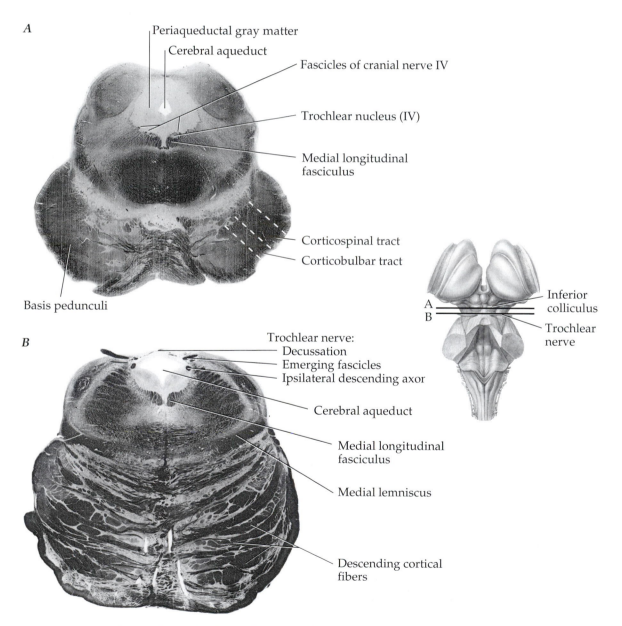

A. Periaqueductal gray matter
Cerebral aqueduct
Fascicles of cranial nerve IV
Trochlear nucleus (IV)
Medial longitudinal fasciculus
Corticospinal tract
Corticobulbar tract
Basis pedunculi

Inferior colliculus
Trochlear nerve

B. Trochlear nerve:
Decussation
Emerging fascicles
Ipsilateral descending axor
Cerebral aqueduct
Medial longitudinal fasciculus
Medial lemniscus
Descending cortical fibers

Figure 11–9. **A.** Myelin-stained section through the caudal midbrain at the level of the trochlear nucleus. **B.** Myelin-stained section through the rostral pons at the level of exiting trochlear nerve fibers. The inset shows planes of section in *A* and *B.*

The Descending Cortical Fibers Break Up Into Small Fascicles in the Pons

In the caudal midbrain the descending cortical fibers, including the corticobulbar and corticospinal tracts, are together within the basis pedunculi (Figure 11–9A). At the next caudal level, in the isthmus of the pons, the cortical projection becomes fragmented into innumerable small fascicles (Figure 11–9B). The isthmus level of the pons is also the level of emergence of the trochlear nerve. The cell bodies of trochlear nerve axons are located rostrally in the trochlear nucleus in the caudal midbrain (Figure 11–9A).

The Trigeminal Motor Nucleus Is Medial to the Main Trigeminal Sensory Nucleus

The most rostral component of the branchiomeric motor column is the **trigeminal motor nucleus** (Figures 11–1 and 11–10). The mediolateral organization of motor and sensory nuclei (see Chapter 3) is revealed by the location of trigeminal motor nucleus: medial to the main trigeminal sensory nucleus. Identifying the **trigeminal root fibers** in Figure 11–10 helps to distinguish the trigeminal sensory from motor nuclei.

The Fibers of the Facial Nerve Have a Complex Trajectory Through the Pons

The pontine section shown in Figure 11–11A cuts through portions of the facial nerve. The axons leave the facial nucleus and follow a path toward the floor of the fourth ventricle (Figure 11–11B). These fibers of the facial nerve are not seen in Figure 11–11A because they do not course in discrete and straight fascicles.

As the facial nerve fibers approach the ventricular floor, they first ascend close to the midline. Next, the fibers sweep around the medial, dorsal, and rostral aspects of the **abducens nucleus,** which contains motor neurons innervating the lateral rectus muscle, which abducts the eye (ie, looking away from the nose). This component is termed the **genu** of the facial nerve and, with the abducens nucleus, forms the **facial colliculus,** a surface landmark on the pontine floor of the fourth ventricle (Figure 11–11, inset). The facial nerve fibers then run ventrally and caudally to exit the pons at the **pontomedullary junction.** In addition to the axons of branchiomeric motor neurons, the facial nerve also contains visceral motor axons from the superior salivatory nucleus that innervate the **pterygopalatine** and **submandibular** ganglia. The pterygopalatine ganglion innervates lacrimal glands and the nasal mucosa.

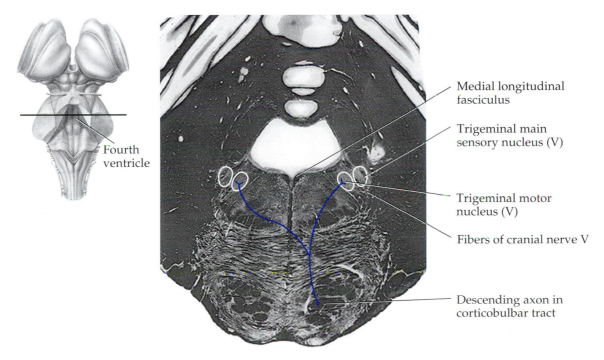

Fourth ventricle

Medial longitudinal fasciculus

Trigeminal main sensory nucleus (V)

Trigeminal motor nucleus (V)

Fibers of cranial nerve V

Descending axon in corticobulbar tract

Figure 11–10. Myelin-stained transverse section through the pons at the level of the trigeminal main sensory and motor nuclei. The inset shows the plane of section.

The submandibular ganglion innervates submandibular and sublingual salivary glands.

The vascular supply to the pons is derived by separate paramedian, short circumferential, and long circumferential branches of the basilar artery (see Figure 4–3B2). At the level of the pons in Figure 11–11, the **anterior inferior cerebellar artery (AICA)** is the long circumferential branch. The more rostral pontine levels (Figures 11–9B and 11–10) also receive their blood supply from branches of the basilar artery.

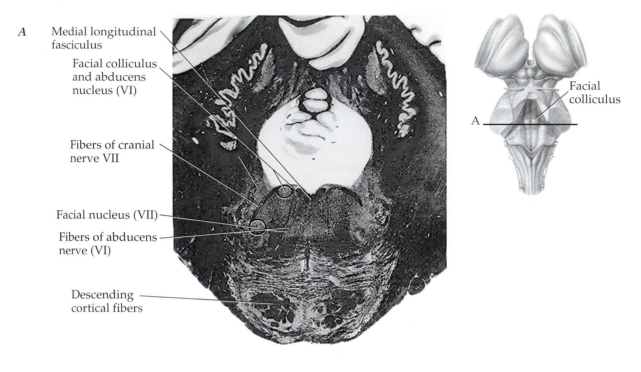

A

Medial longitudinal fasciculus

Facial colliculus and abducens nucleus (VI)

Fibers of cranial nerve VII

Facial nucleus (VII)

Fibers of abducens nerve (VI)

Descending cortical fibers

Facial colliculus

A

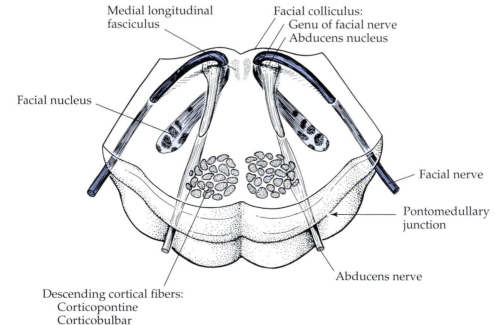

B

Medial longitudinal fasciculus

Facial colliculus:
Genu of facial nerve
Abducens nucleus

Facial nucleus

Facial nerve

Pontomedullary junction

Abducens nerve

Descending cortical fibers:
Corticopontine
Corticobulbar
Corticospinal

Figure 11–11. **A.** Myelin-stained transverse section through the pons at the level of the genu of cranial nerve VII. **B.** The three-dimensional course of the facial nerve in the pons. The inset shows the plane of section in **A.** (**B,** *Adapted from Williams PL, Warwick R: Functional Neuroanatomy of Man. W. B. Saunders, 1975.*)

The Glossopharyngeal Nerve Enters and Exits From the Rostral Medulla

The myelin-stained section through the rostral medulla is through the glossopharyngeal nerve root (Figure 11–12A). The motor axons of the glossopharyngeal nerve originate from neurons in two nuclei: Motor neurons innervating striated muscle are located in the rostral portion of the **nucleus ambiguus** (motor neurons that innervate the stylopharyngeus muscle);

autonomic motor neurons are located in the inferior salivatory nucleus (parasympathetic preganglionic neurons that innervate the otic ganglion). The otic ganglion innervates the parotid gland for salivation.

From a clinical perspective, the glossopharyngeal nerve can be considered a sensory nerve because a unilateral lesion does not produce frank motor dysfunction (either somatic or visceral motor) on clinical examination. Recall that the glossopharyngeal nerve also contains gustatory and viscerosensory afferent

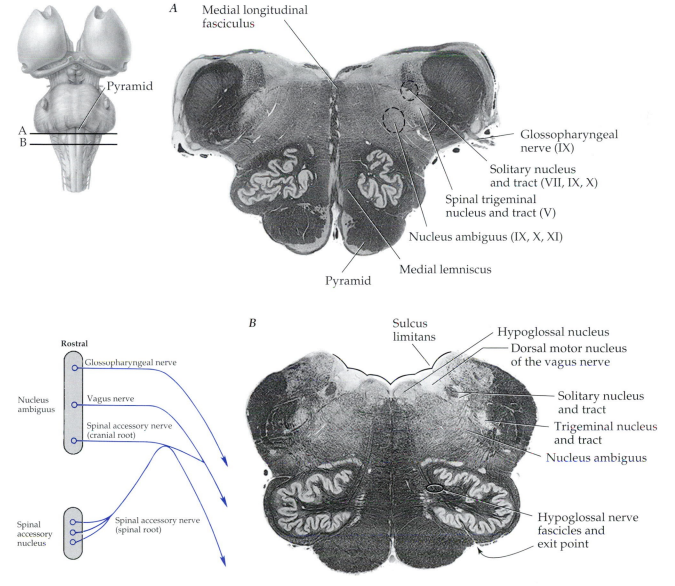

Figure 11–12. **A.** Myelin-stained transverse section at the level of exiting fibers of the glossopharyngeal (IX) nerve. **B.** Myelin-stained transverse section through the hypoglossal nucleus in the medulla. Top inset shows planes of section in **A** and **B.** Bottom inset shows the rostrocaudal organization of the nucleus ambiguus and spinal accessory nucleus.

fibers that terminate in the solitary nucleus as well as somatic sensory afferents that terminate in the trigeminal spinal nucleus (see Figure 11–12B).

A Level Through the Midmedulla Reveals the Locations of Six Cranial Nerve Nuclei

The three cranial nerve motor nuclei in the midmedulla—the hypoglossal nucleus, the dorsal motor nucleus of vagus, and the nucleus ambiguus—are medial to the three sensory nuclei at this level—the solitary, vestibular, and spinal trigeminal nuclei (Figure 11–12B). The cranial nerve sensory and motor nuclei are roughly separated by the sulcus limitans (Figure 11–12B). The hypoglossal and vagal nuclei are immediately beneath the floor of the fourth ventricle, whereas the nucleus ambiguus is deeper within the medulla (Figure 11–12B; see also Figure 11–14). The precise location of the nucleus ambiguus cannot be determined in myelin-stained sections; its approximate location is indicated in Figure 11–12B.

Infarction in the Territory of Different Arterial Branches Interrupts the Function of Specific Cranial Nerve Nuclei and Brain Stem Paths

In the medulla, different cranial nerve nuclei receive their arterial supply from specific branches of the vertebral-basilar system (Figure 11–13; see Figure 6–11). The medial portion of the medulla is supplied by branches of the main portion of the **vertebral artery.** This region contains the hypoglossal nucleus, the medial lemniscus, and the pyramid. Infarction of this region of the medulla produces three deficits. First, tongue muscles are paralyzed on the side of the lesion because the **hypoglossal motor neurons and axons** are destroyed. Second, tactile sensation, vibration sense, and limb proprioception sense on the side opposite the lesion are impaired because the **medial lemniscus** is affected. Third, muscles of the limb on the side opposite the lesion are weak because corticospinal axons in the **pyramid** are affected.

The dorsolateral portion of the medulla is supplied by the **posterior inferior cerebellar artery (PICA)** (Figure 11–13). Six key sensory and motor signs, which comprise the **lateral medullary,** or **Wallenberg, syndrome,** can be produced when the territory of this artery becomes infarcted. Among these signs, three are associated with damage to different cranial nerve nuclei:

- Difficulty in swallowing and hoarseness result from lesions of the **nucleus ambiguus.** An associated change, the loss of the gag reflex, is due either to lesions of the nucleus ambiguus (the efferent limb of the reflex) or to loss of pharyngeal sensation (cranial nerve IX) (the afferent limb).
- **Vertigo** (an illusion of a whirling movement; sometimes described as dizziness) and **nystagmus** (involuntary rhythmical oscillation of the eyes) are produced by **vestibular nuclear** lesions (see Chapter 12).
- Loss of pain and temperature senses on the ipsilateral face is due to lesions of the **spinal trigeminal nucleus and tract.**

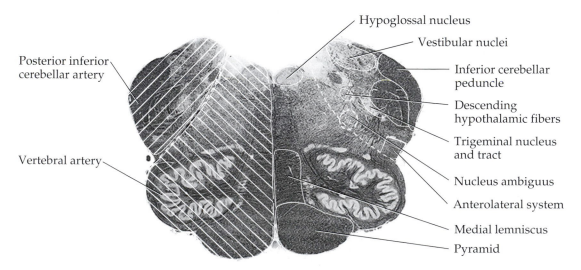

Hypoglossal nucleus
Vestibular nuclei
Inferior cerebellar peduncle
Descending hypothalamic fibers
Trigeminal nucleus and tract
Nucleus ambiguus
Anterolateral system
Medial lemniscus
Pyramid

Posterior inferior cerebellar artery
Vertebral artery

Figure 11–13. Arterial supply of the medulla. Occlusion of the posterior inferior cerebellar artery produces a complex set of neurological deficits, termed the lateral medullary, or Wallenberg, syndrome (see Chapter 6). Occlusion of the vertebral artery can produce a discrete set of limb sensory and motor signs.

The remaining signs result from damage to ascending or descending pathways that course through the dorsolateral medulla:

- Reduced pain and temperature senses on the contralateral limbs and trunk reflect lesion of the **anterolateral system.**
- Ipsilateral limb **ataxia** (jerky or uncoordinated movements) is due to lesions of the **inferior cerebellar peduncle** (see Chapter 13).
- **Horner syndrome** results from damage to descending hypothalamic axons that regulate the sympathetic nervous system. (The precise location of these axons in the dorsolateral medulla is not known.) Horner syndrome consists of **pupillary constriction** due to unopposed actions of parasympathetic pupillary constrictors; **pseudoptosis** due to weakness of the tarsal muscle, a smooth muscle that assists the action of the levator palpebrae muscle (ptosis is drooping of the upper eyelid due to levator palpebrae muscle weakness); **reddening** of facial skin due to loss of sympathetic vasoconstrictor activity and resulting vasodilation; and **impaired sweating** due to loss of sympathetic control of the sweat glands.

The Spinal Accessory Nucleus Is Located at the Junction of the Spinal Cord and Medulla

The **pyramidal decussation** marks the boundary between the spinal cord and medulla (Figure 11–14B).

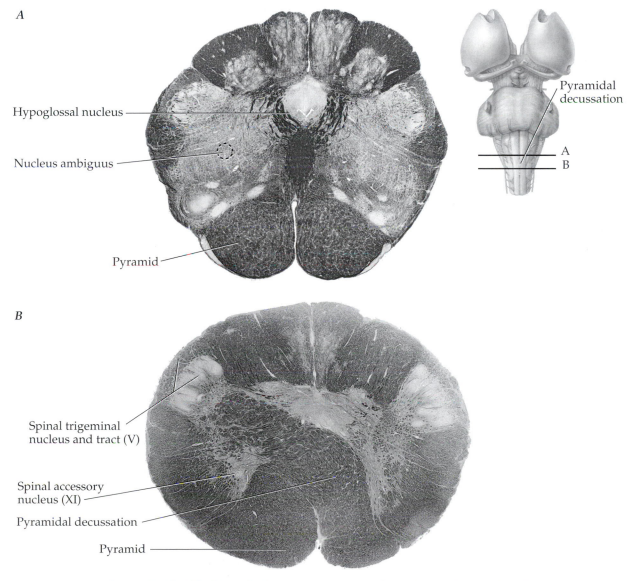

A

Hypoglossal nucleus

Nucleus ambiguus

Pyramid

Pyramidal decussation

A

B

B

Spinal trigeminal nucleus and tract (V)

Spinal accessory nucleus (XI)

Pyramidal decussation

Pyramid

Figure 11–14. Myelin-stained transverse sections through the mid-medulla (*A*) and spinal cord–medulla junction (*B*). The inset shows planes of section in *A* and *B*.

The **spinal accessory nerve** contains axons of motor neurons whose cell bodies are located in the **spinal accessory nucleus** (Figure 11–14B). Recall that these motor neurons innervate the sternocleidomastoid muscle and the upper part of the trapezius muscle. Comparison of this section with the one through the cervical enlargement (eg, see Figure AII–5) reveals the similarity in location of the spinal accessory nucleus, on the one hand, and the ventral horn motor nuclei, on the other.

Summary

There are three separate columns of cranial nerve motor nuclei (Figure 11–1), from medial to lateral: somatic skeletal motor, branchiomeric motor, and autonomic.

Somatic Skeletal Motor Nuclei

The somatic skeletal motor column is the most medial motor column. It comprises four nuclei, each of which contains motor neurons that innervate striated muscle derived from the **occipital somites.** The **oculomotor nucleus** (1) (Figures 11–6, 11–8, and 11–9) contains motor neurons whose axons course in the **oculomotor (III) nerve** and innervate the following extraocular muscles: **medial rectus, superior rectus, inferior rectus,** and **inferior oblique.** The oculomotor nucleus also innervates the **levator palpebrae superioris muscle.** The **trochlear nucleus** (2), via the **trochlear (IV) nerve,** innervates the **contralateral superior oblique muscle;** the **abducens nucleus** (3), via the **abducens (VI) nerve,** innervates the **lateral rectus muscle.** The **hypoglossal nucleus** (4) gives rise to axons that course in the **hypoglossal (XII) nerve** and innervate tongue muscles (Figures 11–1 and 11–12). The hypoglossal nucleus is the only nucleus of this column that receives a projection from the primary motor cortex.

Branchiomeric Motor Nuclei

The branchiomeric motor column is displaced ventrally from the floor of the fourth ventricle (Figures 11–1, 11–3, and 11–4). It contains three nuclei, each of which innervates striated muscles derived from the branchial arches. The **trigeminal motor nucleus** (1) (Figures 11–4 and 11–10) innervates the muscles of **mastication** via the **trigeminal (V) nerve.** This nucleus receives a bilateral projection from the motor cortex.

The **facial nucleus** (2) (Figures 11–1 and 11–11) innervates the muscles of **facial expression.** The axons of facial motor neurons course in the **facial (VII) nerve.** Facial motor neurons that innervate lower face muscles receive a contralateral projection from the primary motor cortex. Motor neurons innevating upper facial muscles receive weak bilateral projections from the primary motor cortex but dense projections from premotor areas (Figure 11–4). The **nucleus ambiguus** (3) innervates the muscles of the **pharynx** and **larynx** predominantly via the **vagus (X) nerve** and to a lesser extent via the **glossopharyngeal (IX) nerve** and the cranial root of the **spinal accessory (XI) nerve** (Figure 11–4). The **spinal accessory nucleus** (spinal root) is in line with the nucleus ambiguus but is not part of the branchiomeric motor column. It innervates the sternocleidomastoid and trapezius muscles via the **spinal accessory (XI) nerve** (Figures 11–1 and 11–14B).

Autonomic Nuclei

The autonomic motor column contains four nuclei (Figure 11–1). Each nucleus contains **parasympathetic preganglionic neurons** (Figure 11–6). The **Edinger-Westphal nucleus** (1) is located in the midbrain (Figures 11–1 and 11–8). Its axons project via the **oculomotor nerve** to the **ciliary ganglion,** where postganglionic neurons innervate the constrictor muscles of the iris and the ciliary muscle. Axons from the **superior salivatory nucleus** (2) (Figures 11–1 and 11–6) course in the **intermediate nerve** (a branch of the **facial nerve**). Via synapses in the pterygopalatine and submandibular ganglia, this nucleus influences the **lacrimal gland** and **glands of the nasal mucosa.** The **inferior salivatory nucleus** (3) (Figures 11–1 and 11–6), via the **glossopharyngeal nerve,** synapses on postganglionic neurons in the **otic ganglion.** From there, postganglionic neurons innervate the **parotid gland.** Axons from the **dorsal motor nucleus of the vagus** (4) (Figures 11–1, 11–6, and 11–12) course in the periphery in the **vagus nerve** and innervate **terminal ganglia** in most of the thoracic and abdominal viscera (proximal to the splenic flexure of the colon).

Related Sources

Brust JCM: The Practice of Neural Science. McGraw-Hill; 2000. (See ch. 3, pp. 27, 29, 36, 37, 39; ch. 12, cases 24, 28, 29, 31; ch. 13, case 39; ch. 14, cases 50, 51, 53, 54; ch. 15, case 57.)

Saper CB: Brain stem modulation of sensation, movement, and consciousness. In Kandel ER, Schwartz JH, Jessell TM (editors): Principles of Neural Science, 4th ed. McGraw-Hill; 2000:889–909.

Saper CB: Brain stem, reflexive behavior, and the cranial nerves. In Kandel ER, Schwartz JH, Jessell TM (editors): Principles of Neural Science, 4th ed. McGraw-Hill; 2000:873–888.

Selected Readings

Aviv J: The normal swallow. In Carrau RL (editor): Comprehensive Management of Swallowing Disorders. Singular Publishing Group; 1999:23–29.

Brodal A: The Cranial Nerves: Anatomical and Anatomico-clinical Correlations. Blackwell Scientific Publications, 1965.

Hamdy S, Rothwell JC: Gut feelings about recovery after stroke: The organization and reorganization of human swallowing motor cortex. Trends Neurosci 1998;21:278–282.

Patten J: Neurological Differential Diagnosis, 2nd ed. Springer-Verlag; 1996:448.

References

Akert K, Glickman MA, Lang W, et al: The Edinger-Westphal nucleus in the monkey. A retrograde tracer study. Brain Res 1980;184:491–498.

Broussard DL, Altschuler SM: Brainstem viscerotopic organization of afferents and efferents involved in the control of swallowing. Am J Med 2000;108(Suppl 4a):79S–86S.

Chung CS, Caplan LR, Yamamoto Y, et al: Striatocapsular haemorrhage. Brain 2000;123:1850–1862.

Ferner H, Staubestand J (editors): Sobota Atlas of Human Anatomy, Vol. 1: Head, Neck, Upper Extremities. Urban & Schwartzenberg, 1983.

Hamdy S, Rothwell JC, Brooks DJ, Bailey D, Aziz Q, Thompson DG: Identification of the cerebral loci processing human swallowing with H$_2$^{15}O PET activation. J Neurophysiol 1999;81:1917–1926.

Jenny AB, Saper CB: Organization of the facial nucleus and corticofacial projection in the monkey: A reconsideration of the upper motor neuron facial palsy. Neurology 1987;37:930–939.

Kidder TM: Esophago/pharyngo/laryngeal interrelationships: Airway protection mechanisms. Dysphagia 1995;10:228–231.

Lowey AD, Saper CB, Yamondis ND: Re-evaluation of the efferent projections of the Edinger-Westphal nucleus in the cat. Brain Res 1978;141:153–159.

Martin RE, Goodyear BG, Gati JS, Menon RS: Cerebral cortical representation of automatic and volitional swallowing in humans. J Neurophysiol 2001;85:938–950.

Martin RE, Sessle BJ: The role of the cerebral cortex in swallowing. Dysphagia 1993;8:195–202.

Miller AJ: Deglutition. Physiol Rev 1982;62:129–184.

Miller AJ: The search for the central swallowing pathway: The quest for clarity. Dysphagia 1993;8:185–194.

Morecraft RJ, Louie JL, Herrick JL, Stilwell-Morecraft KS: Cortical innervation of the facial nucleus in the non-human primate: A new interpretation of the effects of stroke and related subtotal brain trauma on the muscles of facial expression. Brain 2001;124:176–208.

Shaker R: Airway protective mechanisms: Current concepts. Dysphagia 1995;10:216–227.

Thompson ML, Thickbroom GW, Mastaglia FL: Corticomotor representation of the sternocleidomastoid muscle. Brain 1997;120:245–255.

Törk I, McRitchie DA, Rikkard-Bell GC, Paxinos G: Autonomic regulatory centers in the medulla oblongata. In Paxinos G (editor): The Human Nervous System. Academic Press; 1990:221–259.

12

The Vestibular and Oculomotor Systems

DURING TAKEOFF IN A JET, you experience a particularly salient function of the vestibular system: sensing body acceleration. Although perception of signals from the vestibular sensory organs occurs only under special circumstances, this system is operating continuously by controlling relatively automatic movements, such as maintaining balance.

The oculomotor system controls the extraocular muscles, which move the eyes. Eye movement must be precisely controlled in order to position the image of an object of interest over the fovea, the portion of the retina that provides the greatest visual acuity (see Chapter 7). This chapter examines the vestibular and oculomotor systems together because they share many brain stem neural circuits, especially the circuitry underlying the vestibuloocular reflexes. These reflexes help to stabilize an object's image on the retina during head movements. Consider your ability to maintain gaze on a friend's face in a crowded airport terminal as you run toward her. Your head bobs up and down, and from side to side, but you can maintain fixation effortlessly. This is accomplished automatically by the coordinated actions of the vestibular system, for detecting head motion, and the oculomotor system, for making compensatory eye movements. In addition, the medial descending motor pathways (see Chapter 10) assist in this action by adjusting head position. This happens without conscious awareness, apart from knowing where to fixate your gaze.

From a clinical perspective the vestibular and oculomotor systems are also very tightly linked. An important part of testing the integrated functions of the brain stem involves careful assessment of a person's ability to coordinate eye movement during head motion. This chapter also completes the examination of the cranial nerve nuclei, through which greater knowledge of brain stem regional anatomy will emerge. Such knowledge is essential for clinical problem solving, for example, in identifying the locus of central nervous system damage. Because each of the cranial nerve nuclei has a clearly identifiable sensory or motor function, the clinician can thoroughly test the integrity of such functions.

FUNCTIONAL ANATOMY OF THE VESTIBULAR SYSTEM

Vestibular receptors sense head motion, both linear—such as that experienced during fast acceleration in an elevator or a jet—and angular—such as during turning. These receptors are located in five peripheral vestibular organs (Figure 12–1): the three **semicircular canals,** which signal angular acceleration, and the **utricle** and **saccule,** which signal linear acceleration. These receptor organs project to the vestibular nuclei, located in the medulla and pons (Figure 12–2A). The vestibular sensory organs are contained within the **membranous labyrinth,** which is filled with **endolymph** (see Chapter 8).

Vestibular receptor cells are hair cells, like auditory receptors, located in specialized regions of the semicircular canals (termed ampullae) (Figure 12–1, inset) and the saccule and utricle (termed maculae). The hair cells of the semicircular canals are covered by a gelatinous mass (termed the cupula) into which the stereocilia embed. Angular head movement induces the endolymph within the canals to flow, displacing the

gelatinous mass, which in turn deflects the hair cell stereocilia. The utricle and saccule also have a gelatinous covering over hair cells in their maculae. Calcium carbonate crystals, embedded in the gelatin, rest on the stereocilia. Linear acceleration causes the crystals to deform the gelatinous mass, thereby deflecting the stereocilia. The saccule and utricle are sometimes called the **otolith organs** because *otolith* is the term for the calcium carbonate crystals. The semicircular canals, utricle, and saccule each have a different orientation with respect to the head, thereby conferring selective sensitivity to head movement in different directions. Vestibular hair cells are innervated by bipolar neurons, whose cell bodies are located in the **vestibular ganglion.** The axons of these bipolar neurons travel to the brain stem in the **vestibular division** of **cranial nerve VIII** and terminate in the **vestibular nuclei** (Figure 12–2A).

An Ascending Pathway From the Vestibular Nuclei to the Thalamus Is Important for Perception and Orientation

A small ascending thalamocortical projection from the vestibular nuclei is important in the conscious awareness of head motion, balance, and orientation. Originating from the superior, lateral, and medial vestibular nuclei, this path ascends bilaterally to sev-

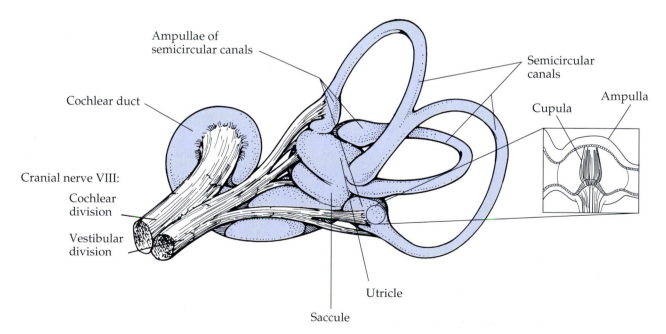

Figure 12–1. The peripheral auditory and vestibular structures and innervation by the cochlear and vestibular divisions of cranial nerve VIII. The upper inset shows the ampulla of one of the semicircular canals.

eral sites within and around the **ventral posterior nucleus** of the thalamus (Figure 12–2A, B). Three major sites within the parietal lobe and insular cortex receive this information (Figure 12–2, inset). The vestibular cortex in (1) **area 3a** (part of the primary somatic sensory cortex) is thought to participate in head position and neck motor control, whereas the areas in the (2) **posterior parietal lobe** and (3) **insular cortex** play roles in the sensing of body orientation and the orientation of the visual world.

The Vestibular Nuclei Have Functionally Distinct Efferent Projections for Axial Muscle Control and Perception

Two descending motor pathways originate from the vestibular nuclei, which form a major portion of the **medial descending motor pathways.** The **lateral vestibulospinal tract,** which begins at the **lateral vestibular nucleus,** descends ipsilaterally in the white matter to all spinal levels (Figure 12–2A,C). This pathway is crucial for controlling posture and balance. Recall from Chapter 10 that even though a particular tract may have a unilateral projection, the medial descending pathways collectively exert a bilateral influence on axial muscle control. The **medial vestibulospinal tract,** which starts primarily at the **medial vestibular nucleus,** descends bilaterally in the white matter but only to the cervical and upper thoracic spinal cord (Figure 12–2A,C). The medial vestibulospinal tract plays a role in controlling head position.

■ FUNCTIONAL ANATOMY
OF THE OCULOMOTOR SYSTEM
AND THE CONTROL OF GAZE

The position and movement of the eyes are controlled voluntarily and by vestibular reflexes. There are five types of eye movements:

- **Saccades** are rapid movements that shift the fovea to an object of interest.
- **Smooth pursuit movements** are slow and are used for tracking a moving object.
- **Vergence movements** (either convergent or divergent) ensure that the image of an object of interest falls on the same place on the retina of each eye.
- **Vestibuloocular reflexes** use information from the semicircular canals to compensate for head motion by adjusting eye position to maintain the direction of gaze.

- **Optokinetic reflexes** use visual information to supplement the effects of the vestibuloocular reflex.

With the exception of vergence, all eye movements are conjugate: The eyes move in tandem at the same speed and in the same direction. Vergence movements are disconjugate; the eyes move in opposite directions.

Each eye is controlled by six muscles, which operate as three functional pairs, with antagonistic actions (Figure 12–3). The lateral and medial rectus muscles move the eye horizontally, abducting (looking away from the nose) and adducting (looking toward the nose), respectively. The superior and inferior rectus muscles elevate and depress the eyes, particularly when the eye is abducted. Finally, the superior and inferior oblique muscles depress and elevate the eye, especially when the eye is adducted.

The Extraocular Motor Neurons Are Located in Three Cranial Nerve Motor Nuclei

The **oculomotor nucleus** contributes most of the axons of the **oculomotor (III) nerve,** which exits the rostral midbrain. The oculomotor nucleus (Figure 12–4) innervates four of the six extraocular muscles: **medial rectus, inferior rectus, superior rectus,** and **inferior oblique** (Figure 12–3). This nucleus also innervates the **levator palpebrae superioris muscle,** an eyelid elevator.

The other two extraocular motor nuclei are the trochlear and abducens nuclei (Figure 12–4). Motor neurons in the **trochlear nucleus** give rise to the fibers in the **trochlear (IV) nerve,** which innervate the **superior oblique muscle** (Figure 12–3). This cranial nerve is the only one that exits from the dorsal brain stem surface. The trochlear nerve is further distinguished because all of its axons **decussate** within the central nervous system. The **abducens nucleus** (Figure 12–4) contains the motor neurons that project their axons to the periphery through the **abducens (VI) nerve.** Abducens motor neurons innervate the **lateral rectus muscle** (Figure 12–3). Unlike spinal and other cranial nerve motor neurons, extraocular motor neurons are not controlled by the primary motor cortex.

Voluntary Eye Movement Direction Is Controlled by Neurons in the Frontal Lobe and the Parietal-Temporal-Occipital Association Cortex

Saccades are triggered by neurons in the **frontal eye field,** a portion of cytoarchitectonic area 8. This

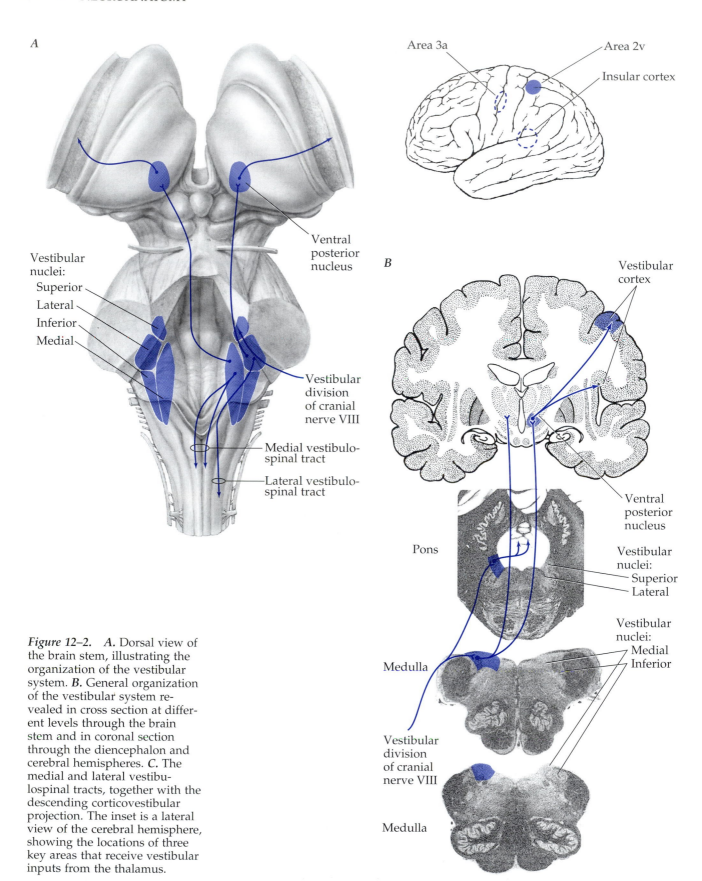

A

Area 3a

Area 2v

Insular cortex

Vestibular nuclei:
Superior
Lateral
Inferior
Medial

Ventral posterior nucleus

Vestibular division of cranial nerve VIII

Medial vestibulo-spinal tract

Lateral vestibulo-spinal tract

B

Vestibular cortex

Ventral posterior nucleus

Vestibular nuclei:
Superior
Lateral

Vestibular nuclei:
Medial
Inferior

Pons

Medulla

Vestibular division of cranial nerve VIII

Medulla

Figure 12–2. *A.* Dorsal view of the brain stem, illustrating the organization of the vestibular system. *B.* General organization of the vestibular system revealed in cross section at different levels through the brain stem and in coronal section through the diencephalon and cerebral hemispheres. *C.* The medial and lateral vestibulospinal tracts, together with the descending corticovestibular projection. The inset is a lateral view of the cerebral hemisphere, showing the locations of three key areas that receive vestibular inputs from the thalamus.

c

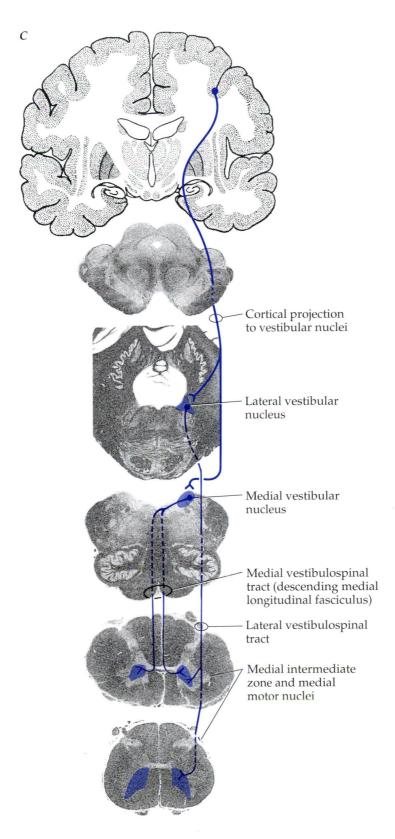

Cortical projection
to vestibular nuclei

Lateral vestibular
nucleus

Medial vestibular
nucleus

Medial vestibulospinal
tract (descending medial
longitudinal fasciculus)

Lateral vestibulospinal
tract

Medial intermediate
zone and medial
motor nuclei

cortical territory receives subcortical inputs from the basal ganglia and cerebellum, transmitted via thalamic neurons. The frontal eye field projects to the **superior colliculus** (Figure 12–5A). The axons of these frontal lobe projection neurons descend within the **anterior limb** and **genu of the internal capsule** to the brain stem. Collicular neurons, in turn, project to distinct regions of the pontine and midbrain reticular

A

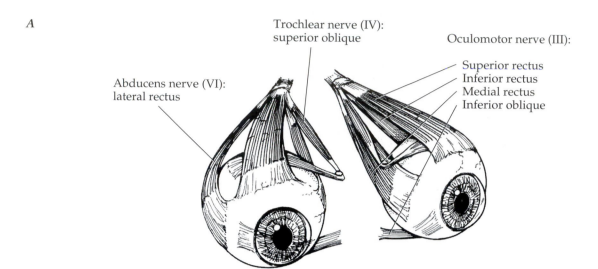

Trochlear nerve (IV):
superior oblique

Oculomotor nerve (III):

Abducens nerve (VI):
lateral rectus

Superior rectus
Inferior rectus
Medial rectus
Inferior oblique

B

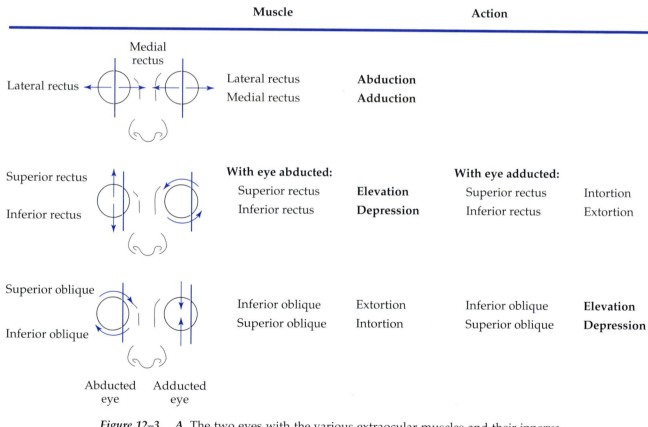

	Muscle	Action		
Lateral rectus	Lateral rectus	**Abduction**		
Medial rectus	Medial rectus	**Adduction**		
	With eye abducted:		**With eye adducted:**	
Superior rectus	Superior rectus	**Elevation**	Superior rectus	Intortion
Inferior rectus	Inferior rectus	**Depression**	Inferior rectus	Extortion
Superior oblique	Inferior oblique	Extortion	Inferior oblique	**Elevation**
Inferior oblique	Superior oblique	Intortion	Superior oblique	**Depression**

Abducted   Adducted
eye   eye

Figure 12–3. **A.** The two eyes with the various extraocular muscles and their innervation patterns. Not shown is the levator palpebrae, an eyelid elevator innervated by cranial nerve III. The extraocular muscles of both eyes operate as three functional pairs. The lateral and medial rectus muscles move the eye horizontally. The superior and inferior rectus muscles elevate and depress the eye, respectively (particularly when the eye is abducted). Finally, the inferior and superior oblique muscles elevate and depress the eye but to a greater extent when the eye is adducted. **B.** The mechanical actions of the extraocular muscles.

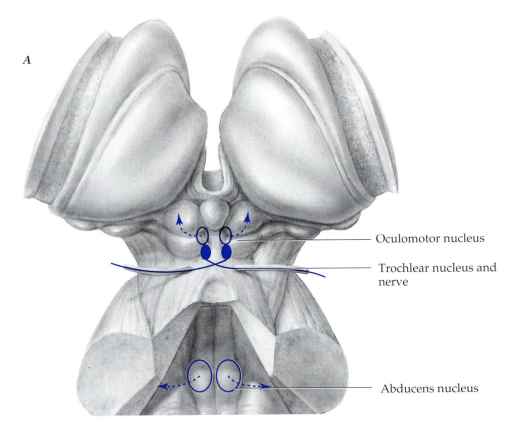

Oculomotor nucleus

Trochlear nucleus and nerve

Abducens nucleus

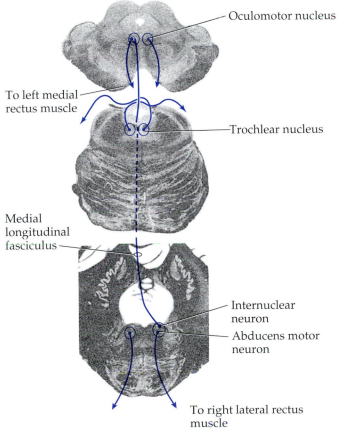

Oculomotor nucleus

To left medial rectus muscle

Trochlear nucleus

Medial longitudinal fasciculus

Internuclear neuron

Abducens motor neuron

To right lateral rectus muscle

Figure 12–4. Extraocular muscle control. *A.* View of the dorsal brain stem, showing the locations of the oculomotor nuclei (open ovals) and trochlear nuclei (filled ovals) and depicting the course of the trochlear nerve within the brain stem. *B.* Transverse sections through the oculomotor, trochlear, and abducens nuclei. Axon of internuclear neuron travels in the contralateral medial longitudinal fasciculus.

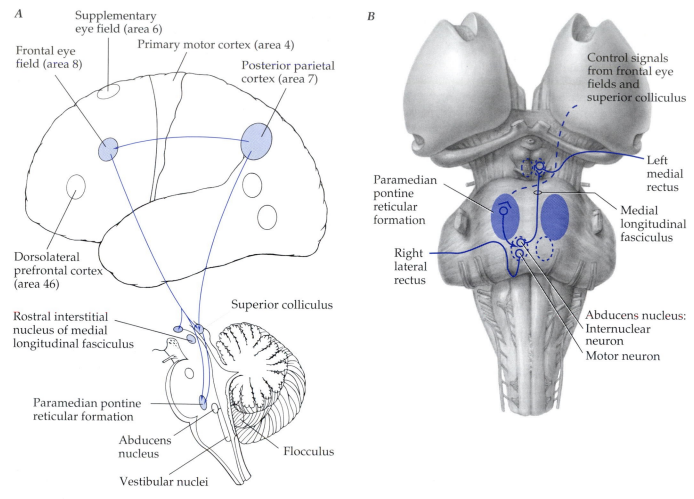

Figure 12–5. **A.** Lateral view of the cerebral cortex and midsagittal view of the brain stem show the approximate location of structures involved in controlling saccadic eye movements. **B.** Ventral surface of the brain stem, diencephalon, and basal ganglia, showing the circuit for producing conjugate horizontal saccades to the right.

formation that directly control saccades through their monosynaptic connections to extraocular motor neurons. The frontal eye fields also project directly to these two reticular formation zones. Horizontal saccades are controlled primarily by neurons in the **paramedian pontine reticular formation** (Figure 12–5B). These neurons process control signals and project to the abducens nucleus. The abducens nucleus is more than a motor nucleus because, in addition to containing lateral rectus motor neurons, it also contains **internuclear neurons** (Figure 12–5B). Signals from the paramedian pontine reticular formation trigger horizontal saccades by directly exciting lateral rectus motor neurons in the abducens nucleus and, via the internuclear neurons, indirectly exciting medial rectus motor neurons in the oculomotor nucleus. For vertical

eye movements the **rostral interstitial nucleus of the medial longitudinal fasciculus** in the midbrain reticular formation is essential (Figure 12–5A). Neurons in this nucleus coordinate the muscles that produce vertical eye movements (Figure 12–3B). A portion of the **posterior parietal cortex** within area 7 participates in saccade generation through its role in visual attention: You must first attend to a stimulus before looking at it. This region projects through the **posterior limb of the internal capsule** to the superior colliculus.

Smooth pursuit movements have a remarkably different control circuit, one that involves higher-order **cortical visual areas** implicated in visual motion perception and the **cerebellum** (Figure 12–6). The cortical control of smooth pursuit eye movements begins in the middle temporal (also termed V5) and middle

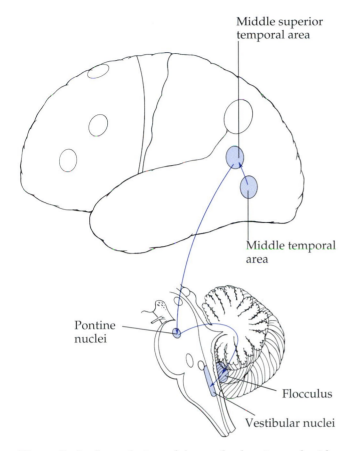

Middle superior
temporal area

Middle temporal
area

Pontine
nuclei

Flocculus

Vestibular nuclei

Figure 12–6. Lateral view of the cerebral cortex and mid-sagittal view of the brain stem show the approximate location of structures involved in controlling smooth pursuit eye movements.

superior temporal visual areas (see Figure 6–9). From the cortex, axons descend in the posterior limb of the internal capsule to engage a brain stem and cerebellar circuit comprising the **pontine nuclei,** the **flocculus** (a portion of the cerebellum; see Chapter 13), and the **vestibular nuclei** (Figure 12–6). All three extraocular nuclei receive input from the vestibular nuclei; the vestibular axons course in the **medial longitudinal fasciculus** (MLF). Axons in the MLF originating from the vestibular nuclei are also especially important in stabilizing eye position when the head is moved (see next section).

The Vestibuloocular Reflex Maintains Direction of Gaze During Head Movement

Stable fixation can be maintained on an object during head movement because the vestibular system generates eye movement control signals that compensate for head movements. For example, horizontal

rightward movement of the head generates leftward conjugate movement of the eyes (Figure 12–7A). This movement is produced by excitation of left lateral rectus motor neurons and right medial rectus motor neurons. The lateral and medial rectus motor neurons are directly activated by vestibular neurons (Figure 12–7B). In addition, the medial rectus motor neurons are indirectly activated by the internuclear neurons in the left abducens nucleus (Figure 12–7B, thin line). Although not shown in Figure 12–7B, the circuit for vestibuloocular control also ensures that the mechanical action of the muscle that moves the eye, termed the agonist muscle, is not impeded by contraction of the antagonistic muscles (the muscles whose mechanical action is opposite that of the agonist muscle). This process occurs through inhibitory connections with the motor neurons of antagonistic muscles. For example, when the left lateral rectus motor neurons are excited, the left medial rectus motor neurons are inhibited.

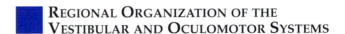

REGIONAL ORGANIZATION OF THE VESTIBULAR AND OCULOMOTOR SYSTEMS

Vestibular Nerve Fibers Project to the Vestibular Nuclei and the Cerebellum

Vestibular hair cells are innervated by the peripheral processes of vestibular bipolar neurons, the cell bodies of which are located in the **vestibular ganglion.** The central processes of these bipolar neurons, which form the **vestibular division** of **cranial nerve VIII,** course along with the cochlear division and enter the brain stem at the lateral pontomedullary junction. Axons in the vestibular division terminate on neurons in the four **vestibular nuclei** (Figure 12–8). Some vestibular axons project directly to the cerebellum (see Chapter 10). In fact, the vestibular sensory neurons are the only primary sensory neurons that have this privileged access to the cerebellum because of the special role of the vestibular system in controlling eye, limb, and trunk movements.

The Vestibular Nuclei Have Functionally Diverse Projections

The vestibular nuclei occupy the floor of the fourth ventricle in the dorsolateral medulla and pons (Figure 12–2A). This region is termed the **cerebellopontine angle.** There are four separate vestibular nuclei: inferior, medial, lateral, and superior (Figure 12–8). The **posterior inferior cerebellar artery** (PICA) supplies

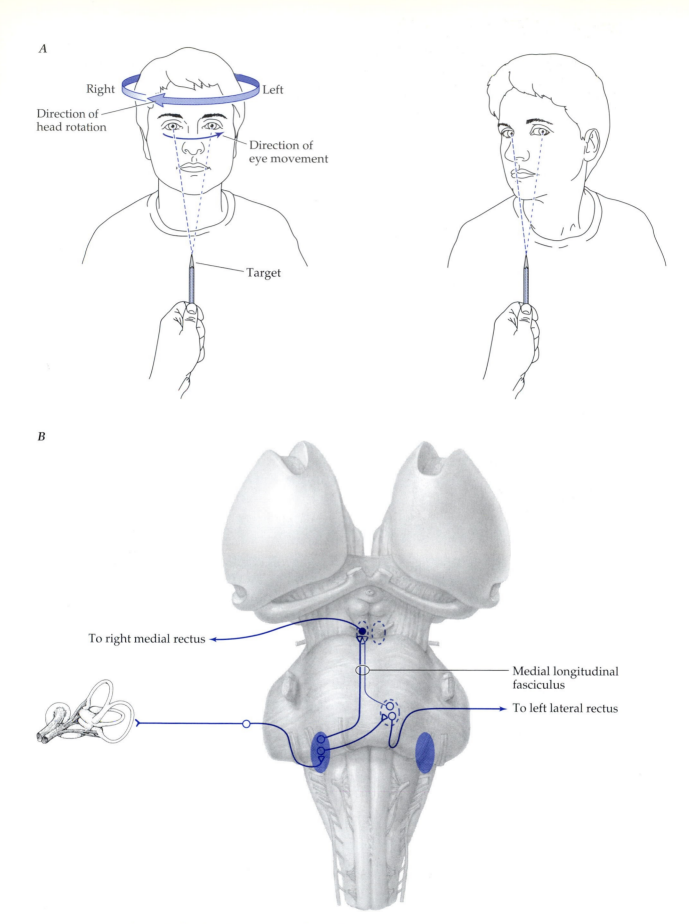

Figure 12–7. Vestibuloocular reflex. **A.** When the head turns to the right, the eyes compensate by turning an equal amount to the left. **B.** Ventral view of the brain stem, diencephalon, and basal ganglia, showing the circuit for the vestibuloocular reflex for the head turning to the right.

Labels in figure:

A
Right — Left
Direction of head rotation
Direction of eye movement
Target

B
To right medial rectus
Medial longitudinal fasciculus
To left lateral rectus

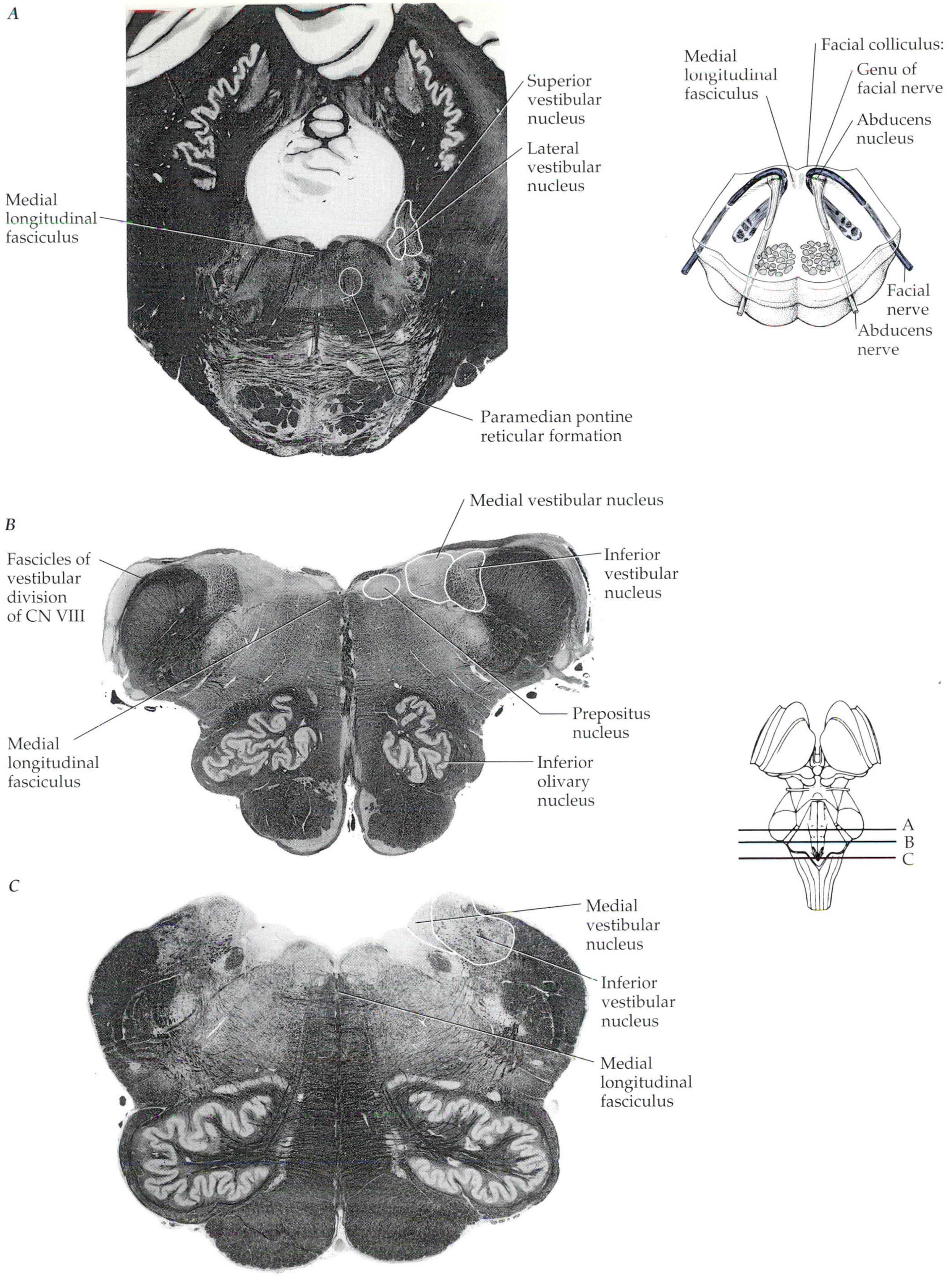

A

Medial longitudinal fasciculus

Superior vestibular nucleus

Lateral vestibular nucleus

Paramedian pontine reticular formation

Medial longitudinal fasciculus

Facial colliculus:
Genu of facial nerve
Abducens nucleus

Facial nerve
Abducens nerve

B

Medial vestibular nucleus

Fascicles of vestibular division of CN VIII

Inferior vestibular nucleus

Prepositus nucleus

Inferior olivary nucleus

Medial longitudinal fasciculus

C

Medial vestibular nucleus

Inferior vestibular nucleus

Medial longitudinal fasciculus

A
B
C

Figure 12–8. Myelin-stained transverse sections through the caudal pons (*A*), at the level of the cochlear nuclei (*B*), and medial vestibular nuclei (*C*). The top inset shows the three-dimensional course of the facial and abducens nerves in the pons. The bottom inset shows the planes of section. (*Top inset, Adapted from William PL, Warwick R: Functional Neuroanatomy of Man. W. B. Saunders, 1975.*)

blood to the vestibular nuclei (see Chapter 4). Occlusion of this artery can produce **vertigo,** an illusion of movement—typically whirling—of the patient or his or her surroundings.

The vestibular nuclei have extensive interconnections with components of the nuclear complex on the same and opposite sides that are important in the basic processing of vestibular signals. There are three sets of vestibular projections: descending spinal projections, connections within the brain stem, and ascending thalamic projections (see section below on thalamocortical relationships).

The Vestibular Nuclei Have Descending Spinal Projections for Controlling Axial Muscles

Together, the cerebellar projections of the primary and secondary vestibular neurons are essential for maintaining balance and head position by controlling axial and girdle muscles via the vestibulospinal tracts. The **lateral vestibulospinal tract** is an ipsilateral descending pathway that projects to all levels of the spinal cord. It originates from neurons in the **lateral vestibular nucleus** (also termed **Deiters' nucleus**). The **medial vestibulospinal tract,** a bilateral tract that descends only as far as the cervical segments, originates primarily from neurons in the **medial vestibular nucleus,** with a lesser contribution from the **superior** and **inferior vestibular nuclei.** The lateral vestibulospinal tract is important in maintaining balance, which involves neck, back, hip, and leg muscles. The medial vestibulospinal tract is important in neck muscle control. Both the lateral (despite its name) and medial vestibulospinal tracts are part of the medial descending motor pathways. Their axons descend medially in the spinal white matter and terminate medially in the spinal gray matter to control axial and proximal muscles (Figure 12–9).

Vestibuloocular Reflexes Are Organized by Neurons in the Vestibular and Prepositus Nuclei

The **vestibular nuclei** participate in the reflex stabilization of eye movements, the **vestibuloocular reflex.** As discussed earlier, in this reflex, movements of the eyes compensate for head movements (Figure 12–7). Vestibular axons projecting to the extraocular motor nuclei travel in the MLF (Figures 12–8B and 12–10). Neurons in the vestibular nuclei have complex connections to multiple extraocular nuclei to coordinate particular muscle actions, such as the medial rectus

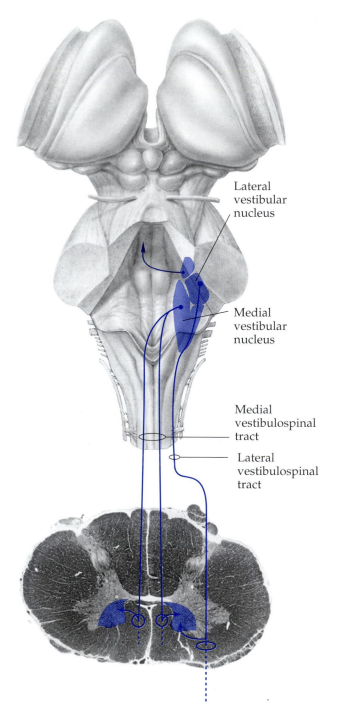

Lateral
vestibular
nucleus

Medial
vestibular
nucleus

Medial
vestibulospinal
tract

Lateral
vestibulospinal
tract

Figure 12–9. Paths of the vestibulospinal tracts are shown on the ventral view of the brain stem. The paths intersect the medial and ventromedial portions of the spinal white matter. Note how both pathways project into the medial motor nuclei.

muscle on one side and the lateral rectus on the other (Figure 12–7B).

The **prepositus nucleus** is located close to the midline in the rostral medulla, just beneath the ventricular floor (Figure 12–8B). Because of its location this nucleus

Figure 12–10. Myelin-stained sagittal sections through the medial longitudinal fasciculus (*A*) and abducens nucleus (*B*).

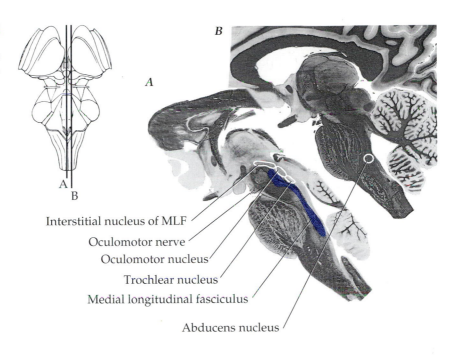

Interstitial nucleus of MLF

Oculomotor nerve

Oculomotor nucleus

Trochlear nucleus

Medial longitudinal fasciculus

Abducens nucleus

can be mistaken for the hypoglossal nucleus. The prepositus nuclei play a key role in maintaining static eye position.

The Extraocular Motor Nuclei Are Located in the Pons and Midbrain

The oculomotor and trochlear nuclei are located close to the midline, and the abducens nucleus is a bit farther from the midline laterally (Figure 12–10). The rostrocaudal course of the MLF also can be followed on the parasagittal section close to the midline (Figure 12–10A).

The **abducens nucleus** (Figures 12–8A and 12–10B) contains the motor neurons that innervate the **lateral rectus muscle.** The nucleus is located just beneath the floor of the fourth ventricle and is partially encircled by facial motor axons on their way to the periphery (Figure 12–8A). The abducens nerve fibers course toward the ventral brain stem surface and exit the pons at the pontomedullary junction, medial to the facial nerve (Figure 12–8, inset). Lesion of the abducens nerve paralyzes the ipsilateral lateral rectus muscle and results in the inability to abduct that eye (see next section).

Trochlear motor neurons, found in the **trochlear nucleus** (Figures 12–10A and 12–11A), innervate the **superior oblique muscle** contralateral to its origin. The nucleus is located in the caudal midbrain at the level of the inferior colliculus, nested within the MLF. Trochlear motor axons course caudally along the lateral margin of the cerebral aqueduct and fourth ven-

tricle, in the **periaqueductal gray matter.** The axons decussate in the rostral pons (Figure 12–11B), dorsal to the cerebral aqueduct, and emerge from the dorsal brain stem surface. This pontine level is also termed the isthmus because it is narrower than adjacent caudal and rostral levels. Lesion of the trochlear nerve paralyzes the superior oblique muscle, resulting in slight outward rotation of the eye (or extortion) because of the unopposed action of the inferior oblique muscle. The eye elevates slightly because of the unopposed action of the superior rectus muscle. A patient with this lesion compensates by tilting his or her head away from the side of the paralyzed muscle.

The oculomotor nucleus innervates the medial, inferior, and superior rectus muscles; the inferior oblique muscle; and the levator palpebrae superioris muscle. The motor axons run in the oculomotor nerve, coursing through the red nucleus and basis pedunculi en route to exiting into the interpeduncular fossa (Figure 12–12B). Oculomotor nerve damage produces a "down and out" resting eye position ipsilaterally, resulting from the unopposed actions of the lateral rectus muscle (producing the outward position) and the superior oblique muscle (producing the downward position).

The levator palpebrae superioris muscle is an eyelid elevator. It is assisted by the **tarsal muscle,** a smooth muscle under sympathetic nervous system control. Conditions that impair the functions of the sympathetic nervous system (see Chapter 15) can produce a mild drooping of the eyelid (pseudoptosis) resulting from weakness of the tarsal muscle. True ptosis is produced by weakness of the levator palpebrae muscle,

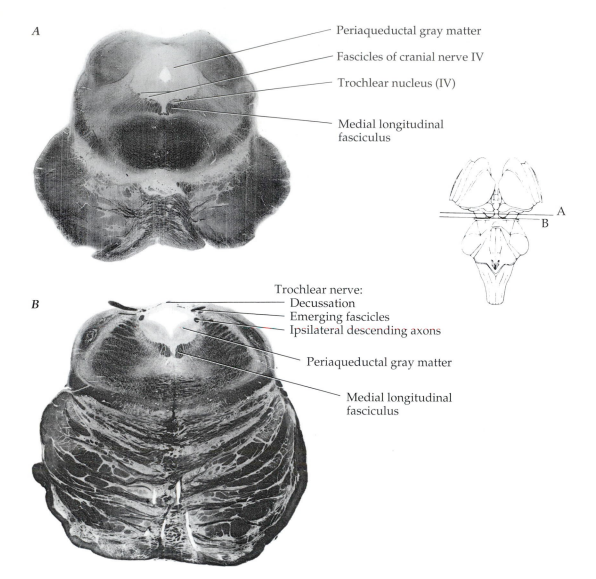

A

Periaqueductal gray matter

Fascicles of cranial nerve IV

Trochlear nucleus (IV)

Medial longitudinal
fasciculus

A
B

B

Trochlear nerve:
Decussation
Emerging fascicles
Ipsilateral descending axons

Periaqueductal gray matter

Medial longitudinal
fasciculus

Figure 12–11. *A.* Myelin-stained section through the caudal midbrain, at the level of the trochlear nucleus. *B.* Myelin-stained section through the rostral pons, at the level of exiting trochlear nerve fibers.

the principal eyelid elevator. This effect can result from third nerve lesions or neuromuscular diseases, such as myasthenia gravis, an autoimmune disease that attacks the neuromuscular junction.

The superior colliculus is an essential brain stem structure for controlling saccadic eye movements (Figures 12–10 and 12–12B). Receiving inputs directly from cortical eye movement control centers in the parietal and frontal lobes, neurons in the deep layers of the superior colliculus project to the paramedian pontine reticular formation in the pons (for controlling horizontal saccades) and to the interstitial nucleus of the MLF in the midbrain (for vertical saccades).

Knowledge of regional midbrain anatomy is clinically important because the ventral midbrain produces

a complex set of neurological deficits that disrupt eye movement control, facial muscle function, and limb movements. Branches of the **posterior cerebral artery** supply the ventral midbrain, and when these branches become occluded the oculomotor nucleus, the third nerve, and the **basis pedunculi** are affected. In addition to producing the "down and out" eye position because of third nerve involvement, this damage results in limb and lower facial muscle weakness on the contralateral side because of involvement of the corticospinal and corticobulbar tracts in the basis pedunculi. Limb tremor can also occur due to damage of the red nucleus and nearby axons. The third nerve also contains the axons of the **Edinger-Westphal nucleus** (Figure 12–12; see Figure 11–8), which con-

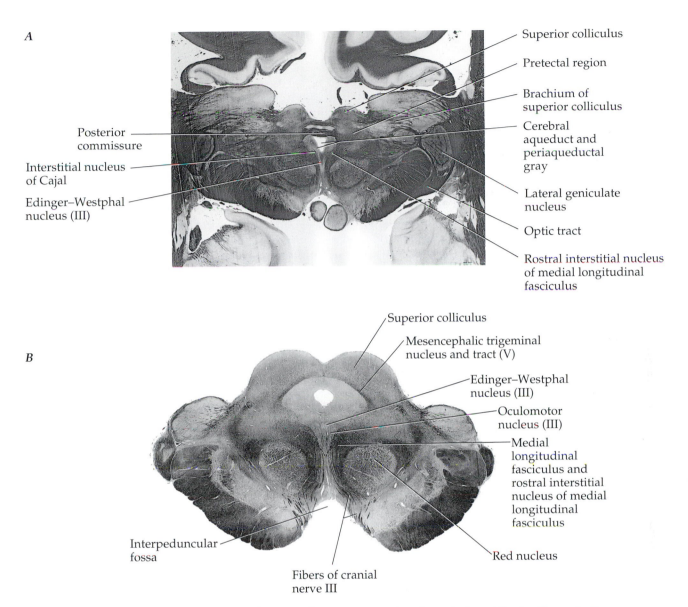

A

Posterior commissure

Interstitial nucleus of Cajal

Edinger–Westphal nucleus (III)

Superior colliculus

Pretectal region

Brachium of superior colliculus

Cerebral aqueduct and periaqueductal gray

Lateral geniculate nucleus

Optic tract

Rostral interstitial nucleus of medial longitudinal fasciculus

B

Superior colliculus

Mesencephalic trigeminal nucleus and tract (V)

Edinger–Westphal nucleus (III)

Oculomotor nucleus (III)

Medial longitudinal fasciculus and rostral interstitial nucleus of medial longitudinal fasciculus

Red nucleus

Interpeduncular fossa

Fibers of cranial nerve III

Figure 12–12. *A.* Myelin-stained transverse section through the midbrain-diencephalic juncture. *B.* Myelin-stained transverse sections through the rostral midbrain, at the level of the superior colliculus.

strict the pupil. Damage to these axons results in pupillary dilation because of the unopposed action of the sympathetic pupillary dilator fibers.

Rostral Midbrain Neurons Organize Vertical Saccades

The rostral midbrain, close to the junction with the diencephalon, contains the interstitial nucleus of the MLF (Figures 12–10A and 12–12A). This nucleus organizes vertical eye movements through its connections with the oculomotor and trochlear nuclei. The **pretec-**

tal nuclei are also located at this level (Figure 12–12A). This nucleus receives visual information from axons coursing in the brachium of superior colliculus and transmits this information bilaterally to neurons in the Edinger-Westphal nucleus. The decussating axons of pretectal neurons course in the **posterior commissure.** The **interstitial nucleus of Cajal,** which is thought to help coordinate eye and head movements, is located at this level. This nucleus projects axons to the spinal cord, for axial muscle control, and to the contralateral interstitial nucleus of Cajal (via the posterior commissure), for coordinating eye and axial muscle control bilaterally.

Eye Movement Control Involves the Integrated Functions of Many Brain Stem Structures

As discussed earlier, horizontal eye movements are controlled by signals from the frontal eye fields and superior colliculus to the paramedian pontine reticular formation (Figure 12–5B). These signals coordinate the actions of the lateral and medial rectus muscles. Lesions at different sites in the circuit for controlling horizontal eye movements produce distinct defects (Figure 12–13). A lesion of the abducens nerve produces paralysis of the ipsilateral **lateral rectus muscle,** thereby preventing ocular abduction on the same side (Figure 12–13, lesion 1). The unopposed action of the medial rectus muscle can sometimes cause the affected eye to be adducted at rest (not shown in figure).

Deficits after an abducens nerve lesion differ from those after a lesion of the abducens nucleus (Figure 12–13, lesion 2). As with the nerve lesion, the ipsilateral eye cannot be abducted because of destruction of the lateral rectus motor neurons. Here, too, the resting position of the eye may be adducted because of the unopposed action of the medial rectus muscle. The nuclear lesion has a second effect: The patient cannot contract the **contralateral medial rectus muscle** on horizontal gaze and hence cannot gaze in the same direction as the side of the lesion. This is called a **lateral gaze palsy,** and it occurs because the lesion also destroys the **internuclear neurons** that coordinate the lateral and medial rectus muscles (Figure 12–5B).

A more rostral lesion of the MLF, which spares the lateral rectus motor neurons but damages the axons of

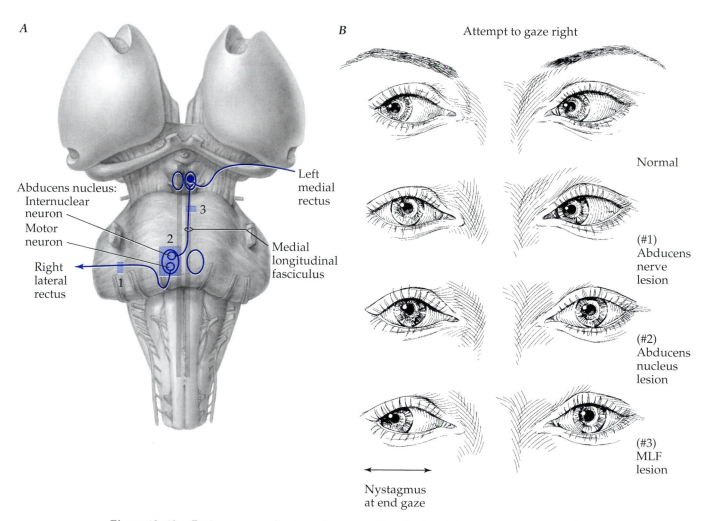

Figure 12–13. Brain stem mechanisms for controlling horizontal eye movements. *A.* Circuit for coordinating eye movements. The blue blocks indicate sites of lesion, producing the movement deficits shown in *B. B.* The four pairs of eyes illustrate eye position when an individual is asked to look to the right: (*from top to bottom row*) normal control of eyes, with a lesion on the right abducens nerve (lesion 1), with a lesion of the right abducens nucleus (lesion 2), and with a left medial longitudinal fasciculus lesion (lesion 3).

the internuclear neurons, produces **internuclear ophthalmoplegia** (Figure 12–13, lesion 3; at level of the pons in Figure 12–11B). This lesion is characterized, on lateral gaze away from the side of the MLF lesion, by the lack of (or reduced) ability to contract the ipsilateral medial rectus muscle and thereby adduct that eye. In addition, **nystagmus** (rhythmic oscillation of the eyes) occurs (more pronounced in the abducting

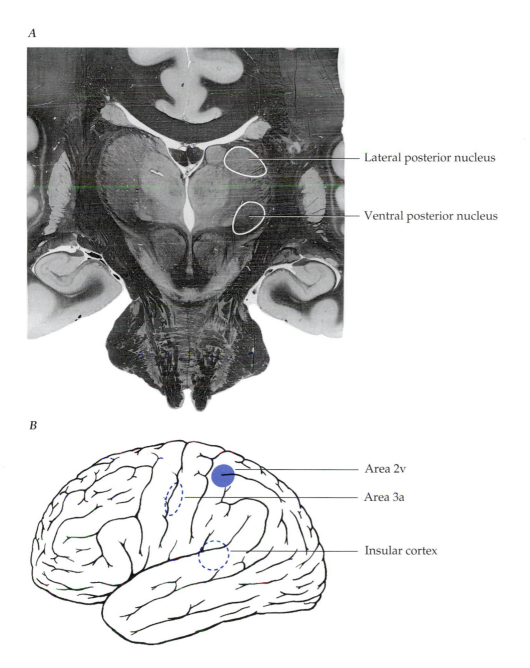

A

Lateral posterior nucleus

Ventral posterior nucleus

B

Area 2v

Area 3a

Insular cortex

Figure 12–14. Vestibular thalamus and cortex. *A.* Myelin-stained transverse section, showing the lateral posterior and ventral posterior nuclei, where ascending vestibular pathways terminate. *B.* A key vestibular cortical area is located in the caudal part of the insular cortex. The inset shows vestibular areas on the lateral surface of the cortex.

eye) as a result of involvement of the axons of vestibular neurons, which also course in the MLF. Internuclear ophthalmoplegia is a common neurological sign in patients with multiple sclerosis, a demyelinating disease. It is due to damage of the internuclear neuron axons in the MLF.

For lesions at sites 2 and 3 (Figure 12–13), a clever way to verify that the affected medial rectus muscle is not paralyzed is to demonstrate that the patient can converge both eyes to view an object at close distance. This eye movement requires activation of both medial rectus muscles. The neural mechanisms that coordinate convergence involve the **visual cortex** and **midbrain** integrative centers, not the internuclear cells of the abducens nucleus.

The Ventral Posterior Nucleus of the Thalamus Transmits Vestibular Information to the Parietal and Insular Cortical Areas

The vestibular nuclei project bilaterally to the **thalamus.** This ascending projection originates from the medial, lateral, and superior vestibular nuclei and travels within the brain stem tegmentum but not in the MLF.

The principal thalamic target of the ascending vestibular projection is the **ventral posterior nucleus** (Figures 12–2A,B; and 12–14). Although this nucleus is familiar as a somatic sensory relay, it serves other functions. The rostral region of the nucleus, adjacent to the ventral lateral nucleus (for motor control; see Chapter 10), receives vestibular input and projects to area 3a of the somatic sensory cortex. This cortical area integrates information from muscle and joint receptors with vestibular information. More dorsal and posterior parts of the ventral posterior nucleus and adjoining nuclei also receive vestibular information but project to the posterior parietal lobe and the insular cortex (Figure 12–14). These vestibular cortical areas—as well as several other regions in the frontal and temporal lobes—are interconnected to form a network. This network integrates information about head motion with information from somatic sensory receptors in the muscles and joints for the perception of the body's orientation in space; this information is used to control posture. Neural activity in the vestibular cortical network is also thought to be important both in the normal perception of body acceleration and when vestibular function becomes disturbed and vertigo is experienced.

The vestibular cortical areas have descending projections to the vestibular nuclei. The organization of this system is similar to the indirect pathways from the frontal motor areas, such as the cortico-reticulo-spinal pathway (see Figure 10–1). The corticovestibular areas, through their projections to the vestibular nuclei, can participate in the control of posture and balance.

Multiple Areas of the Cerebral Cortex Function in Eye Movement Control

Eye movements are not controlled by the primary motor cortex but rather by multiple regions in the frontal and parietal lobes. The **frontal eye fields,** corresponding to a portion of area 8, are the principal frontal lobe regions. Distinct populations of neurons in this area participate in the control of both saccadic and smooth pursuit movements. The neurons involved in saccadic control project to the superior colliculus, the paramedian pontine reticular formation, and the interstitial nucleus of the MLF, as described earlier. Neurons involved in smooth pursuit project to the pontine nuclei which project to the cerebellum (Figure 12–8).

Two other frontal lobe areas contain neurons important for saccadic eye movements, the supplementary eye fields and the dorsolateral prefrontal cortex. The frontal lobe eye movement control centers work together with neurons in the caudate nucleus, a component of the basal ganglia (see Chapter 14). The parietal lobe site important for saccadic eye movements is located in area 7. This region receives visual information from the "where" pathway (see Figure 7–16). Two nearby areas, the middle temporal and middle superior temporal, which are also part of the where pathway, transmit visual information for guiding pursuit movements.

Summary

Vestibular System

Peripheral Vestibular Sensory Organs

There are five vestibular sensory organs: the three **semicircular canals,** the **utricle,** and the **saccule** (Figure 12–1). Receptor cells, located in specialized regions of the vestibular apparatus, are innervated by the distal processes of bipolar neurons located in the **vestibular ganglion.** The central processes of these bipolar neurons form the **vestibular division** of cranial nerve VIII (Figure 12–1). These fibers terminate in the vestibular nuclei, located beneath the floor of the fourth ventricle in the rostral medulla and caudal pons (Figure 12–2A).

Vestibular Nuclei and Their Projections

Four separate vestibular nuclei are located in the medulla and pons: the **inferior vestibular nucleus,** the **medial vestibular nucleus,** the **lateral vestibular nucleus,** and the **superior vestibular nucleus** (Figures 12–2A and 12–8). Neurons within the superior, lateral, and medial vestibular nuclei give rise to an ascending pathway to several sites within and around the **ventral posterior nucleus** of the thalamus (Figures 12–2A, B; and 12–14). Three major sites within the parietal lobe and insular cortex receive this information (Figures 12–2 and 12–14): (1) **area 3a,** which is thought to participate in head position and neck motor control, and (2) the **posterior parietal lobe** and (3) the **insular cortex,** which play roles in the sensing of body orientation and the orientation of the visual world.

There are two vestibulospinal tracts. The **lateral vestibulospinal tract,** which descends to all spinal levels, originates from neurons within the **lateral vestibular nucleus** (Figure 12–9). This pathway is important for balance and posture. The **medial vestibulospinal tract,** which originates primarily from neurons within the **medial vestibular nucleus** (Figure 12–9), descends only to the cervical spinal cord. This pathway is important in controlling head position for gaze. Vestibulospinal tract neurons terminate on motor neurons that innervate **proximal limb** and **axial muscles** as well as on interneurons that synapse on these motor neurons.

Oculomotor System

Extraocular Muscles

Each eye is controlled by six muscles, which operate as three functional pairs, with antagonistic actions (Figure 12–3). The **lateral** and **medial rectus muscles** move the eye horizontally, abducting (looking away from the nose) and adducting (looking toward the nose), respectively. The **superior** and **inferior rectus muscles** elevate and depress the eyes, respectively, but particularly when the eye is abducted. Finally, the **superior** and **inferior oblique muscles** depress and elevate the eye, especially when the eye is adducted.

Extraocular Motor Nuclei

The **oculomotor nucleus** innervates the **medial, inferior,** and **superior rectus muscles;** the **inferior oblique muscle;** and the **levator palpebrae superioris muscle.** The motor axons course in the oculomotor nerve (Figures 12–4, 12–10A, and 12–12B). Motor neurons in the **trochlear nucleus** give rise to the fibers in the **trochlear (IV) nerve,** which innervate the **superior oblique muscle** (see Figures 12–3, 12–10, and 12–11). This is the only cranial nerve that contains decussated axons and exits from the dorsal brain stem surface.

The **abducens nucleus** contains the motor neurons that project their axons to the periphery through the **abducens (VI) nerve** and innervate the **lateral rectus muscle** (Figures 12–3 and 12–8).

Brain Stem Centers for Eye Movement Control and Extraocular Cortical Areas

Saccadic eye movements are controlled by neurons in the **frontal eye fields** (Figure 12–5A) that project to the **superior colliculus** (Figures 12–5B and 12–10) and to the pontine and midbrain reticular formation (Figure 12–5A). The cortical axons descend in the **anterior limb of the internal capsule.** Neurons in the **paramedian pontine reticular formation** (Figure 12–8) coordinate horizontal saccades through their projections to lateral rectus motor neurons and **internuclear neurons** in the abducens nucleus (Figure 12–8), which project to medial rectus motor neurons in the oculomotor nucleus (Figures 12–10 and 12–12B). Neurons in the **interstitial nucleus of the MLF** (Figures 12–10 and 12–12A) control vertical saccades. **Smooth pursuit eye movements** are also controlled by neurons in the frontal eye fields but through connections with the **pontine nuclei, cerebellum,** and **vestibular nuclei** (Figures 12–6 and 12–8).

Related Sources

Brust JCM: The Practice of Neural Science. McGraw-Hill; 2000. (See ch. 3, pp. 19, 32; ch. 10, cases 12, 14; ch. 12, case 19; ch. 14, cases 52, 55; ch. 15, case 58.)

Goldberg M: The control of gaze. In Kandel ER, Schwartz JH, Jessell TM (editors): Principles of Neural Science, 4th ed. McGraw-Hill; 2000:782–800.

Goldberg M, Hudspeth AJ: The vestibular system. In Kandel ER, Schwartz JH, Jessell TM (editors): Principles of Neural Science, 4th ed. McGraw-Hill; 2000:801–815.

Melvill Jones G: Posture. In Kandel ER, Schwartz JH, Jessell TM (editors): Principles of Neural Science, 4th ed. McGraw-Hill; 2000:816–831.

Selected Readings

Büttner U, Büttner-Ennever JA: Present concepts of oculomotor organization. In Büttner-Ennever JA (editor): Neuroanatomy of the Oculomotor System. Elsevier Science Publishers; 1988:3–164.

Büttner-Ennever JA: A review of otolith pathways to brainstem and cerebellum. Ann N Y Acad Sci 1999;871:51–64.

Fukushima K: Corticovestibular interactions: Anatomy, electrophysiology, and functional considerations. Exp Brain Res 1997;117:1–16.

Guldin WO, Grusser OJ: Is there a vestibular cortex? Trends Neurosci 1998;21:254–259.

Patten J: Neurological Differential Diagnosis, 2nd Ed. Springer-Verlag; 1996:446.

Pierrot-Deseilligny C, Gaymard B: Eye movements. In Kennard C (editor): Clinical Neurology. Churchill Livingstone; 1992:27–56.

References

Akbarian S, Grusser OJ, Guldin WO: Thalamic connections of the vestibular cortical fields in the squirrel monkey (Saimiri sciureus). J Comp Neurol 1992;326:423–441.

Büttner-Ennever JA, Henn V: An autoradiographic study of the pathways from the pontine reticular formation involved in horizontal eye movements. Brain Res 1976;108:155–164.

Karnath HO, Ferber S, Dichgans J: The neural representation of postural control in humans. Proc Natl Acad Sci USA 2000;97:13931–13936.

Kokkoroyannis T, Scudder CA, Balaban CD, Highstein SM, Moschovakis AK: Anatomy and physiology of the primate interstitial nucleus of Cajal I. Efferent projections. J Neurophysiol 1996;75:725–739.

Lang W, Büttner-Ennever JA, Büttner U: Vestibular projections to the monkey thalamus: An autoradiographic study. Brain Res 1979;177:3–17.

Lobel E, Kleine JF, Bihan DL, Leroy-Willig A, Berthoz A: Functional MRI of galvanic vestibular stimulation. J Neurophysiol 1998;80:2699–2709.

Shiroyama T, Kayahara T, Yasui Y, Nomura J, Nakano K: Projections of the vestibular nuclei to the thalamus in the rat: A Phaseolus vulgaris leucoagglutinin study. J Comp Neurol 1999;407:318–332.

Simpson JI: The accessory optic system. Annu Rev Neurosci 1984;7:13–41.

13

The Cerebellum

T**HE CEREBELLUM PLAYS A KEY ROLE** in movement by regulating the functions of the motor pathways. When this major brain structure is damaged, movements that were smooth and steered accurately become uncoordinated and erratic. Important insights into the general role of the cerebellum in motor control can be gained by considering its connections with other brain regions. The cerebellum receives information from virtually all other components of the limb and extraocular motor systems, from the spinal cord and brain stem, and from most of the sensory systems. The cerebellum is poised to compare information about the intention of an upcoming movement, by receiving information from the motor pathways, with what actually occurs, by receiving information from sensory systems. Research has shown that the cerebellum may compute control signals to correct for differences between intent and action. The cerebellum, in turn, provides the major input to the brain stem and cortical pathways for limb, trunk, and eye movement control.

The cerebellum also receives information from areas of the central nervous system that do not play a direct role in movement control, such as the parietal association cortex and the limbic association cortex. How is this finding reconciled with an important role in movement control? The association cortex and other nonmotor areas help in the planning of movements—for example, by allowing an individual's motivation state to influence when and where he or she moves. However, the cerebellum serves nonmotor functions, too. Indeed, cerebellar damage can also produce impairments in language, decision making, and affect that cannot be attributed to motor defects.

GROSS ANATOMY OF THE CEREBELLUM

Because the three-dimensional organization of the cerebellum is so complex (Figure 13–1), rivaling that of the cerebral cortex, its gross anatomy is considered before its functional organization. Located dorsal to the pons and medulla (Figure 13–2A), the cerebellum is separated from the overlying cerebral cortex by a tough flap in the dura, the **cerebellar tentorium** (see Figure 4–15). The inferior surface of the cerebellum

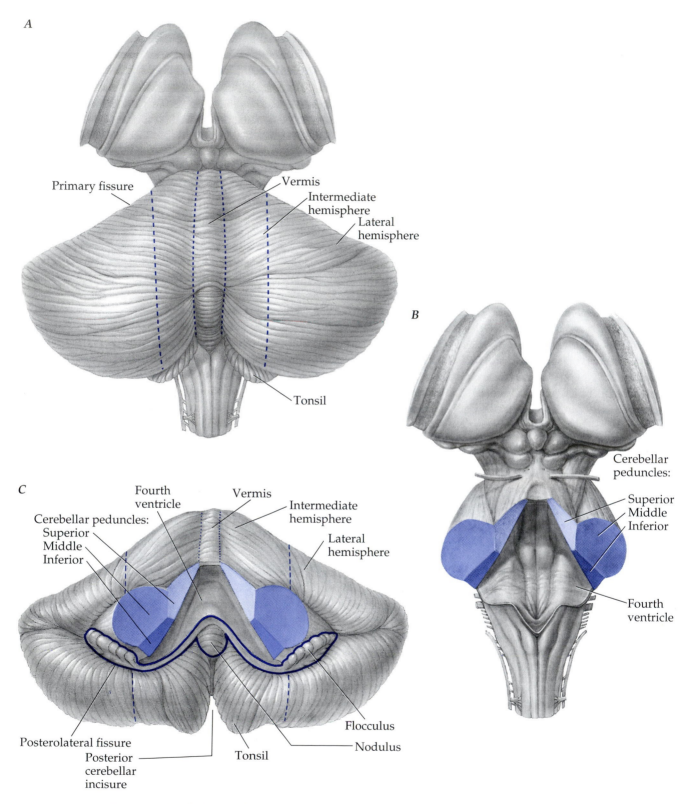

A

Primary fissure

Vermis

Intermediate hemisphere

Lateral hemisphere

Tonsil

B

Cerebellar peduncles:

Superior
Middle
Inferior

Fourth ventricle

C

Fourth ventricle

Vermis

Intermediate hemisphere

Lateral hemisphere

Cerebellar peduncles:
Superior
Middle
Inferior

Posterolateral fissure

Posterior cerebellar incisure

Tonsil

Flocculus

Nodulus

Figure 13–1. *A.* Dorsal view of the brain stem and cerebellum. The border between the vermis and intermediate and lateral parts of the cerebellar hemisphere are shown. These three parts of the cerebellar cortex also correspond to functional subdivisions. *B.* The three cerebellar peduncles are revealed when the cerebellum is removed. *C.* The cerebellum, viewed from the ventral surface.

Figure 13–2. *A.* Midsagittal cut through the brain, revealing the cerebellar vermis. The inset shows the 10 cerebellar lobules. Lobules I through V comprise the anterior lobe, VI through IX comprise the posterior lobe, and X comprises the flocculonodular lobe. *B.* Schematic transverse section through the pons and cerebellum, illustrating the location of the deep cerebellar nuclei. The plane of *B* is shown as the dashed line in *A.*

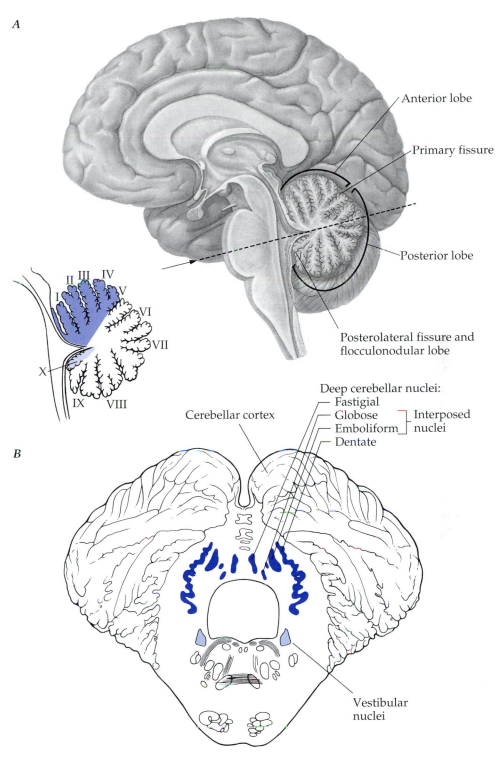

is incompletely divided by the **posterior cerebellar incisure.**

The cerebellum comprises an outer cortex containing neuronal cell bodies overlying a region that contains predominantly myelinated axons. The cerebellar cortex contains an extraordinary number of neurons, rivaling that of the rest of the brain, and a rich array of neuron types (see below). Two prominent neurons are the projection neurons of the cerebellum, the **Purkinje cells,** and a class of cerebellar interneurons, **granule cells.** Most cerebellar neurons belong to this interneuron class.

Two shallow grooves running from rostral to caudal divide the cerebellar cortex into the **vermis,** located along the midline, and **two hemispheres** (Figure 13–1A, C). This anatomical distinction marks the specific functional divisions of the cerebellar cortex (see below). Like the cerebral cortex, the cerebellar cortex is highly convoluted. These characteristic folds, termed **folia,** are equivalent to the gyri of the cerebral cortex. They vastly increase the amount of cerebellar cortex that can be packed into the posterior cranial fossa.

The cerebellar cortex is organized into groups of folia, termed **lobules,** that are separated from one another by fissures. In a section through the vermis, the lobules appear to radiate from the apex of the roof of the fourth ventricle (Figure 13–2A, inset). Anatomists recognize ten lobules, whose nomenclature is used largely by specialists studying the cerebellum. Two fissures are particularly deep and divide the various lobules into **three lobes** (Figures 13–1 and 13–2A). The **primary fissure** separates the **anterior lobe** from the **posterior lobe.** The anterior lobe is important in the control of limb and trunk movements, whereas the posterior lobe may be somewhat more important in movement planning and in the nonmotor functions of the cerebellum. The **flocculo-nodular lobe** is separated from the posterior lobe by the **posterolateral fissure.** This lobe consists of the **nodulus,** located on the midline (ie, the vermis), and the two **flocculi,** on either side. The flocculonodular lobe plays a key role in maintaining balance and controlling eye movement.

Beneath the cerebellar cortex is the **white matter,** which contains axons coursing to and from the cortex (Figure 13–2). The branching pattern of the white matter of the cerebellum inspired early anatomists to refer to it as the **arbor vitae** (Latin for "tree of life"); hence, the name *folia* (Latin for "leaves") rather than *gyri* is used to describe the convolutions. Embedded within the white matter of the cerebellum are four bilaterally paired nuclei: the **fastigial nucleus,** the **globose nucleus,** the **emboliform nucleus,** and the **dentate nucleus.** These nuclei, also called **deep cerebellar nuclei,** are shown in the schematic transverse section through the pons and cerebellum (Figure 13–2B). The globose and emboliform nuclei are collectively termed the **interposed nuclei.** The deep cerebellar nuclei are key elements in the neural circuit of the cerebellum (see below).

Axons projecting to and from the cerebellum course through the **peduncles** (Figure 13–1B, C): The **superior cerebellar peduncle** contains mostly efferent axons, the **middle cerebellar peduncle** contains only afferent axons, and the **inferior cerebellar peduncle** contains both afferent and efferent axons. An alternate

nomenclature is often used for the cerebellar peduncles in the clinical and scientific literature. The superior cerebellar peduncle is also called the brachium conjunctivum; the middle cerebellar peduncle, the brachium pontis; and the inferior cerebellar peduncle, the restiform body. The various peduncles are distinguished in Figure 13–1B,C because each one has been given a different cut surface in the drawing. Three distinct peduncles would not be apparent had a single cut been drawn.

■ FUNCTIONAL ANATOMY OF THE CEREBELLUM

All Three Functional Divisions of the Cerebellum Display a Similar Input-Output Organization

The cerebellum has three functional divisions, named for their major sources of information. Each division consists of a portion of the cerebellar cortex and one or more nuclei (Figures 13–1 and 13–3):

- The **spinocerebellum,** which receives highly organized somatic sensory inputs from the spinal cord, is important in controlling the posture and movements of the trunk and limbs. This division, however, also receives information from structures other than the spinal cord. The spinocerebellum comprises the **vermis;** the adjoining **intermediate hemisphere,** of both the anterior and posterior lobes; and the **fastigial** and **interposed nuclei.**
- The **cerebrocerebellum,** which receives input indirectly from the cerebral cortex, participates in the planning of movement. This division consists of the **lateral hemisphere,** in both the anterior and posterior lobes, and the dentate nucleus.
- The **vestibulocerebellum,** which receives input from the **vestibular labyrinth,** helps in maintaining balance and controlling head and eye movements. This cerebellar division corresponds to the **flocculonodular lobe.** There is no deep cerebellar nucleus for the vestibulocerebellum. Instead, the vestibular nuclei serve a similar role (see below).

Animal studies and clinical findings suggest that the cerebrocerebellum and vermis of the posterior lobe may play a role in the nonmotor functions of the cerebellum.

Each functional division of the cerebellar cortex has a similar generalized pattern of connections. How-

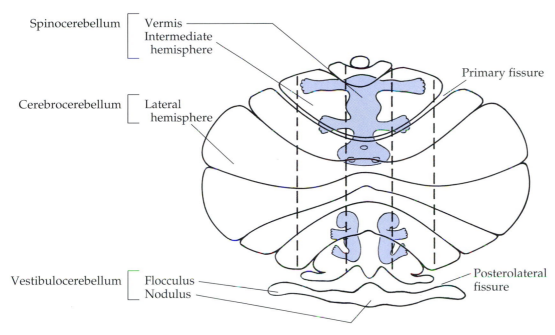

Figure 13–3. The three functional divisions are shown in schematic view of the cerebellum. The topographic organization of somatic sensory inputs to the spinocerebellum is also shown. These inputs are somatotopically organized. Visual, auditory, and vestibular inputs are directed predominantly to the "head" areas.

ever, each division differs from the others with respect to the specific input sources and the specific structures to which it projects. Figure 13–4 shows the basic organizational plan of the cerebellar functional divisions. There are two major sets of inputs to the cerebellum, and with some exceptions, both sets of inputs are directed to neurons in the deep nuclei (or vestibular nuclei) and cortex. The output of the cerebellum originates from the deep nuclei (or vestibular nuclei for the vestibulocerebellum).

The Spinocerebellum Projects to the Lateral and Medial Motor Systems

The **spinocerebellum** is important in the control of body musculature (Figures 13–5A and 13–6). It is somatotopically organized: The vermis and the intermediate hemisphere control axial muscles and limb muscles, respectively (Figure 13–5A). This mediolateral somatotopic arrangement recalls the somatotopic organization of the ventral horn, where medial motor neurons innervate **axial** and **proximal limb muscles,** and those located laterally innervate more **distal muscles** (see Figure 10–2).

The **spinocerebellar tracts** transmit somatic sensory information from the limbs and trunk to the spinocerebellum. Four spinocerebellar tracts can be distin-

guished on the basis of (1) the kind of information they transmit, (2) whether their axons decussate in the spinal cord, and (3) whether they provide information about the upper or lower half of the body (Figure 13–6; Table 13–1). The **dorsal spinocerebellar** and **cuneocerebellar tracts** transmit **somatic sensory information,** primarily from mechanoreceptors (ie, large-diameter primary afferent fibers), such as those that innervate muscle spindles (see Table 5–1). The dorsal spinocerebellar tract originates from **Clarke's nucleus** and transmits sensory information from the leg and lower trunk. By contrast, the cuneocerebellar tract originates from the **accessory cuneate nucleus.** It transmits sensory information from the arm and upper trunk. The spinocerebellar and cuneocerebellar tracts both project to the ipsilateral cerebellum, via the **inferior cerebellar peduncle** (Figure 13–6). Axons in these tracts synapse on neurons in the fastigial and interposed nuclei as well the cerebellar cortex.

The **ventral** and **rostral spinocerebellar tracts**—for the lower and upper halves of the body—are thought to transmit **internal feedback signals** for correcting inaccurate movements rather than somatic sensory information. These pathways, which originate from neurons in ventral regions of the spinal gray matter, receive information from the motor pathways as well as sensory information from the afferent fibers. Their axons decussate in the spinal cord and enter the cerebellum primarily through the superior cerebellar

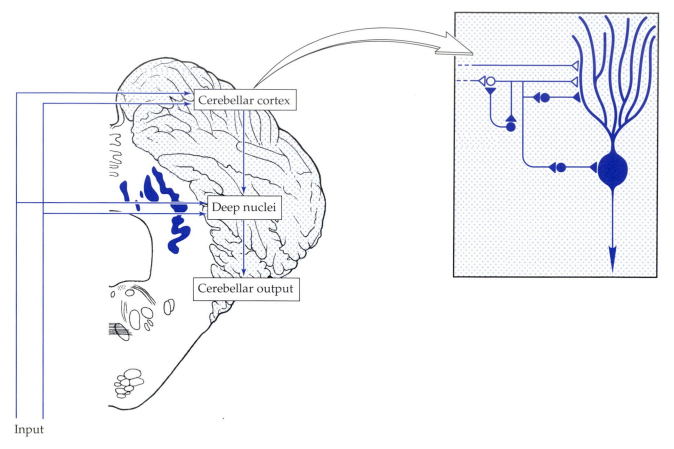

Figure 13–4. Key features of the input-output organization of the cerebellum. The inset shows the complex circuitry of the cerebellum (see Figure 13–11 for explanation).

Input

peduncle. Once in the cerebellum, some axons decussate again and terminate in the ipsilateral cerebellum, resulting in a small "doubly crossed" contingent (see Box 13–1). The **trigeminocerebellar pathways** originate from the **spinal trigeminal nucleus,** principally from parts of the interpolar and oral nuclei (see Figure 6–5). It is not known whether the same organization exists for the trigeminal pathways.

These cerebellar input pathways are important in motor control, whereas ascending pathways to the thalamus and the primary somatic sensory cortex are important in perception. Somatic sensory information is projected to the spinocerebellum in a somatotopic fashion (Figure 13–5A). The vermis receives somatic sensory information primarily from the head, neck, and trunk; the intermediate hemisphere receives signals from the limbs. Within each of these zones, information from a particular part is represented at multiple sites, and conversely, a single site represents different parts of a body region. Termed **fractured somatotopy,** this organization is thought to be important in bringing together information from different parts of the limbs, trunk, or head for coordinating movements. In addition, the vermis receives a direct projection from pri-

mary **vestibular** sensory neurons, as well as **visual** and **auditory** input relayed by brain stem nuclei.

As their names reveal, these are direct pathways from the spinal cord to the cerebellum. In addition, there are indirect routes from the spinal cord to the cerebellum that synapse in the reticular formation or the inferior olivary nuclear complex. Information transmitted by these indirect pathways is subject to more extensive processing and may play more complex roles in movement than information transmitted by the direct pathways.

The two cortical components of the spinocerebellum project to two deep cerebellar nuclei: The **vermis** projects to the **fastigial nucleus,** and the **intermediate hemisphere** projects to the **interposed nuclei** (Figure 13–6). These deep nuclei influence motor neurons primarily through their projections onto the descending pathways. The fastigial nucleus projects most of its axons through the **inferior cerebellar peduncle** to brain stem nuclei that give rise to **medial descending pathways,** the reticulospinal and vestibulospinal tracts (Figure 13–7A). The fastigial nucleus also has a small ascending projection, via a thalamic relay in the ventrolateral nucleus, to the cells of origin of the ventral corticospinal tract in primary and premotor cortical areas.

Figure 13–5. Salient features of the inputs to the three functional divisions of the cerebellum and their outputs. *A.* Spinocerebellum and cerebrocerebellum. *B.* Vestibulocerebellum.

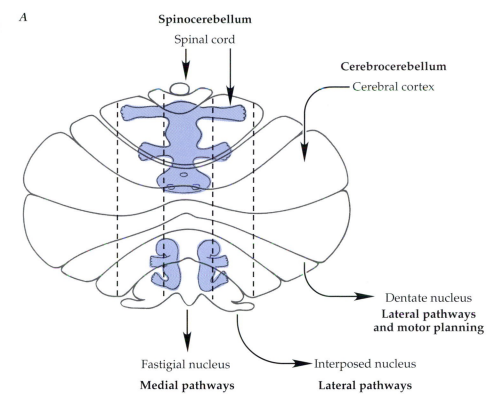

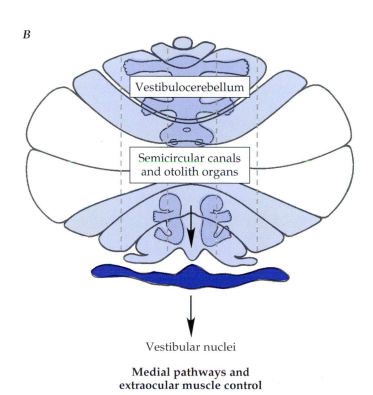

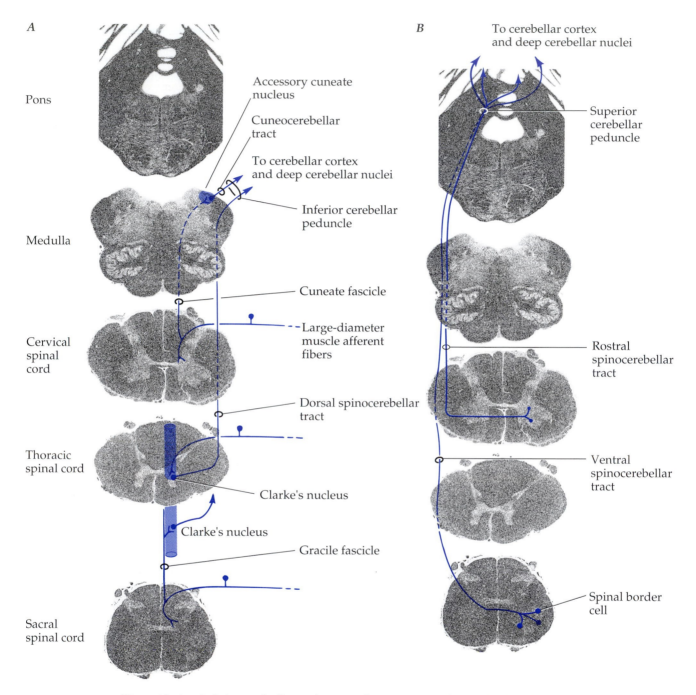

Figure 13–6. **A.** Spinocerebellar pathways relaying sensory feedback (dorsal spinocerebellar and cuneocerebellar tracts). **B.** Spinocerebellar pathways relaying information about the amount of activity in descending pathways (ventral spinocerebellar tract).

This efferent projection exits through the superior cerebellar peduncle. The interposed nuclei project through the **superior cerebellar peduncle** to the magnocellular component of the red nucleus and, via the ventrolateral nucleus of the thalamus, to motor areas of the frontal lobe (Figure 13–7B). These components of the motor systems give rise to the **lateral descending pathways:** the rubrospinal and lateral corticospinal tracts.

The Cerebrocerebellum Projects to Premotor and Association Cortical Areas

The **cerebrocerebellum** (Figures 13–3 and 13–5A) is primarily involved in the planning of movement and is interconnected with diverse regions of the **cerebral cortex.** The afferent and efferent connections of the cerebrocerebellum are illustrated in Figure 13–8. The

Table 13–1. Spinocerebellar pathways.

Pathway	Information	Origin	Body parted	Decussation
Dorsal spinocerebellar	Somatic sensory	Clarke's nucleus	Leg, lower trunk	Uncrossed
Cuneocerebellar	Somatic sensory	Accessory cuneate	Arm, upper trunk	Uncrossed
Ventral spinocerebellar	Internal feedback signals	Ventral horn neurons	Leg, lower trunk	Crossed
Rostral spinocerebellar	Internal feedback signals	Ventral horn neurons	Arm, upper trunk	Crossed

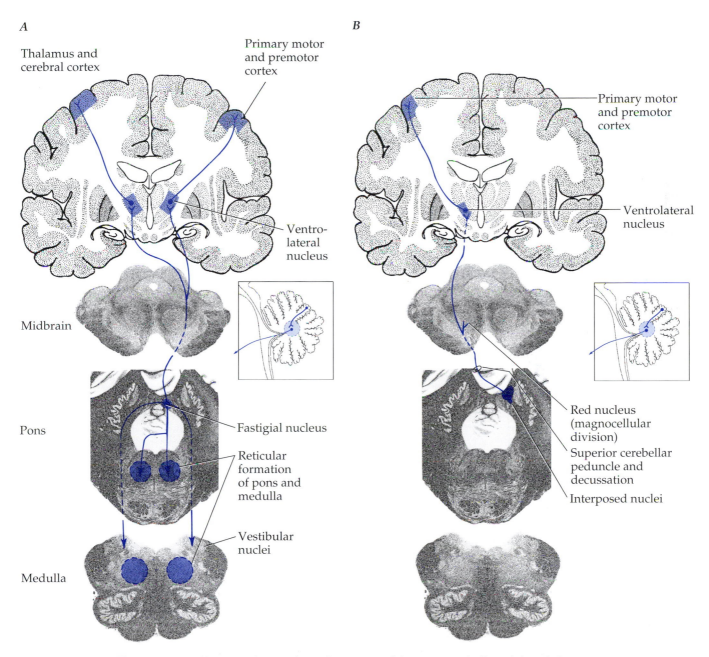

Figure 13–7. Efferent pathways from the vermis of the spinocerebellum (*A*) and the intermediate hemisphere (*B*). Note that the ascending projection of the fastigial nucleus to the thalamus is much smaller than the descending projection to the pons and medulla. Insets show projections from the cerebellar cortex to the fastigial nucleus (*A*) and the interposed nuclei (*B*).

A

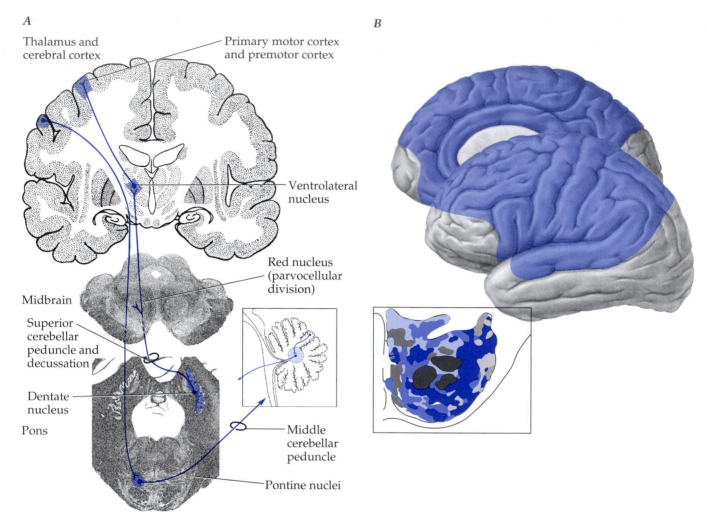

Figure 13–8. *A.* Afferent and efferent connections of the cerebrocerebellum. Note that the major input to the pontine nuclei is from large areas of the cerebral cortex, although input from only a single site is shown. *B.* Most cortical regions project to the cerebellum (blue), via the pontine nuclei (see inset). Different cortical areas project to distinct sets of pontine nuclei (different shades of blue and gray). The black areas correspond to descending cortical axons. The inset shows a semischematic view of the ventral pons of the rhesus monkey. *(Adapted from Schmahmann JD, Pandya DN: The cerebrocerebellar system. Int Rev Neurobiol 1997;41:31–60.)*

major input to the cerebrocerebellum is from the **contralateral cerebral cortex,** not only from the motor areas but also from the sensory and association areas (Figure 13–8B). This projection is relayed by neurons in the **pontine nuclei** (Figure 13–8B, inset). The pontine nuclei, in turn, project to the contralateral cerebellar cortex through the **middle cerebellar peduncle.** The efferent projection from the cortex of the cerebrocerebellum is to the **dentate nucleus,** the largest and most lateral of the deep nuclei. Most neurons in the dentate nucleus project their axons to two main sites. The first site is the ventrolateral nucleus, the motor relay nucleus of the thalamus. The second site is the **red nucleus;** however, it projects to the **parvocellular**

division of the red nucleus, not to the magnocellular division. Whereas the magnocellular portion of the red nucleus gives rise to the rubrospinal tract (see Chapter 10), the parvocellular division projects to the ipsilateral **inferior olivary nucleus,** a major source of input to the cerebellum (see below).

Recent functional imaging and clinical studies in humans suggest that the most ventrolateral and posterior portion of the dentate nucleus participates in nonmotor functions, including cognition, emotions, and language. There may be a distinctive anatomical correlate for the role of the dentate nucleus in higher brain functions. In the monkey, where anatomical tracer studies can be conducted, a portion of the dentate nucleus is analogous to the ventrolateral dentate in the human. This portion in the monkey projects, via parts of the ventrolateral nucleus, to the **prefrontal association cortex.** This region of the frontal lobe is involved in **working memory,** the temporary storing of information that is used to plan and shape upcoming behaviors. A small cluster of dentate neurons also project, via the ventrolateral nucleus, to the posterior parietal association cortex. This area is at the interface of visual perception, attention, and motor action. Thus, the cerebrocerebellum has the connections to mediate several higher brain functions.

The Vestibulocerebellum Projects to Brain Stem Centers for Controlling Eye and Head Movements

The **vestibulocerebellum** is crucial for controlling gaze, through the combined control of eye and head movements (Figures 13–3 and 13–5B). This cerebellar division receives information from **primary vestibular afferents** and secondary vestibular neurons in the

vestibular nuclei. In fact, the vestibular afferents are the only primary sensory neurons that project directly to the cerebellum. The cortical component of the vestibulocerebellum projects to the vestibular nuclei: the medial, inferior, and superior vestibular nuclei (Figure 13–9). These vestibular nuclei play a role in neck muscle control, via the **medial vestibulospinal tract,** as well as eye movement control, via fibers in the **medial longitudinal fasciculus** to extraocular motor nuclei.

■ REGIONAL ANATOMY OF THE CEREBELLUM

The rest of this chapter examines the regional anatomy of the cerebellum and associated nuclei and tracts. The cellular constituents and synaptic connections of the cerebellum are among the best understood of the central nervous system. Sections through key levels are used here to illustrate locations of the cerebellar peduncles, afferent and efferent pathways, and the deep cerebellar nuclei.

Figure 13–9. Afferent and afferent connections of the vestibulocerebellum. The inset shows the structure of the inner ear. The otolith organs provide the major input to the vestibulocerebellum (see Figure 12–1).

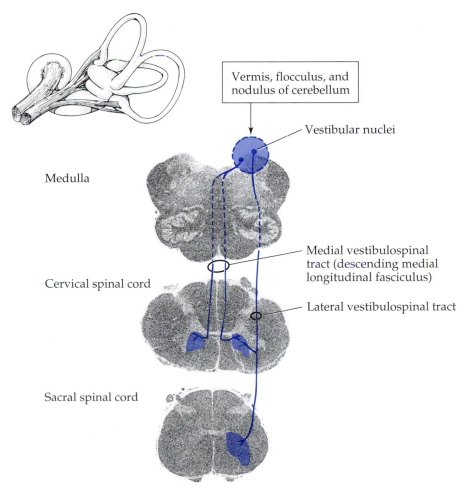

Vermis, flocculus, and nodulus of cerebellum

Vestibular nuclei

Medulla

Cervical spinal cord

Medial vestibulospinal tract (descending medial longitudinal fasciculus)

Lateral vestibulospinal tract

Sacral spinal cord

The Intrinsic Circuitry of the Cerebellar Cortex Is Similar for the Different Functional Divisions

The cerebellar cortex consists of three cell layers, progressing from its external surface inward (Figure 13–10): the **molecular layer,** the **Purkinje layer,** and the **granular layer,** which is adjacent to the white matter. The cerebellar cortex contains five types of neurons, and they each have a different laminar distribution (Table 13–2): (1) Purkinje cell, (2) granule cell, (3) basket cell, (4) stellate cell, and (5) Golgi cell. The cellular organization of the cerebellar cortex is considered in a stepwise fashion in Figure 13–11, beginning with the two major classes of excitatory inputs.

Climbing and Mossy Fibers Are the Two Major Excitatory Inputs to the Cerebellar Cortex

Climbing fibers originate entirely from the **inferior olivary nuclear complex** (see Figure 13–15). The cell bodies of **mossy fibers** are located primarily in the spinal cord (see Figure 13–14) and in three brain stem nuclear groups: pontine nuclei (see Figure 13–16), vestibular nuclei (see Figures 13–15 and 13–16), and nuclei of the reticular formation (see Figure 13–15).

The **Purkinje cell** (Figure 13–12) is the target of the climbing fibers and, via an interneuron, the mossy fibers. The Purkinje cell is the only type of neuron whose axon projects from the cerebellar cortex; it is

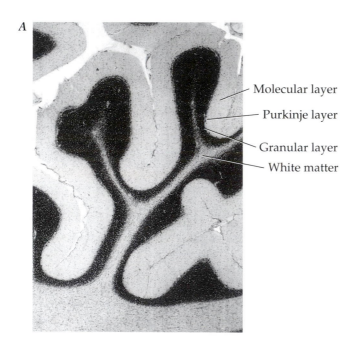

A

— Molecular layer

— Purkinje layer

— Granular layer

— White matter

Figure 13–10. Nissl-stained section through the cerebellar cortex. *A.* Low-power view. *B.* High-power view.

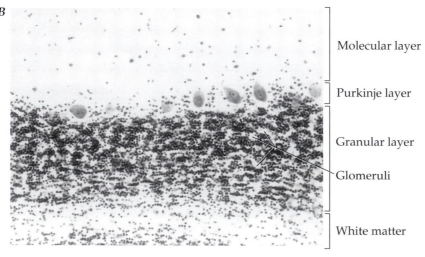

B

Molecular layer

Purkinje layer

Granular layer

Glomeruli

White matter

Table 13–2. Neurons of the cerebellar cortex.

Cell type	Synaptic action	Laminar distribution	Postsynaptic target
Projection Neuron			
Purkinje	Inhibitory	Purkinje	Deep nuclei vestibular nuclei
Interneurons			
Granule	Excitatory	Granular	Purkinje, stellate, basket, and Golgi neurons
Basket	Inhibitory	Molecular	Purkinje neurons
Stellate	Inhibitory	Molecular	Purkinje neurons
Golgi	Inhibitory	Granular	Granule neurons

located in the Purkinje layer. Climbing fibers make multiple synapses with one Purkinje cell, forming one of the strongest excitatory connections in the central nervous system. A remarkable degree of specificity is found in the connections of climbing fibers and Purkinje cells: Each Purkinje cell receives input from a single climbing fiber. Individual climbing fibers make contact with no more than about 10 Purkinje cells.

In contrast to climbing fibers, mossy fibers first synapse on **granule cells**—the only excitatory interneurons in the cerebellum. Located in the granular layer (Figure 13–10), granule cells have an axon that ascends through the Purkinje layer into the molecular layer. Here the axon bifurcates to form the **parallel fibers,** which synapse on Purkinje cells (Figure 13–11A) and other cerebellar interneurons. One parallel fiber will synapse with thousands of Purkinje cells, and each Purkinje cell receives synapses from thousands of parallel fibers. Unlike the climbing fiber, which makes multiple synaptic contacts with the Purkinje cell, the parallel fiber makes only a few synapses with each Purkinje cell.

The paucity of parallel fiber synaptic contacts on the Purkinje cell reflects the orientation of Purkinje cell dendrites to the parallel fibers. Briefly, the Purkinje cell dendritic tree (Figures 13–11 and 13–12) is planar and oriented orthogonal to the long axis of the folium in which it is located (much like coins stacked on top of one another). The parallel fiber courses at a right angle to the dendritic plane of the Purkinje cell (ie, parallel to the long axis of the folium). The fiber makes only a few contacts with a single Purkinje cell as the axon passes through the dendritic tree. As a consequence of the difference in the number of synaptic contacts, the strength of parallel fiber input to a Purkinje cell is much less than that of climbing fiber input. It has been suggested that the efficacy of parallel fiber input onto a given Purkinje cell is increased immediately after Purkinje cell activation by a climbing fiber.

Purkinje Cell Axons Synapse on Neurons of the Deep Cerebellar Nuclei and Vestibular Nuclei

Purkinje cells of the spinocerebellum and cerebrocerebellum project their axons through the cerebellar white matter to synapse on neurons in the deep cerebellar nuclei (Figure 13–11B). To reach the vestibular nuclei, Purkinje axons of the vestibulocerebellum travel through the inferior cerebellar peduncle. The Purkinje cell is an inhibitory projection neuron: When it discharges it hyperpolarizes the neurons in the deep cerebellar nuclei or vestibular nuclei with which it synapses. How then can neurons in the deep cerebellar nuclei and vestibular nuclei fire action potentials when they are inhibited by Purkinje cells? For the deep cerebellar nuclei, recall that the climbing fibers as well as many mossy fibers (from the spinal cord and reticular formation) have a direct excitatory synaptic connection (Figure 13–4). (Anatomical data suggest that most mossy fibers from the pontine nuclei bypass the deep nuclei, synapsing only in the cortex.) It is thought that these direct inputs to the deep nuclear cells increase their excitability and help to maintain their background neuronal activity at a high level. For the vestibular nuclei, direct excitatory inputs from vestibular afferents help to maintain a high background level of activity. Also, intrinsic cell membrane properties, such as high resting inward ionic currents, help to maintain high levels of activity in these neurons. The high levels of neural activity in the deep nuclear and vestibular neurons is then reduced, or "sculpted," by the inhibitory actions of the Purkinje cells.

Cerebellar Cortical Interneurons Inhibit Purkinje and Granule Cells

Purkinje cells are in turn inhibited by two groups of interneurons (Figure 13–11C): **stellate cells,** located

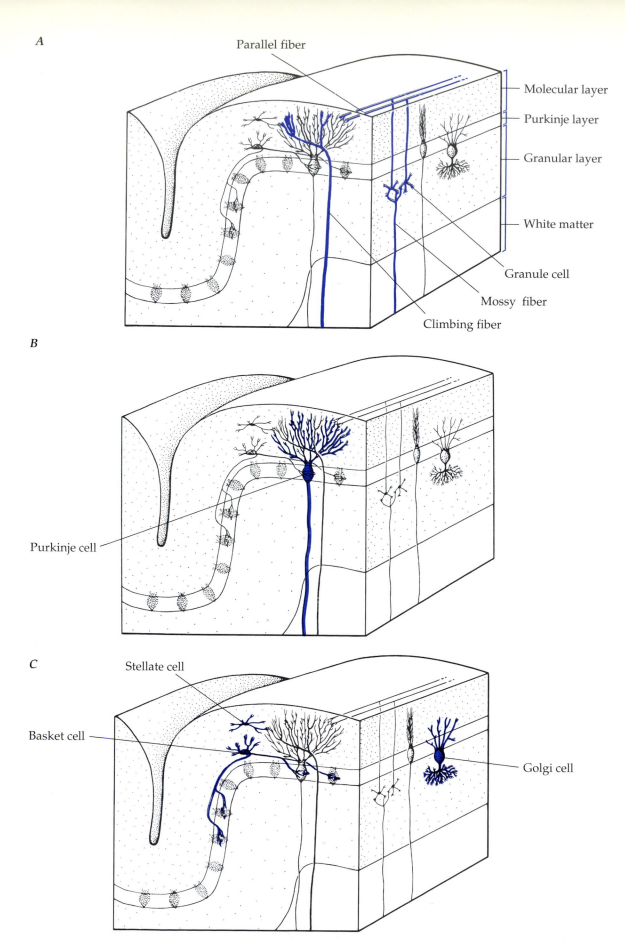

A

Parallel fiber

Molecular layer

Purkinje layer

Granular layer

White matter

Granule cell

Mossy fiber

Climbing fiber

B

Purkinje cell

C

Stellate cell

Basket cell

Golgi cell

Figure 13–11. The circuitry of the cerebellar cortex is illustrated in a stepwise fashion. **A.** There are two major excitatory inputs to the cerebellum: climbing fibers and mossy fibers. Whereas the climbing fibers synapse directly on Purkinje cells, the mossy fibers first synapse on granule cells, which in turn give rise to the parallel fibers, which synapse on Purkinje cells. **B.** Purkinje cells are the output neurons of the cerebellum. **C.** There are three types of inhibitory interneurons: Golgi cells, basket cells, and stellate cells.

initiation zone, at the axon hillock of the Purkinje cell, as well as the high density of synaptic contacts. In contrast, the stellate cell synapse is located on the distal dendrites, far from the axon hillock; hence, the degree of inhibition it produces on Purkinje cells is much less than that of the basket cell. Whereas the inhibitory actions of basket cells can turn off the firing of Purkinje cells, stellate cell inhibition affects only the integration of synaptic actions locally, in the region of its terminals on the distal dendrites of Purkinje cells.

The **Golgi** interneuron inhibits the granule cell (Figure 13–11C). This inhibitory synapse is made in the granular layer, in a complex structure termed the **cerebellar glomerulus** (Figure 13–13). The cerebellar glomerulus consists of two presynaptic elements, the **mossy fiber terminal** and the **Golgi cell axon,** and one main postsynaptic element, the **granule cell dendrite.** The mossy fiber terminal is also termed the mossy fiber rosette because of the configuration of its enlarged terminal. Synaptic glomeruli ensure specificity of connections because this entire synaptic complex is contained within a **glial capsule.** The mossy fiber terminals are located in the clear zones seen under high power in the Nissl-stained section of the cerebellar cortex (Figure 13–10B). An inventory of the synaptic action of the interneurons of the cerebellar cortex demonstrates that all but the granule cell are inhibitory (Table 13–2). Even the projection neuron of the cerebellar cortex, the Purkinje cell, is inhibitory.

The rest of this chapter follows the input and output pathways of the cerebellum by examining sections through the spinal cord, brain stem, thalamus, and cerebral hemispheres.

Spinal Cord and Medullary Sections Reveal Nuclei and Paths Transmitting Somatic Sensory Information to the Cerebellum

Clarke's nucleus and the accessory cuneate nucleus are the principal nuclei that relay somatic sensory information to the spinocerebellum. **Clarke's nucleus** is found in the medial portion of the intermediate zone of the spinal cord gray matter (lamina VII) (Figure 13–14). This nucleus forms a column with a limited rostrocaudal distribution (Figure 13–6A). In the human, Clarke's nucleus spans the **eighth cervical segment** (C8) to approximately the **second lumbar segment** (L2) and relays somatic sensory information from the lower limb and lower trunk. Most of the mechanoreceptive fibers that synapse in Clarke's nucleus course medially around the cap of the dorsal horn and through the ipsilateral dorsal column en route to their termination site (Figure 13–14). Afferent

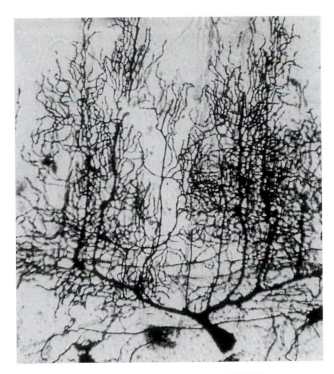

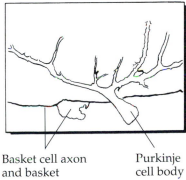

Basket cell axon and basket   Purkinje cell body

Figure 13–12. Golgi-stained section of the human cerebellar cortex, showing a Purkinje cell and basket axons. The inset shows a schematic of the Purkinje cell body, proximal dendrites, basket cell axon, and basket synapse on an adjacent (unstained) Purkinje cell.

in the outer portion of the molecular layer, and **basket cells,** located close to the border between the molecular and Purkinje layers. These neurons receive their predominant input from the parallel fibers.

The locations of the synaptic terminals of the basket and stellate cells on the Purkinje cells are different, which is important functionally in determining the strength of inhibition. The basket cell synapse is located on the Purkinje cell body, forming a dense meshwork, or "basket," of inhibitory synaptic contacts (Figure 13–12). The basket cell synapse is one of the strongest central nervous system inhibitory synapses. This strength results from its proximity to the spike

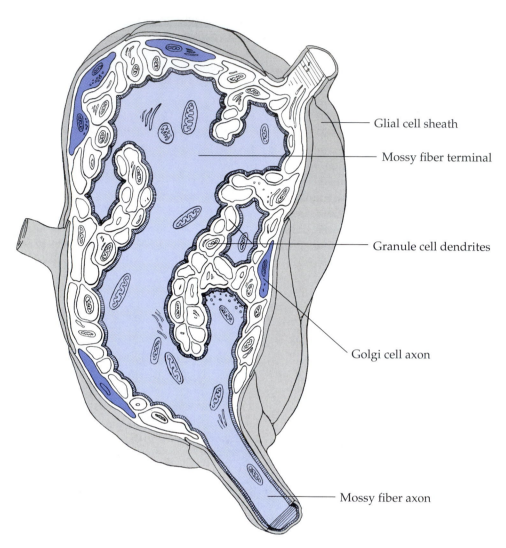

Glial cell sheath

Mossy fiber terminal

Granule cell dendrites

Golgi cell axon

Mossy fiber axon

Figure 13–13. The cerebellar glomerulus consists of two presynaptic elements, the mossy fiber terminal and Golgi cell axon, and one main postsynaptic element, the granule cell dendrite. These neural elements are ensheathed by glial cells. *(Based on Eccles JC, Ito M, Szentágothai J: The Cerebellum as a Neuronal Machine. Springer-Verlag, 1967.)*

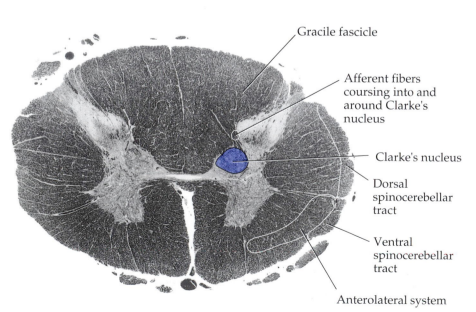

Gracile fascicle

Afferent fibers coursing into and around Clarke's nucleus

Clarke's nucleus

Dorsal spinocerebellar tract

Ventral spinocerebellar tract

Anterolateral system

Figure 13–14. Myelin-stained transverse sections through the lumbar spinal cord. Clarke's nucleus is tinted blue.

fibers arriving over dorsal roots caudal to the second lumbar segment first ascend in the **gracile fascicle** (Figure 13–6A). Then they leave the white matter to terminate in Clarke's nucleus. Clarke's nucleus gives rise to the **dorsal spinocerebellar tract,** which ascends in the outermost portion of the ipsilateral lateral column (Figure 13–14). The other pathway from the lower limb, the **ventral spinocerebellar tract,** is lateral to the ascending fibers of the anterolateral system (Figure 13–14). The ventral spinocerebellar tract originates from diverse neurons in the ventral horn, including a group within the motor nuclei. These neurons are termed the **spinal border cells** because they are located at the margin of the gray matter and white matter. The ventral spinocerebellar tract is a crossed pathway.

The dorsal spinocerebellar tract enters the cerebellum via the **inferior cerebellar peduncle** (Figure 13–15). The ventral spinocerebellar tract continues to ascend within the brain stem and enters the cerebellum via the **superior cerebellar peduncle** (see Figure 13–18).

The caudal medulla contains the **accessory cuneate nucleus** (Figure 13–15), which is rostral to the cuneate nucleus. (The accessory cuneate nucleus is also termed the lateral cuneate nucleus and the external cuneate nucleus.) The accessory cuneate nucleus relays somatic sensory information from the upper trunk and upper limb to the cerebellum, not for perception but for controlling movements. Recall that the cuneate nucleus is important in transmitting somatic sensory information to the thalamus for perception (see Chapter 5). To reach the accessory cuneate nucleus, afferent

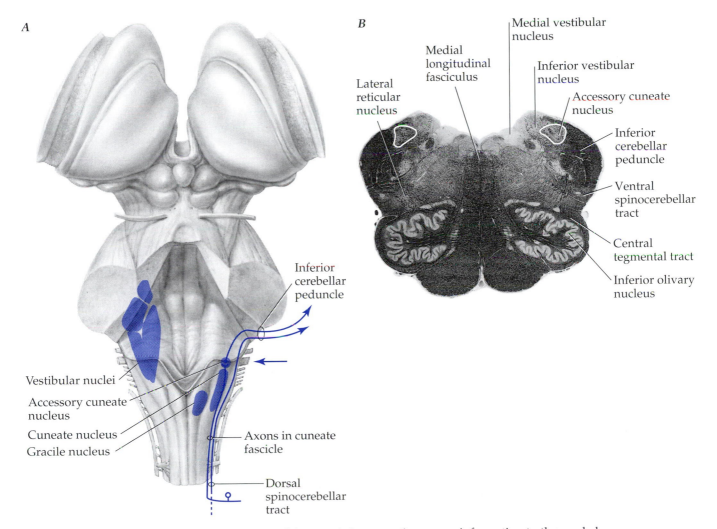

Figure 13–15. Brain stem nuclei transmitting somatic sensory information to the cerebellum. **A.** Key pathways for information from the dorsal spinocerebellar and cuneocerebellar tracts. **B.** Myelin-stained transverse section through the medulla, at the level of the accessory cuneate nucleus. The arrow in **A** indicates the plane of section in **B.**

fibers from the upper trunk and arm first course rostrally within the cervical spinal cord in the **cuneate fascicle** of the dorsal column (Figure 13–15A). Similar to the dorsal spinocerebellar tract, the cuneocerebellar projection courses in the **inferior cerebellar peduncle.**

The Inferior Olivary Nucleus Is the Only Source of Climbing Fibers

The inferior olivary nucleus, from which all **climbing fibers** originate, is a collection of three subnuclei (see Figure AII–8) that have somewhat different connections. It forms an elevation on the ventral surface of the medulla termed the **olive.** The inferior olivary nucleus consists of a convoluted sheet of neurons surrounded by the axons of the central tegmental tract, which originated from the parvocellular division of the red nucleus (see below). Neurons in the inferior olivary nucleus are electrically coupled, resulting in a synchrony of action among local groups of olivary neurons.

Dorsal to the inferior olivary nucleus is the **lateral reticular nucleus,** which gives rise to a mossy fiber projection to the cerebellum. The lateral reticular nucleus receives sensory information from mechanoreceptors of the limbs and trunk as well as information from the motor cortex, by axons of the corticospinal tract. Like neurons of the ventral spinocerebellar tract, the lateral reticular nucleus is thought to participate in correcting for movement errors.

The Vestibulocerebellum Receives Input From Primary and Secondary Vestibular Neurons

The **vestibular nuclei** are located in the rostral medulla and caudal pons (Figure 13–15A). Purkinje cells of the flocculonodular lobe send their axons primarily to these nuclei, rather than to the deep cerebellar nuclei, as do Purkinje cells in other regions of the cerebellum. (Exceptions exist, and the axons of some Purkinje cells of the flocculonodular lobe project to the fastigial nucleus. Similarly, some Purkinje cells of a small portion of the vermis of the posterior lobe project to the vestibular nuclei.)

The vestibular nuclei give rise to major spinal pathways, the vestibulospinal tracts (see Chapters 10 and 12). The flocculonodular lobe projects to the medial, inferior, and superior vestibular nuclei. These nuclei—especially the medial vestibular nucleus—give rise to the medial vestibulospinal tract, for coordinating head

and eye movements. The fastigial nucleus projects primarily to the lateral vestibular nucleus, which gives rise to the lateral vestibulospinal tract, for controlling axial muscles to maintain balance and posture. The vestibular nuclei also contribute to the **medial longitudinal fasciculus** (Figures 13–15B, 13–16, and 13–17B), which plays a key role in eye muscle control through projections to the extraocular motor nuclei (see Chapter 12). Thus, the vestibulocerebellum has direct control of head and eye position via its influence on the vestibular nuclei.

The vestibular nuclei may be the anatomical equivalent of the deep cerebellar nuclei of the vestibulocerebellum because they share two similarities in the sources of afferent input. First, both groups of nuclei receive a projection from the inferior olivary nucleus. Other than the vestibular nuclei, deep cerebellar nuclei, and cerebellar cortex, no other structure receives a projection from the inferior olivary nucleus. Second, neurons in the vestibular nuclei and the deep cerebellar nuclei are monosynaptically inhibited by Purkinje cells.

The Pontine Nuclei Provide the Major Input to the Cerebrocerebellum

The pontine nuclei (Figures 13–16 and 13–17B3, B4) relay input from the cerebral cortex to the cerebrocerebellum. Virtually the entire cerebral cortex projects to the pontine nuclei. The densest projections arise from the somatic sensory and motor regions: (1) the **premotor areas (area 6)** (including the premotor cortex on the lateral cortical surface and the supplementary motor area on the medial surface; see Figure 10–6), (2) the **primary motor cortex (area 4),** (3) the **primary somatic sensory cortex (areas 1, 2, and 3),** and (4) the **higher-order somatic sensory cortex (area 5).** Abundant projections also arise from association cortex in the parietal, frontal, and temporal lobes (which serve cognition and other higher brain functions) and from parts of the limbic cortical areas (which play important roles in emotions).

Corticopontine neurons originate in layer V of the cerebral cortex, the same layer that gives rise to the corticospinal and corticobulbar neurons. The descending axons course within the internal capsule and basis pedunculi to synapse in the pontine nuclei (see below). The axons of neurons of the pontine nuclei decussate in the pons and enter the cerebellum via the **middle cerebellar peduncle** (Figures 13–16 and 13–17B4). (The trapezoid body, which is the pontine auditory decussa-

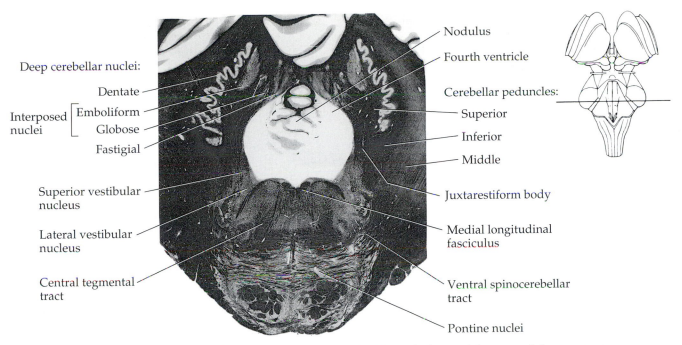

Deep cerebellar nuclei:
- Dentate
- Interposed nuclei { Emboliform / Globose }
- Fastigial

Superior vestibular nucleus

Lateral vestibular nucleus

Central tegmental tract

Nodulus

Fourth ventricle

Cerebellar peduncles:
- Superior
- Inferior
- Middle

Juxtarestiform body

Medial longitudinal fasciculus

Ventral spinocerebellar tract

Pontine nuclei

Figure 13–16. Myelin-stained transverse section through the caudal pons and deep cerebellar nuclei. The inset shows the plane of section.

tion, is dorsal to the decussating pontine nucleus axons [Figure 13–16].)

The Deep Cerebellar Nuclei Are Located Within the White Matter

The deep cerebellar nuclei can be identified in the transverse section through the pons and cerebellum shown in Figure 13–17, from medial to lateral: fastigial, globose, emboliform, and dentate nuclei. Recall that the globose and emboliform nuclei collectively are termed the interposed nuclei. The efferent projections of the deep nuclei course through the inferior and superior cerebellar peduncles.

The fastigial, interposed, and dentate nuclei have differential projections that reflect their functions in maintaining balance, controlling limb movement, and planning movement, respectively. The major targets of the output of the fastigial nucleus are nuclei in the pons and medulla. These fastigial efferent axons course in a particular portion of the inferior cerebellar peduncle termed the **juxtarestiform body** (Figure 13–16). This descending fastigial projection terminates in the vestibular nuclei and the reticular formation, two components of the medial descending pathways

that control balance and posture. The ascending projections from the deep nuclei course in the **superior cerebellar peduncle** (Figure 13–18).

The Superior Cerebellar Peduncle Decussates in the Caudal Midbrain

The superior cerebellar peduncle is dorsal to the pons, and farther rostrally it is located within the pontine **tegmentum** (Figure 13–17A). The **decussation** of the superior cerebellar peduncle is located primarily in the caudal midbrain, at the level of the inferior colliculus (Figure 13–17A, B2). The ascending axons of the interposed nuclei synapse in the **magnocellular division** of the red nucleus. The rubrospinal tract originates primarily from neurons in this division of the red nucleus. Many neurons of the dentate nucleus synapse in the **parvocellular division** of the red nucleus (Figures 13–17B1 and 13–18). The parvocellular division, which is much larger than the magnocellular division, sends its axons to the ipsilateral inferior olivary nucleus via the **central tegmental tract** (Figures 13–15B, 13–16, and 13–17B). The ascending projection from the dentate nucleus to the red nucleus and thalamus can be followed in the oblique section

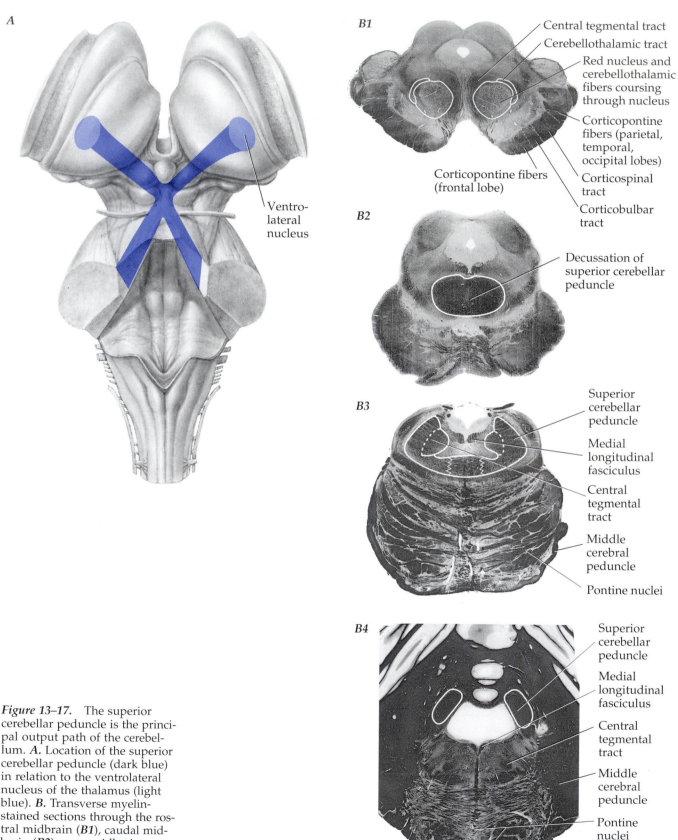

A

Ventro-
lateral
nucleus

B1
Central tegmental tract
Cerebellothalamic tract
Red nucleus and
cerebellothalamic
fibers coursing
through nucleus
Corticopontine
fibers (parietal,
temporal,
occipital lobes)
Corticospinal
tract
Corticobulbar
tract

Corticopontine fibers
(frontal lobe)

B2
Decussation of
superior cerebellar
peduncle

B3
Superior
cerebellar
peduncle

Medial
longitudinal
fasciculus

Central
tegmental
tract

Middle
cerebral
peduncle

Pontine nuclei

B4
Superior
cerebellar
peduncle

Medial
longitudinal
fasciculus

Central
tegmental
tract

Middle
cerebral
peduncle

Pontine
nuclei

Figure 13–17. The superior cerebellar peduncle is the principal output path of the cerebellum. *A.* Location of the superior cerebellar peduncle (dark blue) in relation to the ventrolateral nucleus of the thalamus (light blue). *B.* Transverse myelin-stained sections through the rostral midbrain (*B1*), caudal midbrain (*B2*), pons-midbrain junction (isthmus, *B3*), and rostral pons (*B4*).

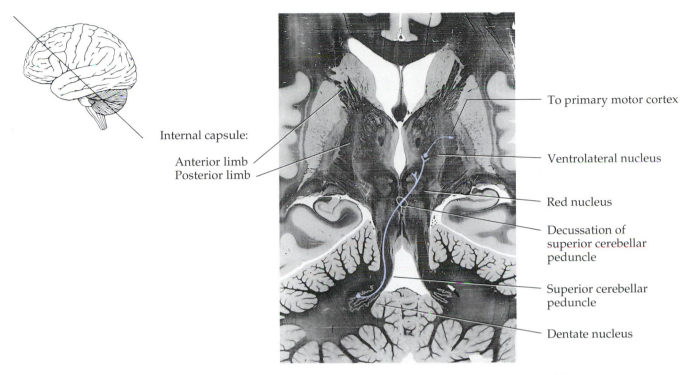

Internal capsule:

Anterior limb
Posterior limb

To primary motor cortex

Ventrolateral nucleus

Red nucleus

Decussation of
superior cerebellar
peduncle

Superior cerebellar
peduncle

Dentate nucleus

Figure 13–18. Myelin-stained oblique section through the cerebellum, brain stem, and cerebral hemispheres. The path of the cerebellothalamic tract from the dentate nucleus to the ventrolateral nucleus and the path to the parvocellular red nucleus are shown. The inset shows the plane of section.

shown in Figure 13–18. This section is cut along the long axis of the superior cerebellar peduncle and complements the drawing shown in Figure 13–17A.

The descending corticopontine projection courses in the basis pedunculi. The corticopontine projection (Figure 13–17B1) from the frontal lobe is located in the medial basis pedunculi, whereas the projection from the parietal, temporal, and occipital lobes descends laterally. The corticospinal and corticobulbar fibers (see Chapters 10 and 11) are flanked between these two contingents of corticopontine fibers.

The Ventrolateral Nucleus Relays Cerebellar Output to the Premotor and Primary Motor Cortical Areas

Collectively the projections from the deep cerebellar nuclei to the thalamus are termed the **cerebellothalamic tract.** This tract courses directly through the red nucleus and also surrounds the nucleus, forming a dense ring of myelinated fibers (Figure 13–17B1).

The portion of the thalamus that receives cerebellar input and transmits this information to the motor areas of the frontal lobe is the **ventrolateral nucleus.** The ventrolateral nucleus (Figure 13–19) is difficult to identify. One clue that makes identification a bit easier is the presence of the **thalamic fasciculus.** This band of myelinated fibers contains axons of the cerebellothalamic tract as well as axons of the basal ganglia projection to the thalamus (see Chapter 14).

The ventrolateral nucleus is large and has many component divisions that have distinctive connections, primarily with the **frontal lobe** but also to the parietal lobe. The interposed and dentate nuclei project to the part of the ventrolateral nucleus that relays information to the **primary motor cortex (area 4)** and the **premotor cortex (lateral area 6).** In addition, the dentate nucleus projects to other parts of the ventrolateral nucleus that transmit information to the prefrontal cortex and posterior parietal cortex. The projections from the dentate nucleus interdigitate with but do not overlay the terminations from the interposed nuclei. Box 13–1 considers projections from the cerebellar nuclei from a clinical perspective.

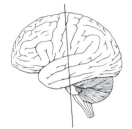

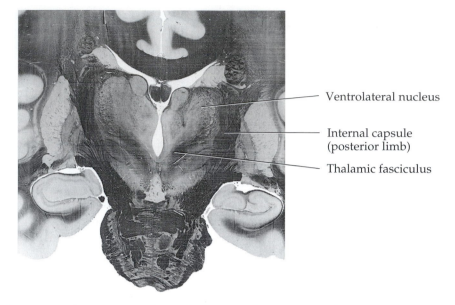

— Ventrolateral nucleus

— Internal capsule (posterior limb)

— Thalamic fasciculus

Figure 13–19. Myelin-stained coronal section through the ventrolateral nucleus. The inset shows the plane of section.

Box 13–1. *Damage to the Cerebellum Produces Neurological Signs on the Same Side as the Lesion*

There are three classic signs of cerebellar damage: ataxia, nystagmus, and tremor. **Ataxia** is inaccuracy in the speed, force, and distance of movement. In reaching for an object, a patient with cerebellar damage overshoots or undershoots the target. Ataxia of gait produces staggering and lurching. Ataxia is due to impairments in interjoint coordination. **Nystagmus** is a rhythmic involuntary oscillation of the eyes. **Tremor** is involuntary oscillation of the limbs or trunk.

Cerebellar tremor is characteristically present when the patient is trying to perform an accurate reaching movement, such as touching the examiner's finger or bringing a forkful of food to the mouth. Ataxia and nystagmus typically occur after damage to cerebellar inputs, such as the spinocerebellar

tracts or the inferior cerebellar peduncle (see below). In contrast, tremor is more often a consequence of damage to the cerebellar output pathways, such as the superior cerebellar peduncle. However, combinations of signs typically occur with damage to the cerebellum depending on the site and size of the lesion.

Knowledge of the anatomy of the descending projection pathways is crucial for understanding why unilateral cerebellar damage typically produces **ipsilateral motor signs.** Ipsilateral signs occur because both the cerebellar efferent projections and the descending pathways (ie, the targets of cerebellar action) are both crossed. The combined decussations result in a system of connections that is "doubly crossed" (Figure 13–20). Damage to cerebellar input from the spinal cord

also produces ipsilateral signs because the principal spinocerebellar pathways, the dorsal spinocerebellar and cuneocerebellar tracts, ascend ipsilaterally. Thus, whether damage occurs to cerebellar inputs or outputs, or to the cerebellum itself, neurological signs are present on the ipsilateral side.

Occlusion of the **posterior inferior cerebellar artery (PICA),** which produces infarction of the **inferior cerebellar peduncle,** also results in ipsilateral signs. Two key signs related to this infarction are nystagmus (also a consequence of damage to the vestibular nuclei) and ataxia. These are the cerebellar signs associated with the **lateral medullary,** or **Wallenberg, syndrome.** Somatic sensory deficits are also present with PICA occlusion because infarction of the dorsolateral

Box 13–1 (continued).

medulla interrupts ascending fibers of the anterolateral system (see Chapter 5) as well as the trigeminal spinal tract and nucleus (see Chapter 6).

Although the principal signs of cerebellar damage are motor, patients with cerebellar damage may also have behavioral impairments that cannot be attributed to a primary motor impairment. This phenomenon has been described as the cerebellar "cognitive affective syndrome." The syndrome is characterized by impairments in executive functions (eg, planning behaviors), abstract reasoning, visuospatial reasoning, and working memory. Some patients have personality changes, with a blunting of affect. This syndrome is more prominent in patients with posterior lobe and vermal lesions. These changes could be due to impairments in processing information from diverse cortical regions—such as association areas, including limbic association cortex—and damage to cerebellar regions that project to the dorsolateral prefrontal cortex.

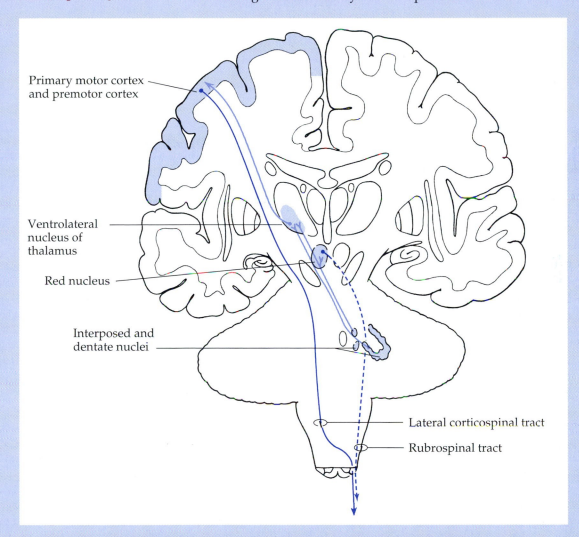

Figure 13–20. The "doubly crossed" arrangement of the efferent projections of the cerebellum. Note that the cerebellar projection to the magnocellular division of the red nucleus is from the interposed nuclei (globose and emboliform nuclei), and the projection to the parvocellular division originates in the dentate nucleus. (*Adapted from Carpenter MB, Sutin J: Human Neuroanatomy. Williams & Wilkins, 1983.*)

Labels in figure:
- Primary motor cortex and premotor cortex
- Ventrolateral nucleus of thalamus
- Red nucleus
- Interposed and dentate nuclei
- Lateral corticospinal tract
- Rubrospinal tract

Summary

Cerebellar Gross Anatomy

The cerebellar cortex overlies the white matter (Figures 13–1 and 13–10A). The cerebellar cortex contains numerous **folia,** which are grouped into three **lobes** (Figures 13–1 and 13–2): the **anterior lobe,** the **posterior lobe,** and the **flocculonodular lobe.** Embedded within the white matter of the cerebellum are four bilaterally paired deep nuclei, from medial to lateral (Figure 13–2B): the **fastigial nucleus,** the **globose nucleus,** the **emboliform nucleus,** and the **dentate nucleus.** The globose and emboliform nuclei are collectively termed the **interposed nuclei.**

Cerebellar Cortex

The cerebellar cortex consists of three cell layers, from the cerebellar surface to the white matter (Figure 13–10): **molecular, Purkinje,** and **granular layers.** Five neuron classes are found in the cerebellar cortex (Figures 13–10 and 13–11; Table 13–2): (1) **Purkinje cells** (Figures 13–11A and 13–12), the **projection neurons** of the cerebellum—which are **inhibitory;** (2) **granule cells,** the only **excitatory interneurons** in the cerebellum; and the (3) **basket,** (4) **stellate,** and (5) **Golgi cells**—the three **inhibitory interneurons** (Figures 13–11 and 13–12; Table 13–2).

Cerebellar Afferents

Two principal classes of afferent fibers reach the cerebellum: **climbing fibers** (Figures 13–4 and 13–11), which are the axons of neurons of the **inferior olivary nuclei** (Figure 13–15B), and **mossy fibers,** which originate from numerous sources, including the **pontine nuclei** (Figure 13–16), **reticular formation nuclei, vestibular nuclei** (Figures 13–15 and 13–16), and **spinal cord** (Figure 13–14). Climbing and mossy fiber inputs are directed to both the deep cerebellar nuclei and the cerebellar cortex (Figure 13–4); but some mossy fiber sources do not project to the deep nuclei. The climbing fibers make monosynaptic connections with the Purkinje cells; the mossy fibers synapse on granule cells, which in turn synapse on Purkinje cells via their **parallel fibers.** The Purkinje cells project from the cerebellar cortex to the deep nuclei (Figure 13–16) and the vestibular nuclei (Figure 13–15).

Cerebellar Functional Divisions

The cerebellum is divided into three functional regions (Figures 13–3 and 13–5): the spinocerebellum, the cerebrocerebellum, and the vestibulocerebellum. The **spinocerebellum** (Figures 13–5A, 13–6, and 13–7), which is important in posture and limb movement, is subdivided into two cortical regions that also have functional counterparts: The medial **vermis** subserves control of **axial and girdle muscles,** and the **intermediate hemisphere** controls **limb muscles.** The principal inputs to the spinocerebellum originate from the spinal cord. Somatic sensory information from the leg and lower trunk is transmitted to the cerebellum by the **dorsal spinocerebellar tract** (Figure 13–6A), via **Clarke's nucleus,** and from the upper trunk, arm, and neck, by the **cuneocerebellar tract,** via the **accessory cuneate nucleus** (Figure 13–15). The **ventral spinocerebellar tract** (Figure 13–6B) transmits information about internal feedback signals from the leg, and the **rostral spinocerebellar tract** transmits information from the arm (Table 13–1). Purkinje cells of the vermis project to the **fastigial nucleus** (Figures 13–5A and 13–16), which influences **medial descending pathways:** the reticulospinal, vestibulospinal, and ventral corticospinal tracts. The projection to the lower brain stem is via the **inferior cerebellar peduncle** (Figure 13–15B), and the thalamic projection is via the **superior cerebellar peduncle** (Figure 13–17). The **intermediate hemisphere** projects to the interposed nuclei (Figures 13–14 through 13–16), which in turn influence the **lateral descending pathways:** the rubrospinal and lateral corticospinal tracts. All projections from the spinocerebellum course through the superior cerebellar peduncle.

The **cerebrocerebellum** (Figure 13–5A) plays a role in planning movements; its cortical component is the **lateral hemisphere.** The cerebral cortex projects to the **pontine nuclei** (Figures 13–16 and 13–17B3, B4), which provide the main input to the cerebrocerebellum. Purkinje cells of this functional division project to the **dentate nucleus** (Figure 13–16). From there, dentate neurons project to the contralateral **parvocellular red nucleus** (Figure 13–17A) and the **ventrolateral nucleus** of the thalamus (Figures 13–18 and 13–19), both via the **superior cerebellar peduncle.** The principal projections of the ventrolateral nucleus are to the **primary motor cortex (area 4)** and the **premotor cortex (lateral area 6).** The dentate nucleus also projects, via the thalamus, to the prefrontal association cortex.

The **vestibulocerebellum** (Figures 13–5B and 13–9) is important in eye and head movement control; the cortical component corresponds anatomically to the **flocculonodular lobe.** It receives input from the **vestibular nuclei** and **primary vestibular afferents** and projects back to the vestibular nuclei via the **inferior cerebellar peduncle** (Figure 13–15).

Related Sources

Brust JCM: The Practice of Neural Science. McGraw-Hill; 2000. (See ch. 10, case 14; ch. 12, cases 33, 34.)

Ghez C, Krakhauer J: The organization of movement. In Kandel ER, Schwartz JH, Jessell TM (editors): Principles of Neural Science, 4th ed. McGraw-Hill; 2000:653–673.

Ghez C, Thach WT: The cerebellum. In Kandel ER, Schwartz JH, Jessell TM (editors): Principles of Neural Science, 4th ed. McGraw-Hill; 2000:832–852.

Selected Readings

Glickstein M, Yeo C: The cerebellum and motor learning. J Cogn Neurosci 1990;2:69–80.

Jueptner M, Weiller C: A review of differences between basal ganglia and cerebellar control of movements as revealed by functional imaging studies. Brain 1998;121:1437–1449.

Leiner HC, Leiner AL, Dow RS: Cognitive and language functions of the human cerebellum. Trends Neurosci 1993; 16:444–447.

Middleton FA, Strick PL: Dentate output channels: Motor and cognitive components. Prog Brain Res 1997;114:553–566.

Schmahmann JD: An emerging concept. The cerebellar contribution to higher function. Arch Neurol 1991;48:1178–1187.

Schmahmann JD, Pandya DN: The cerebrocerebellar system. Int Rev Neurobiol 1997;41:31–60.

Schmahmann JD, Sherman JC: The cerebellar cognitive affective syndrome. Brain 1998;121:561–579.

Thach WT, Goodkin HP, Keating JG: The cerebellum and the adaptive coordination of movement. Annu Rev Neurosci 1992;15:403–442.

References

Allen G, Buxton RB, Wong EC, Courchesne E: Attentional activation of the cerebellum independent of motor involvement. Science 1997;275:1940–1943.

Angevine JB Jr., Mancall EL, Yakovlev PI: The Human Cerebellum: An Atlas of Gross Topography in Serial Sections. Little, Brown, 1961.

Clower DM, West RA, Lynch JC, Strick PL: The inferior parietal lobule is the target of output from the superior colliculus, hippocampus, and cerebellum. J Neurosci 2001; 21:6283–6291.

Dietrichs E, Walberg F: Cerebellar nuclear afferents—Where do they originate? Anat Embryol 1987;177:165–172.

Eccles JC, Ito M, Szentágothai J: The Cerebellum as a Neuronal Machine. Springer-Verlag, 1967.

Hoover JE, Strick PL: The organization of cerebellar and basal ganglia outputs to primary motor cortex as revealed by retrograde transneuronal transport of herpes simplex virus type 1. J Neurosci 1999;19:1446–1463.

Kim SS-G, Ugurbil K, Strick PL: Activation of cerebellar output nucleus during cognitive processing. Science 1994; 265:949–951.

Levisohn L, Cronin-Golomb A, Schmahmann JD: Neuropsychological consequences of cerebellar tumour resection in children: Cerebellar cognitive affective syndrome in a paediatric population. Brain 2000;123:1041–1050.

Massion J: Red nucleus: Past and future. Behav Brain Res 1988;28:1–8.

Matsushita M, Hosoya Y, Ikeda M: Anatomical organization of the spinocerebellar system in the cat, as studied by retrograde transport of horseradish peroxidase. J Comp Neurol 1979;184:81–106.

Middleton FA, Strick PL: Anatomical evidence for cerebellar and basal ganglia involvement in higher cognitive function. Science 1994;266:458–461.

Schell GR, Strick PL: The origin of thalamic inputs to the arcuate premotor and supplementary motor areas. J Neurosci 1984;4:539–560.

Schmahmann JD: From movement to thought: Anatomic substrates of the cerebellar contribution to cognitive processing. Human Brain Mapping 1996;4:174–198.

Schmahmann JD, Pandya DN: Course of the fiber pathways to pons from parasensory association areas in the rhesus monkey. J Comp Neurol 1992;326:159–179.

Stein JF, Glickstein M: Role of the cerebellum in visual guidance of movement. Physiol Rev 1992;72:967–1017.

14

The Basal Ganglia

THE BASAL GANGLIA ARE A COLLECTION of subcortical nuclei that have captured the fascination of clinicians for well over a century because of the remarkable range of behavioral dysfunction associated with basal ganglia disease. Movement control deficits are among the key signs, ranging from the tremor and rigidity of Parkinson disease and the writhing movements of Huntington disease to the bizarre tics of Tourette syndrome. These clinical findings suggest that one important set of basal ganglia functions is control of motor actions. How do the basal ganglia fit into an overall view of the organization of the motor systems? Unlike the motor cortex, which has direct connections with motor neurons, the basal ganglia influence movements by acting on the descending pathways similar to the cerebellum.

In addition to producing movement control deficits, basal ganglia disease can also impair intellectual capacity, suggesting an important role in cognition. Dementia is an early disabling consequence of Huntington disease and can be present in patients with advanced stages of Parkinson disease. The basal ganglia have also been linked with emotional function, playing a role in aspects of drug addiction and psychiatric disease.

Although the basal ganglia are still among the least understood of all brain structures, their mysteries are now yielding to modern neurobiological techniques for elucidating neurochemistry and connections. For example, the basal ganglia contain virtually all of the major neuroactive agents that have been discovered in the various divisions of the central nervous system. Although the reason for this biochemical diversity remains elusive, such knowledge can be used to treat some forms of basal ganglia disease. Indeed, the discovery that the brains of patients with Parkinson disease are deficient in the neuroactive agent dopamine quickly led to the development of drug replacement therapy. Knowledge about connections of the basal ganglia with the rest of the brain has led to a major revision of the traditional views of basal ganglia organization and function. Discoveries about basal ganglia circuitry and pathways have even led to therapeutic neurosurgical and neurophysiological procedures.

This chapter first considers the constituents of the basal ganglia and their three-dimensional shapes. Next, their functional organization is surveyed, emphasizing the role of the basal ganglia in movement control. (Chapter 16 revisits the basal ganglia in relation to emotions.) Finally, this chapter examines the regional anatomy of the basal ganglia using a series of slices through the cerebral hemispheres and brain stem.

FUNCTIONAL ANATOMY OF THE BASAL GANGLIA

Separate Components of the Basal Ganglia Process Incoming Information and Mediate the Output

On the basis of their connections, the components of the basal ganglia can be divided into three categories: input nuclei, output nuclei, and intrinsic nuclei.

The **input nuclei** receive afferent connections from brain regions other than the basal ganglia and in turn project to the intrinsic and output nuclei. The **output nuclei** project to regions of the diencephalon and brain stem that are not part of the basal ganglia. The connections of the **intrinsic nuclei** are largely restricted to the basal ganglia.

The general organization of the basal ganglia from input to output is shown in Figure 14–1. The **striatum** is the input nucleus of the basal ganglia, receiving afferent projections from the cerebral cortex. Three subnuclei comprise the striatum: the **caudate nucleus,** which participates in eye movement control and cognition; the **putamen,** which participates in control of limb and trunk movements; and the **nucleus accumbens,** which participates in emotions. The striatum has a complex shape (Figure 14–2A). The caudate nucleus has a C-shape, with three components: head, body, and tail (Figure 14–2). The putamen, when viewed from its lateral surface, is shaped like a disk.

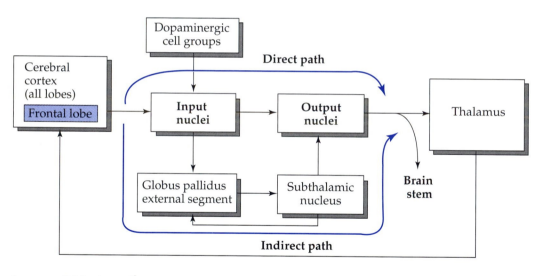

Input nuclei (striatum)[1]

1. Caudate nucleus
2. Putamen[2]
3. Nucleus accumbens

Output nuclei

1. Globus pallidus—internal segment[2]
2. Ventral pallidum
3. Substantia nigra pars reticulata

Intrinsic nuclei

1. Globus pallidus—external segment
2. Subthalamic nucleus
3. Substantia nigra pars compacta
4. Ventral tegmental area

Figure 14–1. (*Top*) Block diagram illustrating the general features of the input-output organization of the basal ganglia. The input nuclei receive their major projections from the entire cerebral cortex, but only the frontal lobe receives output from the basal ganglia, relayed via the thalamus. (*Bottom*) Components of the basal ganglia. (Notes: [1]The striatum is also termed the neostriatum. [2]The putamen and internal and external segments of the globus pallidus together are also termed the lenticular nucleus because their form is similar to that of a lens.)

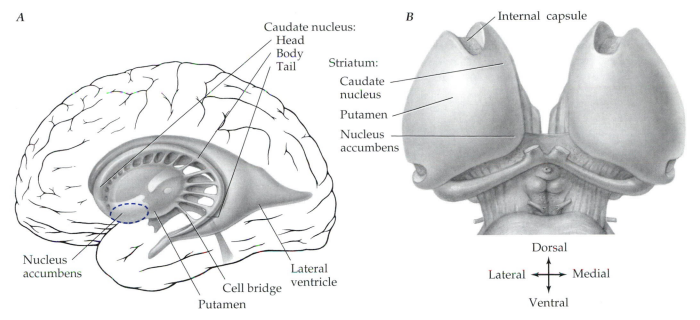

Figure 14–2. A. The striatum in relation to the ventricular system. The striatum consists of the caudate nucleus, putamen, and nucleus accumbens. Only the caudate nucleus has a C-shape, which is similar to that of the lateral ventricle. The nucleus accumbens is located ventromedially, primarily on the medial striatal surface. *B.* Ventral view of the striatum, diencephalon, and midbrain showing how the caudate nucleus, putamen, and nucleus accumbens are continuous ventromedially.

The nucleus accumbens is contiguous with the ventromedial portions of the caudate nucleus and the putamen (Figure 14–2B).

There are three nuclei on the output side of the basal ganglia (Figure 14–1): the **internal segment of the globus pallidus,** the **substantia nigra pars reticulata,** and the **ventral pallidum.** The axons of output nuclei project to thalamic nuclei, which project to different areas of the frontal lobe. These thalamic nuclei include the **ventrolateral nucleus** (a part distinct from the one receiving cerebellar input), the **ventral anterior nucleus,** and the **medial dorsal nucleus.** The output nuclei also project to the **pedunculopontine nucleus** at the junction of the midbrain and pons, which is implicated in limb and trunk control during locomotion, and to the **superior colliculus,** which controls saccadic eye movements. For the components of the basal ganglia that control limb and trunk movements, eye movements, and facial muscles, the path from the striatum to the output nuclei and then to the thalamus and brain stem promotes the production of movements. This circuit is termed the **direct path** of the basal ganglia (Figure 14–1; see Figure 14–5A).

The basal ganglia have four intrinsic nuclei: the **external segment of the globus pallidus,** the **subthalamic nucleus,** the **substantia nigra pars compacta,** and the **ventral tegmental area.** Their connections are closely related to the input and output nuclei. The external segment of the globus pallidus and the sub-

thalamic nucleus are part of a basal ganglia circuit that receives input from other basal ganglia nuclei and in turn projects back. The path from the striatum to these two intrinsic nuclei comprises the **indirect path** of the basal ganglia, which inhibits the production of movements (Figure 14–1; see Figure 14–5B). The substantia nigra pars compacta and the ventral tegmental area contain dopaminergic neurons that project to the striatum (see Figure 2–2B1).

Various Components of the Basal Ganglia Are Separated by Axons of the Internal Capsule

Learning the numerous components and subdivisions of the basal ganglia is a challenge. During development, axons coursing to and from the cerebral cortex in the internal capsule divide many basal ganglia components into separate nuclei, thereby increasing the complexity of the nomenclature. These internal capsule axons incompletely divide the striatum into the three components, leaving behind **cell bridges** (Figure 14–2A).

The internal capsule also separates the internal segment of the globus pallidus and the substantia nigra pars reticulata, similar to the striatal cell bridges (see below). In humans, cells of the substantia nigra pars reticulata and internal segment of the globus pallidus are scattered between each other within the internal capsule. In addition to being part of the same structure but separated by the internal capsule, the morphology, neurotransmitter content, and connections of neurons in the internal segment of the globus pallidus and the substantia nigra pars reticulata are similar.

Parallel Circuits Course Through the Basal Ganglia

The connections of the basal ganglia are remarkably specific. Anatomical "loops" have been identified from separate cortical regions, through different parts of the basal ganglia and thalamic nuclei, to distinct areas of the frontal lobe. Three important points relate to the general organization of these neural circuits:

1. Each of the loops originates from multiple cortical regions that have similar general functions.
2. Each loop passes through different basal ganglia and thalamic nuclei, or separate portions of the same nucleus.
3. The cortical targets of the loops are separate portions of the **frontal lobe.**

Each loop is thought to mediate a different set of functions. Although many parallel loops originate from various cortical areas, anatomical and physiological studies have begun to focus on four such loops (Figure 14–3): the skeletomotor, oculomotor, prefrontal cortex, and limbic loops. The **skeletomotor loop** plays important roles in the control of facial, limb, and trunk musculature (Figure 14–3A1). Inputs originate from the primary somatic sensory and frontal motor areas and project back to the frontal motor areas (Figure 14–3B). Experiments in rhesus monkeys suggest that separate circuits within the skeletomotor loop pass through different parts of the globus pallidus and ultimately terminate in different premotor and motor areas. The **oculomotor loop** plays a role in the control of saccadic eye movements. Key inputs derive from the frontal eye field, which is important in the production of rapid conjugate eye movements through brain stem projections, and the posterior parietal association cortex, which processes visual information for controlling the speed and direction of eye movements (Figure 14–3A2). The output of this loop is to the frontal eye movement control centers (Figure 14–3B; see Chapter 12). More is known about the organization of these two movement control loops than about the other two loops.

The **prefrontal cortex loop** plays a role in cognition and executive behavioral functions, such as strategic planning of behavior. Receiving inputs from diverse association areas, this loop projects to the dorsolateral prefrontal cortex (Figure 14–3A3, B). Though principally involved in thought and reasoning and in the highest level of organizing goal-directed behaviors, the prefrontal cortex has relatively direct connections with premotor areas involved in movement planning.

The **limbic loop** participates in the motivational regulation of behavior and in emotions. The term *limbic* derives from the limbic system, the brain system that comprises the principal structures for emotions. The limbic association cortex and the hippocampal formation provide the major input to the limbic loop. The limbic loop engages the most distinct set of basal ganglia circuits: the **ventral striatum**—which includes the nucleus accumbens and ventromedial portions of the caudate nucleus and putamen—and the **ventral pallidum** (Figure 14–3A4). The limbic association cortex in the anterior cingulate gyrus is the major frontal lobe recipient of the output of the limbic loop (Figure 14–3B).

In organizing behavior, the various parallel circuits of the basal ganglia appear to have distinct functions. For example, when you reach for a glass of water, the limbic loop may play a role in the initial decision to move. This decision is biased by thirst. The prefrontal cortex loop seems to play a key role in formulating a goal plan, for example, how, where, and when to reach for the water. The oculomotor and skeletomotor loops are thought to assist in the programming and execution of the particular behaviors to achieve the goal. For example, these loops may coordinate eye and limb movements to accurately direct your hand to the glass.

Integration across the numerous parallel basal ganglia circuits must take place. For example, how can the limbic loop influence motor behavior, such as reaching for a cup of coffee, if its connections always remain distinct from those of the motor loops? Basal ganglia research is beginning to point to a second organization whereby interactions occur among circuits. Two mechanisms may be important. First, the dendrites of striatal neurons can extend beyond their own loops into adjacent loops, thereby receiving information from more diverse cortical areas. Second, striatal neurons in all of the loops project back to the substantia nigra pars compacta. The terminals of axons comprising the different loops may converge on nigral dopaminergic neurons and interneurons and, thus, be sites for integration.

Knowledge of Basal Ganglia Connections and Neurotransmitters Provides Insight Into Their Function in Health and Disease

Although the loops through the basal ganglia help to shape thoughts, emotions, and motor behaviors, it is not known how information is transformed as it passes through different basal ganglia nuclei. Nevertheless, important insights into the function of the basal ganglia can be gained by examining the kinds of neuroactive compounds present in the various basal ganglia nuclei and the patterns of neuronal connections.

Basal Ganglia Contain Diverse Neurotransmitters and Neuromodulators

Many neurotransmitters and **neuromodulatory** substances are present in the various basal ganglia nuclei (Figure 14–4). The excitatory neurotransmitter **glutamate** is used by corticostriatal neurons (the major input to the basal ganglia), thalamic neurons that project to the striatum, and the projection neurons of the subthalamic nucleus. The major neurotransmitter of the basal ganglia is γ-aminobutyric acid, or **GABA,** which is **inhibitory.** In the striatum, GABA is located in the projection neurons, the **medium spiny neurons.** The axons of these neurons, which have abundant dendritic spines (see Figure 1–1), project to the two segments of the globus pallidus and the substantia nigra pars reticulata. Medium spiny neurons also contain neuropeptides, with two distinct neuron classes containing either **enkephalin** or **substance P** and **dynorphin.** Projection neurons of the internal and external segments of the globus pallidus and the substantia nigra pars reticulata also contain GABA. Thus, the output of the basal ganglia, similar to that of the cerebellar cortex, is inhibitory. The significance of this common synaptic organization is not yet apparent.

Neurons in the substantia nigra pars compacta and the ventral tegmental area contain **dopamine.** The term *substantia nigra,* which means black substance, derives from the presence of the black pigment **neuromelanin,** a polymer of the catecholamine precursor dihydroxy-phenylalanine (or dopa), which is contained in the neurons in the pars compacta. In the movement disorder **Parkinson disease,** the midbrain dopaminergic neurons are destroyed and striatal dopamine is profoundly reduced (see below). Replacement therapy using a precursor to dopamine, L-**dopa,** leads to a dramatic improvement in the neurological signs of this disease. Not surprisingly, neuromelanin is not present in the substantia nigra pars compacta of Parkinson patients. Dopaminergic neurons in other parts of the central nervous system are also destroyed. Dopamine loss in the basal ganglia, however, apparently produces the most debilitating neurological signs.

Acetylcholine is another common neurotransmitter in the basal ganglia. It is present in striatal interneurons, where it is an important neurotransmitter in the function of **local neuronal circuits.**

Parkinson Disease Is a Hypokinetic Movement Disorder Whereas Hemiballism Is a Hyperkinetic Disorder

In Parkinson disease, with its loss of striatal dopamine, there is a major impairment in initiating movements, termed **akinesia,** and a reduction in the extent and speed of movements, called **bradykinesia.** These are called **hypokinetic signs** because movements become impoverished. In addition, patients exhibit a resting **tremor,** and when an examiner moves their limbs, a characteristic stiffness or **rigidity** can be noted.

Researchers recently acquired an important tool in the study of Parkinson disease. They discovered that a certain kind of synthetic heroin produces a permanent clinical syndrome in humans that is remarkably similar to Parkinson disease. This substance contains the neurotoxin MPTP (1-methyl-4-phenyl-1,2,3,6-tetrahydropyridine), which is a meperidine derivative that kills the dopaminergic neurons of the substantia nigra pars compacta (as well as other dopaminergic neurons in the central nervous system). When monkeys are given MPTP, they too develop parkinsonian signs, including akinesia, bradykinesia, rigidity, and tremor.

In contrast to Parkinson disease, which is a hypokinetic disorder because movements are slowed, **Huntington disease** is a hyperkinetic disorder. In most patients, Huntington disease presents during midlife. One **hyperkinetic sign** of this disorder is **chorea,** which is characterized by involuntary rapid and random movements of the limbs and trunk. Patients with Huntington disease also develop dementia. Huntington disease is inherited as an autosomal dominant disorder. The Huntington gene is located on the short arm of chromosome 4 and codes for a protein, huntingtin, whose function is not known. Mutant huntingtin is thought to act within the nucleus of neurons to produce degeneration. Although neurodegeneration is widespread in Huntington disease, pathological changes occur earliest in striatal neurons that contain enkephalin, which are part of the indirect path (Figure 14–5B).

Another hyperkinetic disorder is **hemiballism.** This remarkable clinical disturbance occurs after vascular lesion of the **subthalamic nucleus.** As its name suggests, hemiballism causes patients to make uncontrollable, rapid **ballistic** (or flinging) movements of the contralateral limbs. These movements are produced by motion at proximal limb joints, such as the shoulder and elbow. Involuntary distal limb movements, such as writhing of the hand, or **athetosis,** may also occur. Box 14–1 presents a model for understanding some of

A 1. Skeletomotor loop

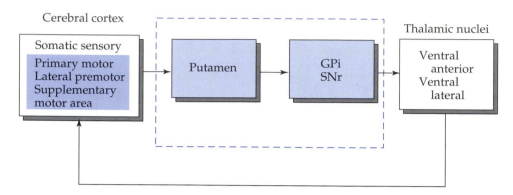

2. Oculomotor loop

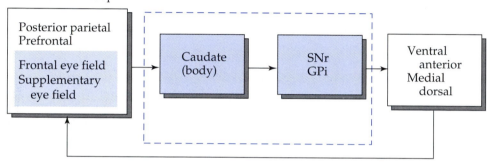

3. Prefrontal cortex loop

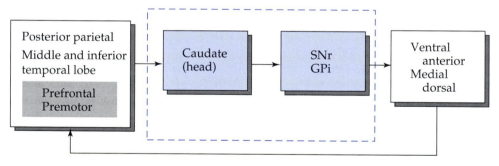

4. Limbic loop

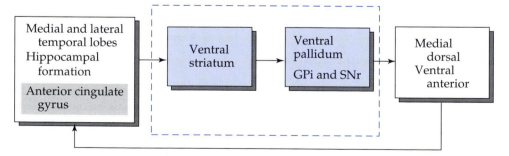

Figure 14–3. There are four principal input-output loops through the basal ganglia. **A.** Block diagrams illustrating the general organization of the loops. (1) Skeletomotor loop, (2) oculomotor loop, (3) prefrontal cortex loop, and (4) limbic loop. (Abbreviations: GPi, internal segment of the globus pallidus; SNr, substantia nigra pars reticulata.)

B

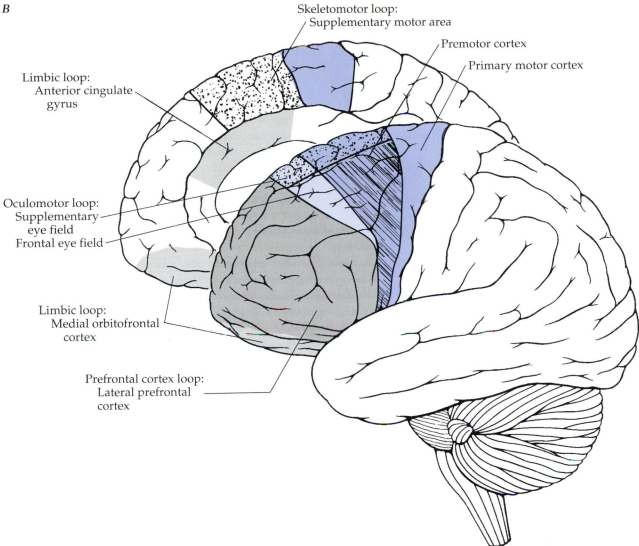

Skeletomotor loop:
Supplementary motor area

Premotor cortex

Primary motor cortex

Limbic loop:
Anterior cingulate
gyrus

Oculomotor loop:
Supplementary
eye field
Frontal eye field

Limbic loop:
Medial orbitofrontal
cortex

Prefrontal cortex loop:
Lateral prefrontal
cortex

Figure 14–3 Continued. **B.** Lateral and medial views of the cerebral cortex, illustrating the approximate location of the target regions in the frontal lobe. The medial orbitofrontal cortex is ventral to the lateral prefrontal cortex and is tinted light gray.

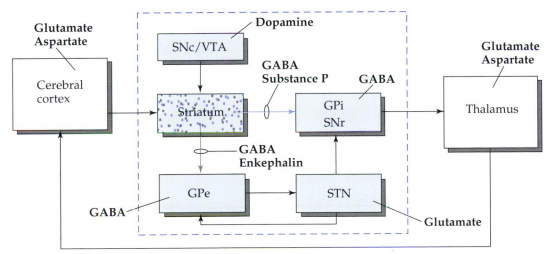

Glutamate
Aspartate

Dopamine

SNc/VTA

GABA
Substance P

GABA

Cerebral
cortex

Striatum

GPi
SNr

Glutamate
Aspartate

Thalamus

GABA
Enkephalin

GPe

STN

GABA

Glutamate

Figure 14–4. The neurotransmitters of the basal ganglia (boldface labels) are shown in relation to the organization of basal ganglia circuits. Neurons in the striatum that contain GABA and substance P (blue) give rise to the direct path, projecting to the internal segment of the globus pallidus. Neurons that contain GABA and enkephalin (gray) give rise to the indirect path and project to the external segment of the globus pallidus. (Abbreviations: GABA, γ-aminobutyric acid; GPe, external segment of the globus pallidus; GPi, internal segment of the globus pallidus; SNc, substantia nigra pars compacta; SNr, substantia nigra pars reticulata; STN, subthalamic nucleus; VTA, ventral tegmental area.)

A Direct path

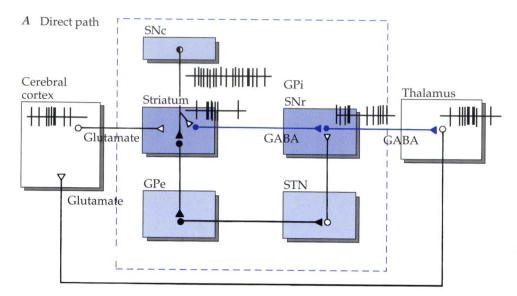

B Indirect path

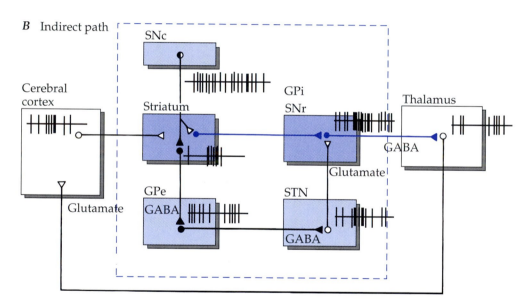

Figure 14–5. Functional basal ganglia circuits in health and disease. Summary of the direct (*A*) and indirect (*B*) paths of the basal ganglia. Filled neuronal cell bodies and terminals indicate inhibitory actions, and open cell bodies indicate excitatory actions. Schematic action potential records are shown by each structure. The vertical line is an action potential; the horizontal line is the baseline. Neural activity for each circuit can be followed, beginning with a phasic excitatory input from the cortex and the resulting phasic change in the thalamus.

the hypokinetic and hyperkinetic signs of movement disorders in terms of the circuitry and biochemistry of the basal ganglia.

REGIONAL ANATOMY OF THE BASAL GANGLIA

The rest of this chapter examines the regional anatomy of the parts of the brain that contain the components and associated nuclei of the basal ganglia. This examination begins with a horizontal slice through the cerebral hemispheres and diencephalon because it permits visualization of the various components of the internal capsule, which form major sub-

cortical landmarks. From there, the chapter moves on to coronal slices. In addition to explaining the regional anatomy of the basal ganglia, this discussion also provides an overall view of the deep structures of the cerebral hemispheres.

The Anterior Limb of the Internal Capsule Separates the Head of the Caudate Nucleus From the Putamen

In horizontal section, the **internal capsule** is shaped like an arrowhead pointed toward the midline (Figure 14–6). The internal capsule contains ascending thalamocortical fibers and descending cortical fibers. The

Figure 14–5 Continued.
Changes in activity in the circuits are shown for hypokinetic (*C1*) and hyperkinetic (*C2*) neurological signs. The thickness of the lines indicates relative changes in the number of neurons and strength of connections. Thicker means stronger connections and more activity; thinner means fewer and weaker connections. Schematic neural responses are also shown. Unlike A and B, which are the neural responses to discrete cortical input signals, the responses in C1 and C2 reflect changes in continuous activation patterns produced by disease. These paths follow only tonic changes in neural activation, because phasic changes are not well characterized. (Abbreviations: GPe, external segment of the globus pallidus; GPi, internal segment of the globus pallidus; SNc, substantia nigra pars compacta; SNr, substantia nigra pars reticulata; STN, subthalamic nucleus.) (*Adapted from Haber SN: Neurotransmitters in the human and nonhuman primate basal ganglia. Human Neurobiology 1986;5:159–168.*)

C1 Hypokinetic

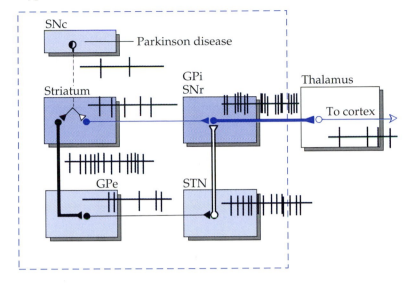

C2 Hyperkinetic

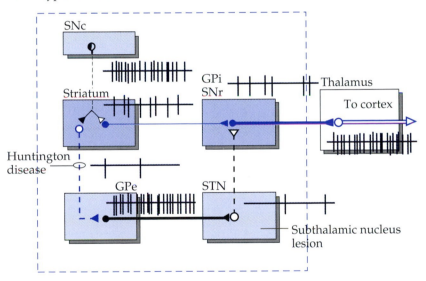

three main segments of the internal capsule are the **anterior limb;** the **posterior limb;** and the **genu,** which connects the two limbs (Figure 14–6; see also Chapter 2). A three-dimensional view of the internal capsule is shown in Figure 14–7, with the striatum drawn in schematically. Whereas the putamen and nucleus accumbens are lateral to the internal capsule, the caudate nucleus is medial to it. Complementing the three main segments of the internal capsule are the retrolenticular and sublenticular portions (Figure 14–7). They are named for their locations with respect to the **lenticular nucleus,** which comprises the putamen and globus pallidus.

The anterior limb separates the **head of the caudate nucleus** from the **putamen** (Figure 14–6). This limb contains axons projecting to and from the prefrontal association cortex and the various premotor cortical areas. The posterior limb separates the **putamen** and the **globus pallidus** (lenticular nucleus) from the **thalamus** and **body and tail of the caudate nucleus** (Figure 14–6). The posterior limb contains the corticospinal tract as well as the projections to and from the somatic sensory areas in the parietal lobe. The genu contains the corticobulbar tract. Only coronal sections through the posterior limb cut through the thalamus.

Box 14–1. Knowledge of the Intrinsic Circuitry of the Basal Ganglia Helps to Explain Hypokinetic and Hyperkinetic Signs

Scientists have begun to study disordered movement control during basal ganglia disease in terms of two sets of connections in the skeletomotor loop (Figure 14–3A1), termed the **direct** and **indirect paths** (Figure 14–5A,B). These paths have antagonistic effects on basal ganglia output: The direct path promotes movements, and the indirect path inhibits movements.

Projection neurons of the putamen in the direct path synapse on neurons in the **internal segment of the globus pallidus,** which project to the ventrolateral and ventral anterior nuclei of the thalamus. This circuit contains two inhibitory neurons, in the putamen and globus pallidus. Thus, a brief period of cortical excitation of the putamen (see neural responses in boxes marked cerebral cortex and striatum; Figure 14–5A) is transformed into an inhibitory message (pause in neural activity) in the internal segment of the globus pallidus because striatal neurons are inhibitory. However, because the output of the internal segment of the globus pallidus is also inhibitory, the amount of inhibition of the thalamus from the internal segment of the globus pallidus is reduced. Inhibition of an inhibitory signal is termed **disinhibition;** functionally, this double negative is equivalent to excitation. The thalamic response shown is transiently released from inhibition and fires a burst of action potentials. In a motor behavior such as reaching for a glass of water,

neurons in premotor areas, as well as corticospinal tract neurons in primary motor cortex, are thought to be excited by the actions of the direct path.

The indirect path has the opposite effect on the thalamus and cerebral cortex as the direct path. Putamen neurons of the indirect path, which are inhibitory because they contain GABA, project to the **external segment of the globus pallidus.** Excitation of the striatal neurons inhibits the external segment of the globus pallidus (pause in action potentials). Because the output of the external segment of the globus pallidus is inhibitory, indirect path neurons of the putamen disinhibit the subthalamic nucleus (burst of action potentials). This disinhibition will excite the internal segment of the globus pallidus and substantia nigra pars reticulata (which are both inhibitory) and thereby increase the strength of the inhibitory output signal directed to the thalamus.

Dopamine excites striatal neurons of the direct path and inhibits striatal neurons of the indirect path. Despite these different actions on striatal neurons, the effect of dopamine on either path is to reduce the inhibitory output of the basal ganglia, thereby reducing inhibition of the thalamus. This effect promotes movement generation by the thalamocortical circuits.

The power of this model is that it helps to explain the mechanisms of some **hypokinetic** and **hyperkinetic signs** seen in basal ganglia disease. Dopamine is deficient in Parkinson disease, which produces

hypokinetic signs. Reduced striatal dopamine in Parkinson disease would be expected to diminish the excitatory effects of the direct path on cortical motor areas and enhance the inhibitory effects of the indirect path (Figure 14–5C1). Together these effects would drastically reduce the thalamic signals to the cortex. For the premotor and motor cortical areas, this would reduce cortical outflow along the corticospinal and corticobulbar tracts and reduce production of motor behaviors (ie, hypokinesia).

In hyperkinetic disorders, the opposite changes take place (Figure 14–5C2): There are enhanced excitatory effects of the indirect path on the cortex. (Note that the output of the substantia nigra pars compactor may be normal.) In Huntington disease, recent studies suggest that striatal neurons of the indirect path, which contain both GABA and enkephalin, are lost (low neural response). This cell loss would result in greater thalamic outflow to the cortex by decreasing striatal inhibition of the external segment of the globus pallidus. Hemiballism, another hyperkinetic disorder, is produced by a subthalamic nucleus lesion. This nucleus normally exerts an excitatory action on the internal segment of the globus pallidus. When the subthalamic nucleus becomes lesioned, the internal segment of the globus pallidus would be expected to inhibit the thalamus less (thin dashed line), thereby increasing outflow to the cerebral cortex.

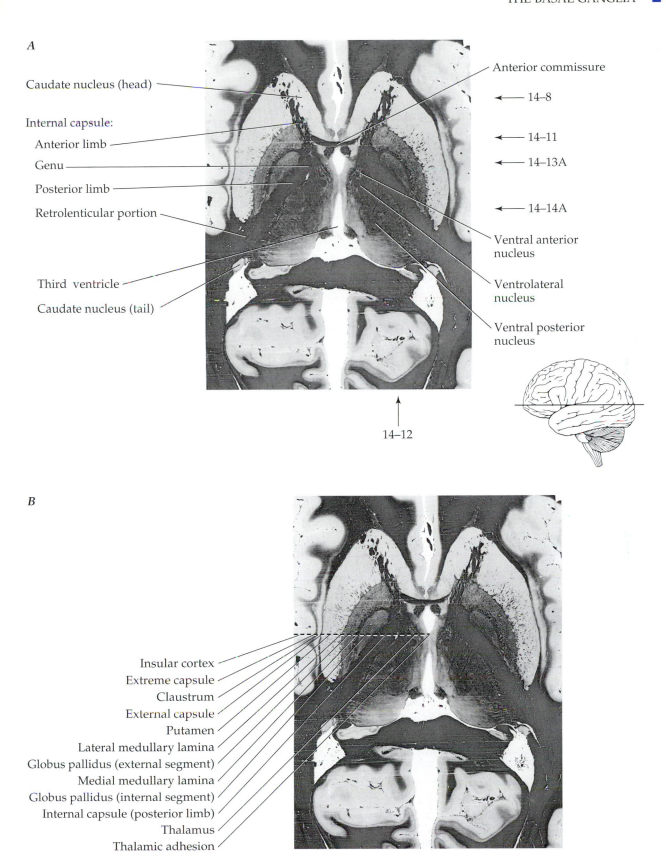

A

Caudate nucleus (head)

Internal capsule:

Anterior limb

Genu

Posterior limb

Retrolenticular portion

Third ventricle

Caudate nucleus (tail)

Anterior commissure

← 14–8

← 14–11

← 14–13A

← 14–14A

Ventral anterior nucleus

Ventrolateral nucleus

Ventral posterior nucleus

14–12

B

Insular cortex
Extreme capsule
Claustrum
External capsule
Putamen
Lateral medullary lamina
Globus pallidus (external segment)
Medial medullary lamina
Globus pallidus (internal segment)
Internal capsule (posterior limb)
Thalamus
Thalamic adhesion

Figure 14–6. Deep structures of the cerebral hemispheres and the diencephalon. *A.* Myelin-stained horizontal section through the cerebral hemispheres. The locations of sections illustrated in Figures 14–8, 14–11, 14–12, 14–13, and 14–14A are indicated. *B.* Structures encountered along a path from the lateral brain surface to the midline.

Retrolenticular and
sublenticular portions

Posterior limb

Caudate nucleus

Genu

Anterior
limb

Putamen

Nucleus
accumbens

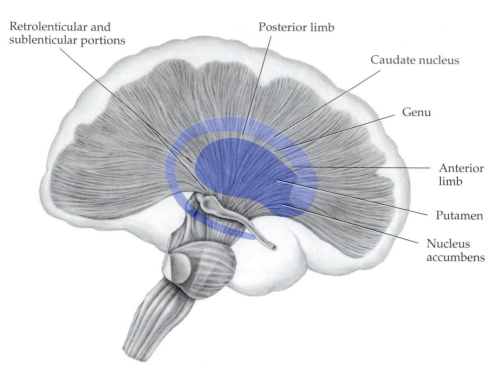

Figure 14–7. Three-dimensional view of the internal capsule of the right hemisphere. The striatum is shown in blue. The caudate nucleus (light blue) is medial to the internal capsule, and the putamen and nucleus accumbens (dark blue) are lateral. (*Adapted from Carpenter MB, Sutin J: Human Neuroanatomy. Williams & Wilkins, 1983.*)

Figure 14–6 also shows the locations of major structures of the cerebral hemispheres and diencephalon. A useful exercise for examining regional anatomy is to identify the various deep structures, beginning laterally and proceeding toward the midline. The sequence of these structures is labeled on Figure 14–6B:

1. **Insular cortex.** Contains part of the cortical representations for taste, viscerosensations, and vestibular function and is an important region for processing pain.
2. **Extreme capsule.** Thin lamina of white matter that contains corticocortical association fibers.
3. **Claustrum.** Thin sheet of neurons that are reciprocally and topographically connected with the cerebral cortex.
4. **External capsule.** Thin sheet of white matter that contains corticocortical association fibers.
5. **Putamen.** Component of the striatum important in movement control.
6. **Lateral medullary lamina.** Axons that separate the putamen from the external segment of the globus pallidus.
7. **External segment of the globus pallidus.** Projects to the subthalamic nucleus.
8. **Medial medullary lamina.** Separates the external and internal segments of the globus pallidus.
9. **Internal segment of the globus pallidus.** Projects to the thalamus and pedunculopontine nucleus.

10. **Posterior limb of the internal capsule.** Contains descending corticospinal axons as well as other descending fibers and ascending thalamocortical fibers.
11. **Thalamus.** Contains the principal sensory and motor relay nuclei for the cerebral cortex.
12. **Thalamic adhesion.** A small portion of the thalamus that physically adheres to its counterpart on the contralateral side, spanning the third ventricle.

An important feature of the complex three-dimensional structure of the caudate nucleus can be identified in Figure 14–6. Because the caudate nucleus has a C-shape, it can be seen in two locations in this section. The head of the caudate nucleus is located rostromedially, and the tail of the caudate nucleus is located caudolaterally. (The body of the caudate nucleus is dorsal to the plane of section.) In certain coronal sections the caudate nucleus is also seen in two locations (dorsomedially and ventrolaterally) (see below).

Cell Bridges Link the Caudate Nucleus and the Putamen

A coronal slice through the anterior limb of the internal capsule reveals the three components of the striatum (Figure 14–8): the **caudate nucleus** (at this level, the head of the caudate nucleus); the **putamen;**

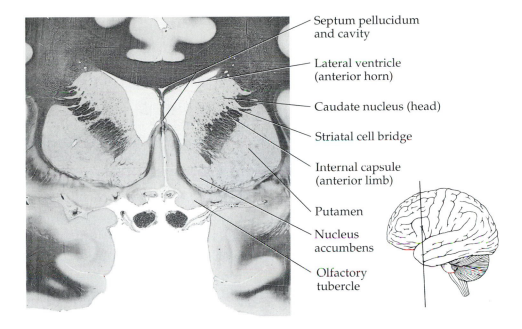

Figure 14–8. Myelin-stained coronal section through the head of the caudate nucleus. The inset shows the plane of section.

Septum pellucidum and cavity

Lateral ventricle (anterior horn)

Caudate nucleus (head)

Striatal cell bridge

Internal capsule (anterior limb)

Putamen

Nucleus accumbens

Olfactory tubercle

and the **nucleus accumbens.** Although the internal capsule courses between the caudate nucleus and the putamen, **striatal cell bridges** link the two structures. These cell bridges are a reminder that, in the developing brain (see Chapter 3), axons coursing to and from the cortex incompletely divide the group developing neurons in the floor of the lateral ventricle that give rise to the striatum. The nucleus accumbens, together with the ventromedial portions of the caudate nucleus and putamen (Figure 14–8), comprise the **ventral striatum,** the striatal component of the limbic loop (Figure 14–3A4). (The olfactory tubercle is sometimes included within the ventral striatum; it is located on the basal surface of the forebrain. A portion of the tubercle receives olfactory inputs.)

The **septum pellucidum** is a thin connective tissue membrane that forms the medial walls of the anterior horn and body of the lateral ventricles (Figure 14–8). Between the two septa is a cavity in which fluid may accumulate. The cavity is large in the fetus, and it can be imaged noninvasively using ultrasound. Normal variation exists in the size of the cavity in mature brains. However, the cavity is consistently large in certain pathological conditions, for example, in the brains of boxers who have dementia pugilistica, a degenerative condition similar to Parkinson disease.

The Striatum Has a Compartmental Organization

In myelin-stained sections the three striatal components appear identical and homogeneous. Histochem-

ical staining also demonstrates similarities in the overall appearance of the striatum. For example, each striatal component stains positive for the enzyme **acetylcholinesterase,** a marker for the neurotransmitter **acetylcholine** (Figure 14–9A), or **enkephalin** (Figure 14–9B).

Histochemical staining, however, also reveals a striking lack of homogeneity in which neurotransmitters and neuromodulators have a nonuniform distribution within local regions of the components of the striatum. For acetylcholinesterase, a **matrix** of tissue that contains a higher concentration surrounds patches, also called **striasomes,** of low concentration (Figure 14–9A). Enkephalin, as well as numerous other neuroactive substances present in the striatum, also has a patchy distribution (Figure 14–9B). The functional significance of striatal compartmentalization has remained elusive and is among the most important of the many unresolved questions concerning basal ganglia organization. Recent experimental findings have shown that neurons in the matrix and striasomal compartments have different connections. The striasomes receive their major cortical input from the limbic association cortex and project to the substantia nigra pars compacta.

The projections of cortical neurons also have a nonuniform distribution to local striatal regions. This distribution is shown (for the rhesus monkey) in Figure 14–9C for projections from the prefrontal association cortex to the head of the caudate nucleus. Other studies have shown that the unlabeled regions receive projections from other cortical association areas, such as the posterior parietal cortex.

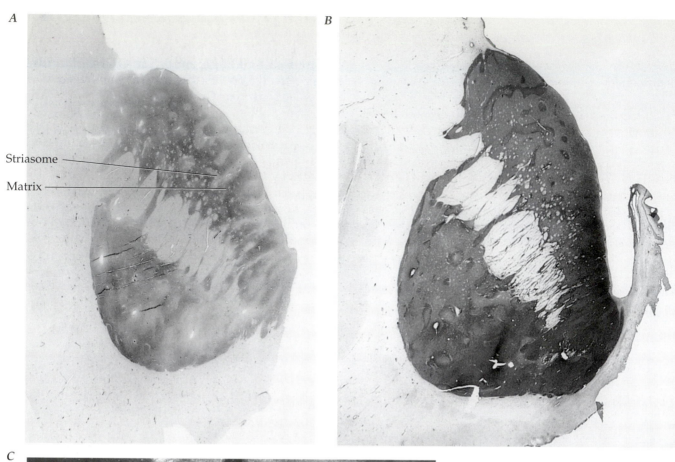

Striasome

Matrix

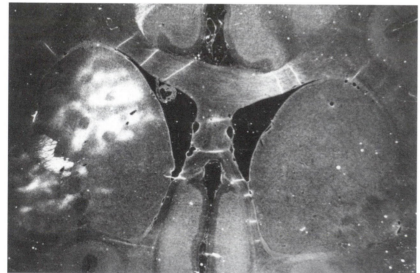

Figure 14–9. Histochemical localization of acetylcholinesterase (*A*) and enkephalin (*B*) in the human striatum. *C.* Autoradiograph of the cerebral hemispheres, showing the patchy distribution of labeled corticostriatal axon terminals in the head of the caudate nucleus of the rhesus monkey. In the center of the figure is the corpus callosum, with the cingulate gyri above and the anterior horns of the lateral ventricles below. As in the human, the head of the caudate nucleus bulges into the anterior horn of the lateral ventricle. Radioactive tracer, consisting of a mixture of ^{3}H proline and ^{3}H leucine, was injected into the prefrontal cortex. Tracer was incorporated into cortical neurons and transported anterogradely to their axons and terminals. This process resulted in an intricate pattern of labeling in the caudate nucleus. Axons were labeled in the white matter, including in the corpus callosum, because the tracer labels callosal neurons as well as a variety of descending projection neurons. (*A and* **B,** *Courtesy of Dr. Suzanne Haber, University of Rochester School of Medicine.* **C,** *Courtesy of Dr. Patricia Goldman-Rakic; Goldman-Rakic PS: Neuronal plasticity in primate telencephalon: Anomalous projections induced by prenatal removal of frontal cortex. Science 1978;202:768–770.*)

*The Head of the Caudate Nucleus
Is a Radiological Landmark*

The head of the caudate nucleus bulges into the anterior horn of the lateral ventricle (Figure 14–8). This can be seen on a magnetic resonance imaging (MRI) scan of a normal individual (Figure 14–10, right). Gross changes in the structure of the caudate nucleus in a patient with Huntington disease also can be seen (Figure 14–10, left). Patients with Huntington disease exhibit a loss of **medium spiny neurons.** This cell loss begins in the caudate nucleus and dorsal putamen. Because these neurons constitute more than three quarters of striatal neurons, in patients with Huntington disease the characteristic bulge of the head of the caudate nucleus into the lateral ventricle is absent.

The External Segment of the Globus Pallidus and the Ventral Pallidum Are Separated by the Anterior Commissure

The external segment of the globus pallidus, as discussed earlier, is an intrinsic basal ganglia nucleus that sends its axons to the subthalamic nucleus. The ventral pallidum is the output nucleus for the limbic loop. The external segment of the globus pallidus and the ventral pallidum are separated by the **anterior commissure** (Figure 14–11). This commissure, like the corpus callosum, interconnects regions of the cerebral cortex of either hemisphere. Unlike the corpus callosum, which connects wide regions of the frontal, parietal, occipital, and posterior temporal lobes, the anterior commissure interconnects specific regions: the

Figure 14–10. Magnetic resonance imaging scans of brain slices through the head of the caudate nucleus of a patient with Huntington disease (*left*). Note that the head of the caudate nucleus is smaller in the patient with Huntington disease compared with a normal individual (*right*). The imaging planes and locations of the scans in *A* and *B* are similar to the planes of section and locations of the myelin-stained sections in Figures 14–8 and 14–6, respectively. (*Courtesy of Dr. Susan Folstein.*)

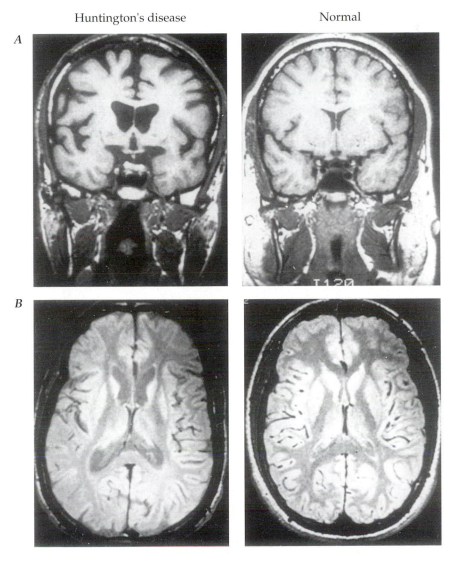

Huntington's disease   Normal

A

B

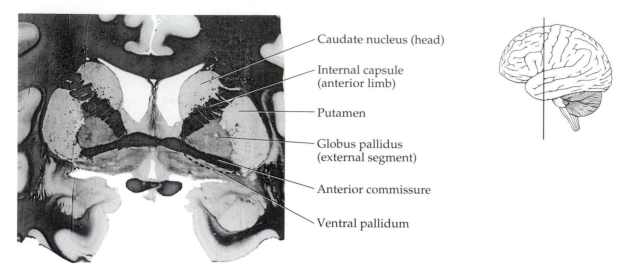

- Caudate nucleus (head)
- Internal capsule (anterior limb)
- Putamen
- Globus pallidus (external segment)
- Anterior commissure
- Ventral pallidum

Figure 14–11. Myelin-stained coronal section through the external segment of the globus pallidus and ventral pallidum. The inset shows the plane of section.

anterior temporal lobes (see Chapter 16), the **amygdaloid nuclear complex,** and several **olfactory structures** (see Chapter 9). Figure 14–12, a parasagittal section through the internal segment of the globus pallidus, shows that the ventral pallidum extends to the ventral brain surface.

The Ansa Lenticularis and the Lenticular Fasciculus Are Output Paths of the Internal Segment of the Globus Pallidus

Two major laminae separate components of the basal ganglia (Figure 14–13A). The **lateral medullary lamina** separates the external segment of the globus pallidus from the putamen, and the **medial medullary lamina** separates the internal and external segments of the globus pallidus. The internal segment of the globus pallidus is a major output of the basal ganglia. Neurosurgeons have been able to produce a lesion (by electrocoagulation) in the internal segment of the globus pallidus in patients with particularly severe Parkinson disease that does not respond well to drug therapy. By eliminating the abnormal output of the basal ganglia, this surgical procedure, termed **pallidotomy,** appears to help the remaining portions of the motor systems to function better. A neurophysiological procedure that has a similar beneficial effect is to implant a stimulating electrode within the internal segment of the globus pallidus and deliver high-frequency electrical stimulation. This appears to "jam" the circuitry and ameliorate the parkinsonian signs. Electrical stimulation in the region of the globus pallidus is also effective for treating other movement disorders. Neurons of the internal segment of the

globus pallidus project their axons to the thalamus (and brain stem, see below). These axons course in two anatomically separate pathways: the **lenticular fasciculus** and the **ansa lenticularis.** The axons of the lenticular fasciculus course directly through the internal capsule, but these axons are not clearly visualized until they collect medial to the internal capsule (Figure 14–13B).

The internal capsule appears to be a barrier for fibers of the ansa lenticularis; these fibers course around it to reach the thalamus (Figure 14–13A,B). The ansa lenticularis and lenticular fasciculus converge beneath the thalamus and join fibers of the cerebellothalamic tract to form the **thalamic fasciculus** (Figure 14–13B). An alternate nomenclature for lenticular and thalamic fasciculi is sometimes used. The lenticular fasciculus is also termed **Forel's field H2,** and the thalamic fasciculus is called **Forel's field H1.** A third Forel's field, termed **H,** is the region ventromedial to field H1 and is continuous with the tegmentum of the midbrain.

The three major thalamic targets of the output nuclei of the basal ganglia (see Figure 14–3A) can be identified in Figures 14–12 through 14–14: the **medial dorsal nucleus,** the **ventrolateral nucleus,** and the **ventral anterior nucleus.** Most of the fibers of the deep cerebellar nuclei also terminate in the ventrolateral nucleus but in a separate portion than axons from the basal ganglia. Two intralaminar thalamic nuclei (see Chapter 2), the **centromedian** and **parafascicular nuclei,** are anatomically closely related to the basal ganglia because they provide a major direct input to the striatum. These thalamic nuclei also project to the frontal lobe, which is the cortical target of the basal ganglia. Because the intralaminar nuclei have widespread cortical projections, they are diffuse-projecting thalamic nuclei and not relay nuclei.

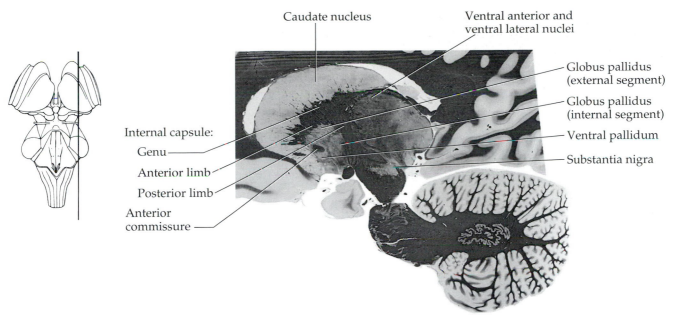

Figure 14–12. Myelin-stained parasagittal section through various components of the basal ganglia. The inset shows the plane of section.

Although GABA is present in both structures, the neuropeptide content of the internal segment of the globus pallidus is different from that of the external segment (Figure 14–15). **Substance P** is contained within the terminals of striatal neurons of the direct path and, therefore, is in greater abundance in the **internal segment of the globus pallidus.** By contrast, **enkephalin** is in striatal neurons of the indirect path and is restricted largely to the **external segment of the globus pallidus.**

Lesion of the Subthalamic Region Produces Hemiballism

Ventral to the thalamus is the subthalamic region, which consists of a disparate collection of nuclei. Two major nuclei in this poorly understood brain region are the **subthalamic nucleus** and **zona incerta** (Figure 14–14A). A lesion of the subthalamic nucleus produces **hemiballism** (see Box 14–1), characterized by ballistic movements of the contralateral limbs. By examining patients who have experienced small vascular accidents in this area, researchers know that the subthalamic nucleus is somatotopically organized. Damage to one portion may involve the upper limb, and damage to the other portion may involve the lower limb. The connections of the subthalamic nucleus are complex. Receiving input from the external segment of the globus pallidus as well as from the motor cortex, the subthalamic nucleus projects back to the **external and internal segments of the globus pallidus** (Figure

14–14B). The subthalamic nucleus is also a target of brain electrical stimulation, where activation of its excitatory output circuitry can have beneficial effects in Parkinson disease. The subthalamic nucleus is also reciprocally connected with the ventral pallidum.

Very little is known of the function of the zona incerta, a nuclear region interposed between the subthalamic nucleus and the thalamus. The zona incerta receives projections from a variety of sources, including the spinal cord and cerebellum. Many of the neurons in the zona incerta contain GABA and have diffuse cortical projections.

The Substantia Nigra Contains Two Anatomical Divisions

The posterior limb of the internal capsule separates the internal segment of the globus pallidus from the substantia nigra, a separation that can be seen in parasagittal (Figure 14–12) and coronal sections (Figure 14–14A). The **substantia nigra pars reticulata,** which is adjacent to the basis pedunculi, contains GABA (Figure 14–4). The substantia nigra pars reticulata, like the internal segment of the globus pallidus, also projects to the thalamus and pedunculopontine nucleus (see below). In addition, the substantia nigra projects to the superior colliculus (Figure 14–16A), which is important in controlling **saccadic eye movements** (see Chapter 12).

The other division of the substantia nigra is the **substantia nigra pars compacta,** which consists of neurons containing dopamine. The projection of these

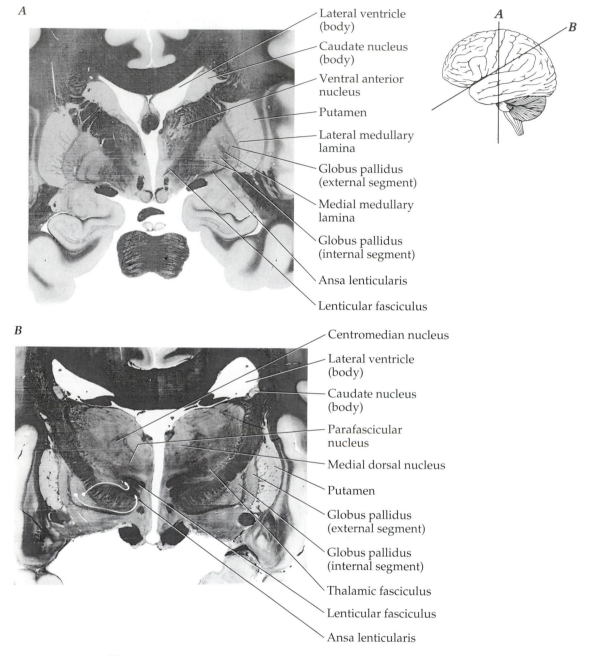

A

Lateral ventricle (body)
Caudate nucleus (body)
Ventral anterior nucleus
Putamen
Lateral medullary lamina
Globus pallidus (external segment)
Medial medullary lamina
Globus pallidus (internal segment)
Ansa lenticularis
Lenticular fasciculus

A
B

B

Centromedian nucleus
Lateral ventricle (body)
Caudate nucleus (body)
Parafascicular nucleus
Medial dorsal nucleus
Putamen
Globus pallidus (external segment)
Globus pallidus (internal segment)
Thalamic fasciculus
Lenticular fasciculus
Ansa lenticularis

Figure 14–13. Myelin-stained coronal (*A*) and oblique (*B*) sections through the internal and external segments of the globus pallidus. The inset shows the planes of section.

neurons to the striatum forms the **nigrostriatal tract.** Dopaminergic neurons that project to the different striatal regions are topographically organized. The dendrites of dopaminergic neurons—irrespective of their location within the substantia nigra pars compacta—extend into the substantia nigra pars reticulata. This arrangement is thought to be functionally important for integrating information between the various parallel loops. For example, the dopaminergic neurons can receive inputs to their distal and proximal dendrites from diverse sources and in turn influence wide areas of the striatum via their diffuse projections. The activity of many of the substantia nigra pars compacta neurons, shown in animal studies, is related to salient stimuli, such as a tone that predicts receiving a food reward, rather than particular features of the movement the animals perform. This salience reflects inputs from the **amygdala,** which is involved in motivation and emotions, and from the **reticular formation,** which is involved in arousal.

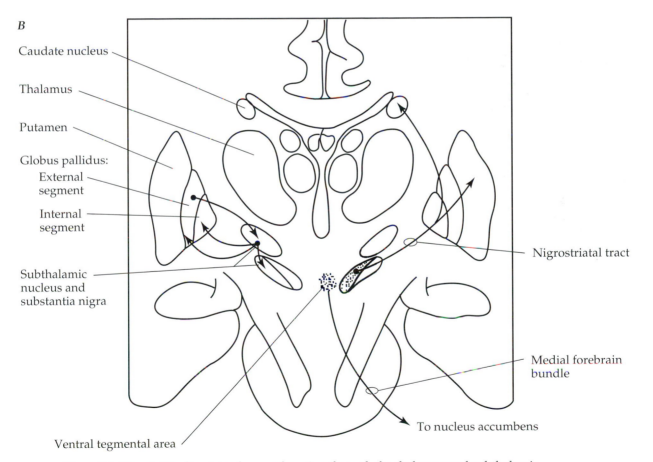

A. Lateral ventricle (body)

Caudate nucleus (body)

Putamen

Globus pallidus (external segment)

Globus pallidus (internal segment)

Caudate nucleus (tail)

Lateral ventricle (inferior horn)

Medial dorsal nucleus

Ventral lateral nucleus

Zona incerta

Subthalamic nucleus

Substantia nigra

Basis pedunculi

B

Caudate nucleus

Thalamus

Putamen

Globus pallidus:
External segment
Internal segment

Subthalamic nucleus and substantia nigra

Nigrostriatal tract

Medial forebrain bundle

To nucleus accumbens

Ventral tegmental area

Figure 14–14. *A.* Myelin-stained coronal section through the thalamus and subthalamic region. The inset shows the plane of section. *B.* Schematic line drawing of the myelin-stained section in *A.* The intrinsic connections of the basal ganglia are shown on the left, and the dopaminergic output is shown on the right.

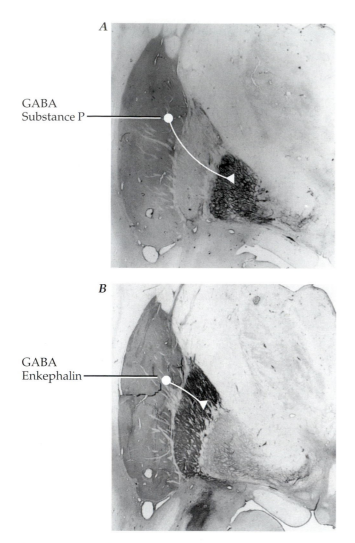

Figure 14–15. Histochemical localization of substance P–like immunoreactivity (*A*) and enkephalin-like immunoreactivity (*B*) in the human globus pallidus. (*Courtesy of Dr. Suzanne Haber, University of Rochester School of Medicine.*)

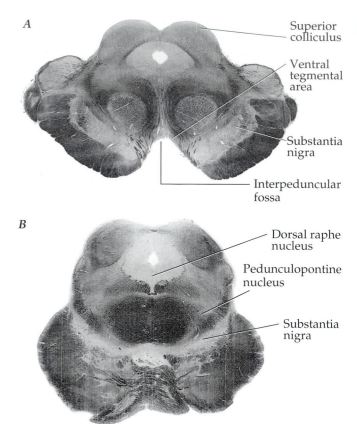

Figure 14–16. Myelin-stained transverse sections through the superior colliculus (*A*) and the inferior colliculus (*B*).

The substantia nigra pars compacta is not the only midbrain region that contains dopamine. The **ventral tegmental area** is dorsomedial to the substantia nigra, beneath the floor of the interpeduncular fossa (Figure 14–16A). Dopaminergic neurons in the ventral tegmental area send their axons to the striatum via the **medial forebrain bundle** (see Chapters 15 and 16) as well as to the frontal lobe (see Figure 2–2B1).

Two other brain stem nuclei are closely associated with the basal ganglia, the **pedunculopontine nucleus,** found at the junction of the pons and midbrain in the reticular formation, and the **dorsal raphe nucleus,** located in the caudal midbrain (Figure 14–16B). The output nuclei of the basal ganglia (the internal segment of the globus pallidus and the substantia nigra pars

reticulata) project to the pedunculopontine nucleus. This is the descending projection of the basal ganglia, and it is thought to play an important behavioral role. The pedunculopontine nucleus has diverse functions, including regulating arousal (through diffuse ascending projections to the thalamus and cortex) and movement control (through reticular formation connections and direct reticulospinal projections). Many of the neurons in this nucleus are **cholinergic,** including those projecting to the thalamus. The dorsal raphe nucleus gives rise to an ascending **serotonergic** projection to the striatum. In addition to projecting to the striatum, the dorsal raphe nucleus has extensive projections to most of the cerebral cortex and to other forebrain nuclei.

The Vascular Supply of the Basal Ganglia Is Provided by the Middle Cerebral Artery

As described in Chapter 4, the vascular supply to the deep structures of the cerebral hemispheres—the **thalamus, basal ganglia,** and **internal capsule**—is provided by branches of the internal carotid artery and the three cerebral arteries. Most of the striatum is supplied by perforating branches of the middle cerebral artery; however, rostromedial regions are supplied by perforating branches of the anterior cerebral artery (see Figures 4–5 and 4–7). Collectively these penetrating branches of the anterior and middle cerebral arteries are termed the **lenticulostriate arteries.** Most of the globus pallidus is supplied by the **anterior choroidal artery,** which is a branch of the internal carotid artery.

Summary

Basal Ganglia Nuclei

The basal ganglia contain numerous component nuclei (Figures 14–1 and 14–2) that can be divided into three groups based on their connections (Figure 14–1): input nuclei, output nuclei, and intrinsic nuclei. The **input nuclei** consist of the **caudate nucleus,** the **putamen,** and the **nucleus accumbens** (Figures 14–2, 14–8, and 14–11) and collectively are termed the **striatum.** The ventromedial portions of the caudate nucleus and putamen, together with the nucleus accumbens, comprise the **ventral striatum.** The **output nuclei** include the **internal segment of the globus pallidus** (Figures 14–12 and 14–14), the **ventral pallidum** (Figures 14–11 and 14–12), and the **substantia nigra pars reticulata** (Figure 14–16). The **intrinsic nuclei** include the **external segment of the globus pallidus** (Figures 14–11 and 14–12), the **subthalamic nucleus** (Figure 14–15), the **substantia nigra pars compacta** (Figure 14–16), and the **ventral tegmental area** (Figure 14–16A).

Basal Ganglia Functional Loops

The basic input-output pathway through the basal ganglia links wide regions of the cerebral cortex with, in sequence, the input nuclei of the basal ganglia (striatum), the output nuclei, the thalamus, and a portion of the frontal lobe (Figures 14–1 and 14–3). There are four key functional loops through the basal ganglia (Figure 14–3): the skeletomotor, oculomotor, prefrontal cortex, and limbic loops. The **skeletomotor** and **oculomotor loops** play important roles in the control of facial, limb, and trunk musculature and extraocular muscles; the **prefrontal cortex loop** may subserve tasks such as cognition and executive behavioral functions; and the **limbic loop** may function in the regulation of behavior and in emotions. The skeletomotor, oculomotor, and prefrontal cortex loops begin in the **somatic sensory, motor,** and **association areas** of the cerebral cortex and pass through the **caudate nucleus** and **putamen** (Fig-

ures 14–2, 14–6, and 14–8). The output nuclei of these loops are the **internal segment of the globus pallidus** (Figures 14–6, 14–12, and 14–13) and the **substantia nigra pars reticulata** (Figures 14–14 and 14–16). They, in turn, synapse in the **ventrolateral, ventral anterior,** and **medial dorsal nuclei** of the thalamus (Figures 14–6A, 14–12, and 14–14). The internal segment of the globus pallidus projects to the thalamus via two pathways: the **ansa lenticularis** and the **lenticular fasciculus** (Figure 14–13B). However, components of the various loops synapse on neurons located in different nuclei or in different portions of the same nuclei. The internal segment of the globus pallidus also projects to the pedunculopontine nucleus, which plays a role in arousal and movement control.

The **limbic loop** begins in the **limbic association cortex.** The **ventral striatum,** which comprises the nucleus accumbens and the ventromedial parts of the caudate nucleus and putamen (Figure 14–8), is the principal input nucleus of the limbic loop; the output and thalamic nuclei of the limbic loop are the **ventral pallidum** (Figure 14–12) and the **medial dorsal nucleus** (Figure 14–14).

The cortical targets of the four loops are (Figure 14–3B) **supplementary motor areas, premotor cortex,** and **primary motor cortex** for the skeletomotor loop; **frontal and supplementary eye fields** for the oculomotor loop; **prefrontal association cortex** for the association loop; and **anterior cingulate gyrus** (and **orbitofrontal gyri**) for the limbic loop.

Intrinsic Basal Ganglia Connections

The intrinsic nuclei have interconnections with the input and output nuclei. Dopaminergic neurons of the **substantia nigra pars compacta** (Figure 14–14) and **ventral tegmental area** project to the **striatum;** dopaminergic neurons of the ventral tegmental area also project directly to parts of the **frontal lobe.** The **external segment of the globus pallidus** projects to the **subthalamic nucleus,** which projects to the **internal** and **external segments of the globus pallidus,** the **substantia nigra pars reticulata** (Figure 14–14B), and the **ventral pallidum.**

Related Sources

Brust JCM: The Practice of Neural Science. McGraw-Hill; 2000. (See ch. 4; ch. 12, cases 35, 36; ch. 16, cases 75–78.)

DeLong MR: The basal ganglia. In Kandel ER, Schwartz JH, Jessell TM (editors): Principles of Neural Science, 4th ed. McGraw-Hill; 2000:853–867.

Selected Readings

Alexander GE, Crutcher MD: Functional architecture of basal ganglia circuits: Neural substrates of parallel processing. Trends Neurosci 1990;13:266–271.

Bergman H, Feingold A, Nini A, et al: Physiological aspects of information processing in the basal ganglia of normal and parkinsonian primates. Trends Neurosci 1998;21: 32–38.

Bolam JP, Hanley JJ, Booth PA, Bevan MD: Synaptic organisation of the basal ganglia. J Anat 2000;196:527–542.

Chesselet MF, Delfs JM: Basal ganglia and movement disorders: An update. Trends Neurosci 1996;19:417–422.

DeLong MR: Primate modes of movement disorders of basal ganglia origin. Trends Neurosci 1990;13:281–285.

Gerfen CR: The neostriatal matrix: Multiple levels of compartmental organization. Trends Neurosci 1992;15:133–139.

Gerfen CR: Molecular effects of dopamine on striatal-projection pathways. Trends Neurosci 2000;23:S64–70.

Graybiel AM: Neurotransmitters and neuromodulators in the basal ganglia. Trends Neurosci 1990;13:244–254.

Haber SN, McFarland NR: The concept of the ventral striatum in nonhuman primates. Ann N Y Acad Sci 1999; 877:33–48.

Jueptner M, Weiller C: A review of differences between basal ganglia and cerebellar control of movements as revealed by functional imaging studies. Brain 1998;121: 1437–1449.

Pahapill PA, Lozano AM: The pedunculopontine nucleus and Parkinson's disease. Brain 2000;123:1767–1783.

Parent A, Sato F, Wu Y, Gauthier J, Levesque M, Parent M: Organization of the basal ganglia: The importance of axonal collateralization. Trends Neurosci 2000;23:S20–27.

Paus T: Primate anterior cingulate cortex: Where motor control, drive and cognition interface. Nat Rev Neurosci 2001;2:417–424.

Special issue on the basal ganglia, Parkinson's disease and levodopa therapy. Trends Neurosci 2000;23:S1–S126.

References

Alheld GF, Heimer L, Switzer RC III: Basal ganglia. In Paxinos G (editor): The Human Nervous System. Academic Press; 1990:483–582.

Bevan MD, Smith AD, Bolam JP: The substantia nigra as a site of synaptic integration of functionally diverse information arising from the ventral pallidum and the globus pallidus in the rat. Neuroscience 1996;75:5–12.

Charara A, Smith Y, Parent A: Glutamatergic inputs from the pedunculopontine nucleus to midbrain dopaminergic neurons in primates: Phaseolus vulgaris-leucoagglutinin anterograde labeling combined with postembedding glutamate and GABA immunohistochemistry. J Comp Neurol 1996;364:254–266.

Goldman-Rakic PS: Neuronal plasticity in primate telencephalon: Anomalous projections induced by prenatal removal of frontal cortex. Science 1978;202:768–770.

Gusella JF, Wexler NS, Conneally PM, et al: A polymorphic DNA marker genetically linked to Huntington's disease. Nature 1983;306:234–238.

Haber SN: Neurotransmitters in the human and nonhuman primate basal ganglia. Human Neurobiology 1986;5:159–168.

Haber SN, Fudge JL, McFarland N: Striatonigrostriatal pathways in primates form an ascending spiral from the shell to the dorsolateral striatum. J Neurosci 2000;20: 2369–2382.

Haber SN, Groenewegen HJ, Grove EA, et al: Efferent connections of the ventral pallidum: Evidence of a dual striato-pallidofugal pathway. J Comp Neurol 1985;235: 322–335.

Haber SN, Watson SJ: The comparative distribution of enkephalin, dynorphin and substance P in the human globus pallidus and basal forebrain. Neuroscience 1985; 4:1011–1024.

Hoover JE, Strick PL: Multiple output channels in basal ganglia. Science 1993;259:819–821.

Hoover JE, Strick PL: The organization of cerebellar and basal ganglia outputs to primary motor cortex as revealed by retrograde transneuronal transport of herpes simplex virus type 1. J Neurosci 1999;19:1446–1463.

Kowianski P, Dziewiatkowski J, Kowianska J, Morys J: Comparative anatomy of the claustrum in selected species: A morphometric analysis. Brain Behav Evol 1999; 53:44–54.

Macchi G, Jones EG: Toward an agreement on terminology of nuclear and subnuclear divisions of the motor thalamus. J Neurosurg 1997;86:670–685.

McFarland N, Haber SN: Organization of thalamostriatal terminals from the ventral motor nuclei in the macaque. J Comp Neurol 2001;429:321–336.

Middleton FA, Strick PL: Anatomical evidence for cerebellar and basal ganglia involvement in higher cognitive function. Science 1994;266:458–461.

Middleton FA, Strick PL: The temporal lobe is a target of output from the basal ganglia. Proc Natl Acad Sci U S A 1996;93:8683–8687.

Middleton FA, Strick PL: Basal ganglia and cerebellar loops: Motor and cognitive circuits. Brain Res Brain Res Rev 2000;31:236–250.

Poirier LJ, Giguère M, Marchand R: Comparative morphology of the substantia nigra and ventral tegmental area in the monkey, cat and rat. Brain Res Bull 1983;11:371–397.

Reiner A, Albin RL, Anderson KD, D'Amato CJ, Penney JB, Young AB: Differential loss of striatal projection neurons in Huntington disease. Proc Natl Acad Sci U S A 1988; 85:5733–5737.

Romanski LM, Giguere M, Bates JF, Goldman-Rakic PS: Topographic organization of medial pulvinar connections with the prefrontal cortex in the rhesus monkey. J Comp Neurol 1997;379:313–332.

Schell GR, Strick PL: The origin of thalamic inputs to the arcuate premotor and supplementary motor areas. J Neurosci 1984;4:539–560.

Schutz W, Romo R: Dopamine neurons of the monkey midbrain: Contingencies of response to stimuli eliciting immediate behavioral reactions. J Neurophysiol 1990;63: 607–624.

Selemon LD, Goldman-Rakic PS: Longitudinal topography and interdigitation of corticostriatal projections in the rhesus monkey. J Neurosci 1985;5:776–794.

Stern CE, Passingham RE: The nucleus accumbens in monkeys (Macaca fascicularis): I. The organization of behaviour. Behav Brain Res 1994;61:9–21.

Yeterian EH, Van Hoesen GW: Cortico-striate projections in the rhesus monkey: The organization of certain cortico-caudate connections. Brain Res 1978;139:43–63.

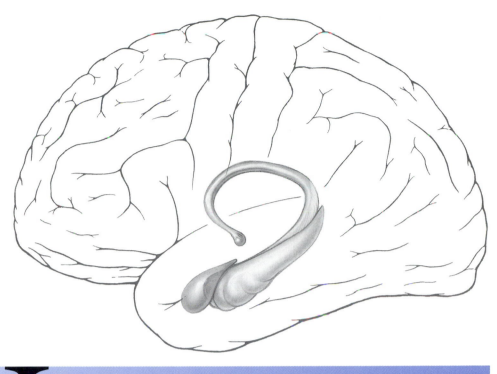

IV Integrative Systems

15

The Hypothalamus and Regulation of Endocrine and Visceral Functions

THE HYPOTHALAMUS IS CRUCIAL FOR MAINTAINING normal organ function and for producing many of the behaviors necessary to meet basic needs such as feeding, drinking, and mating. The hypothalamus thus ensures survival of the individual and its species. Using information about the body's internal state, about emotions, and about critical environmental stimuli, the hypothalamus accomplishes its tasks by controlling hormone production and the functions of the autonomic nervous system. Virtually every body organ depends on the hypothalamus for some aspect of control. Hypothalamic functions also impact cycles of sleep and wakefulness, and when and how much is eaten. In animals the hypothalamus controls sexual responsiveness and maternal care (eg, nursing). It can only be speculated how much of human sexual behavior depends on the hypothalamus. The hypothalamus also helps to organize the body's reactions to disease, such as fever production in response to infection.

The anatomical circuitry underlying the neural control of endocrine and organ functions is beginning to be unraveled, with the aid of techniques for assessing both the projections of hypothalamic neurons and their biochemistry. This chapter first considers neuroendocrine functions and the pituitary gland. Next, the chapter surveys the organization of the autonomic nervous system and examines the control of autonomic function by the hypothalamus. Chapter 16 considers the role of the hypothalamus in motivational and appetitive behavior, along with other brain structures that constitute the limbic system.

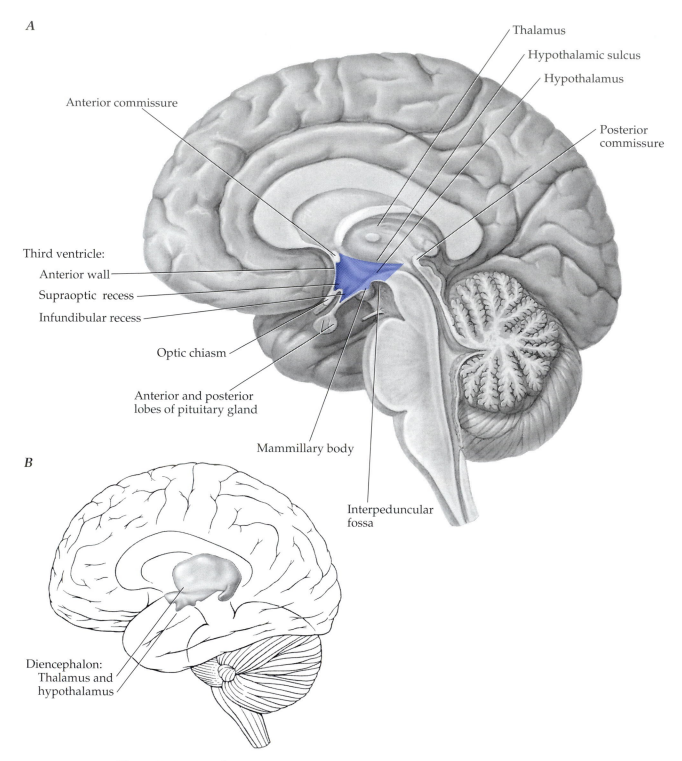

A

Thalamus

Hypothalamic sulcus

Hypothalamus

Posterior commissure

Anterior commissure

Third ventricle:

Anterior wall

Supraoptic recess

Infundibular recess

Optic chiasm

Anterior and posterior lobes of pituitary gland

Mammillary body

Interpeduncular fossa

B

Diencephalon:
Thalamus and
hypothalamus

Figure 15–1. A midsagittal view of the brain, showing key structures in and around the hypothalamus. The inset is a view of the lateral surface of the cerebral hemisphere and brain stem, illustrating the location of the hypothalamus and thalamus.

FUNCTIONAL ANATOMY OF THE NEUROENDOCRINE SYSTEMS

The Hypothalamus Is Divided Into Three Functionally Distinct Mediolateral Zones

The hypothalamus, a key component of the diencephalon, is ventral to the thalamus (Figure 15–1). The third ventricle separates the two halves of the hypothalamus. On its medial, or ventricular, surface the hypothalamus is distinguished from the thalamus by a shallow groove, the **hypothalamic sulcus.** Anteriorly, the hypothalamus extends a bit beyond the anterior wall of the third ventricle (the lamina terminalis; see Chapter 3). The hypothalamus reaches as far caudally as the **mammillary bodies,** paired structures on the ventral hypothalamic surface (Figure 15–2).

The functions of the hypothalamus are organized by projection neurons in discrete nuclei, or small groups of nuclei, that interface with effector systems in other parts of the central nervous system. These hypothalamic nuclei are arranged into three mediolateral zones (Figure 15–3):

1. The **periventricular zone** is the most medial and comprises thin nuclei that border the third ventricle. This zone is important in regulating the release of **endocrine hormones** from the anterior pituitary gland.
2. The **middle zone** serves diverse functions. It contains nuclei that regulate the release of **vasopressin** and **oxytocin** from the posterior pituitary gland. It is also a major site for neurons that regulate the **autonomic nervous system.**

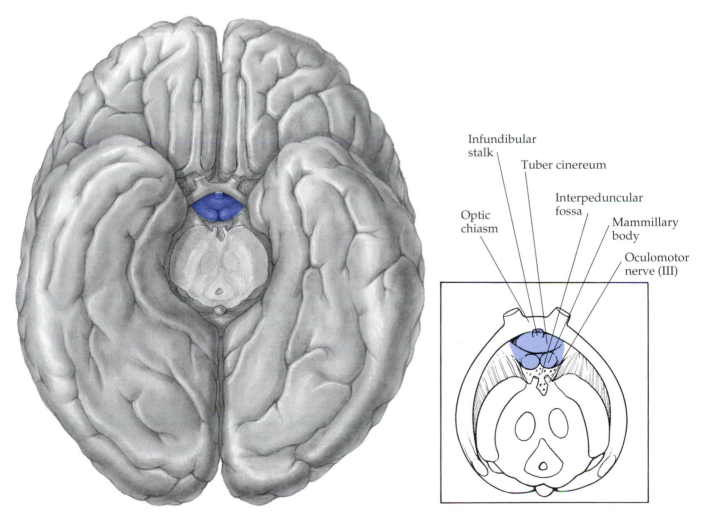

Figure 15–2. The basal surface of the brain. The inset shows the key features of the basal surface of the hypothalamus. The tuber cinereum is a swelling surrounding the base of the infundibular stalk and contains many hypothalamic nuclei that regulate the release of anterior pituitary hormones.

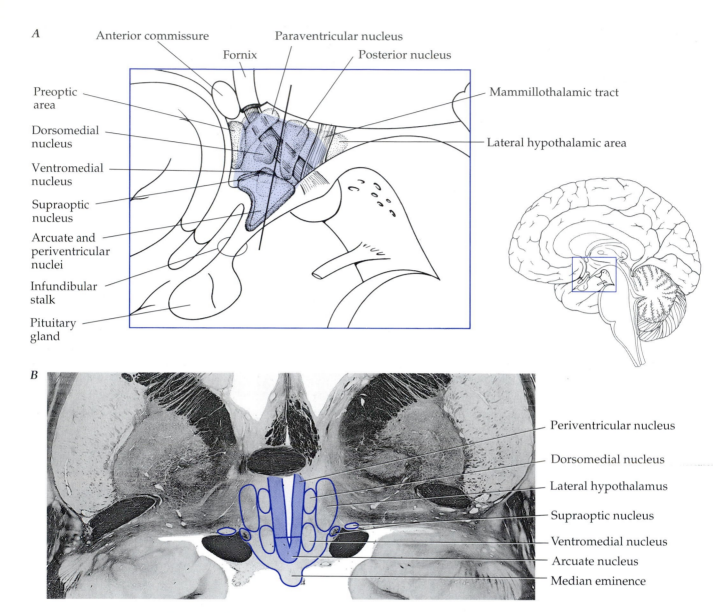

A

Anterior commissure

Fornix

Paraventricular nucleus

Posterior nucleus

Preoptic area

Dorsomedial nucleus

Ventromedial nucleus

Supraoptic nucleus

Arcuate and periventricular nuclei

Infundibular stalk

Pituitary gland

Mammillothalamic tract

Lateral hypothalamic area

B

Periventricular nucleus

Dorsomedial nucleus

Lateral hypothalamus

Supraoptic nucleus

Ventromedial nucleus

Arcuate nucleus

Median eminence

Figure 15–3. **A.** The major nuclei are illustrated in a cutaway view of the hypothalamus. The inset shows the region illustrated in the internal view. Only the locations of the arcuate and periventricular nuclei of this zone are shown. The remaining nuclei form a thin veil beneath the walls and floor of the third ventricle. The middle and lateral zones are the two other hypothalamic zones. The line shows the plane of section in **B. B.** Myelin-stained coronal section through the hypothalamus. The approximate locations of the key hypothalamic nuclei are shown. The periventricular and arcuate nuclei comprise the periventricular zone. The other nuclei form the middle and lateral hypothalamic zones. (**A,** *Adapted from Nauta WJH, Haymaker W: Hypothalamic nuclei and fiber connections. In Haymaker W, Anderson E, Nauta WJH (editors): The Hypothalamus. Charles C. Thomas; 1969:136–209.)*

The body's circadian rhythms are driven by neurons in this zone, as are aspects of the control of wakefulness.

3. The **lateral zone** contains neurons that integrate information from telencephalic structures engaged in emotions and transmit this information to other parts of the brain, as well as to other hypothalamic nuclei. This zone is important in the behavioral expression of emotions. The lateral zone is separated from the medial zone by the **fornix,** a tract that interconnects limbic system structures. The lateral zone is considered in greater detail in Chapter 16.

Separate Parvocellular and Magnocellular Neurosecretory Systems Regulate Hormone Release From the Anterior and Posterior Lobes of the Pituitary

The pituitary gland is connected to the ventral surface of the hypothalamus by the **infundibular stalk** (Figure 15–3A). In humans, two major anatomical divisions of the pituitary gland mediate the release of distinct sets of hormones (Figure 15–4): the **anterior lobe** (also called the adenohypophysis; see Table 15–1) and the **posterior lobe** (or neurohypophysis). A third lobe, the intermediate lobe, although prominent in many simpler mammals, is vestigial in humans.

The anterior and posterior lobes are parts of two distinct neurosecretory systems, and hormone release from these lobes is regulated by different populations of hypothalamic neurons. The anterior lobe is part of the **parvocellular neurosecretory system** (Figure 15–4A). Small-diameter hypothalamic neurons in numerous nuclei regulate hormone release by epithelial secretory cells of the anterior pituitary into the systemic circulation. Parvocellular neurosecretory neurons are located predominantly in nuclei of the **periventricular zone.** By contrast, the posterior lobe is part of the **magnocellular neurosecretory system** (Figure 15–4B).

Here, axons of large-diameter hypothalamic neurons in two nuclei project into the posterior lobe, where peptide hormones are released from their terminals directly onto capillaries of the systemic circulation. Magnocellular neurosecretory neurons are located in the **middle zone.**

Regulatory Peptides Released Into the Portal Circulation by Hypothalamic Neurons Control Secretion of Anterior Lobe Hormones

The process by which the hypothalamus stimulates anterior lobe secretory cells to release their hormones (or to inhibit release) is quite unlike mechanisms of neural action considered in earlier chapters. Rather than synapse on anterior lobe secretory cells, the hypothalamic parvocellular neurosecretory neurons terminate on capillaries of the **pituitary portal circulation** in the floor of the third ventricle (Figure 15–5).

A portal circulatory system is distinguished by the presence of separate **portal veins** interposed between two sets of capillaries. The first set is located in a region termed the **median eminence,** which is part of the proximal infundibular stalk. The portal veins are located in the distal part of the infundibular stalk. The second set of capillaries is found in the anterior

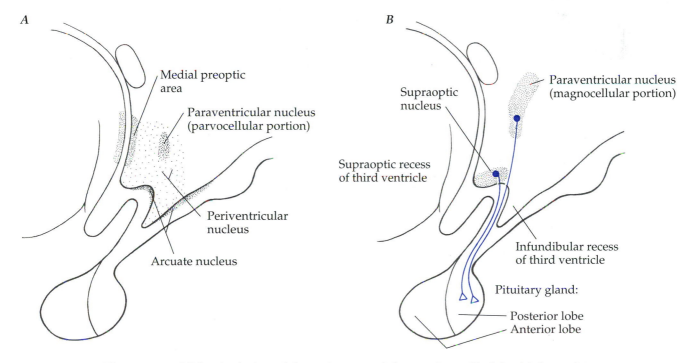

A

Medial preoptic area

Paraventricular nucleus (parvocellular portion)

Periventricular nucleus

Arcuate nucleus

B

Supraoptic nucleus

Paraventricular nucleus (magnocellular portion)

Supraoptic recess of third ventricle

Infundibular recess of third ventricle

Pituitary gland:

Posterior lobe
Anterior lobe

Figure 15–4. Midsagittal view of the region around the anterior wall of the third ventricle, showing the location of neurons of the parvocellular system (*A*). In *B*, neurons constituting the magnocellular system are shown along with the path their axons take to reach the posterior lobe of the pituitary gland.

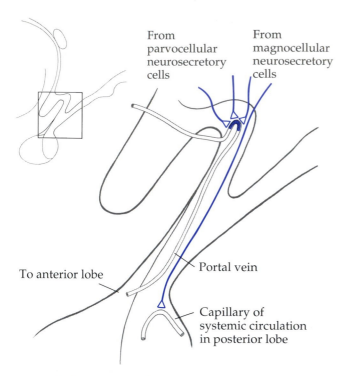

From parvocellular neurosecretory cells

From magnocellular neurosecretory cells

To anterior lobe

Portal vein

Capillary of systemic circulation in posterior lobe

Figure 15–5. The hypothalamus, pituitary gland, and rostral and ventral portions of the third ventricle are shown in this schematic drawing of the midsagittal brain surface. The region indicated by the box is enlarged below to show the organization of the parvocellular and magnocellular neurosecretory systems in relation to the portal circulation. The region of the primary capillaries of the hypophyseal portal system is indicated in dark blue. These vessels derive from the superior hypophyseal arteries, which are branches of the internal carotid and posterior communicating arteries.

pituitary. (In the systemic circulation, such as the vascular supply of the rest of the brain, capillary beds are interposed between arterial and venous systems.)

Parvocellular neurons release chemicals, most of which are peptides, that either promote (**releasing hormones**) or inhibit (**release-inhibiting hormones**) the release of hormones from anterior lobe secretory cells (Table 15–1). Release or release-inhibiting hormones are carried to the anterior lobe in the portal veins (Figure 15–5), where they act directly on epithelial secretory cells.

An analogy can be drawn between the capillaries in the median eminence and the integrative function of spinal motor neurons (see Chapter 10). Separate descending pathways and spinal interneuronal systems synapse on the motor neuron. Thus the motor neuron is the final common pathway for the integration of neuronal information controlling skeletal muscle. The final common pathway for control of anterior lobe hormone release comprises the capillaries of the median eminence. This is because different hypothalamic neurons secrete releasing or release-inhibiting hormones into the capillaries of the median eminence (Figure 15–5), and summation of neurohormones occurs at this vascular site.

The distribution of neurons that project to the median eminence has been examined extensively in rodents. Although these neurons are widespread, the major sources are located in nuclei within the **periventricular zone** (Figures 15–3B and 15–4A). Among the major sources, and the hormones they release, are the following:

- The **arcuate nucleus** contains neurons that release gonadotropin-releasing hormone, luteinizing hormone–releasing hormone, somatostatin, and adrenocorticotropic hormone.
- Neurons in the **periventricular portion** of the **parvocellular nucleus** (which lies along the third ventricle) contain corticotropin-releasing hormone.
- The **periventricular nucleus** provides gonadotropin-releasing hormone, luteinizing hormone–releasing hormone, and dopamine (which inhibits prolactin release).
- The **medial preoptic area** contains parvocellular neurons that secrete luteinizing hormone–releasing hormone.

In addition, there are extrahypothalamic sources of releasing and release-inhibiting neurohormones. For

Table 15–1. Anterior pituitary hormones and substances that control their release.

Anterior pituitary hormones	Releasing hormones (RH)	Release-inhibiting hormones (RIH)
Growth hormone	Growth hormone RH	Growth hormone RIH (somatostatin)
Lutenizing hormone	Gonadotropin RH	
Follicle-stimulating hormone	Gonadotropin RH	
Thyrotropin	Thyrotropin RH (TRH)	Growth hormone RIH (somatostatin)
Prolactin	Prolactin RH, TRH	Prolactin RIH, dopamine
Adrenocorticotropic hormone (ACTH)	Corticotropin RH (CRH)	
Melanocyte-stimulating hormone (MSH)	Melanocyte-stimulating hormone RH	Melanocyte-stimulating hormone RIH

example, the septal nuclei (see Chapter 16) are a source of gonadotropin-releasing hormone. Interestingly, many of these neurohormones are also found in hypothalamic neurons that do not project to the median eminence and in neurons in other regions of the central nervous system. This widespread distribution of neurohormones indicates that they are **neuroactive compounds** at these other sites and not just chemicals that regulate anterior pituitary hormone release.

Individual neurons of the parvocellular system, as in the magnocellular system (see below), may synthesize and release more than one peptide. In certain groups of parvocellular neurons the synthesis of one or another peptide may be regulated by circulating hormones in the blood. This is one way in which environmental factors, such as prolonged exposure to stressful situations, may alter the neurohormonal composition in the portal circulation and thereby influence anterior pituitary hormone release. Note that the blood brain barrier is less of an obstacle in the hypothalamus than in most other brain regions.

Hypothalamic Neurons Project to the Posterior Lobe and Release Vasopressin and Oxytocin

Posterior pituitary hormones are the neurosecretory products of hypothalamic neurons, unlike anterior lobe hormones, which are the products of epithelial secretory cells. **Vasopressin,** a peptide consisting of nine amino acids, has numerous functions. It elevates blood pressure, for example, through its action on vascular smooth muscle. Vasopressin also promotes water reabsorption from the distal tubules of the kidney to reduce urine volume. Another name for vasopressin is **antidiuretic hormone** (sometimes called ADH).

Oxytocin, which has a chemical structure nearly identical to that of vasopressin—differing by amino acids at only two sites—functions primarily to stimulate uterine contractions and to promote ejection of milk from the mammary glands. Although oxytocin is best known for its actions on female organs, there do not seem to be major differences in the numbers and locations of oxytocin-containing neurons in the nervous systems of males and females. Hence, other important actions of this peptide will likely be discovered.

In the hypothalamus, both vasopressin and oxytocin are synthesized primarily in two nuclei, the **paraventricular nucleus** and the **supraoptic nucleus** (Figure 15–4B). Experiments in animals have shown that the paraventricular nucleus comprises at least three distinct cell groups. As described earlier, there are parvocellular neurosecretory neurons in the portion of the nucleus that apposes the third ventricle. Lateral to these neurons are the **magnocellular neurons,** which synthesize and release the two posterior lobe neurohormones, and a third neuron group that gives rise to a descending brain stem and spinal projection for regulating autonomic nervous system functions (see next section). The supraoptic nucleus consists only of magnocellular neurons. The paraventricular and supraoptic nuclei are illustrated in Figure 15–4B, which is a midsagittal view of the hypothalamus.

Both vasopressin and oxytocin are synthesized from larger prohormone molecules. It was once thought that vasopressin was synthesized in one nucleus and oxytocin in the other. With the use of immunocytochemical techniques, however, it has been established that different cells in each nucleus produce one or the other hormone. The prohormone molecules from which vasopressin and oxytocin derive contain additional proteins, called **neurophysins.**

The axons of the paraventricular and the supraoptic magnocellular neurons in the **infundibular stalk** (Figures 15–3A and 15–4B) do not make synaptic contacts with other neurons. Rather, they terminate on **fenestrated capillaries** in the **posterior lobe** of the pituitary (Figure 15–5). (Fenestrations, or pores, make capillaries leaky. Recall that the posterior lobe of the pituitary [see Figure 4–18] is one of the brain regions lacking a blood-brain barrier. Thus, neurohormones can pass freely into the capillaries through the fenestrations.) The process by which these hypothalamic neurons release vasopressin or oxytocin from their terminals into the systemic circulation is similar to the release of neurotransmitters at synapses.

Immunocytochemical studies also have shown that magnocellular neurons, like their parvocellular counterparts, have a complex biochemistry and contain other peptides that act on neurons in the central nervous system and on peripheral organs. These other peptides also may be released into the circulation along with oxytocin or vasopressin and have coordinated actions on diverse structures. Vasopressin itself is an example of a brain peptide that has a diversity of coordinated functions at different sites. For example, it is a blood-borne hormone that influences the function of specific peripheral target organs, such as the kidney, and it is a neuroactive peptide involved in control of the autonomic nervous system (see below).

An understanding of the projections from other brain regions to magnocellular hypothalamic neurons provides insight into how the brain controls neurohormone release. For example, magnocellular neurons that contain vasopressin are important for regulating blood volume. These neurons receive inputs from three sources that each serve a related function.

First, magnocellular neurons receive an indirect projection from the **solitary nucleus.** This pathway conveys **baroreceptor** input from the glossopharyngeal and vagus nerves (see Chapter 6) to the hypothalamus, providing important afferent signals for controlling blood pressure and blood volume.

The second major input source is from the **circumventricular organs.** These structures do not have a blood-brain barrier. Two organs that project to the magnocellular nuclei are the **subfornical organ** and the **organum vasculosum of the lamina terminalis** (see Figure 4–18). As discussed in Chapter 4, the blood-brain barrier is a specific permeability barrier between capillaries in the central nervous system and the extracellular space. This barrier protects the brain from the influence of many neuroactive chemicals circulating in the blood. Having no blood-brain barrier, neurons in these structures are capable of sensing plasma osmolality and circulating chemicals and thereby can regulate blood pressure and blood volume through their hypothalamic projections.

The **preoptic area** provides the third input to the magnocellular neurons. This region is implicated in the central neural mechanisms for regulating the composition and volume of body fluids and thus indirectly affects the control of blood pressure.

■ FUNCTIONAL ANATOMY OF AUTONOMIC NERVOUS SYSTEM CONTROL

The other major role of the hypothalamus is regulating the **autonomic nervous system.** The autonomic nervous system controls several organ systems of the body: cardiovascular and respiratory, gastrointestinal, exocrine, and urogenital. Two divisions of the autonomic nervous system—the **parasympathetic** and **sympathetic nervous systems**—originate from different parts of the central nervous system. Similar to the control of skeletal muscle, visceral control by the sympathetic and parasympathetic systems relies on both relatively simple reflexes, involving the spinal cord and brain stem, and more complex control by higher levels of the central nervous system, including the hypothalamus.

A third division of the autonomic nervous system, the **enteric nervous system,** is located entirely in the periphery. This system provides the intrinsic innervation of the gastrointestinal tract and mediates the complex coordinated reflexes for peristalsis. The enteric nervous system functions independent of the hypothalamus and the rest of the central nervous system.

The next sections review briefly the anatomical organization of the sympathetic and parasympathetic divisions. An understanding of how these autonomic divisions connect to their target organs is essential before considering their higher-order regulation by the hypothalamus.

The Parasympathetic and Sympathetic Divisions of the Autonomic Nervous System Originate From Different Central Nervous System Locations

As discussed in Chapter 11, the innervation of body organs by the sympathetic and parasympathetic systems is fundamentally different from the innervation of skeletal muscle by the somatic nervous system (Figure 15–6). The innervation of skeletal muscle is mediated directly by motor neurons located in spinal and cranial nerve motor nuclei (Figure 15–6A). For autonomic innervation, two neurons link the central nervous system with organs in the periphery: the **preganglionic neuron** and the **postganglionic neuron** (Figure 15–6B; see Figure 11–6).

The cell body of the preganglionic neuron is located in the central nervous system, and its axon follows a tortuous course to the periphery. From the ventral root and through various peripheral neural conduits, the axon of the preganglionic neuron finally synapses on postganglionic neurons in **peripheral ganglia** (Figure 15–6B). A notable exception is the adrenal medulla, which receives direct innervation by preganglionic sympathetic neurons. This exception is related to the fact that adrenal medullary cells, like postganglionic neurons, develop from the neural crest (see Chapter 3).

Two major differences exist in the neuroanatomical organization of the sympathetic and parasympathetic divisions (Figure 15–7). First is the location of the preganglionic neurons in the central nervous system; second is the location of the peripheral ganglia. **Sympathetic preganglionic neurons** are found in the intermediate zone of the spinal cord, between the first thoracic and third lumbar spinal cord segments. Most of the neurons are located in the **intermediolateral nucleus** (Figure 15–6B) (also called the **intermediolateral cell column** because, like Clarke's column, this nucleus has an extensive rostrocaudal organization).

In contrast, **parasympathetic preganglionic neurons** are found in the brain stem and the second through fourth sacral spinal cord segments. The parasympathetic brain stem nuclei were described in Chapter 11 in the discussion of cranial nerve nuclei. Most preganglionic neurons are located in the Edinger-Westphal nucleus, the superior salivatory nucleus, the inferior salivatory nucleus, and the dorsal motor

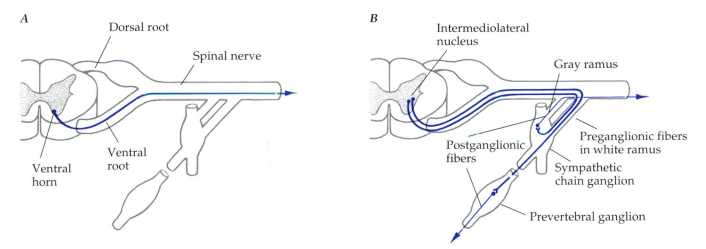

Figure 15–6. **A.** The circuit for peripheral innervation of skeletal muscle. **B.** The innervation of peripheral autonomic ganglia. Preganglionic autonomic neurons are located in the intermediate zone of the spinal cord. Their axons exit the spinal cord through the ventral roots and project to ganglia in the sympathetic trunk (paravertebral ganglia) through the spinal nerves and white rami. The axons of postganglionic neurons in the sympathetic ganglia course to the periphery through the gray rami and spinal nerves. The white and gray rami contain, respectively, the myelinated and unmyelinated axons of preganglionic and postganglionic autonomic neurons. A postganglionic neuron in a prevertebral ganglion is also shown with input from a preganglionic neuron. (**B,** *Adapted from Appenzeller O: Clinical Autonomic Failure: Practical Concepts. Elsevier, 1986.*)

nucleus of the vagus. Others are scattered in the reticular formation. The parasympathetic preganglionic neurons in the sacral spinal cord are found in the intermediate zone, at sites analogous to those of sympathetic preganglionic neurons.

The second major difference in the neuroanatomy of the sympathetic and parasympathetic divisions is the location of the peripheral ganglia in which the postganglionic neurons are located. Parasympathetic ganglia, often called **terminal ganglia,** are located on or near the target organs. In contrast, sympathetic ganglia are found at some distance from the target organs. Postganglionic sympathetic neurons are located in **paravertebral ganglia,** which are part of the sympathetic trunk, and in **prevertebral ganglia** (Figure 15–7).

Hypothalamic Nuclei Coordinate Integrated Responses to Body and Environmental Stimuli via Local Circuits and Descending Visceral Motor Pathways

Most bodily functions necessary for survival have important hypothalamic control. So far this chapter has considered the substrates for hypothalamic control of endocrine hormone release (both anterior and posterior pituitary) and the autonomic nervous system. The hypothalamus also plays a key role in coordinating endocrine and autonomic control, together with somatic motor functions, to produce highly integrated and purposeful responses. The hypothalamus engages in five major functions, each with clear neuroanatomical substrates: (1) regulation of blood pressure and body fluid electrolyte composition, (2) temperature regulation, (3) regulation of energy metabolism, (4) reproductive functions, and (5) organization of a rapid response to emergency situations. For each of these regulatory functions, the hypothalamus senses environmental or body signals and uses this information, first, to organize an appropriate response and, then, to command other brain regions to implement the response. Some signals are remarkably specific, such as **leptin,** a protein whose blood-borne concentration is proportional to body fat content (see Box 15–1), whereas others, such as body temperature, are general. Complex environmental stimuli, such as recognizing a threatening situation, require extensive processing by the cerebral cortex. This information, which is transmitted to the hypothalamus from telencephalic limbic system structures such as the amygdala, can trigger organized and stereotypic behavioral and visceral responses.

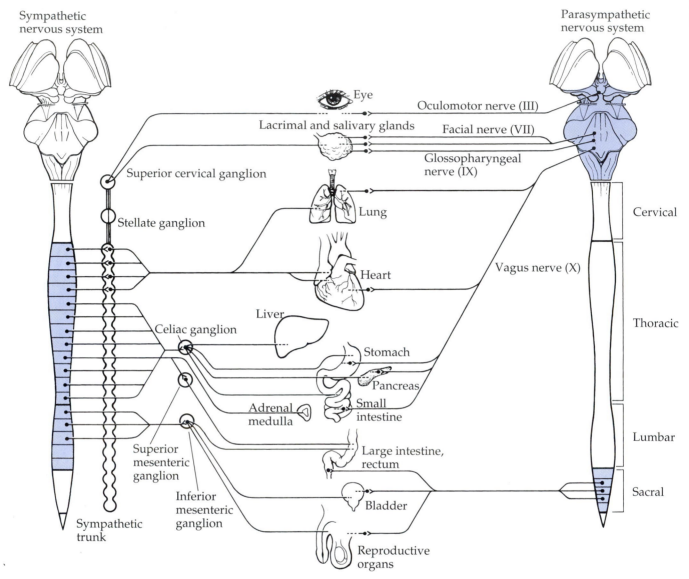

Figure 15–7. Organization of the autonomic nervous system. The sympathetic nervous system is shown at left, and the parasympathetic nervous system is shown at right. Note that the postganglionic neurons for the sympathetic nervous system are located in sympathetic trunk ganglia and prevertebral ganglia (eg, celiac ganglion). The postganglionic neurons for the parasympathetic nervous system are located in terminal ganglia close to the target organ. *(Adapted from Schmidt RF, Thews G (editors): Human Physiology. Springer, 1983.)*

The autonomic nervous system implements important aspects of hypothalamic control of body functions. How does the hypothalamus regulate the functions of the autonomic nervous system? The answer, perhaps surprising, is related to how the brain controls voluntary movement. As discussed in Chapter 10, distinct areas of the cerebral cortex and brain stem nuclei give rise to the descending motor pathways that regulate the excitability of motor neurons and interneurons (Figure 15–8, left). These spinal projections transmit control signals to steer voluntary movements and

regulate spinal reflexes. Visceral motor functions—mediated by the autonomic nervous system—are subjected to a similar control by the brain (Figure 15–8, right). The descending autonomic pathways originate from the hypothalamus and various brain stem nuclei.

The major hypothalamic nucleus for controlling sympathetic and parasympathetic functions is the **paraventricular nucleus** (Figure 15–9). The neurotransmitters used by this pathway include glutamate and the peptides **vasopressin** and **oxytocin,** the same peptides released by the magnocellular neurosecre-

The descending autonomic pathway synapses on brain stem parasympathetic nuclei, such as the dorsal motor nucleus of the vagus, spinal sympathetic neurons in the intermediolateral nucleus of the thoracic and lumbar segments, and spinal parasympathetic neurons in the sacral cord (Figure 15–9).

Other hypothalamic sites contribute axons to the descending visceromotor pathways. These areas include neurons in the lateral hypothalamic zone, the dorsomedial hypothalamic nucleus, and the posterior hypothalamus. In addition, these areas have strong projections to brain stem nuclei. Whereas some of these areas project laterally through the hypothalamus and brain stem, en route to the autonomic nuclei, others project more medially. One such medial hypothalamic path is the **dorsal longitudinal fasciculus** (see Figure 15–19). Throughout its course, the dorsal longitudinal fasciculus travels close to the ventricular system.

In addition to the hypothalamus, numerous brain stem nuclei help to regulate the autonomic nervous system. They do so by projecting to other brain stem nuclei implicated in viscerosensory functions and visceromotor control as well as by projecting directly to brain stem and spinal cord autonomic nuclei:

- The **solitary nucleus** (see Figure 15–19C), in addition to its role in chemosensory mechanisms, has a component that projects to the intermediolateral nucleus. Recall that the solitary nucleus relays viscerosensory information from the glossopharyngeal and vagus nerves to the hypothalamus, as well as to the **parabrachial nucleus** (see Figure 15–19B), the thalamus, and other forebrain structures (see Chapter 6).

- Neurons in the **ventrolateral medulla** (see Figure 15–19C) give rise to an **adrenergic projection** to brain stem and spinal autonomic nuclei. These neurons are thought to play an important role in regulating blood pressure.

- Neurons of the **pontomedullary reticular formation** have strong projections to autonomic preganglionic neurons in the brain stem and spinal cord. Because many of these neurons also project to spinal motor and premotor neurons, they may coordinate complex behavioral responses such as defense reactions that involve both visceral and somatic changes. For example, when you are startled by an unexpected, loud noise, many of your skeletal muscles contract and your blood pressure rises.

- The **raphe nuclei,** which use serotonin as their neurotransmitter, receive strong inputs from the

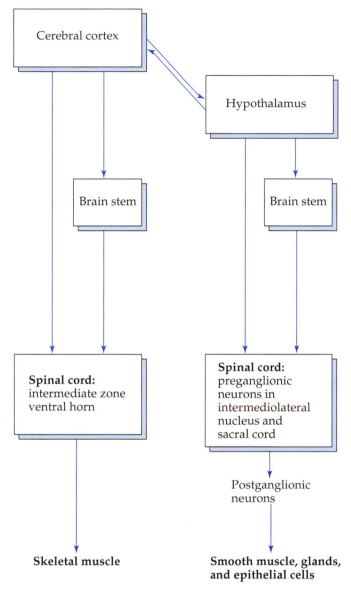

Figure 15–8. Organization of descending pathways controlling voluntary movement (*left*) and visceromotor function (*right*).

tory system. The neurons giving rise to the descending pathway, however, are distinct from those projecting to the posterior pituitary. This pathway descends laterally through the hypothalamus and brain stem. In the hypothalamus, axons course in the **medial forebrain bundle,** which is located in the lateral zone. The descending axons leave the bundle and then run in the **lateral tegmentum** in the midbrain, pons, and medulla (Figure 15–9). As is discussed below, lesions of the lateral brain stem tegmentum can produce characteristic autonomic changes because of damage to these descending hypothalamic axons.

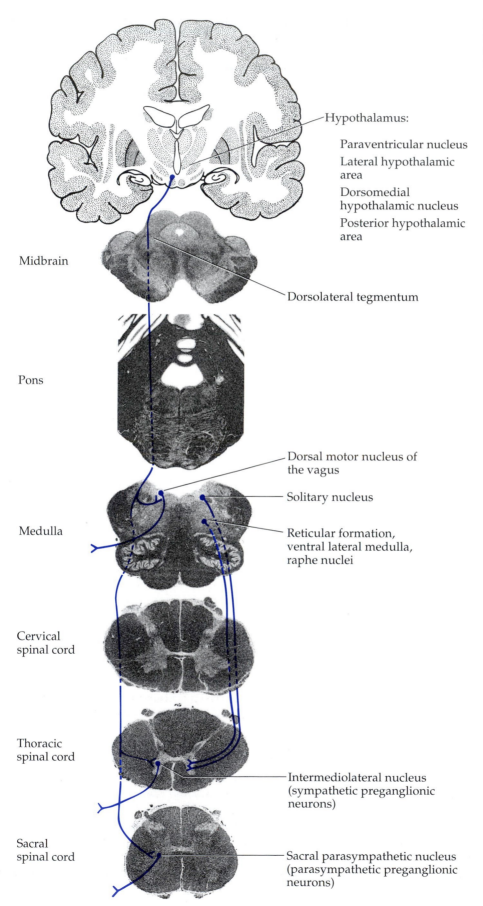

Figure 15–9. Regions of origin, course, and termination sites of descending hypothalamic pathways.

Hypothalamus:

Paraventricular nucleus

Lateral hypothalamic area

Dorsomedial hypothalamic nucleus

Posterior hypothalamic area

Midbrain

Dorsolateral tegmentum

Pons

Dorsal motor nucleus of the vagus

Solitary nucleus

Medulla

Reticular formation, ventral lateral medulla, raphe nuclei

Cervical spinal cord

Thoracic spinal cord

Intermediolateral nucleus (sympathetic preganglionic neurons)

Sacral spinal cord

Sacral parasympathetic nucleus (parasympathetic preganglionic neurons)

hypothalamus and project to spinal and brain stem autonomic nuclei. One function of the raphespinal system is to suppress dorsal horn pain transmission (see Chapter 5) in relation to the individual's emotional state.

REGIONAL ANATOMY OF THE HYPOTHALAMUS

The mediolateral functional organization of the hypothalamus was considered briefly earlier in this chapter. The three zones—periventricular, middle, and lateral—are located at all anterior-posterior levels of the hypothalamus (see Figures 15–11, 15–15, and 15–18). To better explain regional anatomy, this chapter now considers three anterior-to-posterior portions of the hypothalamus and their component nuclei (Table 15–2). Note that the boundaries between these three regions are not precise:

- The **anterior** part of the hypothalamus, located dorsal and rostral to the optic chiasm (see Figure 15–11, inset), includes the preoptic area, with numerous preoptic nuclei.
- The **middle** hypothalamus is between the optic chiasm and the mammillary bodies (see Figure 15–15). This portion contains the infundibular stalk, from which the pituitary gland arises. The magnocellular nuclei are located here, as are many of the parvocellular nuclei, including the arcuate nucleus, and the suprachiasmatic nucleus.
- The **posterior** portion includes the mammillary bodies and the structures dorsal to them (see Figure 15–18).

The Preoptic Area Influences Release of Reproductive Hormones From the Anterior Pituitary

The preoptic area is the most anterior part of the hypothalamus (Figure 15–10). Neurons in the medial preoptic area contain gonadotropin-releasing hormone. These neurons are believed to regulate pituitary reproductive hormone release because they project to the **median eminence.**
Nuclei in the medial preoptic area and anterior hypothalamus of animals show sexual dimorphism (ie, morphological differences in males and females). In the rat, gender affects the size of a sexually dimorphic

Table 15–2. The functions of major hypothalamic nuclei and regions.

Nucleus	Key functions
Anterior Hypothalamus	
Preoptic nuclei:	
Ventrolateral	Sleep-wakefulness
Medial	Parvocellular hormone control
Middle Hypothalamus	
Paraventricular	Magnocellular hormones (oxytocin, vasopressin); parvocellular; direct autonomic control
Supraoptic	Magnocellular hormones (oxytocin, vasopressin)
Arcuate	Parvocellular hormones; visceral functions
Suprachiasmatic	Circadian rhythm
Ventromedial	Appetitive/consummatory behaviors
Dorsomedial	Feeding, drinking, and body weight regulation
Periventricular	Parvocellular hormones
Posterior Hypothalamus	
Mammillary	Memory
Tuberomammillary	Sleep-wakefulness (histamine)
Lateral Hypothalamus	
Lateral hypothalamic and perifornical areas	Various, including arousal, food intake; contain orexin

nucleus as well as the architecture of neurons within the nucleus. Moreover, the size of this nucleus is dependent on perinatal exposure to gonadal steroids. This is an interesting example of how sexual differentiation alters brain morphology. In humans, identification of sexual dimorphism in the hypothalamus and other forebrain regions is controversial, with evidence existing for and against sex differences in the preoptic area and anterior hypothalamus. Part of the problem in identifying sex differences is that the human preoptic area has a complex organization, with numerous small and sometimes poorly differentiated nuclei. One of the nuclei reported to show sexual dimorphism in the human is part of the interstitial nuclei of the anterior hypothalamus, a small nucleus located at the level of the section shown in Figure 15–10.

One function of the lateral preoptic area is in regulating sleep and wakefulness. Damage to the preoptic area and basal forebrain can produce insomnia. Separate populations of neurons in the **ventrolateral**

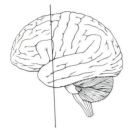

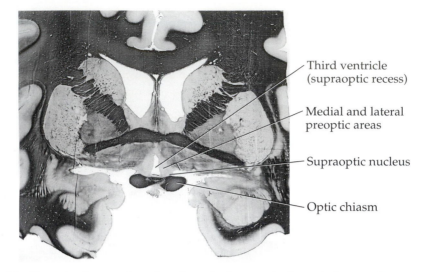

Third ventricle
(supraoptic recess)

Medial and lateral
preoptic areas

Supraoptic nucleus

Optic chiasm

Figure 15–10. Myelin-stained coronal section through the anterior hypothalamus, showing the preoptic area. The inset shows the plane of section.

preoptic area appear to be important in promoting REM (rapid eye movement) and non-REM sleep, through inhibitory connections with other hypothalamic nuclei and brain stem nuclei that promote wakefulness. The preoptic area, along with the posterior hypothalamus, is also involved in thermoregulation. Neural circuits in the preoptic area dissipate heat, through coordinated actions on the autonomic nervous system, to produce vasodilation and increased sweating, and, in animals, on the somatic motor system, to promote panting. By contrast, the posterior hypothalamus is involved in heat conservation (see section on posterior hypothalamus).

The Supraoptic and Paraventricular Nuclei Comprise the Magnocellular Neurosecretory System

The paraventricular and supraoptic nuclei are located in the anterior region (Figures 15–10 and 15–11). These are the two **magnocellular nuclei;** they release vasopressin and oxytocin in the posterior lobe of the pituitary (Figures 15–4A and 15–12). The lobes of the pituitary gland have different developmental histories. The posterior lobe develops from the **neuroectoderm.** In contrast, the anterior and intermediate lobes are of nonneural **ectodermal** origin, developing from a diverticulum in the roof of the developing oral cavity, called **Rathke's pouch.** Early in development the ectodermal and neuroectodermal portions fuse to form a single structure.

The axons from the magnocellular nuclei course through the median eminence, en route to the posterior lobe. However, the axons are segregated in an internal zone of the median eminence from the axons and terminals of the parvocellular neurons, which are located in an external zone. The axons travel down the infundibular stalk to contact systemic capillaries in the posterior lobe. Damage to the infundibular stalk may cut the axons of magnocellular neurosecretory cells as they pass to the posterior pituitary. This damage results in **diabetes insipidus,** in which excessive amounts of urine are produced. Fortunately the condition can be temporary because the cells are capable of forming a new, functional posterior lobe with nearby capillaries.

Recall that the paraventricular nucleus has a complex organization. It contains three major functional subdivisions (Figure 15–13):

1. The **parvocellular division,** apposed to the third ventricle, projects to the median eminence (Figure 15–4A).
2. The **magnocellular division** projects to the posterior lobe (Figure 15–4B).
3. A separate **autonomic division** projects to brain stem and spinal cord nuclei containing autonomic preganglionic neurons (Figure 15–9).

A common feature of paraventricular nucleus biochemistry is that many neurons in each subdivision contain vasopressin or oxytocin. Release of vasopressin or oxytocin at the various target sites of neurons in the paraventricular nucleus may subserve sim-

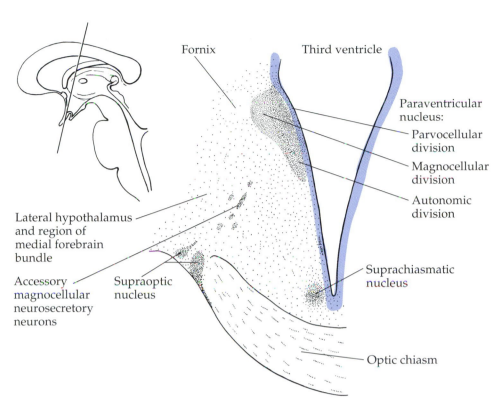

Figure 15–11. Drawing of Nissl-stained section through the anterior hypothalamus (optic chiasm). The blue region corresponds to the periventricular zone. The inset shows the plane of section. (*Adapted from Clarke WEL: Morphological aspects of the hypothalamus. In Clarke WEL, Beattie J, Riddoch G, et al. (editors): The Hypothalamus: Morphological, Functional, Clinical and Surgical Aspects. Oliver & Boyd; 1938:2–68.*)

ilar sets of functions, for example, in regulating blood pressure through sympathetic nervous system control and blood volume by acting on the kidney.

The paraventricular and supraoptic nuclei derive from the same group of embryonic neurons. Their locations in the mature brain reflect the complex migration that neuroblasts often undergo. Accessory magnocellular neurosecretory neurons bridge the gap between the paraventricular and supraoptic nuclei (Figure 15–11).

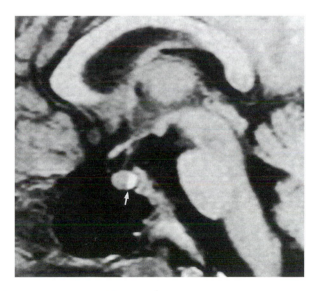

Figure 15–12. A midsagittal magnetic resonance imaging scan through the human pituitary gland. The posterior lobe (*arrow*) produces a bright signal. The thin infundibular stalk connects the basal surface of the hypothalamus with the pituitary. (*From Sartor K: MR Imaging of the Skull and Brain. Springer, 1992.*)

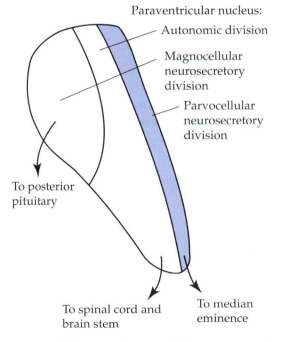

Figure 15–13. Schematic drawing of the paraventricular nucleus and the approximate locations of the three divisions.

The Suprachiasmatic Nucleus Is the Master Clock for Circadian Rhythms

The **suprachiasmatic nucleus** is also located at the level of the magnocellular nuclei (Figure 15–11). Neurons in the suprachiasmatic nucleus act as circadian clocks. They receive a direct projection from the **retina**—the **retinohypothalamic tract**—thereby allowing visual stimuli to synchronize (or reset) the internal clock (or circadian rhythm) of the body. The suprachiasmatic nucleus controls circadian rhythms primarily through local connections with other hypothalamic nuclei that are more directly involved in behavior. One path by which the suprachiasmatic nucleus controls the rhythm of body functions, such as adrenal medullary secretions, is through projections to the paraventricular nucleus. From here, descending projection neurons contact sympathetic preganglionic neurons in the spinal cord, which project to the adrenal medulla. This descending hypothalamic sympathetic pathway also controls circadian release of melatonin from the **pineal gland:** Sympathetic preganglionic neurons synapse on postganglionic neurons in the superior cervical ganglion that project to the pineal. The suprachiasmatic nucleus, through its projections to various hypothalamic nuclei—for example, the arcuate nucleus and the paraventricular nucleus—can control the circadian release of anterior lobe hormones. The clinical significance of normal circadian rhythms and the function of the suprachiasmatic nucleus are just beginning to be appreciated. For example, defects in circadian rhythms are believed to underlie some sleep disorders and certain forms of depression, notably **seasonal affective disorder.**

Parvocellular Neurosecretory Neurons Project to the Median Eminence

The **median eminence,** which contains the primary capillaries of the hypophyseal portal system, is located in the proximal portion of the infundibular stalk (Figure 15–3). The myelin-stained section in Figure 15–14 transects this region, although the median eminence is not differentiated. A midsagittal magnetic resonance imaging (MRI) scan through the pituitary gland is shown in Figure 15–12.

The infundibular stalk connects the basal hypothalamic surface with the pituitary gland. Releasing and release-inhibiting hormones secreted by the parvocellular neurosecretory neurons pass directly into the portal circulation through fenestrations, or pores, in the capillaries of the median eminence. The blood-brain barrier is absent in the median eminence (see Figure 4–18).

The three mediolateral zones are shown in Figure 15–14. The **arcuate nucleus** is located in the periventricular hypothalamic region (Figure 15–15). Parvocellular neurons in the arcuate nucleus contain various releasing and release-inhibiting hormones. In addition, many neurons in the arcuate nucleus contain **β-endorphin,** an endogenous opiate cleaved from the large peptide **proopiomelanocortin.** Some of these

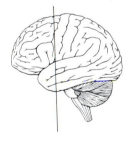
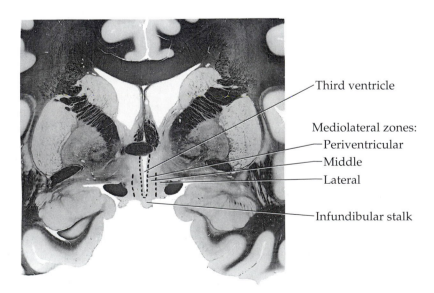

Figure 15–14.   Myelin-stained coronal section through the infundibular stalk. The inset shows the plane of section.

Labels on figure:
- Third ventricle
- Mediolateral zones:
- Periventricular
- Middle
- Lateral
- Infundibular stalk

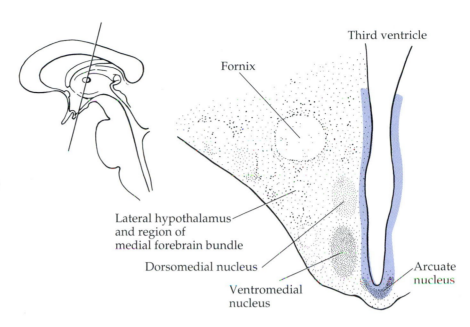

Figure 15–15. Drawing of Nissl-stained section through the middle hypothalamus. The blue region corresponds to the periventricular zone. The inset shows the plane of section. *(Adapted from Clarke WEL: Morphological aspects of the hypothalamus. In Clarke WEL, Beattie J, Riddoch G, et al. (editors): The Hypothalamus: Morphological, Functional, Clinical and Surgical Aspects. Oliver & Boyd; 1938:2–68.)*

Third ventricle

Fornix

Lateral hypothalamus and region of medial forebrain bundle

Dorsomedial nucleus

Ventromedial nucleus

Arcuate nucleus

neurons may play a role in opiate analgesia because they project to the periaqueductal gray matter, where electrical stimulation produces analgesia (see Chapter 5). Neurons in the arcuate nucleus are sensitive to circulating proteins important in the hormonal regulation of metabolism and feeding (Box 15–1). Two other nuclei are located in the middle hypothalamus. The **ventromedial hypothalamic nucleus** (Figure 15–15) receives input from a major limbic system structure, the **amygdala** (see Chapter 16), and is important in regulating appetite and other consummatory behaviors.

The Posterior Hypothalamus Contains the Mammillary Bodies

A section through the posterior hypothalamus reveals the mammillary nuclei (or bodies) (Figures 15–17 and 15–18). Each mammillary body contains two nuclei: the prominent **medial mammillary nucleus** and the smaller lateral mammillary nucleus. Remarkably, the mammillary bodies, the principal components of the posterior hypothalamus, establish virtually no intrahypothalamic connections. By contrast, most other hypothalamic nuclei have extensive intrahypothalamic connections. This shows that the function of the mammillary bodies is unlike that of the other hypothalamic nuclei. They receive their major input from a portion of the hippocampal formation, via the **fornix** (Figure 15–3; see Chapter 16). The efferent projections of the mammillary bodies are carried primarily in the **mammillothalamic tract**, which projects to the anterior nuclei of the thalamus

(see Figure AII–19). The mammillary bodies also have a descending projection to the midbrain and pons, the **mammillotegmental tract.** Whereas the mammillothalamic tract originates from the medial and lateral mammillary nuclei, the mammillotegmental tract originates only from the lateral nucleus. The outputs of the mammillary bodies are considered part of the limbic system and are discussed further in Chapter 16. Another nucleus in the posterior hypothalamus, the **tuberomammillary nucleus,** contains histamine. Like the brain stem monoamine systems, noradrenalin, dopamine, and serotonin, histaminergic neurons in the tuberomammillary nucleus have widespread projections. This system is important in maintaining arousal. Blockade of histamine reduces cortical neuronal responsiveness, and antihistamine therapy in humans typically produces drowsiness.

Other nuclei within the posterior hypothalamus do not contribute in a major way to neuroendocrine function. Rather, this region plays a role in regulating autonomic functions and mediating integrated behavioral responses to environmental stimuli. For example, the posterior hypothalamus is important in conserving body heat, which includes mediation of vasoconstriction and shivering in response to low temperatures.

Neurons in the Lateral Hypothalamic Area Can Have Widespread Effects on Cortical Neuron Function

Many hypothalamic neurons in the lateral zone (Figures 15–11, 15–15, and 15–18) also have wide-

Box 15–1. Neuroanatomical Substrates for Controlling Food Intake, Body Weight, and Metabolism

The hypothalamus is essential for the control of the body's nutritional state. Neurons in the hypothalamus transduce circulating hormones that indicate the metabolic and nutritional state of the organism into a coordinated response that involves changes in cellular metabolism, gastrointestinal physiological changes, and behavior. The arcuate nucleus, the paraventricular nucleus, and the lateral hypothalamic area are thought to be particularly important in different aspects of this control.

Arcuate neurons are sensitive to three circulating hormones that play important roles in the control of feeding: insulin, leptin, and ghrelin (Figures 15–15 and 15–16). Because the blood-brain barrier in the arcuate nucleus is weak compared to most other brain regions, circulating peptides have access to arcuate neurons. **Insulin,** produced by the pancreas, circulates in relation to body energy balance (ie, the difference between energy consumed and energy expended). **Leptin** is produced by adipocytes in proportion to the amount of body fat. Both leptin and insulin are signals that act to inhibit food intake and increase energy expenditure. They are normally both available during times of plenty. Reductions in leptin and insulin, usually signaling anorexia, are stimuli to increase food intake and inhibit energy expenditure. **Ghrelin,** which is produced by enteroendocrine cells of the stomach, promotes feeding. Fasting stimulates its release; therefore, it has the opposite effects of insulin and leptin. In addition, neurons in the **arcuate nucleus** contain peptide neurotransmitters that have strong effects on feeding. For example, neuropeptide Y is contained in arcuate neurons and promotes feeding when injected intracerebrally into laboratory animals. Several other arcuate peptides have potent stimulatory and inhibitory effects on food intake and metabolism.

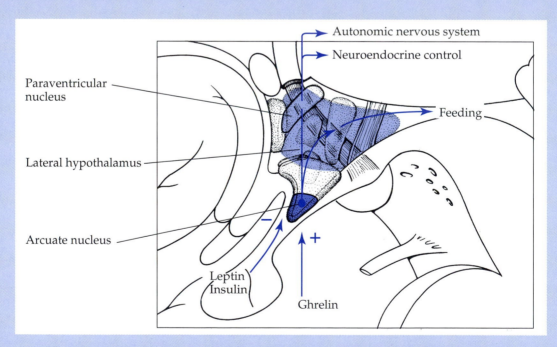

Figure 15–16. Key hypothalamic nuclei for feeding. Neurons in the arcuate nucleus are sensitive to circulating leptin and insulin, which are two peptides that suppress feeding, and ghrelin, which stimulates feeding. Neurons in the arcuate nucleus project directly to the paraventricular nucleus, which controls various autonomic and neuroendocrine functions related to feeding and metabolism. Arcuate neurons also project to the lateral hypothalamus, which plays a role in promoting feeding, such as seeking food.

Box 15–1 (continued).

Although other hypothalamic neurons may also respond to these and similar compounds, two structural features of the arcuate nucleus highlight its important role in feeding: projections to the paraventricular nucleus and the lateral hypothalamic area.

The **paraventricular nucleus** (Figure 15–16) exerts direct control over two aspects of metabolism. First, many parvocellular neurons contain corticotropin- and thyrotropin-releasing hormones, which promote a negative energy balance (ie, increased energy expenditure in relation to consumption). Second, neurons in the paraventricular nucleus have direct projections to parasympathetic preganglionic neurons in the dorsal motor nucleus of the vagus and to sympathetic preganglionic neurons in the intermediolateral cell column in the spinal cord. These projections can regulate gastrointestinal secretions and motility, thereby affecting digestion and absorption.

For controlling the nutritional state of an organism, it is not enough only to control autonomic and endocrine function. Food-seeking behavior also must be stimulated. Another major projection of the arcuate nucleus is to the **lateral hypothalamic area** (Figure 15–16), a region critical for normal food intake. Lesions of this area in laboratory animals can cause reduced food intake and weight loss. The lateral hypothalamus is the only site that contains neurons with two particular peptides that affect food intake: **melanin-concentrating hormone** and **orexin** (also termed hypocretin). These neurons have diverse projections that could engage cortical circuits for organizing feeding behavior. Orexin-containing neurons, through their projections to brain stem arousal systems, also promote arousal (see section on posterior hypothalamus).

spread projections to the cerebral cortex. One population of lateral hypothalamic neurons is particularly intriguing because the neurons contain peptides, termed **orexins** (or hypocretins), that appear to be essential for the proper maintenance of the aroused state. These peptides are found in no other place in the brain. Orexin is implicated in the sleep disorder **narcolepsy.** Humans with this disorder have persistent daytime sleepiness. Oftentimes they experience **cataplexy,** the transient loss of muscle tone without a loss of consciousness. A strain of dogs with narcolepsy has an orexin gene mutation, and transgenic mice in

Figure 15–17. Myelin-stained coronal section through the mamillary bodies. The inset shows the plane of section.

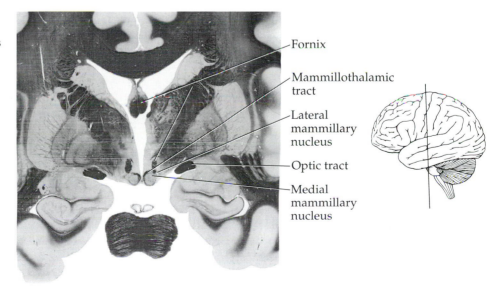

Fornix

Mammillothalamic tract

Lateral mammillary nucleus

Optic tract

Medial mammillary nucleus

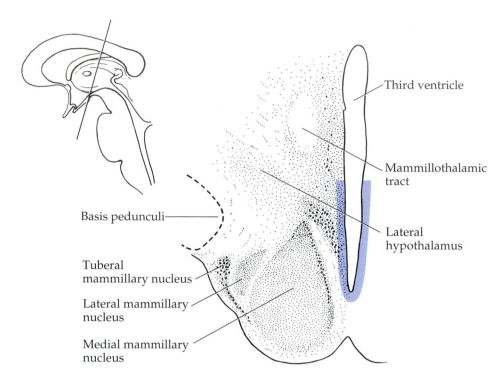

Figure 15–18. Drawing of Nissl-stained section through the posterior hypothalamus (mamillary bodies). The blue region corresponds to the periventricular zone. The inset shows the plane of section. *(Adapted from Clarke WEL: Morphological aspects of the hypothalamus. In Clarke WEL, Beattie J, Riddoch G, et al. (editors): The Hypothalamus: Morphological, Functional, Clinical and Surgical Aspects. Oliver & Boyd; 1938:2–68.)*

which the gene for orexin has been deleted have narcolepsy. It has been suggested that narcolepsy could be an autoimmune disease in which the immune system mistakes orexin receptors for a foreign protein.

Descending Autonomic Fibers Course in the Periaqueductal Gray Matter and in the Lateral Tegmentum

Hypothalamic regulation of the autonomic nervous system is mediated, in part, by direct projections to brain stem parasympathetic nuclei, sympathetic neurons in the intermediolateral nucleus in thoracic and lumbar spinal segments, and parasympathetic neurons in the intermediate zone of the sacral spinal cord. The major path from the hypothalamus taken by the autonomic pathway is through the **medial forebrain bundle** (MFB), which is in the lateral zone. This path is a conduit for axons from diverse sources, including ascending and descending connections between the brain stem, the hypothalamus, and the cerebral hemisphere. Neurons in the lateral zone are not organized into distinct nuclei but are interspersed along the MFB. The MFB becomes dispersed in the brain stem, where the descending autonomic pathway courses in the lateral tegmentum (Figure 15–19A). (The term *medial forebrain bundle* is not applied to the brain stem segment.)

Another hypothalamic pathway, the **dorsal longitudinal fasciculus,** contains ascending viscerosensory and descending fibers. This pathway courses within the gray matter along the wall of the third ventricle, in the midbrain periaqueductal gray matter and the gray matter in the floor of the fourth ventricle. Although diffuse in the diencephalon and midbrain, fibers constituting this pathway can be identified in the pons and in the medulla (in the dorsal portion of the hypoglossal nucleus; Figure 15–19C). The Edinger-Westphal nucleus, which contains parasympathetic preganglionic neurons innervating the ciliary ganglion, is located at this level.

Nuclei in the Pons Are Important for Bladder Control

The dorsal longitudinal fasciculus can be seen within the periventricular gray matter in the pons and medulla (Figure 15–19B,C). The pons is an important site for bladder control, receiving control signals from the preoptic area: Neurons in the **medial preoptic area** project to a cluster of neurons in the dorsolateral pons that trigger **urination.** These neurons project to the parasympathetic bladder motor neurons and interneurons that inhibit urethral sphincter motor neurons. Separate pontine neurons, located laterally and

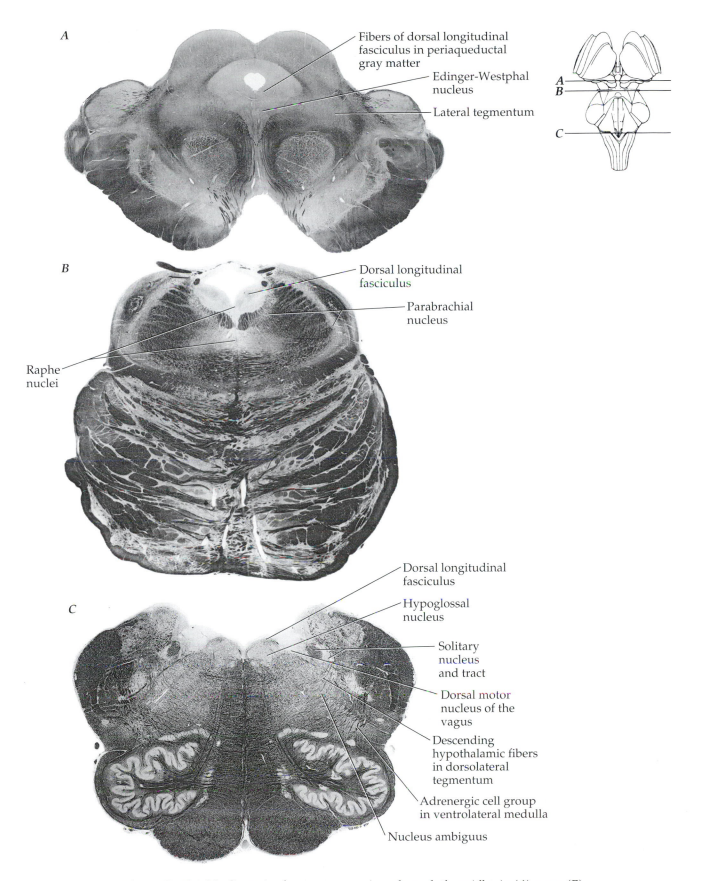

Figure 15–19. Myelin-stained transverse sections through the midbrain (***A***), pons (***B***), and medulla (***C***). The medial forebrain bundle extends into the lateral brain stem, but it is not a discrete tract.

ventrally, that excite urethral sphincter motor neurons are implicated in circuitry to prevent urination (ie, sphincter contraction). A positron emission tomography (PET) scan obtained while a human subject urinated is shown in Figure 15–20A, whereas a scan from a subject who was unable to voluntarily urinate during the scan—presumably because sphincter tone was too high—is shown in Figure 15–20B. These two scans reveal two distinct regions of the lateral pons that control urination. Surprisingly, only the right pons became activated, suggesting cerebral lateralization of this function. Research in laboratory animals and humans is showing a greater number of lateralized visceral functions than previously suspected.

Dorsolateral Brain Stem Lesions Interrupt Descending Sympathetic Fibers

Several key structures for controlling the autonomic nervous system are located in the medulla (Figure 15–19C). The **dorsal motor nucleus of the vagus** contains parasympathetic preganglionic neurons that innervate the various terminal ganglia. This nucleus was considered in Chapter 11. The **solitary nucleus,** considered in Chapter 6, is the major brain stem relay for visceral afferent fibers. Different populations of projection neurons in the solitary nucleus ascend to the parabrachial nucleus (Figure 15–19B) and the hypothalamus and descend to the spinal cord. Adrenergic neurons in the ventrolateral medulla project to the intermediolateral cell column for blood pressure control.

Damage to the dorsolateral pons or medulla can produce **Horner syndrome,** a disturbance in which the functions of the sympathetic nervous system become impaired. Surprisingly, parasympathetic functions are spared (see below). Such damage typically occurs as a consequence of occlusion of the **posterior inferior cerebellar artery** (PICA) (see Figure 4–3B3). The most common signs of Horner syndrome and their causes are as follows:

- **Ipsilateral pupillary constriction** (miosis), resulting from the unopposed action of the pupillary constrictor innervation by the Edinger-Westphal nucleus (see Chapter 11).
- **Partial dropping of the eyelid,** or **pseudoptosis,** produced by removal of the sympathetic control of the smooth muscle (tarsal muscle) assisting the action of the levator palpebrae muscle.
- **Decreased sweating** and **increased warmth and redness of the ipsilateral face,** related to reduced sympathetic control of facial blood flow.

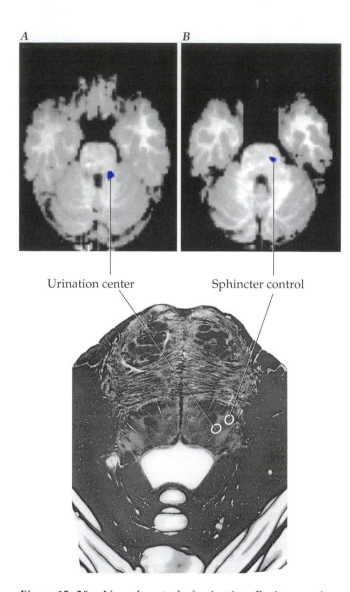

Urination center   Sphincter control

Figure 15–20. Neural control of urination. Positron emission tomography (PET) scans through the rostral pons show activation of two zones that play distinct roles in urination. *A.* The area that excites parasympathetic motor neurons that control muscles of the bladder wall and inhibit the sphincter motor neurons. This scan was obtained while the subject urinated. *B.* The area thought to prevent urination by exciting sphincter motor neurons, which are somatic motor neurons of the ventral horn. This scan was obtained while the subject was asked to urinate but was unable do to so on command. This is presumably because the sphincter muscles were contracting. Pontine control of urination is exerted via axons that travel in the reticulospinal tract. The inset shows the approximate locations of these zones on a transverse myelin-stained section through the pons. The section is inverted to match the orientation of the pons in the PET scans. *(From Blok BF, Willemsen AT, Holstege G: A PET study on brain control of micturition in humans. Brain 1997;120:111–121.)*

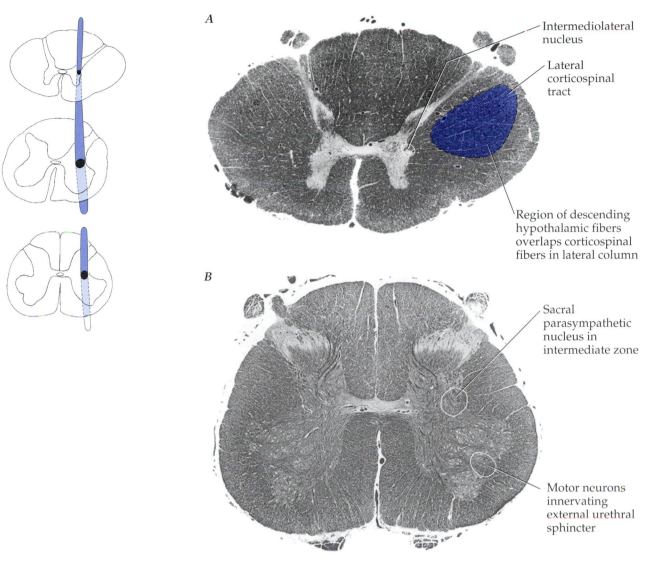

A

Intermediolateral nucleus

Lateral corticospinal tract

Region of descending hypothalamic fibers overlaps corticospinal fibers in lateral column

B

Sacral parasympathetic nucleus in intermediate zone

Motor neurons innervating external urethral sphincter

Figure 15–21. Myelin-stained transverse sections through the thoracic (*A*) and sacral (*B*) spinal cord. The inset shows the columnar configuration of the intermediolateral cell column.

Box 15–2. Lesions in Diverse Locations Can Produce Horner Syndrome

Unfortunately, Horner syndrome alone provides little information to the clinician for localizing the site of a lesion. The syndrome can be produced by a lesion anywhere along the descending autonomic pathway, from the hypothalamus, through the dorsolateral brain stem, to the spinal cord (Figure 15–9). Horner syndrome can also be produced by a lesion in the periphery, where axons of the sympathetic postganglionic neurons course to reach the head. How can the clinician distinguish between damage to one or another level? The answer lies in identifying other neurological signs that may accompany Horner syndrome. For example, a medullary lesion that produces Horner syndrome also will produce other signs associated with the **lateral medullary syndrome** (see Chapter 6; Figure 6–11). Similarly, a spinal cord lesion producing Horner syndrome will also cause paralysis because the descending autonomic pathway is near the axons of the lateral corticospinal tract (Figure 15–21A) (see Chapter 10).

It is not understood why damage to the dorsal motor nucleus of the vagus following PICA occlusion does not produce parasympathetic signs. Perhaps the parasympathetic functions of the nucleus are not well lateralized and the intact side can take over the functions of the damaged side.

Preganglionic Neurons Are Located in the Lateral Intermediate Zone of the Spinal Cord

The descending autonomic fibers from the hypothalamus course in the lateral column of the spinal cord, within the region of the lateral corticospinal tract (Figure 15–21), and terminate in the intermediolateral nucleus (or cell column) of the thoracic and lumbar cord (Figure 15–21A) and the intermediate zone of the second through fourth sacral segments (Figure 15–21B). These sites in the spinal gray matter are where most of the autonomic preganglionic neurons are located. Additional preganglionic neurons are scattered medially in the intermediate zone. At certain thoracic levels the intermediolateral nucleus extends into the lateral column (Figure 15–21A), which explains why this region is sometimes called the **intermediate horn** of the spinal cord gray matter. The inset in Figure 15–21 shows the columnar shape of the intermediolateral nucleus. This organization is similar to that of Clarke's nucleus (see Figure 13–6) and the cranial nerve nuclei (see Figure 6–4). Because important control of the sympathetic nervous system is present in divisions of the central nervous system, it is not surprising that damage at different levels can produce Horner syndrome (Box 15–2).

Summary

General Hypothalamic Anatomy

The hypothalamus regulates the neuroendocrine and autonomic nervous systems. It is a part of the diencephalon. On the midline it is bounded by the **lamina terminalis** rostrally and the **hypothalamic sulcus** dorsally. The lateral boundary is the **internal capsule** (Figure 15–1). The hypothalamus has a mediolateral anatomical and functional organization, with separate **periventricular, medial,** and **lateral zones** (Figure 15–3).

Neuroendocrine Control

Neuroendocrine control by the hypothalamus is mediated by separate **parvocellular** and **magnocellular neurosecretory systems,** which control hormone release from the anterior and posterior pituitary, respectively (Figure 15–4).

Parvocellular neurosecretory neurons (Figure 15–4A) regulate anterior lobe hormone release by secreting **releasing** or **release-inhibiting hormones** (Table 15–1) into the **portal circulation** in the **median eminence** (Figure 15–5). The major parvocellular nuclei, which are largely located in the periventricular zone, are the **periventricular nuclei,** the **arcuate nucleus,** the **paraventricular nucleus** (medial part, only), and the **medial preoptic area.** Additional hypothalamic and extrahypothalamic sites project to the median eminence and release gonadotropin-releasing hormones.

Two nuclei form the magnocellular system: the magnocellular division of the **paraventricular nucleus** and the **supraoptic nucleus** (Figures 15–3, 15–4B, and 15–10). Axons from the magnocellular neurons in these nuclei project into the **infundibular stalk,** which connects the pituitary gland with the brain (Figure 15–3). Their termination site is the posterior lobe, where they release **vasopressin** and **oxytocin** directly into the systemic circulation. Separate neurons in the paraventricular and supraoptic nuclei synthesize either vasopressin or oxytocin (Figure 15–11). Both parvocellular and magnocellular neurons colocalize neuroactive peptides.

Autonomic Nervous System and Visceromotor Functions

The autonomic nervous system has three anatomical components: the **sympathetic division,** the **parasympathetic division,** and the **enteric nervous system,** which is the intrinsic innervation of the gut. For the sympathetic and parasympathetic divisions, two neurons link the central nervous system with their target organs (Figure 15–6B): a **preganglionic neuron,** located in the central nervous system, and a **postganglionic neuron,** located in peripheral ganglia (Figure 15–7). The sympathetic division originates from the spinal cord, between the first thoracic and third lumbar segments (Figure 15–7). Preganglionic neurons of this division are located in the **intermediolateral nucleus** (Figure 15–21A). The parasympathetic division originates from the brain stem and the sacral spinal cord. Four parasympathetic nuclei in the brain stem contain preganglionic neurons (see Chapter 13):

the Edinger-Westphal nucleus, the superior salivatory nucleus, the inferior salivatory nucleus, and the dorsal motor nucleus of the vagus. The lateral intermediate zone of the second through fourth sacral segments contains parasympathetic preganglionic neurons (Figure 15–21B).

Hypothalamic control of the autonomic nervous system is through descending pathways whose axons synapse on preganglionic neurons (Figures 15–8 and 15–9). The major source of this projection is the autonomic division of the **paraventricular nucleus.** This hypothalamic pathway courses in the **medial forebrain bundle** (Figures 15–11 and 15–15), located laterally in the hypothalamus, and its caudal extension in the lateral tegmentum of the brain stem (Figure 15–19) and the lateral column of the spinal cord (Figure 15–21A). Disruption of axons of this pathway at any level can produce **Horner syndrome.** The hypothalamus also projects to other sites important in visceral sensory and motor function: the **parabrachial nucleus,** the **solitary nucleus, raphe nuclei,** and the **reticular formation** (Figure 15–19).

Related Sources

Brust JCM: The Practice of Neural Science. McGraw-Hill; 2000. (See ch. 13, cases 38, 39; ch. 15, cases 61, 62.)

Iversen S, Iversen L, Saper CB: The autonomic nervous system and the hypothalamus. In Kandel ER, Schwartz JH, Jessell TM (editors): Principles of Neural Science, 4th ed. McGraw-Hill; 2000:960–981.

Rechtschaffen A, Siegel J: Sleep and dreaming. In Kandel ER, Schwartz JH, Jessell TM (editors): Principles of Neural Science, 4th ed. McGraw-Hill; 2000:936–947.

Selected Readings

Appenzeller O: Clinical Autonomic Failure: Practical Concepts. Elsevier, 1986.

Bellinger LL, Bernardis LL: The dorsomedial hypothalamic nucleus and its role in injestive behavior and body weight regulation: Lessons learned from lesioning studies. Physiology and Behavior 2002;432–442.

Blok BF, Holstege G: The central nervous system control of micturition in cats and humans. Behav Brain Res 1998; 92:119–125.

Elmquist JK, Maratos-Flier E, Saper CB, Flier JS: Unraveling the central nervous system pathways underlying responses to leptin. Nat Neurosci 1998;1:445–450.

Elmquist JK, Scammell TE, Saper CB: Mechanisms of CNS response to systemic immune challenge: The febrile response. Trends Neurosci 1997;20:565–570.

Fowler CJ: Neurological disorders of micturition and their treatment. Brain 1999;122:1213–1231.

Gershon M: The enteric nervous system. Annu Rev Neurosci 1981;4:227–272.

Holstege G: The emotional motor system in relation to the supraspinal control of micturition and mating behavior. Behav Brain Res 1998;92:103–109.

Roth T, Roehrs T: Disorders of sleep and wakefulness. 948–959.Saper CB, Chou TC, Scammell TE: The sleep switch: Hypothalamic control of sleep and wakefulness. Trends Neurosci 2001;24:726–731.

Schwartz MW, Woods SC, Porte D Jr., Seeley RJ, Baskin DG: Central nervous system control of food intake. Nature 2000;404:661–671.

Siegel JM: Narcolepsy. Sci Am 2000;282:76–81.

Swaab DF, Hofman MA: Sexual differentiation of the human hypothalamus in relation to gender and sexual orientation. Trends Neurosci 1995;18:264–270.

References

Blok BF, Sturms LM, Holstege G: Brain activation during micturition in women. Brain 1998;121:2033–2042.

Blok BF, Willemsen AT, Holstege G: A PET study on brain control of micturition in humans. Brain 1997;120:111–121.

Buijs RM, Van Eden CG: The integration of stress by the hypothalamus, amygdala and prefrontal cortex: Balance between the autonomic nervous system and the neuroendocrine system. In Uylings HBM, Van Eden CG, DeBruin JPC, Feenstra MGP, Pennartz CMA (editors): Progress in Brain Research. Elsevier Science; 2000:117–132.

Cechetto DF, Saper CB: Neurochemical organization of the hypothalamic projection to the spinal cord in the rat. J Comp Neurol 1988;272:579–604.

Clarke WEL: Morphological aspects of the hypothalamus. In Clarke WEL, Beattie J, Riddoch G, et al. (editors): The Hypothalamus: Morphological, Functional, Clinical and Surgical Aspects. Oliver & Boyd; 1938:2–68.

Gerendai I, Halasz B: Asymmetry of the neuroendocrine system. News Physiol Sci 2001;16:92–95.

Herman JP, Cullinan WE: Neurocircuitry of stress: Central control of the hypothalamo-pituitary-adrenocortical axis. Trends Neurosci 1997;20:78–84.

Holstege G: Some anatomical observations on the projections from the hypothalamus to brainstem and spinal cord: An HRP and autoradiographic tracing study in the cat. J Comp Neurol 1987;260:98–126.

Inui A: Feeding and body-weight regulation by hypothalamic neuropeptides—mediation of the actions of leptin. Trends Neurosci 1999;22:62–67.

Inui A: Ghrelin: An orexigenic and somatotrophic signal from the stomach. Nat Rev Neurosci 2001;2:551–560.

Kilduff TS, Peyron C: The hypocretin/orexin ligand-receptor system: Implications for sleep and sleep disorders. Trends Neurosci 2000;23:359–365.

Leander P, Vrang N, Moller M: Neuronal projections from the mesencephalic raphe nuclear complex to the suprachiasmatic nucleus and the deep pineal gland of the golden hamster (Mesocricetus auratus). J Comp Neurol 1998;-399:73–93.

Lechan RM, Nestler JL, Jacobson S: The tuberoinfundibular system of the rat as demonstrated by immunohistochemical localization of retrogradely transported wheat germ agglutinin (WGA) from the median eminence. Brain Res 1982;245:1–15.

Mifflin SW: What does the brain know about blood pressure? News Physiol Sci 2001;16:266–271.

Moore RY: Neural control of the pineal gland. Behav Brain Res 1996;73:125–130.

Mtui EP, Anwar M, Reis DJ, Ruggiero DA: Medullary visceral reflex circuits: Local afferents to nucleus tractus solitarii synthesize catecholamines and project to thoracic spinal cord. J Comp Neurol 1995;351:5–26.

Munch IC, Moller M, Larsen PJ, Vrang N: Light-induced c-Fos expression in suprachiasmatic nuclei neurons targeting the paraventricular nucleus of the hamster hypothalamus: Phase dependence and immunochemical identification. J Comp Neurol 2002;442:48–62.

Nathan PW, Smith RC: The location of descending fibres to sympathetic neurons supplying the eye and sudomotor neurons supplying the head and neck. J Neurol Neurosurg Psychiatry 1986;49:187–194.

Nauta WJH, Haymaker W: Hypothalamic nuclei and fiber connections. In Haymaker W, Anderson E, Nauta WJH (editors): The Hypothalamus. Charles C. Thomas; 1969: 136–209.

Rogers RC, Kita H, Butcher LL, Novin D: Afferent projections to the dorsal motor nucleus of the vagus. Brain Res Bull 1980;5:365–373.

Ruggiero DA, Cravo SL, Arango V, Reis DJ: Central control of the circulation by the rostral ventrolateral reticular nucleus: Anatomical substrates. In Ciriello J, Caverson MM, Polosa C (editors): Progress in Brain Research. Elsevier, 1989.

Ruggiero DA, Cravo SL, Golanov E, Gomez R, Anwar M, Reis DJ: Adrenergic and non-adrenergic spinal projections of a cardiovascular-active pressor area of medulla oblongata: Quantitative topographic analysis. Brain Res 1994;663:107–120.

Saper CB: Organization of cerebral cortical afferent systems in the rat. II. Hypothalamocortical projections. J Comp Neurol 1985;237:21–46.

Saper CB: Hypothalamus. In Paxinos G (editor): The Human Nervous System. Academic Press; 1990:389–413.

Saper CB: Hypothalamic connections with the cerebral cortex. In Uylings HBM, Van Eden CG, DeBruin JPC, Feenstra MGP, Pennartz CMA (editors): Progress in Brain Research. Elsevier Science; 2000:39–47.

Saper CB, Loewy AD, Swanson LW, Cowan WM: Direct hypothalamo-autonomic connections. Brain Res 1976;117:305–312.

Sartor K: MR Imaging of the Skull and Brain. Springer, 1992.

Schmidt RF, Thews G (editors): Human Physiology. Springer, 1983.

Siegel JM: Narcolepsy: A key role for hypocretins (orexins). Cell 1999;98:409–412.

Silverman AJ, Zimmerman EA: Magnocellular neurosecretory system. Annu Rev Neurosci 1983;6:357–380.

Sutcliffe JG, De Lecea L: The hypocretins: Setting the arousal threshold. Nat Rev Neurosci 2002;3:339–349.

Swaab DF, Fliers E, Hoogendijk WJG, Veltman DJ, Zhuo JN: Interaction of prefrontal cortical and hypothalamic systems in the pathogenesis of depression. In Uylings HBM (editor): Progress in Brain Research. Elsevier, 2000.

Swanson LW: Organization of mammalian neuroendocrine system. In Bloom FE (editor): Intrinsic Regulatory Systems of the Brain. American Physiological Society; 1986:317–363.

Swanson LW, Kuypers HGJM: The paraventricular nucleus of the hypothalamus: Cytoarchitectonic subdivisions and organization of projections to the pituitary, dorsal vagal complex, and spinal cord as demonstrated by retrograde fluorescence double-labeling methods. J Comp Neurol 1980;1984:555–570.

Thompson RH, Swanson LW: Organization of inputs to the dorsomedial nucleus of the hypothalamus: A reexamination with Fluorogold and PHAL in the rat. Brain Res Brain Res Rev 1998;27:89–118.

Van Eden CG, Buijs RM: Functional neuroanatomy of the prefrontal cortex: Autonomic interactions. In Uylings HBM, Van Eden CG, DeBruin JPC, Feenstra MGP, Pennartz CMA (editors): Progress in Brain Research. Elsevier Science; 2000:49–62.

Veazey RB, Amaral DG, Cowan MW: The morphology and connections of the posterior hypothalamus in the cynomolgus monkey (*Macaca fascicularis*). II. Efferent connections. J Comp Neurol 1982;207:135–156.

Watson RE Jr., Hoffmann GE, Wiegand SJ: Sexually dimorphic opioid distribution in the preoptic area: Manipulation by gonadal steroids. Brain Res 1986;398:157–163.

16

The Limbic System and Cerebral Circuits for Emotions, Learning, and Memory

THE LIMBIC SYSTEM IS A DIVERSE COLLECTION of cortical and subcortical regions that are crucial for normal human behavior. Who you are—your memories, your unique personality, your thoughts, your emotions—in large measure are determined by the functions of the diverse brain regions that comprise the limbic system. Virtually all psychiatric diseases involve dysfunction of one or more of these structures.

Nineteenth century neurologists and anatomists recognized that damage to particular parts of the human brain were associated with disorders of emotion and memory. These lesions, unlike those of the cerebellum, occipital lobe, or cortical regions around the central sulcus, for example, spared perception and movement. This research led to the understanding that the neural systems for emotions, learning, and memory are distinct from the sensory and motor systems. Hence, the structures for emotions, learning, and memory, and their interconnections, are grouped into a single system, called the limbic system. The term *limbic* derives from the Latin word *limbus* for "border," because many of the structures engaged in emotions, learning, and memory encircle the diencephalon on the medial brain surface and thus are at the border between subcortical nuclei and the cerebral cortex.

However, the more that is understood about the myriad functions of limbic system structures, the less helpful it is to adhere to the notion of a single system. It becomes more meaningful to consider the individual functional systems. As a consequence, the term

377

limbic system is gradually being abandoned in favor of a more functionally descriptive terminology. Nevertheless, the notion of the limbic system has some utility. Brain structures for emotions, learning, and memory have been conserved throughout much of vertebrate evolution, reflecting the common and important need for these functions.

The basic organizational plan of the circuits for emotions, learning, and memory appear to be different from the sensory and motor systems. The different sensory and motor systems consist of structurally and functionally independent regions that are interconnected only at the highest levels of processing. This functional independence makes sense. For example, although perceptions are enriched when information from different modalities is combined, you can nevertheless identify an apple by touch alone or a dog by the sound of a bark. In contrast, circuits for emotions, learning, and memory are highly integrated from the start. This no doubt reflects the fact that emotions depend on the concurrent analysis of diverse sensory information and actions, and therefore are highly integrated behaviors. So, too, are memories. The sight of an old house and children playing in the yard can evoke vivid recollection of times spent during childhood.

This chapter first considers the components of the limbic system in relation to their generalized roles in emotions, learning, and memory. Then the chapter reexamines the same structures from the perspective of their spatial interrelations, their tracts, and their connections.

■ ANATOMICAL AND FUNCTIONAL OVERVIEW OF NEURAL SYSTEMS FOR EMOTIONS, LEARNING, AND MEMORY

The circuits for emotions, learning, and memory have tremendous anatomical and functional diversity (Table 16–1). Two key subcortical structures, the **hippocampal formation** and the **amygdala** (Figure 16–1), form distinct neural circuits that mediate the two major limbic system functions: (1) learning and memory and (2) emotions.

The hippocampal formation and amygdala receive their major inputs from the **limbic association cortex** (Figures 16–2 and 16–3). These cortical areas are the

Table 16–1. Components of the limbic system.

Major brain division	Structure	Component part
Cerebral hemisphere (telencephalon)	Limbic association cortex	Orbitofrontal
		Cingulate
		Entorhinal
		Temporal pole
		Perirhinal
		Parahippocampal
	Hippocampal formation	Hippocampus (Ammon's horn)
		Subiculum
		Dentate gyrus
	Amygdala	Corticomedial
		Basolateral
		Central nucleus[1]
	Ventral striatum	Nucleus accumbens
		Olfactory tubercle
		Ventromedial caudate and putamen
Diencephalon	Thalamus	Anterior nucleus
		Medial dorsal nucleus
		Midline nuclei
	Hypothalamus	Mammillary nuclei
		Ventromedial nucleus
		Lateral hypothalamic area
	Epithalamus[2]	Habenula
Midbrain	Portions of the periaqueductal gray matter and reticular formation	

[1]The bed nucleus of stria terminalis is largely included within the division of the central nucleus.
[2]In addition to the two major divisions of the diencephalon, there is a third division that includes the pineal gland, located along the midline, and the bilaterally paired habenula nuclei.

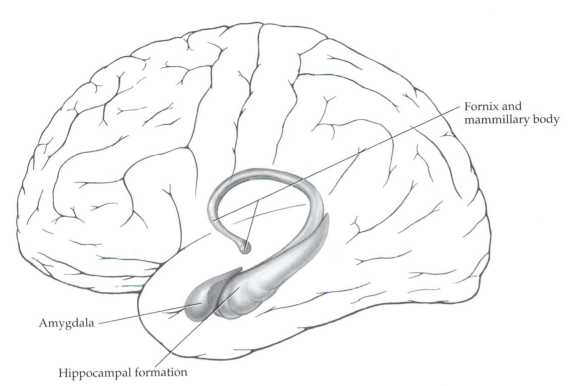

Fornix and
mammillary body

Amygdala

Hippocampal formation

Figure 16–1. Three-dimensional view of the amygdala and the hippocampal formation. The fornix, which is the output pathway of the hippocampal formation, and the mammillary body, a target to which it projects, are also illustrated.

targets of highly processed information from various higher brain regions, including other cortical association areas and higher-order sensory areas.

Hippocampal circuits are engaged in consolidating **explicit memories** (also termed **declarative memories**), such as the conscious recollection of facts, and in forming **spatial memories.** The hippocampal formation works closely with the adjoining **entorhinal cortex** (Figure 16–2), so much so that the two are functionally inseparable. These structures receive complex sensory and cognitive information from the limbic association cortex. Damage to the hippocampal formation or entorhinal cortex, depending on the extent, can result in severe and pervasive **anterograde amnesia.** In this form of amnesia, impairments occur in **semantic memory,** such as knowledge of facts, people, and objects, including new word meaning, and the **episodic memory** of events that have a specific spatial and temporal context, such as meeting a friend last week. By contrast, patients with hippocampal (or medial temporal lobe) damage are capable of remembering procedures and actions (ie, **implicit** or **nondeclarative memory**), and they retain the capacity for a variety of simple forms of learning and memory. The hippocampal formation, together with the prefrontal cortex, is implicated in the pathophysiology of **schizophrenia.**

Amygdala circuits are preferentially involved in emotions and their overt behavioral expressions. The functions of amygdala circuits are therefore similar to the functions originally proposed for the entire limbic system. Like the hippocampal circuits, the amygdala receives extensive information from cortical association areas. This information helps the amygdala learn about the emotional content of an experience. The amygdala influences emotional behaviors directly through its projections to the effector systems of the brain. Conscious feelings are thought to be represented in the cerebral cortex. Consistent with this idea is the observation that the amygdala also has strong cortical projections, both direct and via the thalamus and basal forebrain, that could confer emotional significance to experiences and memories. The amygdala, together with the hypothalamus and ventral striatum (Chapter 14), is strongly implicated in the mood disorders, including **depression** and **anxiety,** and in **substance abuse.**

Considerable overlap exists in some of the connections and functions of the amygdala and hippocampal formation and the other structures they engage. The amygdala is involved in the acquisition, consolidation, and recall of emotional memories. Moreover, several components of the amygdala and hippocampal formation receive olfactory inputs (Chapter 9),

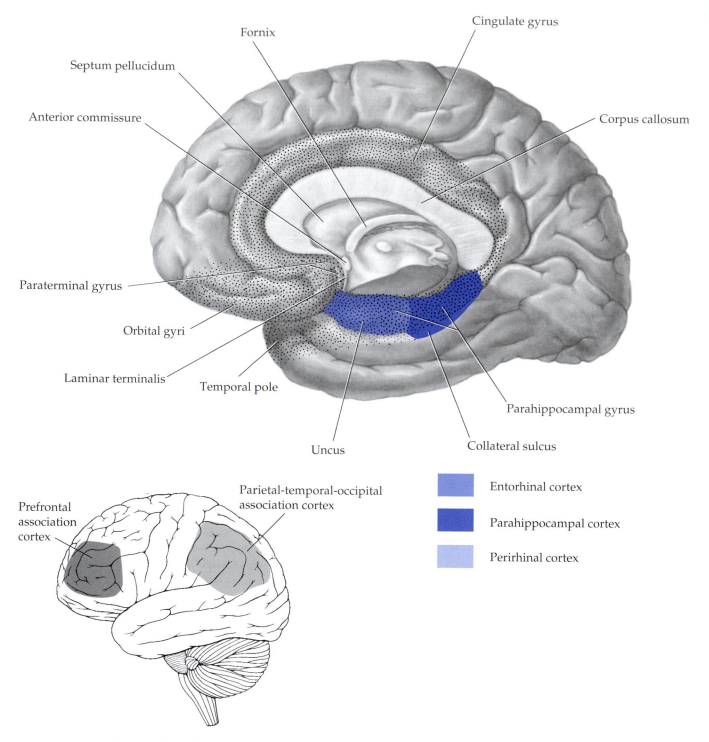

Fornix

Cingulate gyrus

Septum pellucidum

Anterior commissure

Corpus callosum

Paraterminal gyrus

Orbital gyri

Laminar terminalis

Temporal pole

Uncus

Parahippocampal gyrus

Collateral sulcus

Prefrontal association cortex

Parietal-temporal-occipital association cortex

Entorhinal cortex

Parahippocampal cortex

Perirhinal cortex

Figure 16–2. Midsagittal view of the right cerebral hemisphere, with the brain stem removed. The limbic association areas are indicated by the dotted regions. The inset shows the prefrontal association cortex and the parietal-temporal-occipital association cortex.

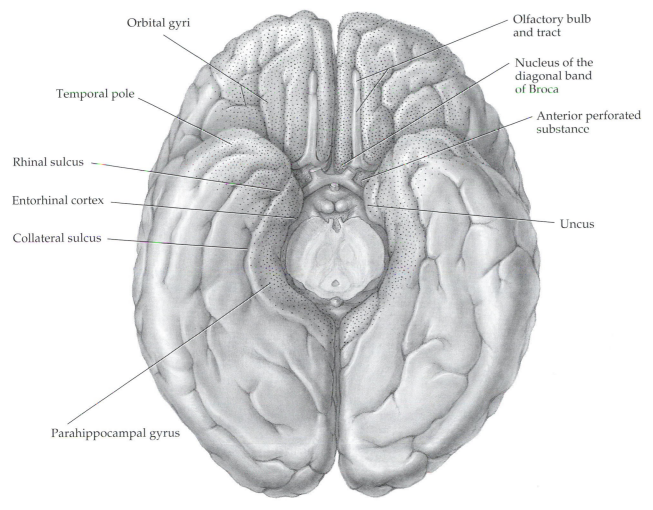

Figure 16–3. Ventral surface of the cerebral hemispheres, showing key components of the limbic association cortex (dotted area) as well as other basal forebrain structures.

possibly reflecting the importance of the sense of smell in emotional behaviors. Many of the limbic system components work together in a more general and integrative way in **cognition.** This role in cognition reflects a major input from cortical association areas to the amygdala and hippocampal circuits.

The Limbic Association Cortex Is Located on the Medial Surface of the Frontal, Parietal, and Temporal Lobes

There are three major cortical association areas: (1) the parietal-temporal-occipital area, (2) the prefrontal association cortex (Figure 16–2, inset), and (3) the limbic association cortex. The limbic association cortex (Figures 16–2 and 16–3) receives information from the higher-order sensory areas and from the two other

major cortical association areas, the prefrontal cortex and the parietal-temporal-occipital association cortex. The limbic association cortex conveys this information to the amygdala and hippocampal formation. The information the amygdala and hippocampal formation receive from the cortex is not the same, however. The amygdala uses sensory information to link particular stimuli, such as seeing an object or hearing a sound, with particular emotions. The amygdala is an important target of the **ventral stream** for object recognition (see Figure 7–16B). By contrast, the hippocampal formation receives more integrated sensory information thought to reflect complex features of the environment, such as spatial relationships. For example, when you see a snake you may feel threatened and fearful. Visual pathways through the ventral portion of the temporal lobe convey information about the snake to the amygdala. The amygdala uses this information to organize your response, both the emotions you feel and your overt behavior to this potential danger. The hippocampal formation is thought to be important in learning the complex environmental setting, or context, in which the snake was seen.

The limbic association cortex consists of morphologically and functionally diverse regions on four sets of gyri on the medial and orbital surfaces of the cerebral hemisphere (Figures 16–2 and 16–3): the cingulate gyrus, the parahippocampal gyrus, the medial orbital gyri, and the gyri of the temporal pole. Together, the **cingulate and parahippocampal gyri** form a C-shaped ring of cortex that partially encircles the corpus callosum, diencephalon, and midbrain (Figure 16–1). The **cingulum** (or cingulum bundle) is a collection of axons that courses in the white matter deep within the cingulate and parahippocampal gyri. Cortical association fibers course in the cingulum and terminate in the parahippocampal gyrus.

Rostral to this cortical ring are the **medial frontal** and **medial orbitofrontal gyri** and the cortex of the **temporal pole.** Functional imaging studies in humans show that neural activity in these areas is, at rest, different in patients with depression or obsessive-compulsive disorders than in healthy control subjects. Certain areas become more active in healthy subjects when they are made to feel anxious. On the ventral brain surface (Figure 16–3), the lateral boundary of the limbic association cortex corresponds approximately to the **collateral sulcus.**

The Hippocampal Formation Plays a Role in Memory Consolidation

Important insights into the function of the hippocampal formation have been obtained by studying the behavior of patients whose medial temporal lobe was either damaged because of a stroke or ablated to ameliorate the symptoms of temporal lobe epilepsy. In one of the most extensively examined cases, this region was removed bilaterally from a patient referred to as H.M. After surgery, H.M. lost the capacity for consolidating short-term memory into long-term memory but retained the memory of events that occurred before the lesion. This loss is attributable to a lesion of the hippocampal formation. More commonly, sometimes after a severe heart attack, patients suffer bilateral damage to the hippocampal formation. This damage results because certain neurons there require consistently high circulating blood oxygen levels. During a heart attack, circulation of blood to the brain can become compromised. These patients develop an amnesic syndrome similar to H.M.'s.

The **hippocampal formation** consists of three components, each with distinctive morphologies and connections (Figure 16–4; Table 16–1): the **dentate gyrus,** the **hippocampus** proper, and the **subiculum.** (The nomenclature of the hippocampal formation is variable, and exactly which components are considered to be part of this structure may differ, depending on the source.) The three components are organized roughly as strips running rostrocaudally within the temporal lobe and together forming a cylinder (Figure 16–4). These strips are initially a flattened sheet located on the brain surface, but during prenatal development they become buried under the cortex (see Figure 16–17). The flat sheet also folds in a complex manner to assume its mature configuration, which resembles a jelly-roll pastry.

The hippocampal formation is involved in the long-term consolidation of information that is thought to reside in the higher-order association areas of the cerebral cortex. A model for the functional organization of the hippocampal formation is based on its anatomical circuitry. Information that is first processed in the higher-order association areas on the lateral surface of the cerebral hemisphere, such as the parietal-temporal-occipital association area, is next processed in the limbic association cortex on the medial temporal lobe. This processing takes place in three key areas: the perirhinal cortex, the parahippocampal cortex, and the entorhinal cortex (Figure 16–2). From here, information is transmitted to the hippocampal formation (see Figure 16–5), where further processing results in changes in the amount or timing of activity of certain populations of neurons. The complex neural responses comprise a "representation" of the memory, which unfortunately is not well understood. Finally, via two sets of return projections to the cortex, which are discussed below, this hippocampal memory representation enables consolidation of explicit and spatial memories in the association areas.

The Hippocampal Formation Has Serial and Parallel Circuits

The hippocampal formation receives its major input from a portion of the **limbic association cortex** termed the **entorhinal cortex** (Figures 16–2, 16–3, and 16–4). This region, located on the parahippocampal gyrus adjacent to the hippocampal formation, collects information from other parts of the limbic association cortex (perirhinal and parahippocampal cortex) as well as from other association areas (Figures 16–5 and 16–6A). Extensive processing of information occurs

Figure 16–4. Schematic view of the hippocampal formation and fornix. The general spatial relations of components of the hippocampal formation, its efferent pathway (fornix), and the entorhinal cortex. The middle portion of the hippocampal formation is shown. This region corresponds approximately to the area defined by the blue trapezoid in the inset. Note that the structures highlighted in the inset are in the left hemisphere, whereas the semischematic hippocampal formation and fornix are in the right hemisphere.

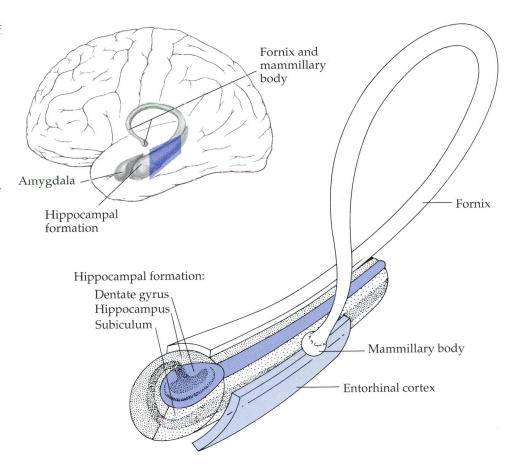

within the hippocampal formation, within a prominent **serial circuit,** in which information is projected in sequential steps (Figure 16–5A, bold arrows). There also is a parallel circuit, in which information from the entorhinal cortex projects directly to each hippocampal component. Combined serial and parallel processing within neural circuits is also a feature of sensory and motor pathways.

The output neurons of the hippocampal formation are pyramidal neurons, similar to the neocortex covering most of the cerebral hemisphere, and they are located in the hippocampus and subiculum. The projection of the dentate gyrus is entirely within the hippocampal formation. Pyramidal neurons have axon collaterals that collect on the surface of the hippocampal formation. Eventually these axons form a compact fiber bundle, the **fornix** (Figures 16–1 and 16–4), which projects to other subcortical telencephalic and diencephalic structures. The hippocampal formation, together with the fornix, has a C-shape. Two output systems can be distinguished within the fornix, from the subiculum and the hippocampus (Figures 16–5B and 16–6B). Although these systems are involved in the cognitive aspects of learning and memory, it is not

yet understood how their functions differ. From the subiculum, axons synapse in the **mammillary bodies** of the hypothalamus (Figures 16–1 and 16–6B). This projection completes an anatomical loop: Via the **mammillothalamic tract,** the mammillary body projects to the **anterior nuclei of the thalamus,** which project to the **cingulate gyrus** (Figure 16–6B). The cingulate gyrus provides information to the entorhinal cortex, which projects to the hippocampal formation. In 1937, James Papez postulated this pathway to play an important role in emotion. It is now known that the circuit named in his honor is part of a complex network of bidirectional connections and that many components of this network play a more important role in memory than emotions. For example, profound memory loss is a key sign of **Korsakoff syndrome.** In this condition, which results from thiamin deficiency accompanying alcoholism, the mammillary bodies and portions of the medial thalamus are destroyed.

From the hippocampus, axons synapse in the **septal nuclei,** located more rostrally in the forebrain (Figure 16–5B). Little is known about the function of septal nuclei in humans. In a fascinating series of experiments

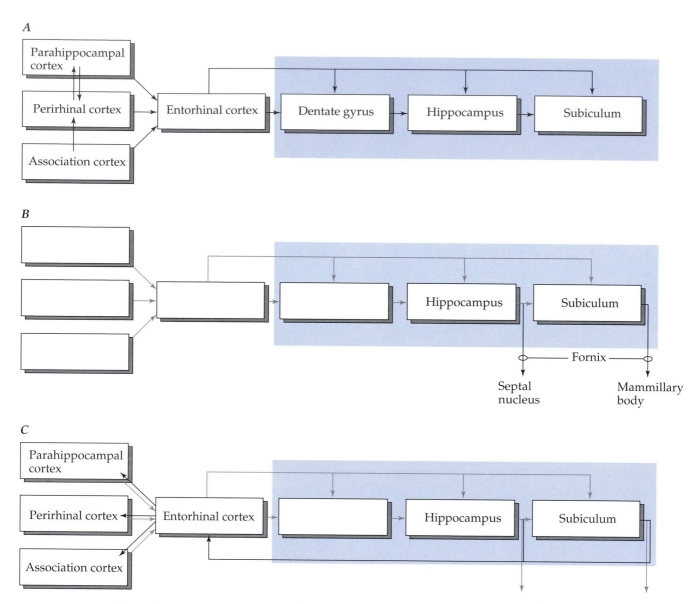

Figure 16–5. Serial and parallel hippocampal circuits. *A.* Cortical inputs to the hippocampal formation. *B.* Subcortical outputs via the fornix. *C.* Cortical projections from the hippocampal formation to the entorhinal cortex, which projects back to the cortical areas from which it received input. The blue boxes enclose the components of the hippocampal formation.

in the early 1950s, laboratory rats, when given the choice of receiving either electrical stimulation of the septal nuclei or food and water, preferred the electrical stimulation. Investigators reasoned that this region is a so-called pleasure center that likely plays an important role in regulating highly motivated behaviors, such as reproductive behaviors or feeding. The septal nuclei give rise to a cholinergic (see Figure 2–2A) and GABA-ergic projection, via the fornix, back to the hippocampal formation. This septal projection is important in regulating hippocampal activity during certain active behavioral states.

The Hippocampal Formation Has Diverse Cortical Projections

The fornix is an extremely large tract, with over one million heavily myelinated axons on each side. This number is comparable to the number of myelinated axons in one medullary pyramid or an optic nerve. Despite its size a major target of axons of the fornix is the ipsilateral mammillary body, whose output is also highly focused, on the **anterior thalamic nuclei.** How can the hippocampal formation, with such a focused subcortical projection, have a generalized

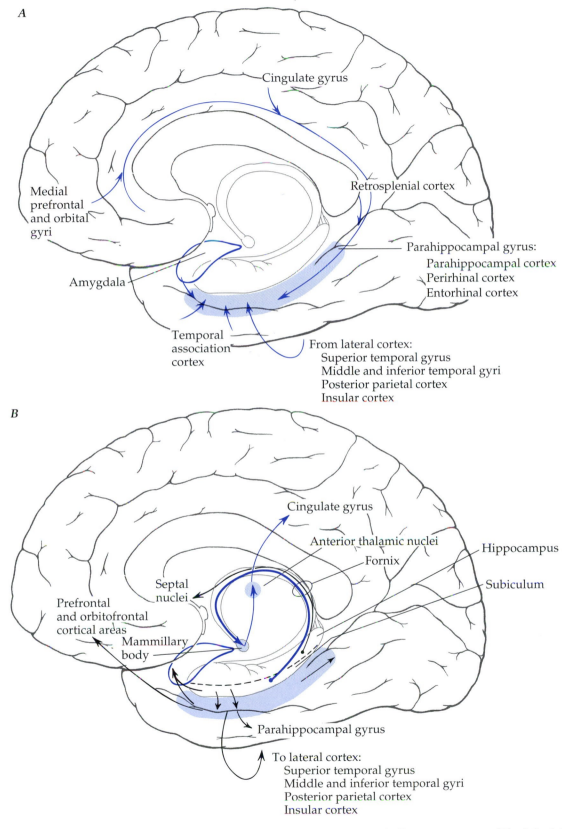

A

Cingulate gyrus

Medial
prefrontal
and orbital
gyri

Retrosplenial cortex

Amygdala

Parahippocampal gyrus:
 Parahippocampal cortex
 Perirhinal cortex
 Entorhinal cortex

Temporal
association
cortex

From lateral cortex:
 Superior temporal gyrus
 Middle and inferior temporal gyri
 Posterior parietal cortex
 Insular cortex

B

Cingulate gyrus

Anterior thalamic nuclei

Fornix

Hippocampus

Septal
nuclei

Subiculum

Prefrontal
and orbitofrontal
cortical areas

Mammillary
body

Parahippocampal gyrus

To lateral cortex:
 Superior temporal gyrus
 Middle and inferior temporal gyri
 Posterior parietal cortex
 Insular cortex

Figure 16–6. Principal afferent connections (*A*) and efferent projections (*B*) of the hippocampal formation. Inputs from the cingulate gyrus and other association areas of the
cerebral cortex are transmitted to the hippocampal formation via the entorhinal cortex, a
portion of the parahippocampal gyrus. Efferent projections from the subiculum and hippocampus to the rostral diencephalon and telencephalon are located in the fornix.

role in memory? One answer is that the fornix is not the only major output of the hippocampal formation. The subiculum and hippocampus also project back to the entorhinal cortex (Figure 16–5C), which has diverse efferent corticocortical connections to the prefrontal cortex, orbitofrontal cortex, parahippocampal gyrus, cingulate gyrus, and insular cortex (Figure 16–6B). Collectively these cortical areas also have widespread projections. Through the divergence of connections emerging from the entorhinal cortex to cortical association areas, the hippocampal formation can influence virtually all association areas of the temporal, parietal, and frontal lobes, as well as some higher-order sensory areas, after as few as three synapses. The divergence in the cortical output of the hippocampal formation parallels the widespread convergence of its inputs, also via the entorhinal cortex, from association areas.

Despite what is known about such connections and circuitry, little insight exists into the mechanisms of hippocampal function. The strength of synaptic connections in parts of this circuit can be modified by neuronal activity, but it is not yet known what infor-

mation is modified and how this synaptic plasticity helps the hippocampus consolidate memory.

The Amygdala Contains Three Major Functional Divisions

The **amygdala** (sometimes termed the amygdaloid complex) is a collection of morphologically, histochemically, and functionally diverse nuclei. Located largely within the rostral temporal lobe (Figure 16–1), the main portion of the amygdala is almond-shaped (*amygdala* is Greek for "almond"). One of its output pathways, however, the **stria terminalis,** and one of its component nuclei, the **bed nucleus of the stria terminalis,** are C-shaped (Figure 16–7). Axons of the other output pathway of the amygdala, the **ventral amygdalofugal pathway,** take a somewhat more direct route to their targets.

The amygdala is key to emotional experiences. What stimuli are responded to, how overt responses to these stimuli are organized, and the internal responses of the body's organs, are all dependent on this subcortical

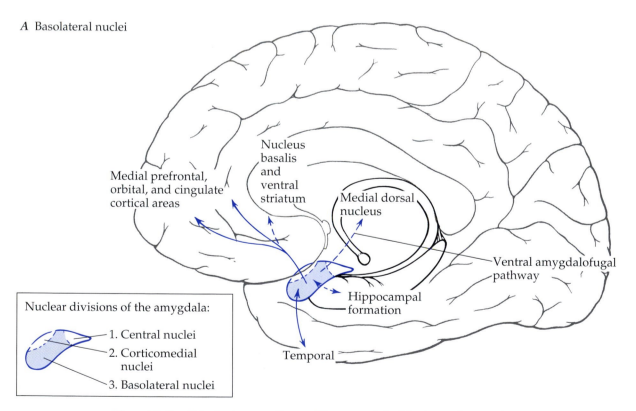

A Basolateral nuclei

Medial prefrontal, orbital, and cingulate cortical areas

Nucleus basalis and ventral striatum

Medial dorsal nucleus

Ventral amygdalofugal pathway

Hippocampal formation

Temporal

Nuclear divisions of the amygdala:
1. Central nuclei
2. Corticomedial nuclei
3. Basolateral nuclei

Figure 16–7.   Principal connections of the amygdala. The inset shows schematically the three divisions of the amygdala. *A.* The basolateral nuclei are reciprocally connected with the cortex of the temporal lobe, including higher-order sensory areas and association cortex. The basolateral amygdala also projects to the medial dorsal nucleus of the thalamus, the basal nucleus, and the ventral striatum.

Figure 16–7 Continued.
B. The central nuclei receive input from the brain stem, especially from visceral afferent relay nuclei (ie, solitary nucleus and parabrachial nucleus). The targets of its efferent projections include the hypothalamus and autonomic nuclei in the brain stem. **C.** The corticomedial nuclei have reciprocal connections with the olfactory bulb and efferent projections via the stria terminalis to the ventromedial nucleus of the hypothalamus.

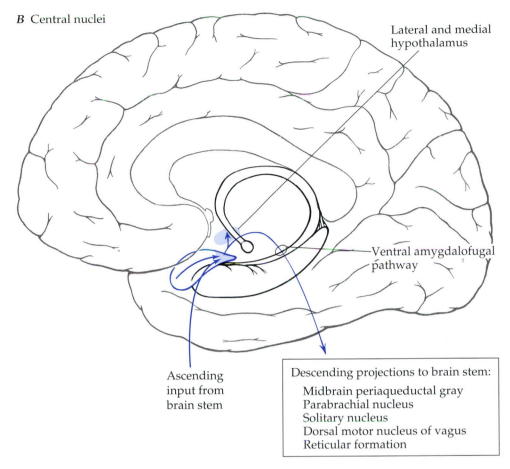

B Central nuclei

Lateral and medial hypothalamus

Ventral amygdalofugal pathway

Ascending input from brain stem

Descending projections to brain stem:
   Midbrain periaqueductal gray
   Parabrachial nucleus
   Solitary nucleus
   Dorsal motor nucleus of vagus
   Reticular formation

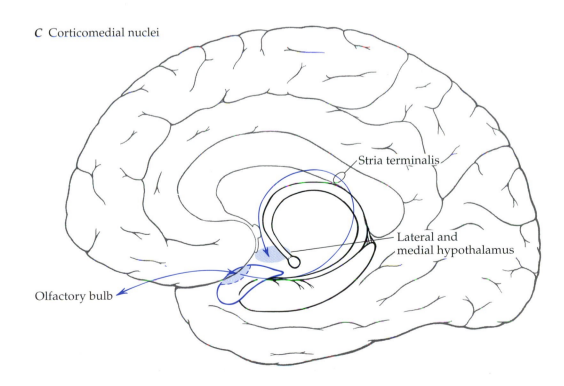

C Corticomedial nuclei

Stria terminalis

Lateral and medial hypothalamus

Olfactory bulb

structure. Following damage to the amygdala, people lose the ability to recognize the affective meaning of facial expression, especially threatening faces. People also fail to recognize the emotional content of speech. Given the defects observed with its damage, it is not surprising that the amygdala is a central figure in emotion regulation, especially in relation to violent behavior. For example, analysis of staring eyes, a vocalization, and body posture can lead to a set of potential emotional outcomes, such as fear or anxiety, and a set of possible actions, such as fleeing or attacking a potential foe. In animals, electrical stimulation of the amygdala, depending on the particular site, can evoke diverse defense reactions and visceral motor responses. The numerous nuclei of the amygdala can be divided into three principal nuclear groups (Figure 16–7): basolateral, central, and corticomedial. Each group has different connections and functions.

The Basolateral Nuclei Are Reciprocally Connected With the Cerebral Cortex

The **basolateral nuclei** (Figure 16–7A) comprise the largest division of the amygdala. These nuclei are thought to attach emotional significance to a stimulus. The basolateral nuclei receive information about the particular characteristics of a stimulus from higher-order sensory cortical areas in the temporal and insular cortical areas and from association cortex. The major efferent connections are directed back to the cerebral cortex, either directly or indirectly. The cortical areas receiving a direct projection from the basolateral amygdala are the limbic association cortex—which includes the cingulate gyrus, temporal pole, and medial orbitofrontal cortex—and the prefrontal cortex. The amygdala also projects directly to the hippocampal formation, which is thought to be important in learning the emotional significance of complex stimuli or the context in which emotionally charged stimuli are experienced. In addition to direct cortical projections, the basolateral division has extensive subcortical projections that give rise, indirectly, to connections to the cortex. Via the **ventral amygdalofugal pathway,** the basolateral amygdala projects to the thalamic relay nucleus for association areas in the frontal lobe, the **medial dorsal nucleus.** It also has a major projection to cholinergic forebrain neurons located in the **basal nucleus** (of Meynert), which itself has widespread cortical projections (see next section and Figure 2–2A). Neurons of the basolateral nuclei also project to the central amygdala nuclei (see below), which are important in mediating behavioral responses to emotional stimuli.

The Central Nuclei Project to Autonomic Control Centers in the Brain Stem and Hypothalamus

The **central nuclei** (Figure 16–7B) mediate emotional responses. In regulating the autonomic nervous system, the central nuclei receive viscerosensory input from brain stem nuclei, in particular the **solitary nucleus** and the **parabrachial nucleus** (see Chapter 6). In turn, the central nuclei project via the **ventral amygdalofugal pathway** to the **dorsal motor nucleus of the vagus** as well as to other brain stem parasympathetic nuclei and nearby portions of the reticular formation. The central nuclei also regulate the autonomic nervous system through projections to the lateral hypothalamus (see Chapter 15). As discussed earlier in this chapter, the central nuclei receive an input from the basolateral nuclei. This is the key path for fear conditioning, which helps to shape responses to emotional stimuli. The central nuclei of the amygdala are also important structures in substance abuse and dependence (Box 16–1).

The Corticomedial Nuclei Are Reciprocally Connected With Olfactory Structures

As discussed in Chapter 9, the corticomedial nuclei receive olfactory information from the olfactory bulb (Figure 16–7C; see Figure 9–11). The piriform cortex, along with the lateral orbitofrontal cortex, is thought to be important in olfactory perception. In animals the corticomedial nuclei are thought to play a role in behaviors triggered by olfactory stimuli, especially sexual responses.

Connections Exist Between Components of the Limbic System and the Effector Systems

The limbic system is difficult to study partly because a bewilderingly large number of interconnections exist between its many structures. What might be the functions of these myriad interconnections? Many of the connections relate to the behavioral expression of emotions. Complex polysynaptic pathways ultimately link limbic system structures with the three effector systems for the behavioral expression of emotion: the endocrine, autonomic, and somatic motor systems (Figure 16–9).

Paths by which the limbic system may influence pituitary hormone secretion involve indirect connections between the amygdala and the periventricular hypothalamus. One such path, for example, involves the projection from the corticomedial amygdala, via the **stria terminalis,** to the **ventromedial nucleus** (Figure 16–7C). This nucleus projects to a key component of the parvocellular neurosecretory system, the **arcuate nucleus** (see Chapter 15).

The visceral consequences of emotions are mediated by direct and indirect connections to nuclei of the autonomic nervous system (Figure 16–9B). As discussed above, the central nuclei project directly to brain stem autonomic centers (Figure 16–7B). The amygdala also affects autonomic function indirectly, through projections to the lateral hypothalamus, which influences autonomic function through neural circuits of the reticular formation and other parts of the hypothalamus. Recall that the hypothalamus, including part of the paraventricular nucleus and the lateral hypothalamus, gives rise to descending pathways that regulate autonomic function (Figure 15–8).

The overt behavioral signs of emotion, such as flight or fight reactions, are mediated by the actions of the limbic system on the **somatic motor systems,** especially the reticulospinal tracts. For example, projections from the hippocampus, septal nuclei, and amygdala to the lateral hypothalamus can influence the reticulospinal system (Figure 16–9C). These connections may be important in triggering stereotypic responses, such as defense reactions and reproductive behaviors. Experimental studies in animals have also shown that the periaqueductal gray matter mediates motor behaviors typical of particular species, such as growling and hissing in carnivores. The periaqueductal gray matter receives inputs from the central amygdala nuclei and the hypothalamus.

The limbic system can also influence somatic motor functions in more complex and behaviorally flexible ways through the **limbic loop of the basal ganglia,** which includes the ventral striatum, ventral pallidum, and thalamic medial dorsal nucleus (Figure 16–8; see Figure 14–3). Cortical inputs to this loop derive from the limbic association areas, hippocampal formation, and basolateral nuclei of the amygdala. As noted in Chapter 14, the output of the limbic loop is to the limbic association areas of the frontal lobe. These areas can influence the planning of movements through projections to premotor areas and possibly the execution of movements through projections to the cingulate motor areas (see Figure 10–6B).

All Major Neurotransmitter Regulatory Systems Have Projections to the Limbic System

The innervation of the limbic system by the major neurotransmitter regulatory systems (see Chapter 2;

Figure 2–2) appears to be particularly important for normal thoughts, moods, and behaviors. This conclusion is based on the observation that many of the drugs used to treat psychiatric illness—the disorders of thought, such as schizophrenia, and of mood, such as depression and anxiety—selectively affect one of the neurotransmitter systems. These neurotransmitter systems have direct and widespread connections with the limbic system:

- The **midbrain dopaminergic** projections originate from the **ventral tegmental area** and the **substantia nigra pars compacta** (see Figure 16–8B); however, the ventral tegmental area influences limbic system structures. Coursing through the **medial forebrain bundle,** the dopaminergic fibers synapse on neurons in various cortical and subcortical structures involved in emotions, learning, and memory: prefrontal association area, medial orbitofrontal cortex, cingulate gyrus, ventral striatum, amygdala, and hippocampal formation. All effective drugs for treating schizophrenia block the actions of a class of dopamine receptor, and drugs that increase dopamine release mimic aspects of schizophrenia. An important hypothesis for the pathophysiology of schizophrenia is that an exaggerated dopamine response in the nucleus accumbens (part of the ventral striatum) can lead to prefrontal cortex dysfunction, which is a key region for organization of thoughts and behaviors. Some schizophrenic individuals exhibit degeneration of medial temporal lobe neural structures, including the **hippocampal formation,** and a consequent increase in the size of the lateral ventricle.
- **Serotonergic** projections to limbic system structures of the telencephalon and diencephalon originate from the **dorsal and median raphe nuclei** (see Figure 16–20B,C). Coursing within three tracts—the medial forebrain bundle, the dorsal longitudinal fasciculus, and the medial longitudinal fasciculus—the ascending serotonergic projection synapses on neurons in the amygdala, hippocampal formation, all areas of the striatum, and cerebral cortex. Drugs that block serotonin reuptake mechanisms are effective in treating mood disorders, including anxiety and obsessive-compulsive disorders.
- The **noradrenergic** projection, which originates from the **locus ceruleus** (see Figure 16–20C), influences the entire cerebral cortex, including the limbic association areas, as well as limbic and other subcortical structures. This system,

Box 16–1. *The Mesocorticolimbic Dopamine System and the Neuroanatomical Substrates of Drug Addiction*

The brain has two major dopamine systems. One originates from the **substantia nigra pars compacta** (Figure 16–8B) and projects primarily to two parts of the striatum, the caudate and the putamen, and less so to the nucleus accumbens. This is termed the **nigrostriatal dopaminergic system.** The other is the **mesocorticolimbic dopaminergic system,** which originates from the **ventral tegmental area** (Figure 16–8B). This system provides the principal dopaminergic innervation of the **nucleus accumbens** (Figure 16–8A; see Figure 16–10), the **amygdala,** and various parts of the cortex, especially the **prefrontal cortex.** The mesocortical dopaminergic axons travel in the **medial forebrain bundle** (Figure 16–8A). Whereas dysfunction of the nigrostriatal system is associated with Parkinson disease, the mesocorticolimbic dopaminergic system is implicated in schizophrenia and depression.

The dopaminergic systems are important in responding to natural rewarding stimuli for survival, such as feeding and reproduction. Dopaminergic neurons do not simply signal the hedonic (ie, subjective experience of pleasure) value of events, because novel negative reinforcing stimuli can also activate the dopaminergic systems. Nevertheless, the mesocorticolimbic dopaminergic system is central to the brain's reward circuit. Most drugs of abuse—such as cocaine, sedative-hypnotics (including ethanol), nicotine, THC (tetrahydrocannabinol, the active compound in marijuana), and opiates—produce an increase in dopamine in several target areas of the mesocorticolimbic dopaminergic system. Several substance-specific mechanisms account for this effect, including decreased reuptake of dopamine at synaptic sites and disinhibition of ventral tegmental neurons so that they can release more dopamine. The nucleus accumbens, which is part of the ventral striatum, is a particularly important area because the reinforcing effects of drugs of abuse are greatly diminished or eliminated when dopamine transmission is blocked there. Another area important for the reinforcing actions of drugs, especially ethanol, is the central nuclear division of the amygdala (see Figure 16–13).

The nucleus accumbens is also a key site for neural interactions responsible for drug reinforcement and the motivation to seek drugs. Release of dopamine in the nucleus accumbens is critically involved in forming the associations between drug-related cues and rewarding experiences. The nucleus accumbens is a striatal component of the limbic loop (see Chapter 14). This loop can provide an emotional context for planning motor behavior. The output nucleus of the limbic loop is the **ventral pallidum,** which projects to the **anterior** and **medial dorsal thalamic nuclei** and then to the **prefrontal cortex** (including the medial orbitofrontal and medial prefrontal cortex) and **cingulate cortex** (Figure 16–8C). The various frontal association areas project to premotor areas to influence movements directly (see Figure 10–1B). This circuit could mediate the flexible responses to cues associated with drug use and abuse.

together with the serotonergic system, may play a role in depression because drugs that ameliorate depression result in elevations of these two monoamines.

• The **cholinergic** projection originates from large neurons near the ventral telencephalic surface. The neurons are found in the **basal nucleus,** the **medial septal nucleus,** and the **nucleus of the diagonal band of Broca** (see Figure 16–11). Additional cholinergic cell groups with widespread cortical projections in the brain stem are found near the **pedunculopontine nucleus** (see Figure 16–20). As discussed in Chapter 14, the pedunculopontine nucleus is an important target of the output nuclei of the basal ganglia. Targets of the cholinergic projection include the entire neocortex (including the limbic association cortex), the amygdala, and the hippocampal formation. **Alzheimer disease,** characterized by progressive dementia, begins with a loss

Box 16–1   (continued).

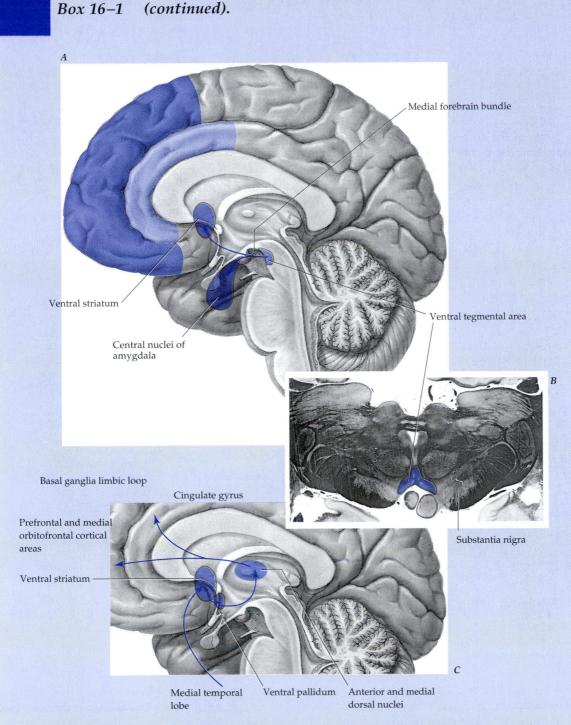

Figure 16–8.   Brain regions important in drug addiction. ***A.*** The ventral tegmental area gives rise to a dopaminergic projection to the amygdala and ventral striatum that is important in various aspects of drug addiction. The ventral tegmental area also projects to the prefrontal cortex. ***B.*** Transverse section through the midbrain-diencephalon junction, showing the location of the ventral tegmental area and substantia nigra, both of which contain dopaminergic neurons. ***C.*** An expanded view of the region containing components of the limbic loop of the basal ganglia.

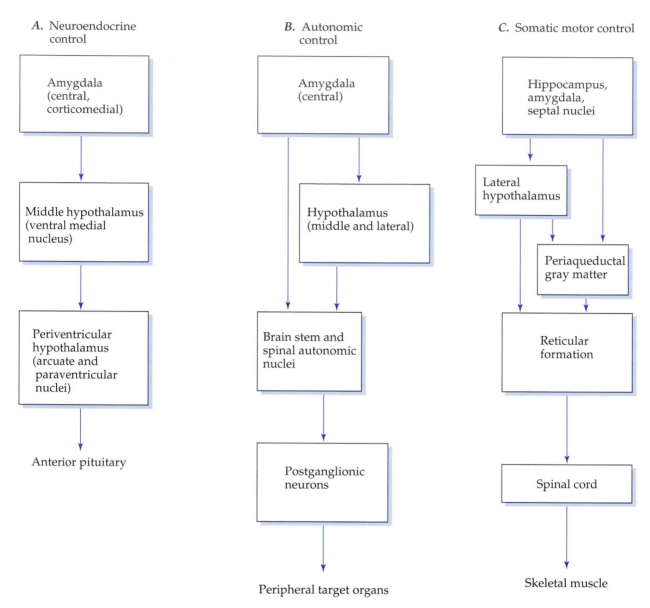

A. Neuroendocrine control

B. Autonomic control

C. Somatic motor control

Figure 16–9. Relations between the limbic system and effector systems. *A.* Neuroendocrine control is mediated by the amygdala via the periventricular hypothalamus. *B.* Autonomic control is mediated by both the amygdala and the lateral hypothalamus, via descending pathways that originate from the central nucleus of the amygdala and the middle and lateral hypothalamus. *C.* Somatic motor control is mediated by relatively direct projections to the reticular formation, for stereotypic behaviors, and through more complex telencephalic and diencephalic circuitry (not shown), for more flexible control.

of these basal forebrain cholinergic neurons. As the disease progresses, other neurotransmitter systems are also affected.

REGIONAL ANATOMY OF NEURAL SYSTEMS FOR EMOTIONS, LEARNING, AND MEMORY

Knowledge of the three-dimensional configuration of individual limbic system structures is essential for understanding their location in two-dimensional slices. As noted earlier in this chapter, three components of the limbic system have a C-shape: (1) the hippocampal formation and its output pathway, the fornix (Figure 16–1), (2) part of the amygdala and one of its pathways, the stria terminalis (Figures 16–1 and 16–7C), and (3) the limbic association cortex, especially the cingulate and parahippocampal gyri (Figure 16–2). As a consequence of their C-shape, a coronal section through the cerebral hemisphere may transect these structures twice: first dorsally and then ventrally. In horizontal sections, C-shaped structures are located rostrally and caudally.

The Nucleus Accumbens and Olfactory Tubercle Comprise Part of the Basal Forebrain

Sections through the rostral forebrain cut through components of the limbic loop of the basal ganglia. The input side of the loop (see Figure 14–3) is the **ventral striatum**, consisting of the **nucleus accumbens**, the olfactory tubercle, and the ventromedial parts of the caudate nucleus and putamen (Figure 16–10). The ventral striatum receives information from all of the nuclear divisions of the amygdala as well as from the hippocampal formation and limbic association cortex. The output nucleus of the limbic loop is the **ventral pallidum** (Figure 16–11), which projects to parts of the **medial dorsal nucleus** of the thalamus (see Figure 16–14B) and from there to the **prefrontal cortex, medial orbitofrontal cortex,** and **anterior cingulate gyrus.** The ventral striatum also has direct projections to the amygdala. Recall that the dorsal parts of the striatum are important in skeletal motor and oculomotor functions and cognition. Their outputs are focused on the internal and external segments of the globus pallidus and the substantia nigra pars reticulata.

Other than receiving olfactory input from the olfactory bulb and tract, little is known of the functions of the **olfactory tubercle.** The olfactory tubercle corresponds to the region on the ventral surface termed the **anterior perforated substance** (Figure 16–3). This is where penetrating branches of the middle and anterior cerebral arteries (the lenticulostriate arteries) enter the basal brain surface to supply parts of the basal ganglia and internal capsule. The slice shown in Figure 16–10 also cuts through the most anterior portions of the cingulate and parahippocampal gyri.

Basal Forebrain Cholinergic Systems Have Diffuse Limbic and Neocortical Projections

The **septal nuclei** are adjacent to the **septum pellucidum** (Figures 16–10 and 16–11), a nonneural structure that separates the anterior horns of the lateral ventricles of the two cerebral hemispheres. Animal studies have revealed that the septal nuclei consist of separate medial and lateral components. In humans the lateral septal nucleus may correspond to neurons located near the ventricular surface, whereas the medial septal nucleus corresponds to those near the septum pellucidum. Moreover, these medial cells are continuous with the gray matter on the medial surface of the cerebral hemisphere, just rostral to the **lamina terminalis.** This region, termed the **paraterminal gyrus** (Figure 16–2), merges with the **nucleus of the diagonal band of Broca,** which is located on the basal forebrain surface (Figure 16–3).

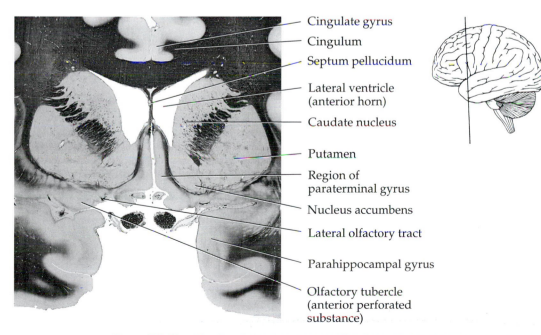

Cingulate gyrus

Cingulum

Septum pellucidum

Lateral ventricle (anterior horn)

Caudate nucleus

Putamen

Region of paraterminal gyrus

Nucleus accumbens

Lateral olfactory tract

Parahippocampal gyrus

Olfactory tubercle (anterior perforated substance)

Figure 16–10. Myelin-stained coronal section through the rostral forebrain. The inset shows the plane of section.

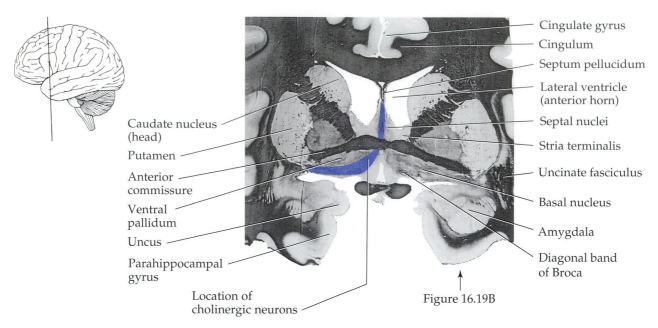

Cingulate gyrus

Cingulum

Septum pellucidum

Lateral ventricle (anterior horn)

Septal nuclei

Stria terminalis

Uncinate fasciculus

Basal nucleus

Amygdala

Diagonal band of Broca

Figure 16.19B

Caudate nucleus (head)

Putamen

Anterior commissure

Ventral pallidum

Uncus

Parahippocampal gyrus

Location of cholinergic neurons

Figure 16–11. Myelin-stained coronal section through the septal nuclei, basal nucleus, and amygdala. The arrow points to the plane of section of this image in Figure 16.19B. The inset shows the plane of section.

The lateral septal nucleus is a target of the projection from the hippocampus, via the fornix. The medial septal nucleus receives its major input from the lateral septal nucleus and projects to three sites: (1) the hippocampal formation, (2) the periaqueductal gray matter and reticular formation, and (3) the habenula, a portion of the diencephalon. The projection to the hippocampal formation, via the fornix, is important in regulating hippocampal neuronal activity. The projection to the periaqueductal gray matter and reticular formation, via the **medial forebrain bundle,** is thought to be important in evoking stereotypic behaviors in response to environmental stimuli. Finally, the projection to the **habenula,** located lateral and ventral to the pineal gland (see Figure AI–7), is part of a circuit with the midbrain medial dopaminergic and serotonergic systems (see Figures 16–8B and 16–20B,C).

The **basal forebrain** is located on the ventral surface of the cerebral hemisphere. It includes the paraterminal gyrus, nucleus of the diagonal band of Broca, and anterior perforated substance. The septal nuclei are continuous with many basal forebrain structures. On Figure 16–3, the basal forebrain is located approximately anterior to and beneath the optic chiasm and tracts. Large neurons are located here that use **acetylcholine** as their principal neurotransmitter. In addition to the medial septal nucleus, cholinergic neurons are located in the nucleus of the diagonal band of Broca and the **basal nucleus** (Figure 16–11). The various cholinergic neurons form a con-

tinuous band, from dorsomedially in the septal nuclei to ventrolaterally in the basal nucleus (Figure 16–11, blue shading). Other large cholinergic neurons are dispersed between the lamina of the globus pallidus and putamen and adjacent to the internal capsule.

The basal forebrain cholinergic neurons (including those in the medial septal nucleus) excite their targets primarily through **muscarinic receptors;** such responses to acetylcholine may facilitate cortical responses to other inputs. These cholinergic neurons, through widespread cortical projections, may also modulate overall cortical excitability.

The Cingulum Courses Beneath the Cingulate and Parahippocampal Gyri

The morphology of many of the limbic association areas differs from that of the rest of the cortex. The principal cortex is **neocortex** (eg, primary somatic sensory cortex or posterior parietal association cortex), which has at least six cell layers (Figure 16–12A). The other type of cortex is allocortex (Figure 16–12B), which has fewer than six layers and is more variable. Allocortex is phylogenetically older than neocortex. For example, parts of the basal forebrain are considered to be allocortex (although named a nucleus). Much of the parahippocampal gyrus is allocortex and so, too, are the hippocampal formation and entorhinal cortex.

Figure 16–12. The neocortex (**A**) has six cell layers, and the allocortex (**B**) has fewer than six layers. The drawing of a Nissl-stained section through the neo-cortex of the human brain is semischematic. The section through the allocortex is of a portion of the hippocampal formation. This is archicortex, and it has three cell layers. (**A,** *Adapted from Brodmann K: Vergleichende Lokalisationslehre der Grosshirnrinde in ihren Prinzipien dargestellt auf Grund des Zellenbaues. Barth, 1909.*)

A   Neocortex

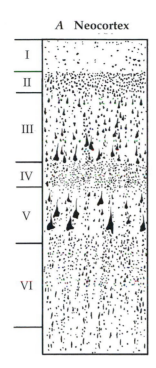

I
II
III
IV
V
VI

B   Allocortex

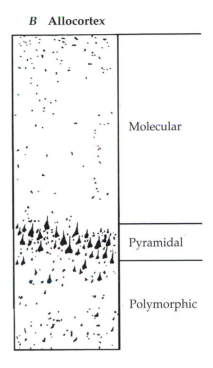

Molecular

Pyramidal

Polymorphic

Two cortical limbic areas, the cingulate and parahippocampal gyri, are seen in a series of coronal sections (Figures 16–10, 16–11, 16–13, 16–14, and 16–15): The cingulate gyrus is located dorsally, and the parahippocampal gyrus is located ventrally. The pathway that connects regions of the orbitofrontal gyri and the cingulate gyrus with the parahippocampal gyrus, including the **entorhinal cortex,** is termed the **cingulum.** This pathway is located beneath the cingulate gyrus (Figure 16–14). Unlike the cingulum, another limbic system cortical association pathway, the **uncinate fasciculus** (Figures 16–11 and 16–13), has a more direct trajectory for interconnecting anterior portions of the temporal lobe with medial orbital gyri of the frontal lobe.

The Three Nuclear Divisions of the Amygdala Are Revealed in Coronal Section

The amygdala is located in the rostral temporal lobe beneath the cortex of the parahippocampal gyrus (Figures 16–11, 16–13, and 16–14A). The amygdala is rostral and slightly dorsal to the hippocampal formation. (Compare the parasagittal section in Figure 16–19B with the drawing in Figure 16–1.) The laterally placed arrow in Figure 16–11 shows the approximate plane of section in Figure 16–19B. The amygdala and the rostral hippocampal formation form the uncus (Figures 16–1, 16–2, and 16–13). Expanding space-

occupying lesions above the tentorium cerebelli (see Figure 4–15), especially those of the temporal lobe, may displace the uncus medially. This **uncal herniation** compresses midbrain structures, ultimately resulting in coma and even death. Initially uncal herniation can compress the oculomotor nerves, which exit from the ventral midbrain surface. This results in third nerve dysfunction, including paralysis of extraocular muscles and loss of pupillary light reflexes.

The three nuclear divisions of the amygdala are schematically depicted in the inset to Figure 16–13. The **corticomedial** division of the amygdala merges with the overlying cortex of the medial temporal lobe. This division receives a major input directly from the **olfactory bulb.** The two other nuclear divisions, **basolateral** and **central,** are also shown. The **bed nucleus of the stria terminalis** is the C-shaped nuclear component of the amygdala. It has connections with brain stem autonomic and visceral afferent nuclei and thus has connections similar to those of the central nuclear division. A portion of the bed nucleus of the stria terminalis is thought to be sexually dimorphic.

The Stria Terminalis and the Ventral Amygdalofugal Pathway Are the Two Output Pathways of the Amygdala

The **stria terminalis** carries output from the amygdala, predominantly from the corticomedial nuclei. In

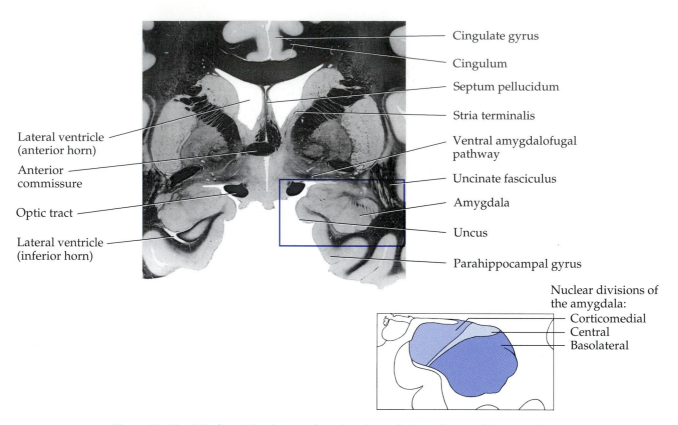

Lateral ventricle (anterior horn)

Anterior commissure

Optic tract

Lateral ventricle (inferior horn)

Cingulate gyrus

Cingulum

Septum pellucidum

Stria terminalis

Ventral amygdalofugal pathway

Uncinate fasciculus

Amygdala

Uncus

Parahippocampal gyrus

Nuclear divisions of the amygdala:
Corticomedial
Central
Basolateral

Figure 16–13. Myelin-stained coronal section through the column of fornix and amygdala. The inset shows the approximate location of the nuclear divisions in the amygdala.

coronal section (Figures 16–11, 16–13, and 16–14), the stria terminalis is medial to the caudate nucleus in the roof of the inferior horn of the lateral ventricle and the floor of the body and anterior horn of the lateral ventricle. In horizontal section (Figure 16–16), it is located rostrally (where the bed nucleus is more prominent) and caudally (where the stria is more prominent) rather than dorsally and ventrally.

The stria terminalis and its bed nucleus have a C-shape, following that of the lateral ventricle and the caudate nucleus. These limbic system structures lie in a shallow groove formed at the junction of the thalamus and the caudate nucleus, termed the terminal sulcus. Running along with the stria terminalis and bed nucleus is the **thalamostriate vein** (or terminal vein), which drains portions of the thalamus and caudate nucleus. The stria terminalis does not stain darkly because its axons are not heavily myelinated. A major target of the axons running in the stria terminalis is the **ventral medial nucleus of the hypothalamus,** which is important in feeding.

The other efferent pathway of the amygdala, the **ventral amygdalofugal pathway** (Figure 16–13), runs ventral to the anterior commissure and globus pallidus (see Chapter 14). The projections of the central and basolateral nuclei course primarily in this effer-

ent pathway. The ventral pathway has four major targets:

1. The **medial dorsal nucleus** of the thalamus (Figures 16–14B and 16–15) links the basolateral amygdala indirectly with the prefrontal and orbitofrontal cortical areas.
2. The **hypothalamus** links the central nuclei of the amygdala with the lateral hypothalamus for autonomic nervous system control and with parvocellular neurons for neuroendocrine control. The central nuclei of the amygdala influence corticotropin hormone release by parvocellular neurosecretory neurons of the paraventricular nucleus (Chapter 15). This control is exerted by disinhibition: GABA-ergic output neurons of the central nuclei synapse on GABA-ergic neurons in the hypothalamus that control the neurosecretory neurons. Disinhibition is an important feature of circuitry in the cerebellar cortex (Chapter 13) and basal ganglia (Chapter 14).
3. The **basal forebrain,** including the ventral striatum and the cholinergic neurons of the basal nucleus and nucleus of the diagonal band of Broca, links the amygdala with the cortex indirectly.

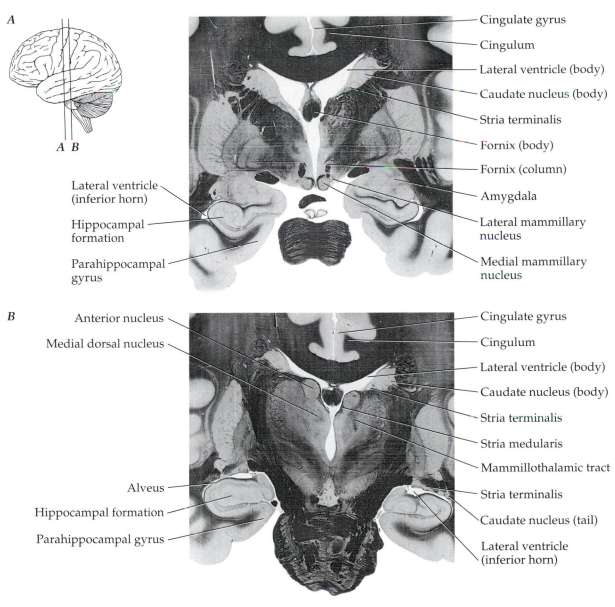

Figure 16–14. Myelin-stained coronal section through the mammillary bodies (**A**) and through the mammillothalamic tract (**B**). In **B**, the mammillothalamic tract is seen on the right side only because the section is asymmetric. The inset shows the planes of section.

4. The **brain stem,** which contains parasympathetic preganglionic nuclei, receives a projection from the central nuclei.

The Hippocampal Formation Is Located in the Floor of the Inferior Horn of the Lateral Ventricle

Coronal sections through the temporal lobe, from rostral to caudal directions, slice first through the amygdala, then through both the amygdala and hippocampal formation, and finally through the hippocampal formation alone. (Figures 16–13 and 16–14 show these rostrocaudal relationships.) The hippocampal formation forms part of the floor of the inferior horn of the lateral ventricle. In coronal section (eg, Figure 16–15) the hippocampal formation is located ventrally and the fornix is located dorsally. In horizontal section (Figure 16–16) the hippocampal formation (which here is quite small) is caudal and the fornix is rostral. As discussed in Chapter 3, the hippocampal formation is dorsal to the corpus callosum early in brain development; later, it is as if it were "dragged" into the temporal lobe. The minuscule portion of the hippocampal formation dorsal to the cor-

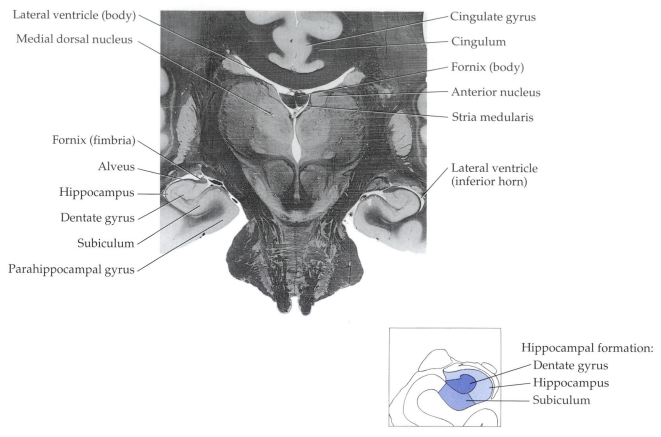

Lateral ventricle (body)
Medial dorsal nucleus
Fornix (fimbria)
Alveus
Hippocampus
Dentate gyrus
Subiculum
Parahippocampal gyrus

Cingulate gyrus
Cingulum
Fornix (body)
Anterior nucleus
Stria medularis
Lateral ventricle (inferior horn)

Hippocampal formation:
Dentate gyrus
Hippocampus
Subiculum

Figure 16–15. Myelin-stained coronal section through the medial dorsal nucleus of the thalamus. The divisions of the hippocampal formation are shown.

pus callosum in the mature brain is termed the indusium griseum (see Figure AII–16).

During development the hippocampal formation also undergoes an infolding into the temporal lobe (Figure 16–17). The simple sequence of the component parts of the temporal lobe, from the parahippocampal gyrus on the lateral surface to the dentate nucleus on the medial surface, becomes more complex later in development. As the **hippocampal sulcus** forms, the dentate gyrus and the subiculum become apposed; the pial surfaces of these two structures fuse, and a hippocampal afferent pathway (the perforant pathway) courses through this fusion (see Figure 16–18B).

The Hippocampal Formation Is Archicortex and Has a Laminar Organization

The hippocampal formation is a primitive form of allocortex, termed **archicortex,** with three principal cell layers (Figure 16–12). (The other type of allocortex is paleocortex, which is primarily olfactory cortex.)

The three divisions of the hippocampal formation—the **dentate gyrus, hippocampus,** and **subiculum**—are shown in the inset in Figure 16–15. Each division has three principal cell layers. The dentate gyrus contains the molecular, granule cell, and polymorphic layers (Figure 16–18A). In the molecular layer are the apical dendrites of granule cells and other processes, but few cell bodies. Granule cells, which are the projection neurons of the dentate gyrus, are in the second layer. Their axons synapse on other neurons of the hippocampal formation. The polymorphic layer contains interneurons. The three layers of the hippocampus and subiculum are analogous to those of the dentate gyrus (Figure 16–18). The important difference is that the granule cell layer is replaced by the pyramidal layer, which contains **pyramidal cells,** the projection neurons of the hippocampus and subiculum.

Pyramidal cells of the entorhinal cortex send their axons to the dentate gyrus to synapse on granule cells. This is the **perforant pathway.** Granule cell axons, termed **mossy fibers,** synapse on pyramidal cells of the CA3 region of the hippocampal formation,

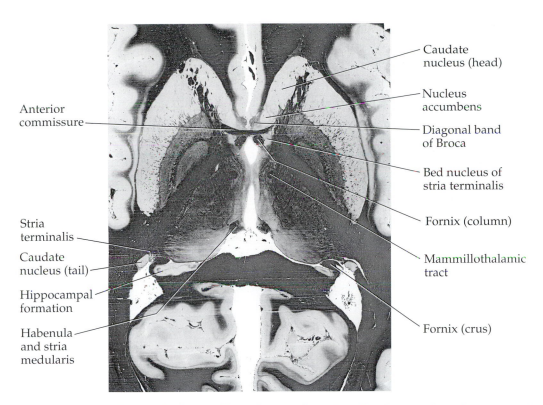

Anterior commissure

Stria terminalis

Caudate nucleus (tail)

Hippocampal formation

Habenula and stria medularis

Caudate nucleus (head)

Nucleus accumbens

Diagonal band of Broca

Bed nucleus of stria terminalis

Fornix (column)

Mammillothalamic tract

Fornix (crus)

Figure 16–16. Myelin-stained horizontal section through the anterior commissure.

which send their axons (called the **Schaefer collaterals**) to pyramidal cells of the CA1 region. (These axon collaterals spare the CA2 region.) The subiculum receives the next projection in the sequence, from the CA1 region, and it projects back to the entorhinal cortex. As described earlier, additional parallel projections from entorhinal cortex are also important (Figure 16–5). It is not known how the myriad connections of the entorhinal cortex and hippocampal formation are organized to play a role in memory consolidation, spatial memory, and other aspects of cognition. However, an important clue exists: The strength of many synapses in the hippocampal formation can be modified under various experimental conditions.

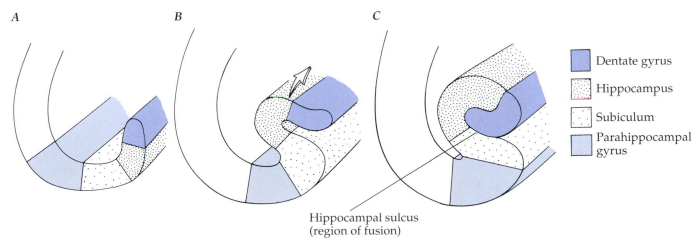

A *B* *C*

Dentate gyrus

Hippocampus

Subiculum

Parahippocampal gyrus

Hippocampal sulcus (region of fusion)

Figure 16–17. Schematic of the hippocampal formation at two stages of development (***A, B***) and in maturity (***C***). (*Adapted from Williams PL, Warwick R: Functional Neuroanatomy of Man. W. B. Saunders, 1975.*)

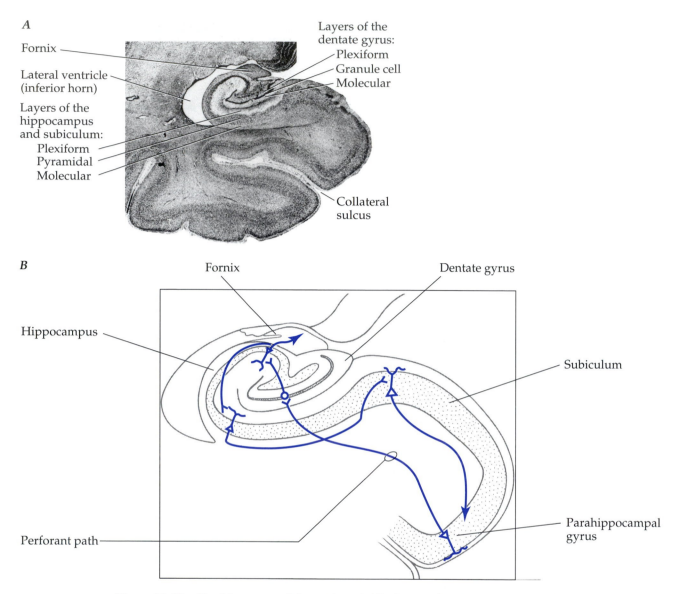

A

Fornix

Lateral ventricle (inferior horn)

Layers of the hippocampus and subiculum:
Plexiform
Pyramidal
Molecular

Layers of the dentate gyrus:
Plexiform
Granule cell
Molecular

Collateral sulcus

B

Fornix

Dentate gyrus

Hippocampus

Subiculum

Perforant path

Parahippocampal gyrus

Figure 16–18. The hippocampal formation. *A.* Nissl-stained section through the human hippocampal formation, parahippocampal gyrus, and ventral temporal lobe. The hippocampus has three cytoarchitectonic divisions. These divisions are abbreviated CA for cornus ammonis, or Ammon's horn. (To early anatomists, the hippocampal formation together with the fornix looked like the horns of a ram.) *B.* The basic circuitry of the hippocampal formation is superimposed on the cytoarchitecture of the hippocampal formation and entorhinal cortex. (**A,** *Courtesy of Dr. David Amaral, State University of New York at Stony Brook.* **B,** *Adapted from Zola-Morgan S, Squire LR, Amaral DG: Human amnesia and medial temporal lobe region: Enduring memory impairment following a bilateral lesion limited to field CA1 of the hippocampus. J Neurosci 1986;6:2950–2967.*)

Pyramidal cells of the hippocampus and subiculum have extrinsic connections, sending their axons to cortical and subcortical targets (Figure 16–6B). The hippocampus and subiculum have extensive "back" projections to the entorhinal cortex that, in turn, project widely to other cortical regions (Figure 16–5). The principal subcortical targets are the mammillary bodies, which receive a projection from pyramidal cells of the subiculum, and the lateral septal nucleus, which receives a projection from the hippocampus. These axons course in the fornix. In addition to extrinsic connections, both sides of the hippocampal formation are interconnected through **commissural neurons** whose axons course in the ventral portion of the fornix.

A Sagittal Cut Through the Mammillary Bodies Reveals the Fornix and Mammillothalamic Tract

Structures that have a C-shape are oriented approximately in the sagittal plane. The sagittal section in Figure 16–19A is located close to the midline and transects the fornix, although not through its entire length. The sagittal section in Figure 16–19B is located farther laterally and cuts through the long axis of the hippocampal formation.

Pyramidal cell axons of the hippocampus and subiculum form the **alveus,** the myelinated envelope sur-

rounding the hippocampal formation (Figure 16–19B). These axons collect on the medial side of the hippocampal formation to form the first of the four anatomical parts of the fornix, termed the **fimbria.** The other three parts—the **crus** (where the axons are separate from the hippocampal formation), the **body** (where the axons from both sides join at the midline), and the **column** (where axons descend toward their targets)—bring the axons of the fornix to neurons in the diencephalon and rostral telencephalon.

The body and column of the fornix can be seen in Figure 16–19A. Note how the column of the fornix descends caudal to the **anterior commissure** to termi-

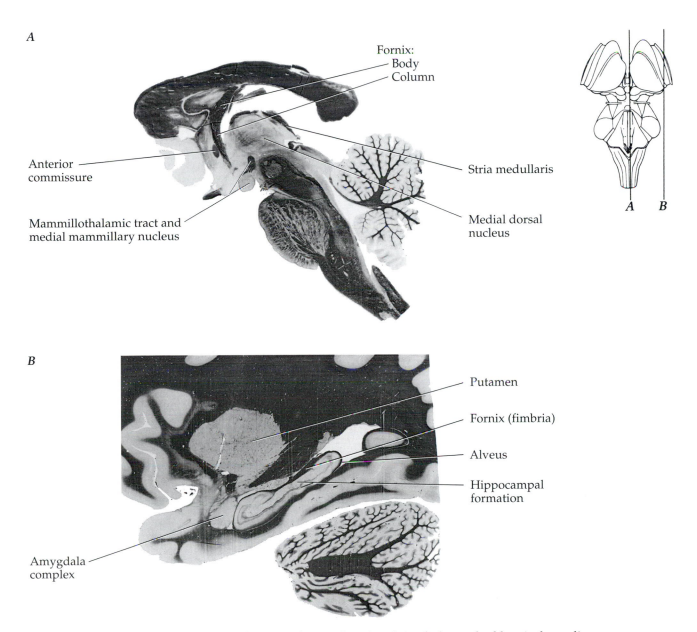

Figure 16–19. ***A.*** Myelin-stained sagittal section through the cerebral hemisphere, diencephalon, and brain stem close to the midline. ***B.*** Parasagittal section through the amygdaloid complex and hippocampal formation.

A

B

C

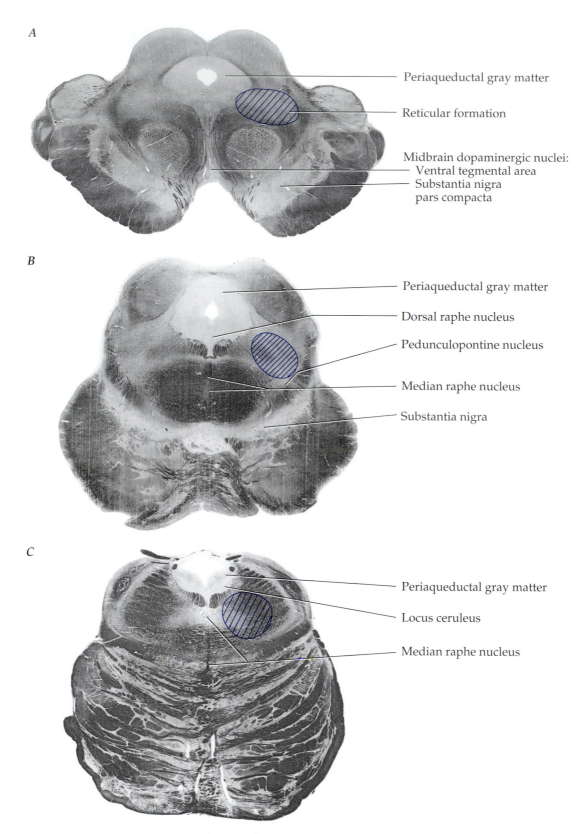

Periaqueductal gray matter

Reticular formation

Midbrain dopaminergic nuclei:
Ventral tegmental area
Substantia nigra
pars compacta

Periaqueductal gray matter

Dorsal raphe nucleus

Pedunculopontine nucleus

Median raphe nucleus

Substantia nigra

Periaqueductal gray matter

Locus ceruleus

Median raphe nucleus

Figure 16–20. Components of the brain stem related to the limbic system. Myelin-stained sections through the rostral midbrain (*A*), caudal midbrain (*B*), and rostral pons (*C*). The reticular formation is indicated by hatched regions.

nate in the **mammillary body;** this is the **postcommissural fornix** (see also Figure 16–16, where the columns of the fornix are caudal to the anterior commissure). The mammillary body comprises the medial and lateral mammillary nuclei (Figure 16–14A), and the fornix terminates in both components. The major output, the **mammillothalamic tract,** originates from both the medial and lateral mammillary nuclei. Axons of the mammillothalamic tract also can be seen leaving the mammillary body in Figure 16–19A. These axons are coursing toward the **anterior thalamic nuclei** (Figure 16–14B). The lateral mammillary nucleus (Figure 16–14A) also gives rise to the **mammillotegmental tract,** which descends to the midbrain and rostral pontine reticular formation.

Fibers of the fornix also terminate in locations other than the mammillary bodies. Some of these fibers terminate directly in the anterior thalamic nuclei; others project to the amygdala and nucleus accumbens. Moreover, rostral to the anterior commissure, the **precommissural fornix,** which is smaller than the postcommissural portion, courses away from the midline. (It cannot be seen in the section in Figure 16–19A.) The precommissural fornix, which contains the axons from both the subiculum and hippocampus, terminates in the lateral septal nucleus. A portion of the **stria medullaris,** which has a predominantly rostrocaudal course, is also revealed in this section (Figure 16–19A). As discussed earlier, the medial septal nucleus projects axons into the stria medullaris. These axons synapse in the habenula (see Figures AI–7 and AII–18).

Nuclei in the Brain Stem Link Telencephalic and Diencephalic Limbic Structures With the Autonomic Nervous System and the Spinal Cord

The **periaqueductal gray matter** and **reticular formation** (Figure 16–20) are thought to be important in the behavioral expression of emotions, such as stereotypic defense reactions or the body's response to stress. Septal neurons project to the midbrain reticular formation via neurons of the **lateral hypothalamus.** Neurons of the lateral hypothalamus are interspersed throughout the **medial forebrain bundle** (see Chapter 15). From these midbrain regions the actions of neurons in wide areas of the reticular formation can be modified by the limbic system. The hypothalamus also projects to the periaqueductal gray matter. Chapter 5 considered the projection of the periaqueductal gray matter to the raphe nuclei (see Figure 5–14), which give rise to a spinal cord projection for regulating pain transmission.

Summary

General Anatomy of the Limbic System

The limbic system comprises a set of structures located predominantly on the medial surface of the cerebral hemisphere (Figures 16–1 and 16–2). The diverse functions of the limbic system include important roles in **learning and memory** and in **emotions**—and their **behavioral** and **visceral consequences.** Many of the structures have a **C-shaped configuration.** The limbic system has three C-shaped components (Figures 16–1 through 16–4): (1) the **limbic association cortex,** (2) the **hippocampal formation** and **fornix,** and (3) part of the **amygdala** (bed of the stria terminalis) and the **stria terminalis.**

Limbic Association Cortex

The limbic cortical areas include the following structures (Figures 16–2 and 16–3): the **medial orbital gyri** of the frontal lobe, the **cingulate gyrus** in the frontal and parietal lobes, the **parahippocampal gyrus** in the temporal lobe, and the cortex of the **temporal pole.** The limbic cortical areas receive input from higher-order sensory areas in the temporal lobe and from the **prefrontal association cortex** and the **parietal-temporal-occipital association area.** The two principal pathways carrying cortical association axons to and from other limbic system structures are the **cingulum** (Figure 16–10) (located beneath the cingulate gyrus; Figure 16–11) and the **uncinate fasciculus** (Figure 16–11). The cytoarchitecture of limbic association cortex differs from that of other cortical regions. The cortex on the external surface of the parahippocampal gyrus lateral to the **collateral sulcus** (Figure 16–3) has at least six layers (**neocortex**), whereas the cortex medial to the sulcus is more variable and typically has fewer than six cell layers (**allocortex**) (Figure 16–12). Cholinergic projections to limbic cortex, the hippocampal formation, and lateral cortical areas originate from the basal forebrain, including the **basal nucleus,** the **nucleus of the diagonal band of Broca,** and the **medial septal nucleus** (Figure 16–11).

Hippocampal Formation

The **hippocampal formation** (Figures 16–1 and 16–4) includes three cytoarchitectonically distinct subdivisions (Figures 16–4 and 16–15): the **dentate gyrus,** the **hippocampus,** and the **subiculum.** The hippocampal formation plays an essential role in consolidation of explicit and spatial memory. The limbic association cortex provides the major input to the hippocampal formation. The **entorhinal cortex,** a specific portion of the rostral parahippocampal gyrus, projects directly to the hippocampal formation (Figures 16–5 and 16–6A). Other portions of the limbic association cortex influence the hippocampal formation indirectly, via the entorhinal cortex. The dentate gyrus, hippocampus, and subiculum are separate processing stages in a sequence of intrinsic connections in the hippocampal formation (Figures 16–5 and 16–18). The flow of information through the hippocampal formation is largely unidirectional.

Hippocampal efferents originate from the subiculum and the hippocampus proper; the dentate gyrus projects only to the hippocampus. Cortical projections from the hippocampus and subiculum terminate in the entorhinal cortex, and from there information is widely distributed throughout the cerebral cortex (Figures 16–5 and 16–6B). Subcortical projections are via the **fornix.** Most of the axons in the fornix are those of **pyramidal cells** of the subiculum and hippocampus. Axons from the **subiculum** synapse in the **mammillary body** (Figures 16–6B, 16–14A, and 16–19A). These axons course in the postcommissural fornix (Figures 16–13 and 16–19A). The mammillary bodies project, via the **mammillothalamic tract** (Figures 16–14A and 16–19A), to the **anterior thalamic nuclei** (Figure 16–14B), which project to the **cingulate gyrus** (Figures 16–2 and 16–10). The hippocampus projects, via the precommissural fornix, to the **lateral septal nucleus** (Figures 16–5B and 16–11). The **medial septal nucleus,** which contains cholinergic and GABA-ergic neurons, projects back to the **hippocampal formation,** via the **fornix.**

Amygdala

The amygdala has three major nuclear divisions (Figures 16–7 and 16–13), which collectively are involved in **emotions** and their **behavioral expression** (Figure 16–7): the basolateral nuclei, the central nuclei, and the corticomedial nuclei. The **basolateral nuclei** receive a major input from the **cerebral cortex** and project to the **medial dorsal nucleus** of the thalamus, the **basal nucleus,** the **ventral striatum,** and back to the **cortex** (temporal, orbitofrontal, and prefrontal association areas). The **central nuclei** are reciprocally connected with **viscerosensory** and **visceral motor nuclei** of the brain stem. They also project to the hypothala-

mus to regulate neuroendocrine functions. The **corticomedial nuclei** receive direct olfactory input. They may play a role in appetitive behaviors and neuroendocrine functions through their projections to the **ventromedial nucleus** of the hypothalamus.

The amygdala has two output pathways: (1) The **stria terminalis** (Figures 16–7C and 16–13), which is C-shaped, carries the efferent projection primarily from the **corticomedial nuclei,** and (2) the **ventral amygdalofugal pathway** (Figure 16–13) carries the efferents from the **central nuclei,** which descend to the **brain stem,** and those from the **basolateral nuclei,** which ascend to the **thalamus,** the **ventral striatum,** and the **basal nucleus** (Figure 16–13). The bed nucleus of the stria terminalis runs along with the stria.

Related Sources

Brust JCM: The Practice of Neural Science. McGraw-Hill; 2000. (See ch. 16, cases 71–74.)

Iversen S, Kupfermann I, Kandel ER: Emotional states and feelings. In Kandel ER, Schwartz JH, Jessell TM (editors): Principles of Neural Science, 4th ed. McGraw-Hill; 2000: 983–997.

Kandel ER: Cellular mechanisms of learning and the biological basis of individuality. In Kandel ER, Schwartz JH, Jessell TM (editors): Principles of Neural Science, 4th ed. McGraw-Hill; 2000:1247–1279.

Kandel ER: Disorders of mood: Depression, mania, and anxiety disorders. In Kandel ER, Schwartz JH, Jessell TM (editors): Principles of Neural Science, 4th ed. McGraw-Hill; 2000:1207–1226.

Kandel ER: Disorders of thought and volition: Schizophrenia. In Kandel ER, Schwartz JH, Jessell TM (editors): Principles of Neural Science, 4th ed. McGraw-Hill; 2000: 1188–1208.

Kandel ER, Kupfermann I, Iversen S: Learning and memory. In Kandel ER, Schwartz JH, Jessell TM (editors): Principles of Neural Science, 4th ed. McGraw-Hill; 2000:1227–1246.

Kandel ER, Kupfermann I, Iversen S: Motivational and addictive states. In Kandel ER, Schwartz JH, Jessell TM (editors): Principles of Neural Science, 4th ed. McGraw-Hill; 2000:998–1013.

Selected Readings

Aggleton JP: The contribution of the amygdala to normal and abnormal emotional states. Trends Neurosci 1993; 16:328–333.

Amaral DG: Emerging principles of intrinsic hippocampal organization. Curr Opin Neurobiol 1993;3:225–229.

Andreasen NC: The mechanisms of schizophrenia. Curr Opin Neurobiol 1994;4:245–251.

Cleghorn JM, Zipursky RB, List SJ: Structural and functional brain imaging in schizophrenia. J Psychiatry Neurosci 1991;16:53–74.

Corkin S: What's new with the amnesic patient H.M.? Nat Rev Neurosci 2002;3:153–160.

Drevets WC: Neuroimaging and neuropathological studies of depression: Implications for the cognitive-emotional features of mood disorders. Curr Opin Neurobiol 2001; 11:240–249.

Hyman SE, Malenka RC: Addiction and the brain: The neurobiology of compulsion and its persistence. Nat Rev Neurosci 2001;2:695–703.

Koob GF, Sanna PP, Bloom FE: Neuroscience of addiction. Neuron 1998;21:467–476.

LeDoux JE: Emotion and the limbic system concept. Concepts in Neuroscience 1991;2:169–199.

LeDoux JE: Emotion, memory and the brain. Sci Am 1994; 270:50–57.

LeDoux JE: Emotion circuits in the brain. Annu Rev Neurosci 2000;23:155–184.

Nestler EJ, Barrot M, DiLeone RJ, Eisch AJ, Gold SJ, Monteggia LM: Neurobiology of depression. Neuron 2002; 34:13–25.

Price JL, Russchen FT, Amaral DG: The limbic region. II: The amygdaloid complex. In Björklund A, Hökfelt T, Swanson LW (editors): Handbook of Chemical Neuroanatomy. Vol. 5. Integrated Systems of the CNS, Part I. Elsevier; 1987:279–388.

Sisodia SS, St George-Hyslop PH: gamma-Secretase, Notch, Abeta and Alzheimer's disease: Where do the presenilins fit in? Nat Rev Neurosci 2002;3:281–290.

References

Amaral DG: Memory: Anatomical organization of candidate brain regions. In Plum F (editor): Handbook of Physiology, Section 1, Vol. 1, Part 2. American Physiological Society; 1987:211–294.

Amaral DG: Introduction: What is where in the medial temporal lobe? Hippocampus 1999;9:1–6.

Amaral DG, Insausti R: Hippocampal formation. In Paxinos G (editor): The Human Nervous System. Academic Press; 1990:711–755.

Andy OJ, Stephan H: The septum of the human brain. J Comp Neurol 1968;133:383–410.

Bietz AJ: Central gray. In Paxinos G (editor): The Human Nervous System. Academic Press; 1990:307–320.

Blanchard C, Blanchard R, Fellous JM, et al: The brain decade in debate: III. Neurobiology of emotion. Braz J Med Biol Res 2001;34:283–293.

Carlsen J, Heimer L: The basolateral amygdaloid complex as a cortical-like structure. Brain Res 1988;441:377–380.

Davidson RJ, Putnam KM, Larson CL: Dysfunction in the neural circuitry of emotion regulation—A possible prelude to violence. Science 2000;289:591–594.

DeOlmos JS: Amygdala. In Paxinos G (editor): The Human Nervous System. Academic Press; 1990:583–710.

Duvernoy HM: The Human Hippocampus: An Atlas of Applied Anatomy. J. F. Bergmann Verlag; 1988:166.

Farnham FR, Ritchie CW, James DV, Kennedy HG: Pathology of love. Lancet 1997;350:710.

Grace AA: Gating of information flow within the limbic system and the pathophysiology of schizophrenia. Brain Res Brain Res Rev 2000;31:330–341.

Grace AA, Bunney BS, Moore H, Todd CL: Dopamine-cell depolarization block as a model for the therapeutic action of antipsychotic drugs. Trends Neurosci 1997;20: 31–37.

Hedren JC, Strumble RG, Whitehouse PJ, et al: Topography of the magnocellular basal forebrain system in the human brain. Journal of Neuropathology and Experimental Neurology 1984;43:1–21.

Herman JP, Cullinan WE: Neurocircuitry of stress: Central control of the hypothalamo-pituitary-adrenocortical axis. Trends Neurosci 1997;20:78–84.

Holstege G: Subcortical limbic system projections to caudal brainstem and spinal cord. In Paxinos G (editor): The Human Nervous System. Academic Press; 1990: 261–286.

Holstege G: The emotional motor system in relation to the supraspinal control of micturition and mating behavior. Behav Brain Res 1998;92:103–109.

Inui A: Feeding and body-weight regulation by hypothalamic neuropeptides—Mediation of the actions of leptin. Trends Neurosci 1999;22:62–67.

Lavenex P, Amaral DG: Hippocampal-neocortical interaction: A hierarchy of associativity. Hippocampus 2000; 10:420–430.

LeDoux JE: Emotion and the amygdala. In Appleton JP (editor): The Amygdala: Neurobiological Aspects of Emotion, Memory, and Mental Dysfunction. Wiley-Liss; 1992: 339–351.

Levitt P: A monoclonal antibody to limbic system neurons. Science 1984;223:299–301.

Meyer-Lindenberg A, Miletich RS, Kohn PD, et al: Reduced prefrontal activity predicts exaggerated striatal dopaminergic function in schizophrenia. Nat Neurosci 2002;5: 267–271.

Millhouse OE, DeOlmos J: Neuronal configurations in lateral and basolateral amygdala. Neuroscience 1983;10: 1269–1300.

Ojemann GA, Schoenfield-McNeill J, Corina DP: Anatomic subdivisions in human temporal cortical neuronal activity related to recent verbal memory. Nat Neurosci 2002; 5:64–71.

Naidich TP, Daniels DL, Haughton VM, et al: Hippocampal formation and related structures of the limbic lobe: Anatomical-MR correlations. Part I. Surface features and coronal sections. Neuroradiology 1987;162: 747–754.

Naidich TP, Daniels DL, Haughton VM, et al: Hippocampal formation and related structure of the limbic lobe: Anatomical-MR correlations. Part II. Sagittal sections. Neuroradiology 1987;162:755–761.

Nauta WJH, Haymaker W: Hypothalamic nuclei and fiber connections. In Haymaker W, Anderson E, Nauta WJH (editors): The Hypothalamus. Charles C. Thomas; 1969: 136–209.

Nieuwenhuys R, Voogd J, van Huijzen C: The Human Central Nervous System: A Synopsis and Atlas, 3rd ed. Springer-Verlag, 1988.

Papez JW: A proposed mechanism of emotion. Archives of Neurology and Psychiatry 1937;38:725–743.

Paus T: Primate anterior cingulate cortex: Where motor control, drive and cognition interface. Nat Rev Neurosci 2001;2:417–424.

Pfefferbaum A, Zipursky RB: Neuroimaging in schizophrenia. Schizophr Res 1991;4:193–208.

Pitkanen A, Savander V, LeDoux JE: Organization of intraamygdaloid circuitries in the rat: An emerging framework for understanding functions of the amygdala. Trends Neurosci 1997;20:517–523.

Price JL, Amaral DG: An autoradiographic study of the projections of the central nucleus of the monkey amygdala. J Neurosci 1981;1:1242–1259.

Swanson LW, Petrovich GD: What is the amygdala? Trends Neurosci 1998;21:323–331.

Talairach J, Tournoux P: Co-planar stereotaxic atlas of the human brain. Georg Thieme Verlag, 1988.

Wiebe S, Blume WT, Girvin JP, Eliasziw M: A randomized, controlled trial of surgery for temporal-lobe epilepsy. N Engl J Med 2001;345:311–318.

Williams PL, Warwick R: Functional Neuroanatomy of Man. W. B. Saunders, 1975.

Zola-Morgan S, Squire LR, Amaral DG: Human amnesia and the medial temporal region: Enduring memory impairment following a bilateral lesion limited to field CA1 of the hippocampus. J Neurosci 1986;6:2950–2967.

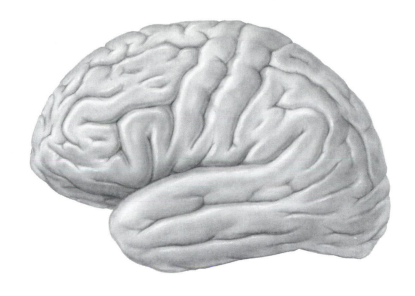

V

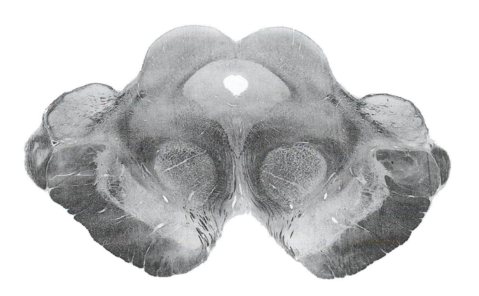

I

ATLAS

Surface Topography of the Central Nervous System

THE SURFACE TOPOGRAPHY ATLAS IS A COLLECTION OF drawings of the brain and rostral spinal cord. The various views are based on specimens and brain models. Key features are labeled on an accompanying line drawing of each view.

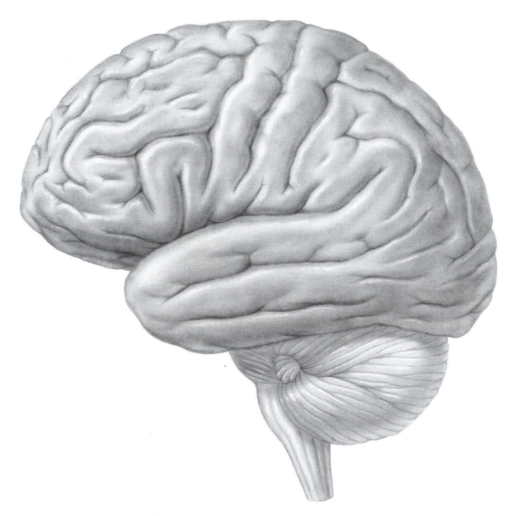

Figure AI–1. Lateral surface of the cerebral hemisphere, brain stem, cerebellum, and rostral spinal cord.

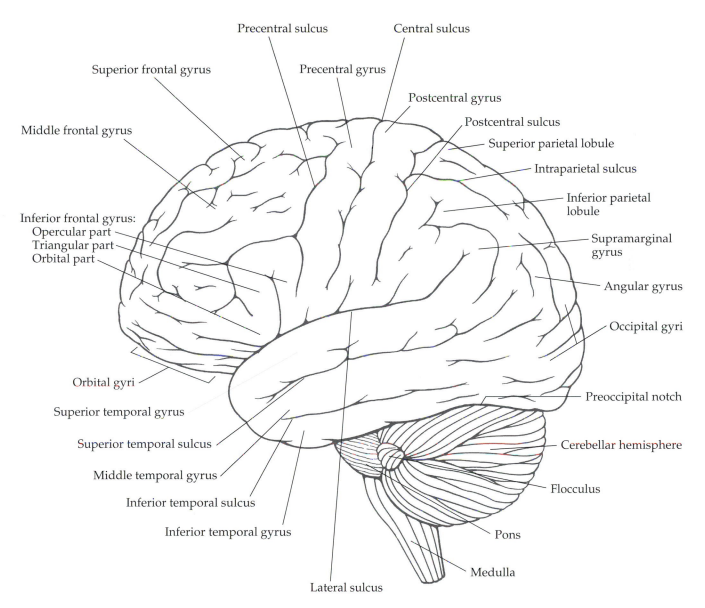

Figure AI–1 Continued.

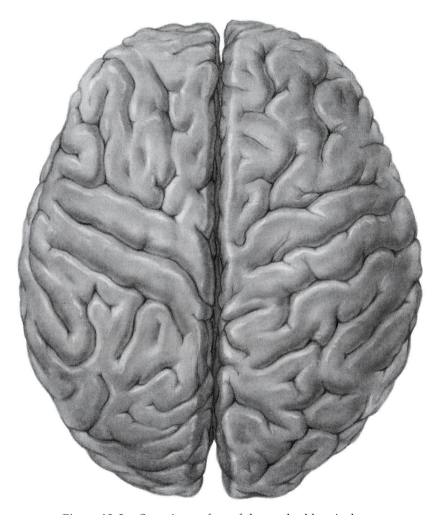

Figure AI–2. Superior surface of the cerebral hemisphere.

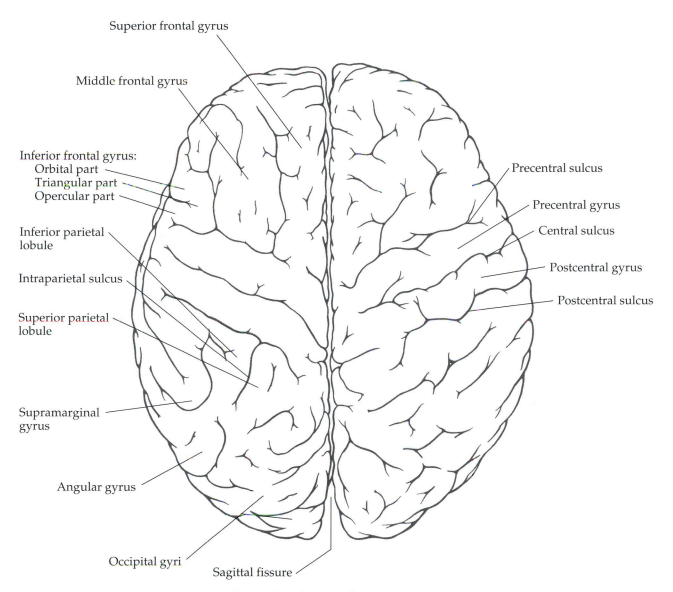

Superior frontal gyrus

Middle frontal gyrus

Inferior frontal gyrus:
  Orbital part
  Triangular part
  Opercular part

Inferior parietal lobule

Intraparietal sulcus

Superior parietal lobule

Supramarginal gyrus

Angular gyrus

Occipital gyri

Sagittal fissure

Precentral sulcus

Precentral gyrus

Central sulcus

Postcentral gyrus

Postcentral sulcus

Figure AI–2 Continued.

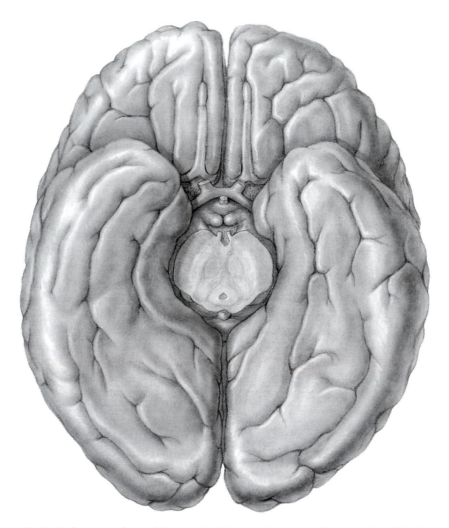

Figure AI–3. Inferior surface of the cerebral hemisphere and diencephalon. The brain stem is transected at the rostral midbrain.

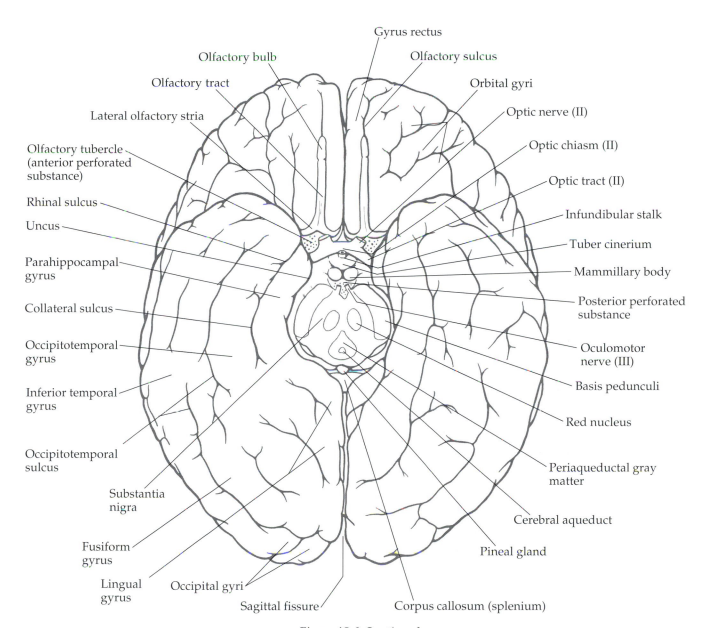

Figure AI–3 Continued.

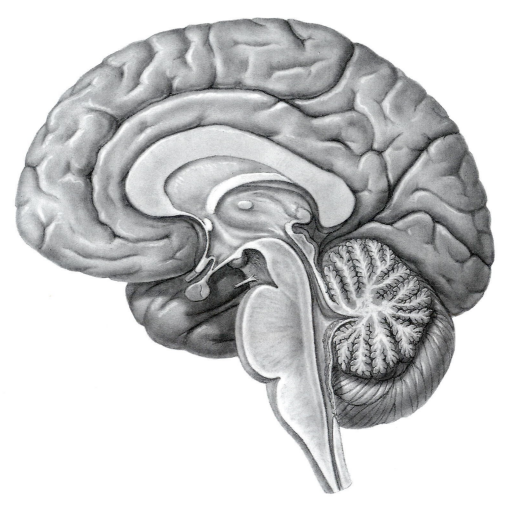

Figure AI–4. Medial surface of the cerebral hemisphere and midsagittal section through the diencephalon, brain stem, cerebellum, and rostral spinal cord.

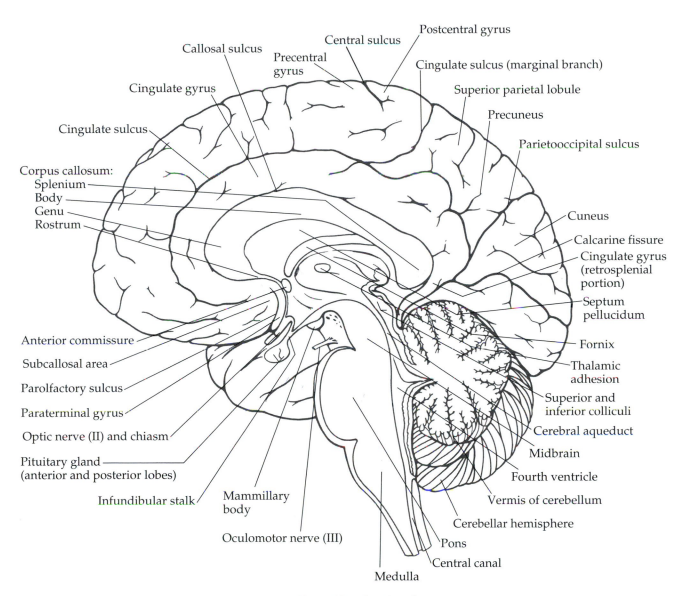

Figure AI–4 Continued.

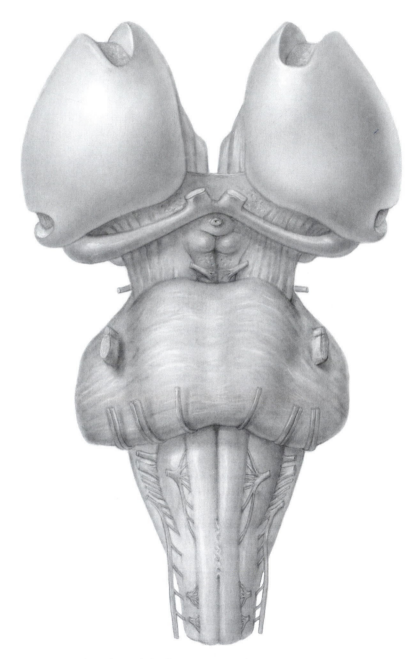

Figure AI–5. Ventral surface of the brain stem and rostral spinal cord. The striatum and diencephalon are also shown.

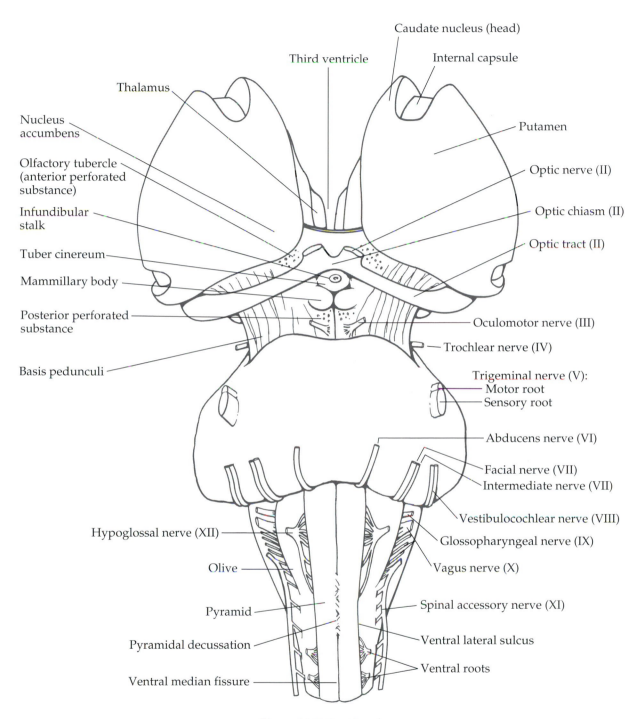

Figure AI–5 Continued.

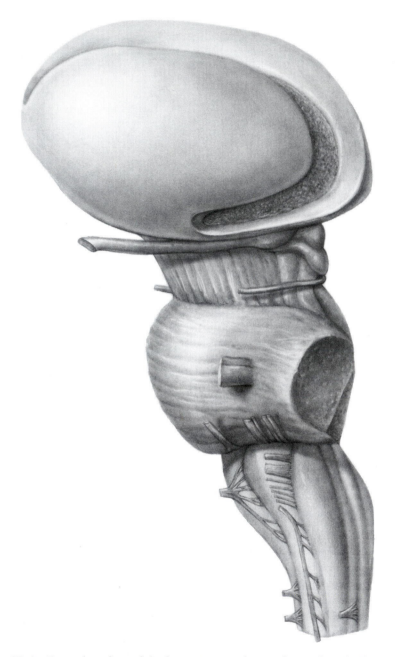

Figure AI–6. Lateral surface of the brain stem and rostral spinal cord. The striatum and diencephalon are also shown.

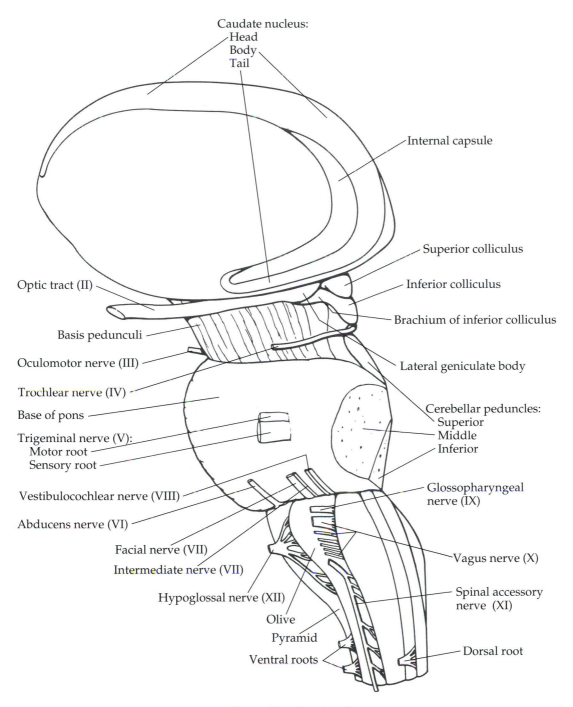

Figure AI–6 Continued.

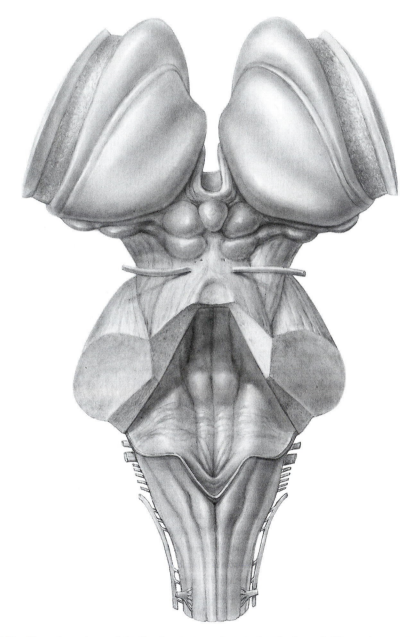

Figure AI–7. Dorsal surface of the brain stem and rostral spinal cord. The striatum and diencephalon are also shown. The cerebellum was removed to reveal the structure of the floor of the fourth ventricle.

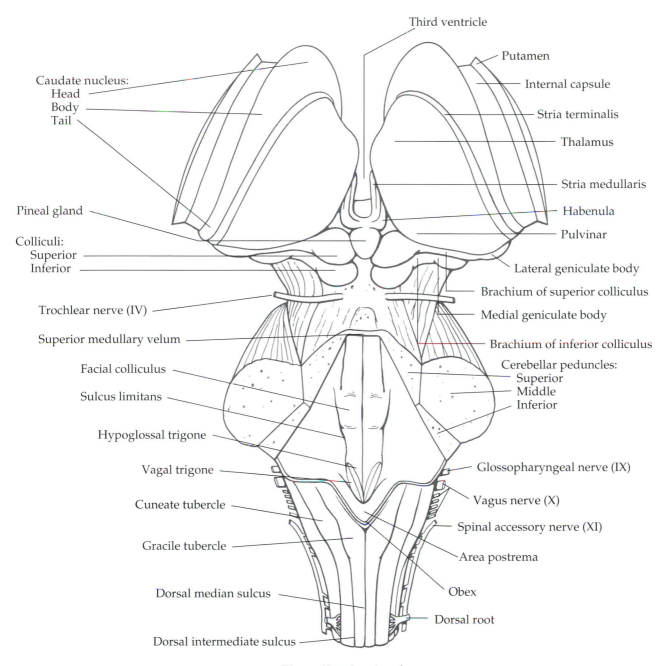

Figure AI–7 Continued.

References

Braak H, Braak E: Architectonics of the Human Telencephalic Cortex. Springer-Verlag, 1976.

Carpenter MB, Sutin J: Human Neuroanatomy. Williams & Wilkins, 1983.

Crosby EC, Humphrey T, Lauer EW: Correlative Anatomy of the Nervous System. Macmillan, 1962.

Ferner H, Staubesand J: Sobotta Atlas of Human Anatomy. Urban & Schwartzenberg, 1983.

Nieuwenhuys R, Voogd J, van Huijzen C: The Human Central Nervous System, 3rd ed. Springer-Verlag, 1988.

Williams PL, Warwick R: Functional Neuroanatomy of Man. W. B. Saunders, 1975.

Zilles K: Cortex. In Paxinos G (editor): The Human Central Nervous System. Academic Press, 1990.

II

ATLAS

Myelin-Stained Sections Through the Central Nervous System

T HE ATLAS OF MYELIN-STAINED SECTIONS THROUGH the central nervous system is in three planes: transverse, horizontal, and sagittal. (See Figure 1–14 for schematic views of these planes of sections.) Transverse sections through the cerebral hemispheres and diencephalon are termed coronal sections because they are approximately parallel to the coronal suture. These sections also cut the brain stem, but parallel to its long axis. In addition, three sections are cut in planes oblique to the transverse and horizontal sections.

In this atlas, each level through the central nervous system is printed without labeled structures as well as with labels on an accompanying photograph (printed at reduced contrast to preserve the essence of the structure). Typically, the border of a structure is indicated either when the structure's location is extremely important for understanding the functional consequences of brain trauma or when the structure is clearly depicted on the section and it is didactically important to emphasize the border. Axons of cranial nerves and primary afferent fibers are indicated by bold lines to distinguish them from the other fibers.

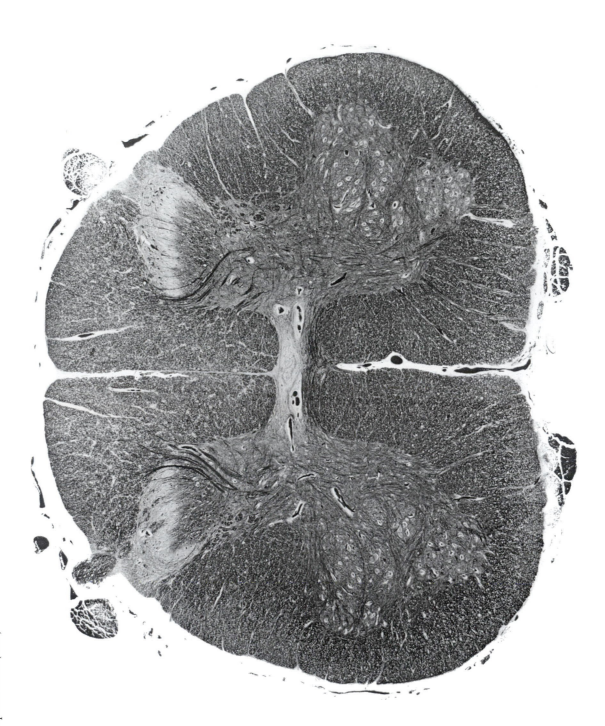

Figure AII-1. Transverse section of the first sacral segment (S1) and of the spinal cord. (×20)

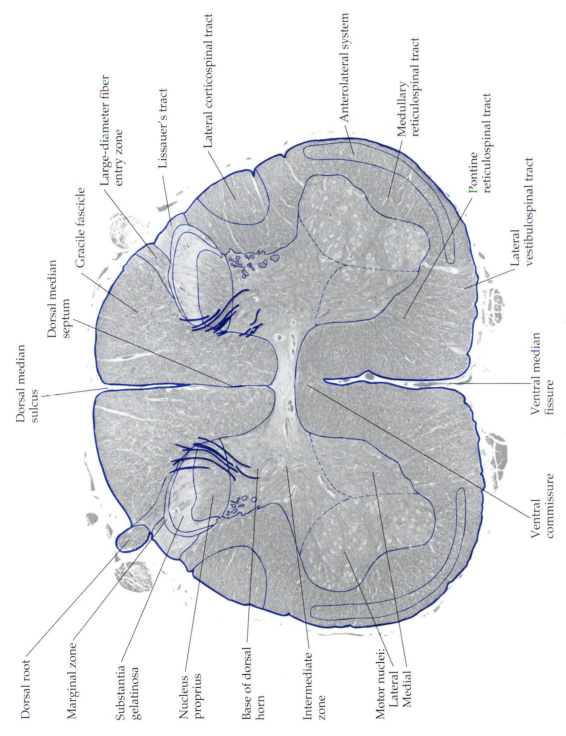

Figure AII–1 Continued.

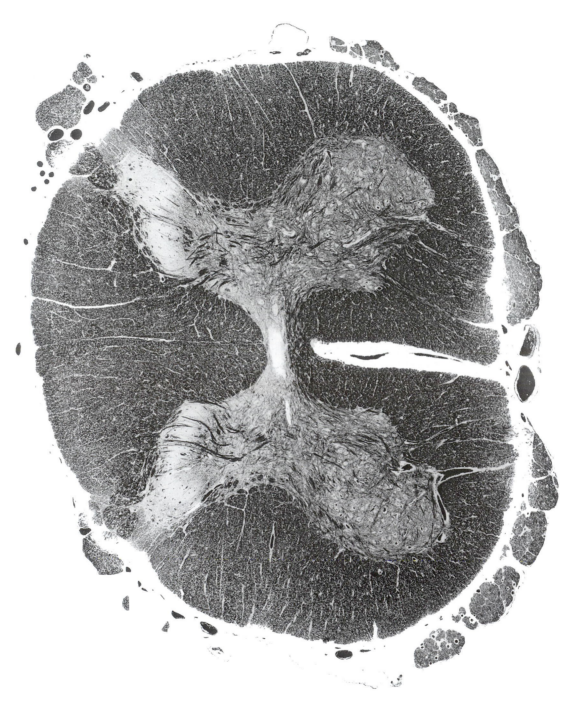

Figure AII-2. Transverse section of the second lumbar segment (L2) of the spinal cord. (×18)

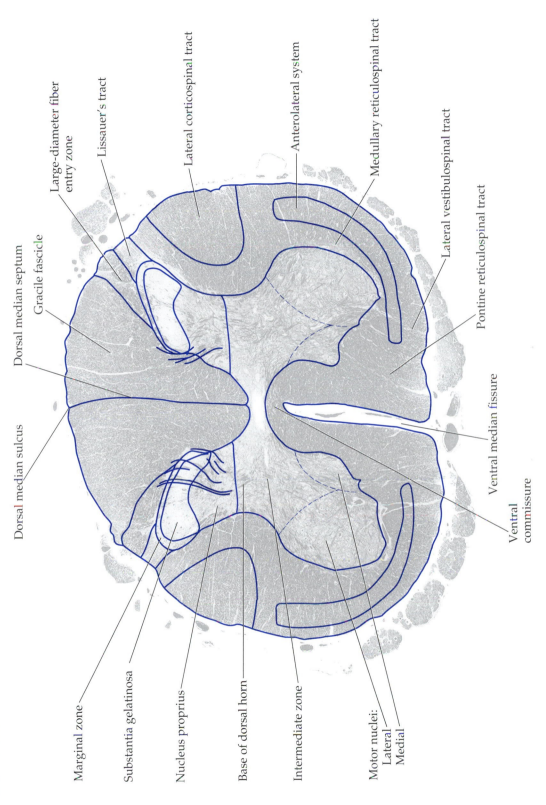

Figure AII–2 Continued.

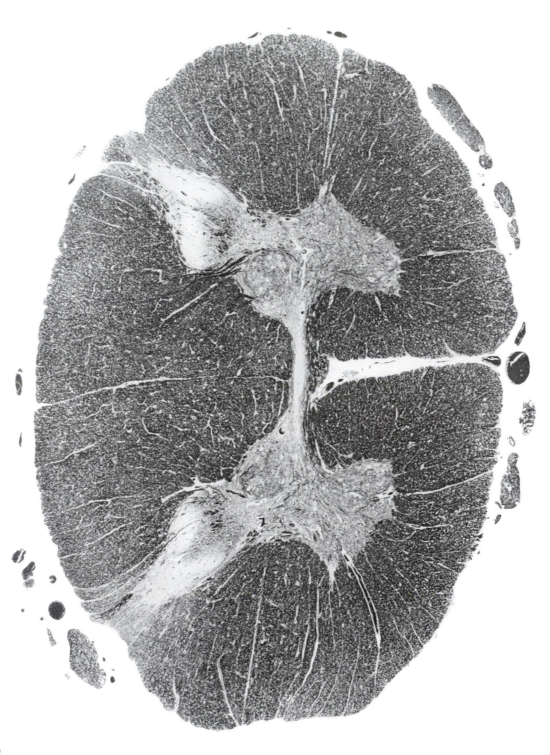

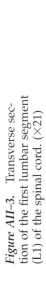

Figure AII–3. Transverse section of the first lumbar segment (L1) of the spinal cord. (×21)

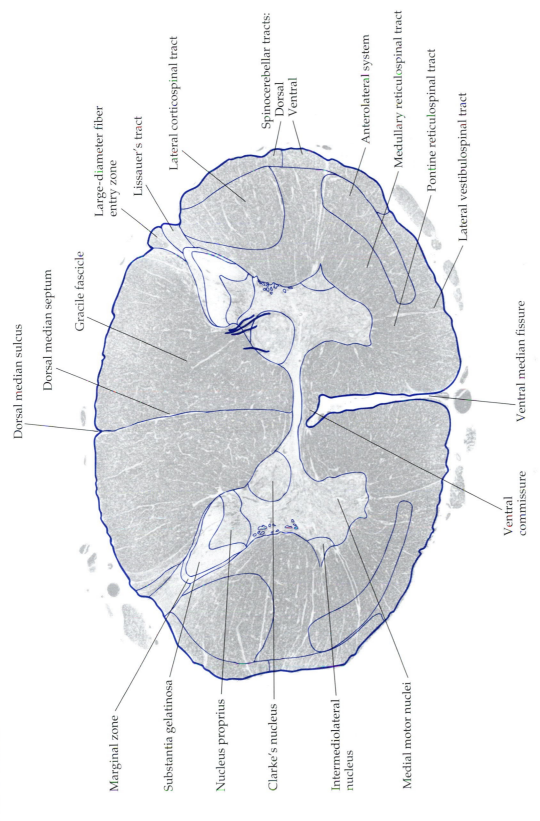

Figure AII-3 Continued.

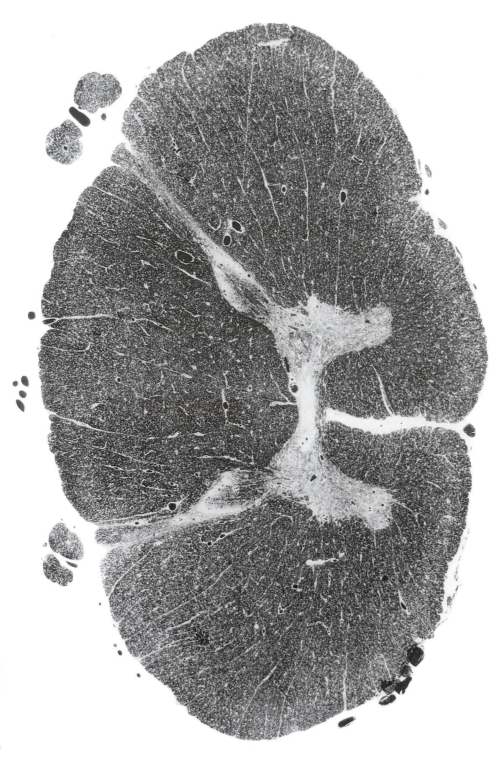

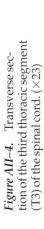

Figure AII–4. Transverse section of the third thoracic segment (T3) of the spinal cord. (×23)

Figure AII–4 Continued.

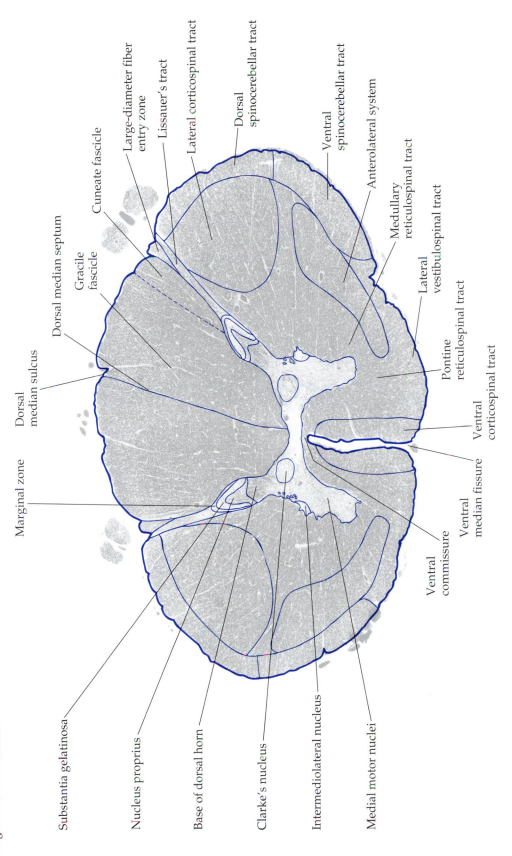

Dorsal median sulcus

Dorsal median septum

Large-diameter fiber entry zone

Lissauer's tract

Lateral corticospinal tract

Dorsal spinocerebellar tract

Ventral spinocerebellar tract

Anterolateral system

Medullary reticulospinal tract

Lateral vestibulospinal tract

Gracile fascicle

Cuneate fascicle

Dorsal median septum

Marginal zone

Dorsal median sulcus

Pontine reticulospinal tract

Ventral corticospinal tract

Ventral median fissure

Ventral commissure

Substantia gelatinosa

Nucleus proprius

Base of dorsal horn

Clarke's nucleus

Intermediolateral nucleus

Medial motor nuclei

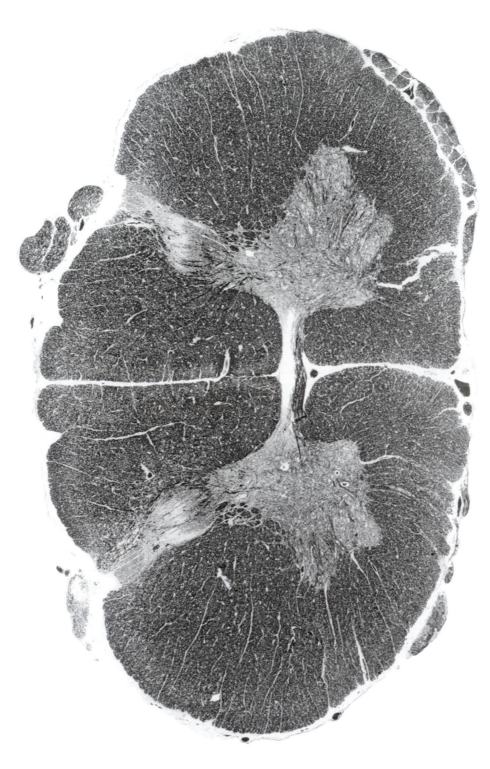

Figure AII-5. Transverse section of the seventh cervical segment (C7) of the spinal cord. (×16)

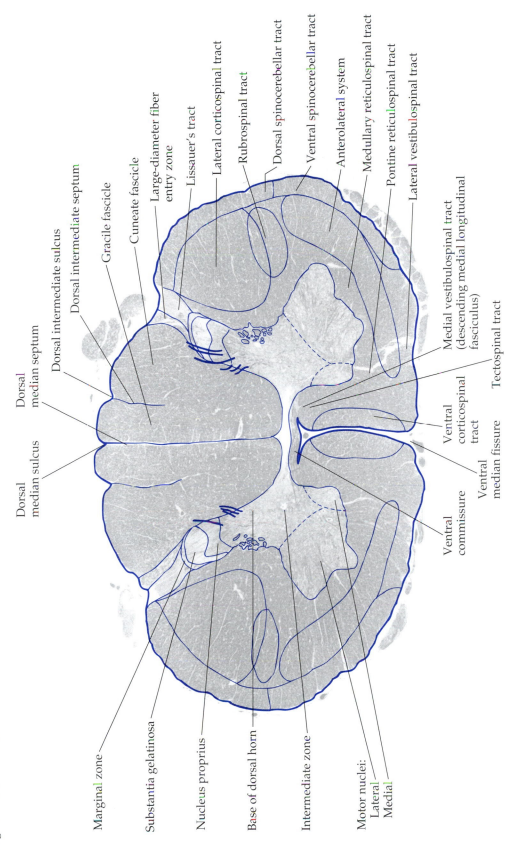

Figure AII–5 Continued.

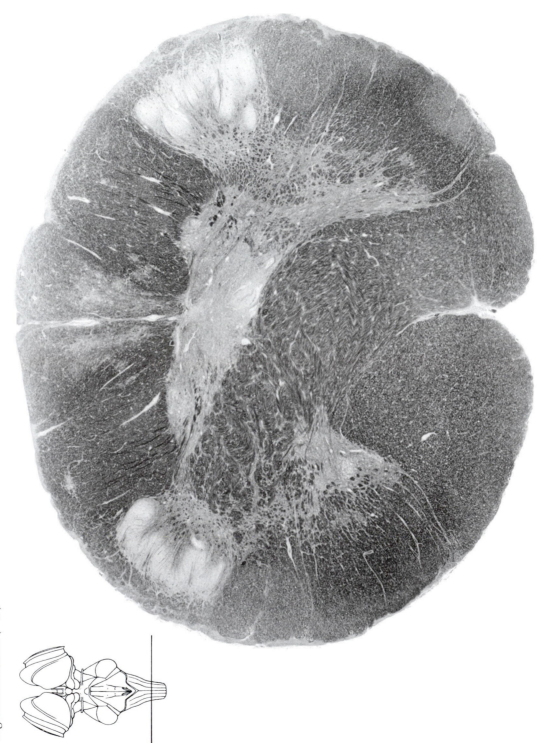

Figure AII-6. Transverse section of the caudal medulla at the level of the pyramidal (motor) decussation and the spinal (caudal) trigeminal nucleus. (×17)

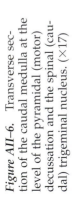

Figure AII–6 Continued.

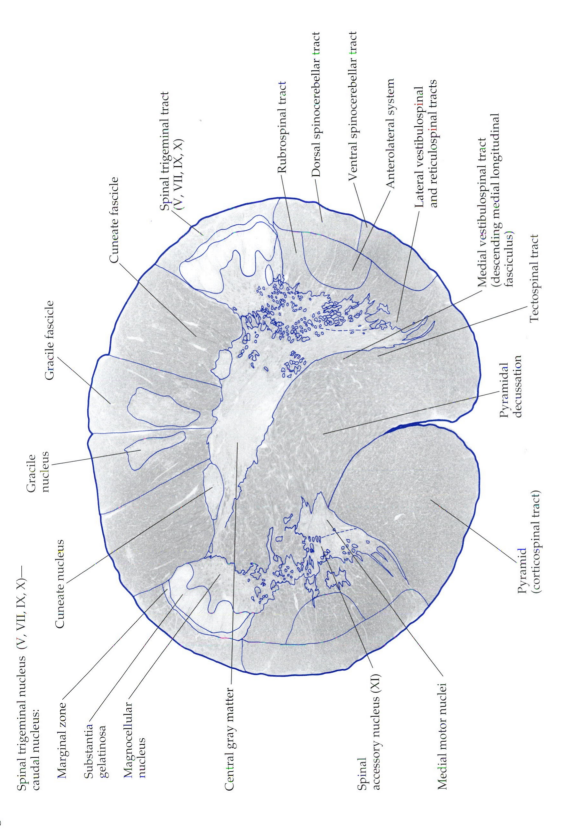

Spinal trigeminal nucleus (V, VII, IX, X)—caudal nucleus:

Marginal zone

Substantia gelatinosa

Magnocellular nucleus

Central gray matter

Spinal accessory nucleus (XI)

Medial motor nuclei

Gracile nucleus

Cuneate nucleus

Gracile fascicle

Cuneate fascicle

Spinal trigeminal tract (V, VII, IX, X)

Rubrospinal tract

Dorsal spinocerebellar tract

Ventral spinocerebellar tract

Anterolateral system

Lateral vestibulospinal and reticulospinal tracts

Medial vestibulospinal tract (descending medial longitudinal fasciculus)

Tectospinal tract

Pyramidal decussation

Pyramid (corticospinal tract)

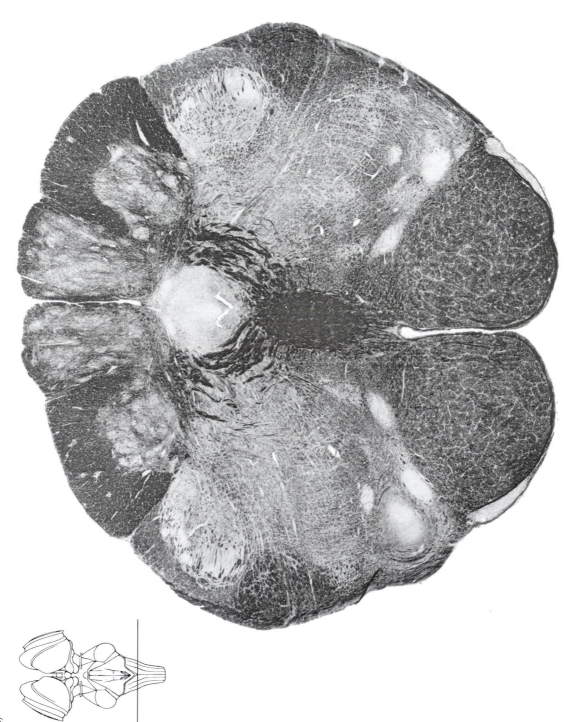

Figure AII-7. Transverse section of the medulla at the level of the dorsal column nuclei and the somatic sensory decussation. (×12)

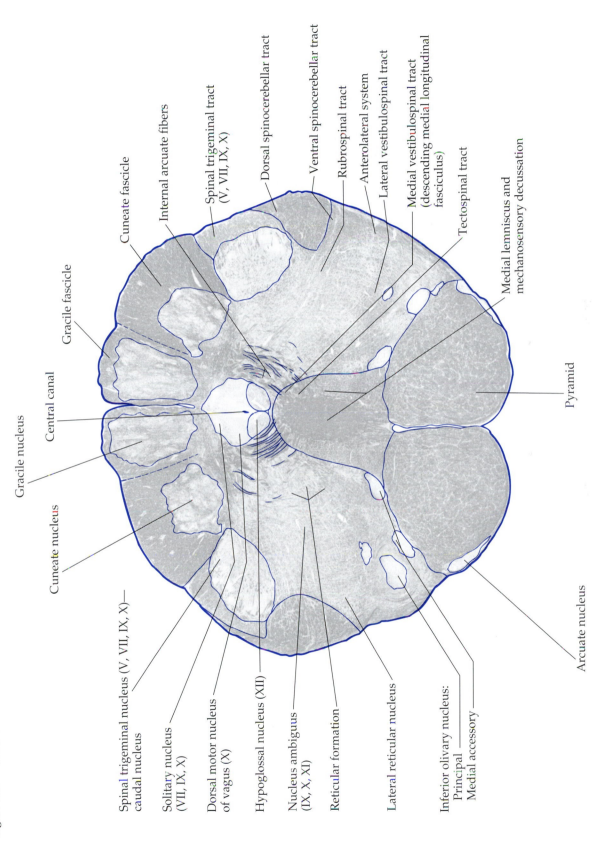

Figure AII–7 Continued.

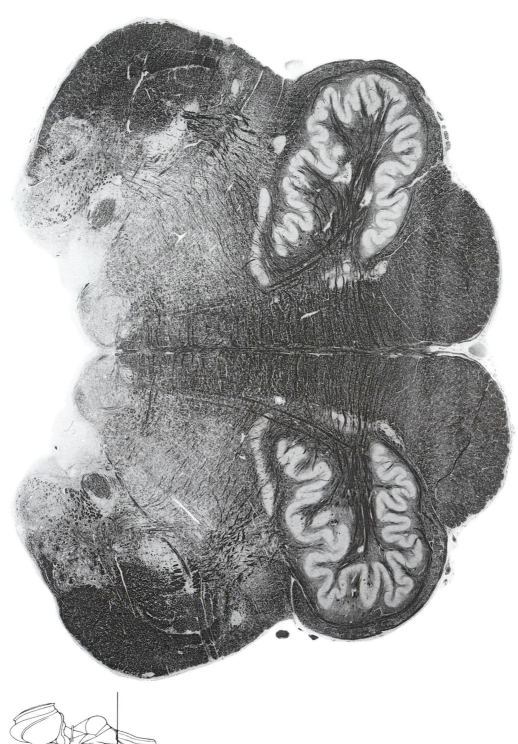

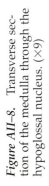

Figure AII–8. Transverse section of the medulla through the hypoglossal nucleus. (×9)

Figure AII–8 Continued.

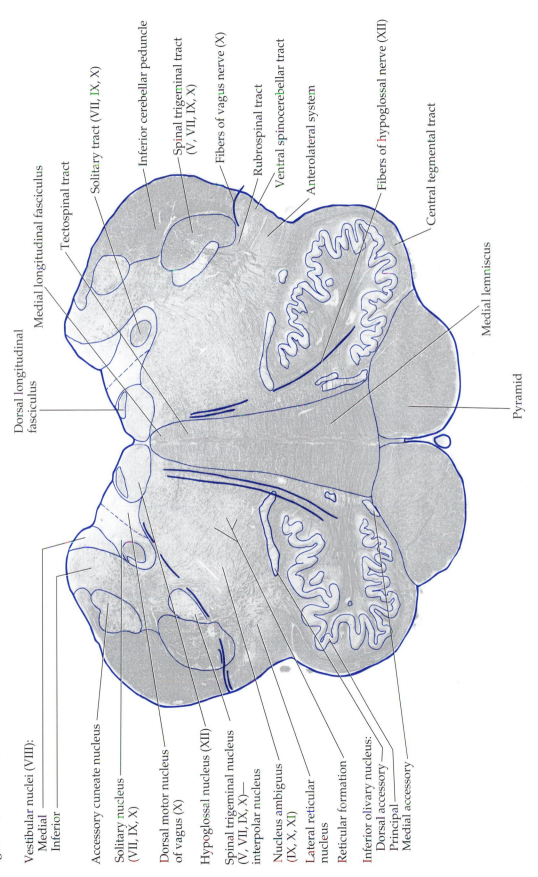

Dorsal longitudinal fasciculus

Medial longitudinal fasciculus

Tectospinal tract

Solitary tract (VII, IX, X)

Inferior cerebellar peduncle

Spinal trigeminal tract (V, VII, IX, X)

Fibers of vagus nerve (X)

Rubrospinal tract

Ventral spinocerebellar tract

Anterolateral system

Fibers of hypoglossal nerve (XII)

Central tegmental tract

Medial lemniscus

Pyramid

Vestibular nuclei (VIII):
Medial
Inferior

Accessory cuneate nucleus

Solitary nucleus (VII, IX, X)

Dorsal motor nucleus of vagus (X)

Hypoglossal nucleus (XII)

Spinal trigeminal nucleus (V, VII, IX, X)—interpolar nucleus

Nucleus ambiguus (IX, X, XI)

Lateral reticular nucleus

Reticular formation

Inferior olivary nucleus:
Dorsal accessory
Principal
Medial accessory

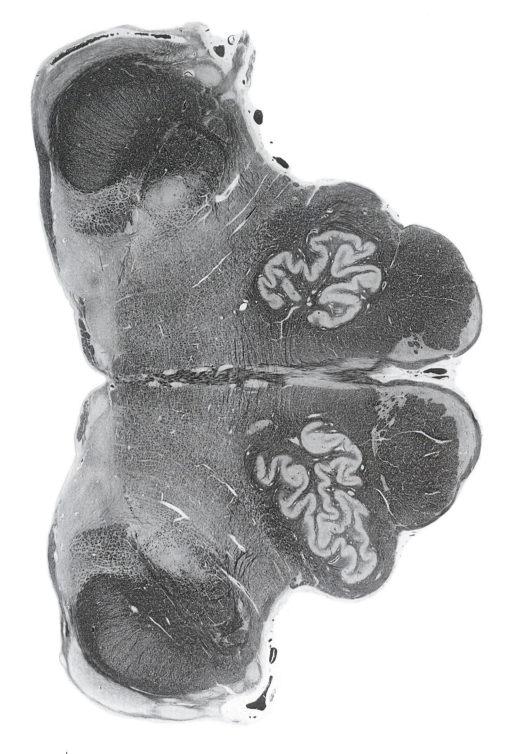

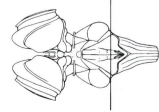

Figure AII–9. Transverse section of the rostral medulla through the cochlear nuclei. (×9)

Figure AII-9 Continued.

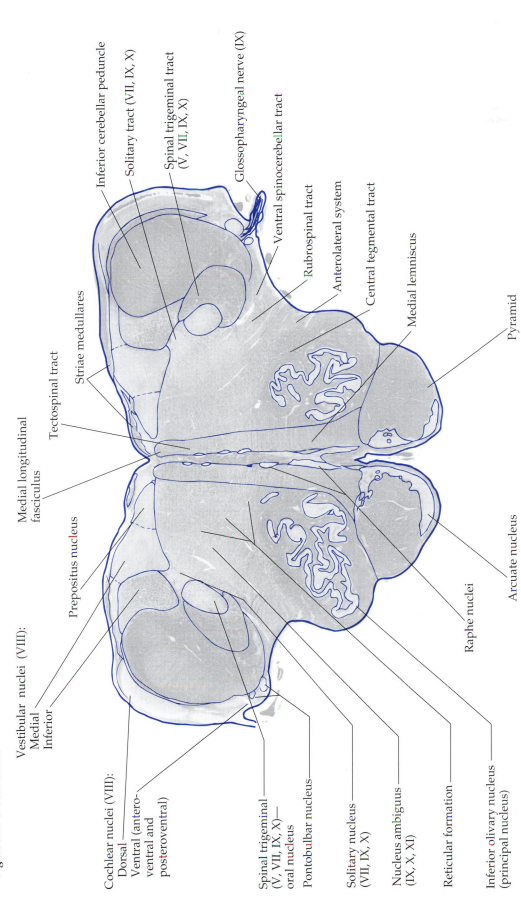

Inferior cerebellar peduncle

Solitary tract (VII, IX, X)

Spinal trigeminal tract (V, VII, IX, X)

Glossopharyngeal nerve (IX)

Ventral spinocerebellar tract

Rubrospinal tract

Anterolateral system

Central tegmental tract

Medial lemniscus

Pyramid

Arcuate nucleus

Raphe nuclei

Striae medullares

Tectospinal tract

Medial longitudinal fasciculus

Prepositus nucleus

Vestibular nuclei (VIII):
Medial
Inferior

Cochlear nuclei (VIII):
Dorsal
Ventral (antero-ventral and posteroventral)

Spinal trigeminal (V, VII, IX, X)—oral nucleus

Pontobulbar nucleus

Solitary nucleus (VII, IX, X)

Nucleus ambiguus (IX, X, XI)

Reticular formation

Inferior olivary nucleus (principal nucleus)

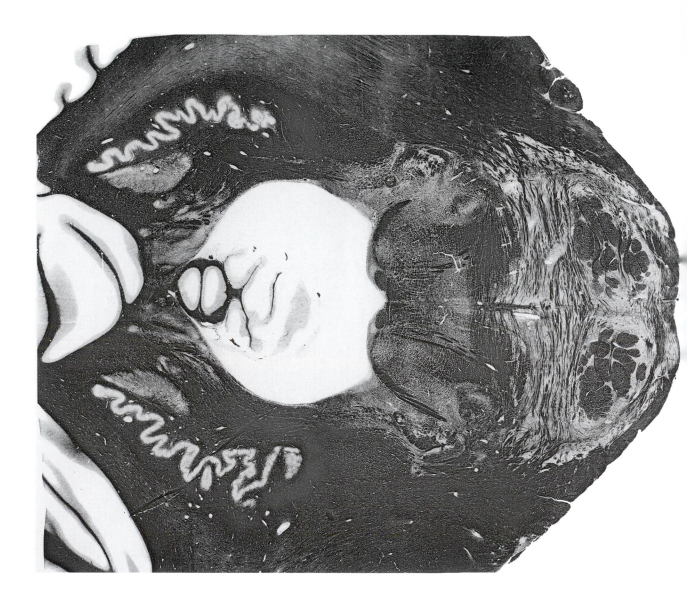

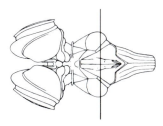

Figure AII–10. Transverse section of the pons at the level of the genu of the facial nerve and the deep cerebellar nuclei. (×4.3)

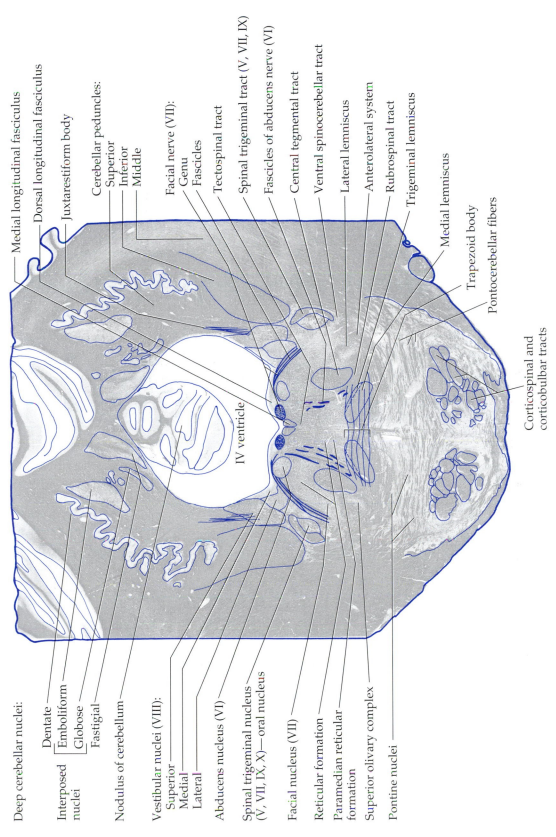

Figure AII–10 Continued.

Deep cerebellar nuclei:
Dentate
Interposed nuclei [Emboliform / Globose
Fastigial
Nodulus of cerebellum

Vestibular nuclei (VIII):
Superior
Medial
Lateral

Abducens nucleus (VI)

Spinal trigeminal nucleus (V, VII, IX, X)—oral nucleus

Facial nucleus (VII)

Reticular formation

Paramedian reticular formation

Superior olivary complex

Pontine nuclei

Medial longitudinal fasciculus

Dorsal longitudinal fasciculus

Juxtarestiform body

Cerebellar peduncles:
Superior
Inferior
Middle

Facial nerve (VII):
Genu
Fascicles

Tectospinal tract

Spinal trigeminal tract (V, VII, IX)

Fascicles of abducens nerve (VI)

Central tegmental tract

Ventral spinocerebellar tract

Lateral lemniscus

Anterolateral system

Rubrospinal tract

Trigeminal lemniscus

Medial lemniscus

Trapezoid body

Pontocerebellar fibers

Corticospinal and corticobulbar tracts

IV ventricle

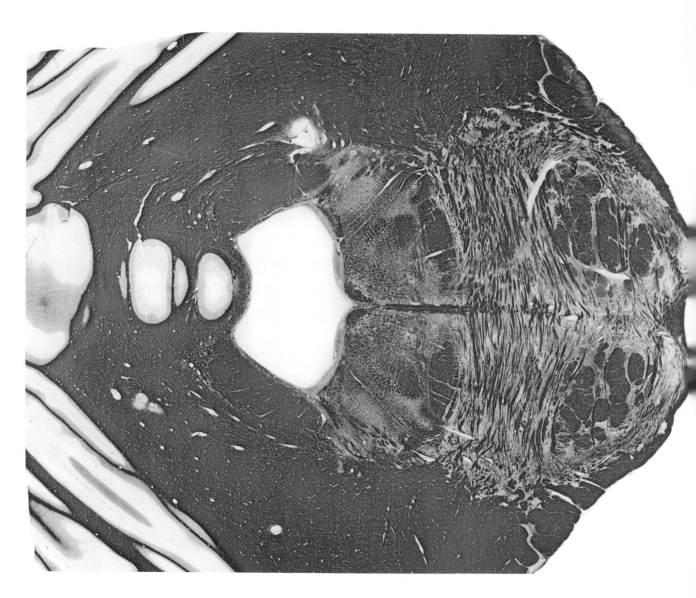

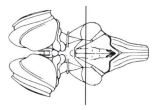

Figure AII–11. Transverse section of the pons through the main trigeminal sensory nuclei. (×10)

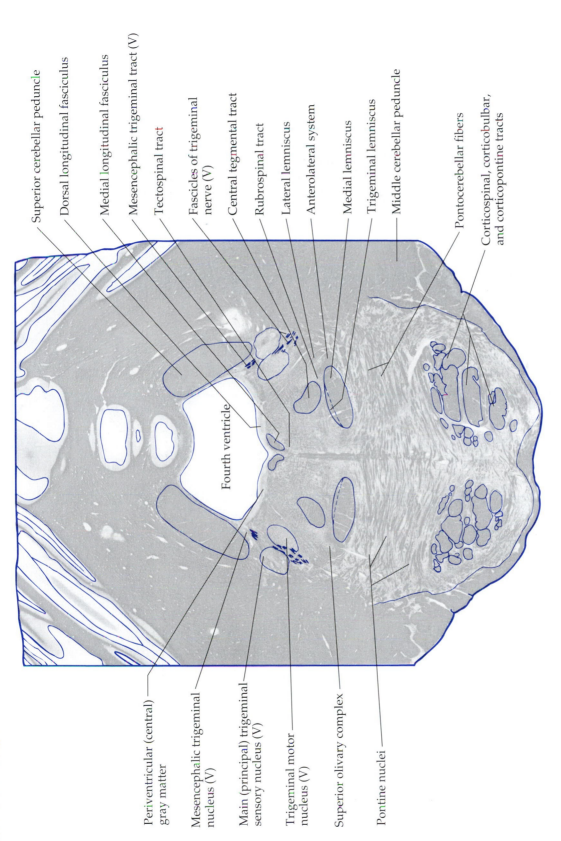

Figure AII–11 Continued.

Superior cerebellar peduncle

Dorsal longitudinal fasciculus

Medial longitudinal fasciculus

Mesencephalic trigeminal tract (V)

Tectospinal tract

Fascicles of trigeminal nerve (V)

Central tegmental tract

Rubrospinal tract

Lateral lemniscus

Anterolateral system

Medial lemniscus

Trigeminal lemniscus

Middle cerebellar peduncle

Pontocerebellar fibers

Corticospinal, corticobulbar, and corticopontine tracts

Fourth ventricle

Periventricular (central) gray matter

Mesencephalic trigeminal nucleus (V)

Main (principal) trigeminal sensory nucleus (V)

Trigeminal motor nucleus (V)

Superior olivary complex

Pontine nuclei

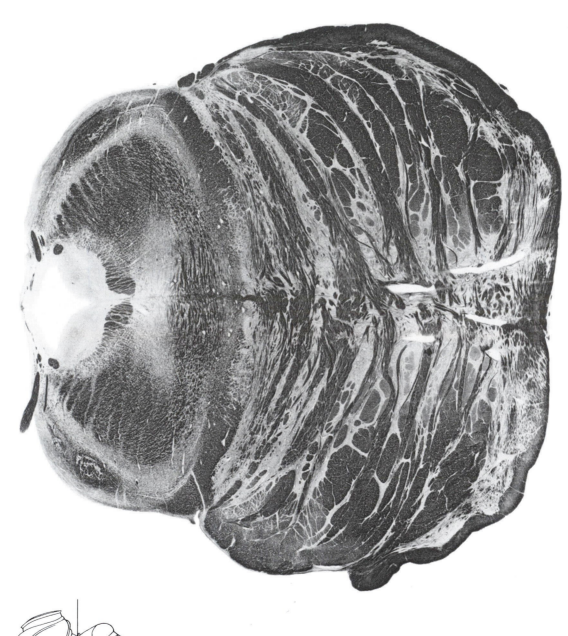

Figure AII–12. Transverse section through the rostral pons (isthmus) at the level of the decussation of the trochlear nerve. (×6)

Figure AII–12 Continued.

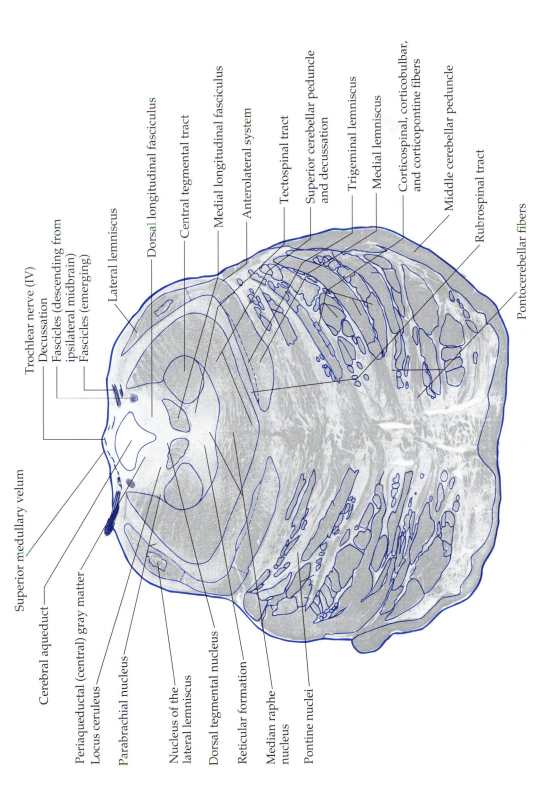

Superior medullary velum

Cerebral aqueduct

Periaqueductal (central) gray matter

Locus ceruleus

Parabrachial nucleus

Nucleus of the lateral lemniscus

Dorsal tegmental nucleus

Reticular formation

Median raphe nucleus

Pontine nuclei

Trochlear nerve (IV)
Decussation
Fascicles (descending from ipsilateral midbrain)
Fascicles (emerging)

Lateral lemniscus

Dorsal longitudinal fasciculus

Central tegmental tract

Medial longitudinal fasciculus

Anterolateral system

Tectospinal tract

Superior cerebellar peduncle and decussation

Trigeminal lemniscus

Medial lemniscus

Corticospinal, corticobulbar, and corticopontine fibers

Middle cerebellar peduncle

Rubrospinal tract

Pontocerebellar fibers

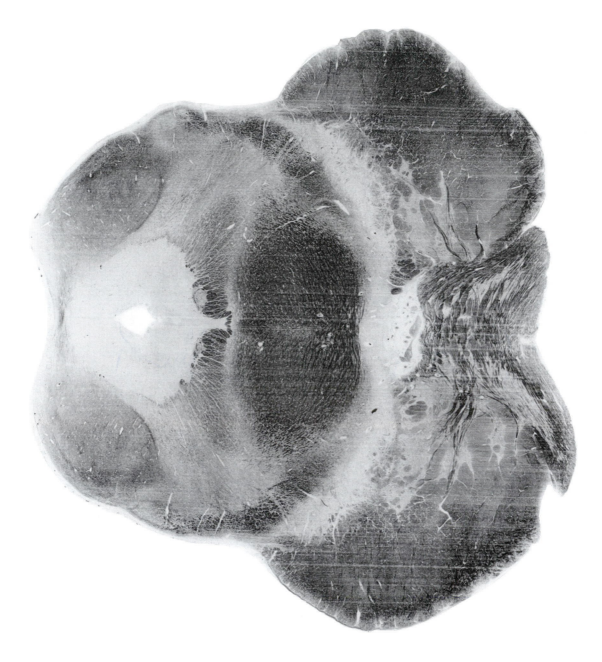

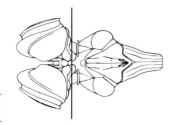

Figure AII–13. Transverse section of the caudal midbrain at the level of the inferior colliculus. (×5.6)

Figure AII–13 Continued.

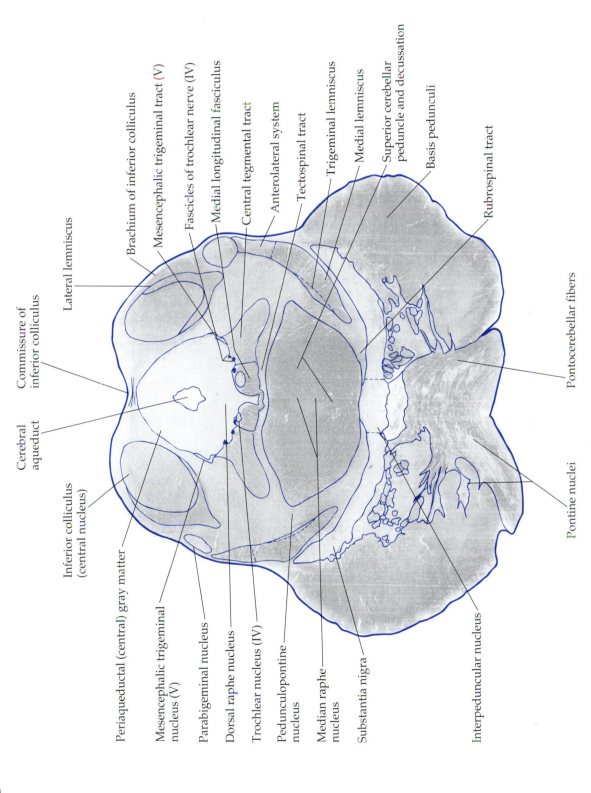

Cerebral aqueduct

Commissure of inferior colliculus

Lateral lemniscus

Brachium of inferior colliculus

Mesencephalic trigeminal tract (V)

Fascicles of trochlear nerve (IV)

Medial longitudinal fasciculus

Central tegmental tract

Anterolateral system

Tectospinal tract

Trigeminal lemniscus

Medial lemniscus

Superior cerebellar peduncle and decussation

Basis pedunculi

Rubrospinal tract

Pontocerebellar fibers

Pontine nuclei

Interpeduncular nucleus

Substantia nigra

Median raphe nucleus

Pedunculopontine nucleus

Trochlear nucleus (IV)

Dorsal raphe nucleus

Parabigeminal nucleus

Mesencephalic trigeminal nucleus (V)

Periaqueductal (central) gray matter

Inferior colliculus (central nucleus)

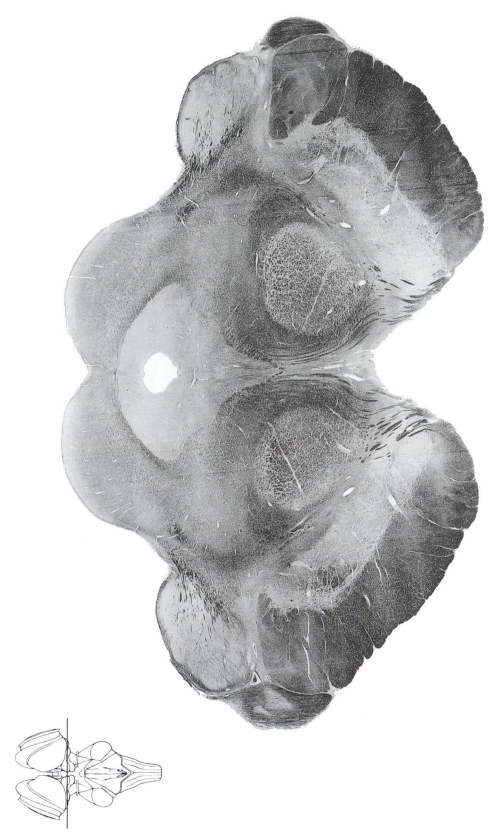

Figure AII-14. Transverse section of the rostral midbrain at the level of the superior colliculus. (×5.0)

Figure AII–14 Continued.

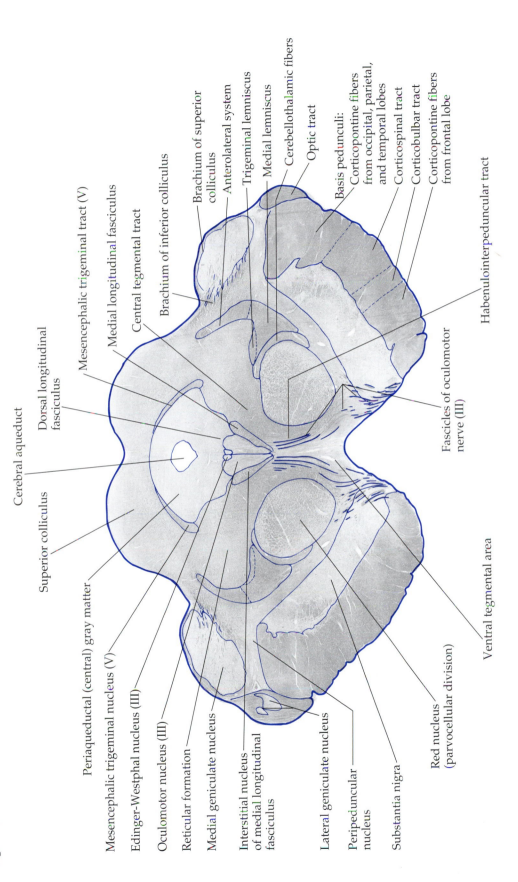

Cerebral aqueduct

Dorsal longitudinal fasciculus

Mesencephalic trigeminal tract (V)

Medial longitudinal fasciculus

Central tegmental tract

Brachium of inferior colliculus

Brachium of superior colliculus

Anterolateral system

Trigeminal lemniscus

Medial lemniscus

Cerebellothalamic fibers

Optic tract

Basis pedunculi:
Corticopontine fibers from occipital, parietal, and temporal lobes

Corticospinal tract

Corticobulbar tract

Corticopontine fibers from frontal lobe

Habenulointerpeduncular tract

Fascicles of oculomotor nerve (III)

Ventral tegmental area

Red nucleus (parvocellular division)

Substantia nigra

Peripeduncular nucleus

Lateral geniculate nucleus

Interstitial nucleus of medial longitudinal fasciculus

Medial geniculate nucleus

Reticular formation

Oculomotor nucleus (III)

Edinger-Westphal nucleus (III)

Mesencephalic trigeminal nucleus (V)

Periaqueductal (central) gray matter

Superior colliculus

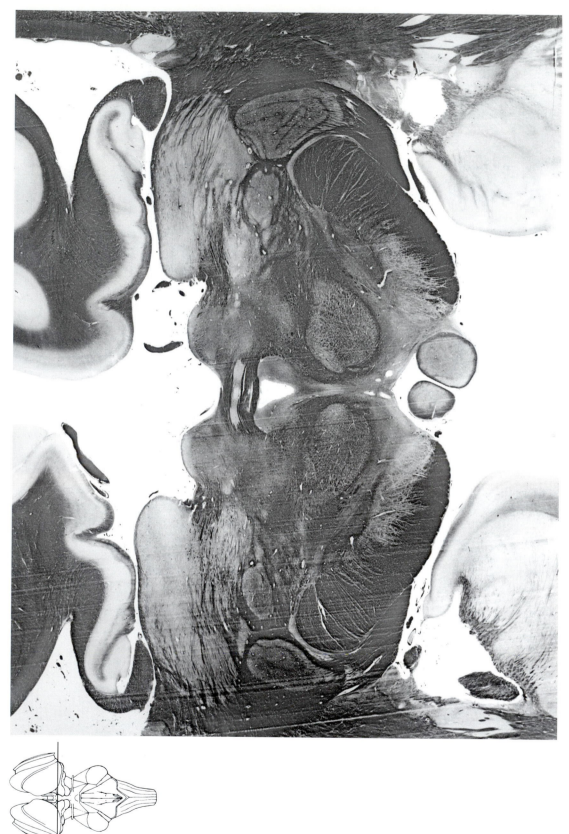

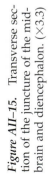

Figure AII-15. Transverse section of the juncture of the midbrain and diencephalon. (×3.3)

Figure AII–15 Continued.

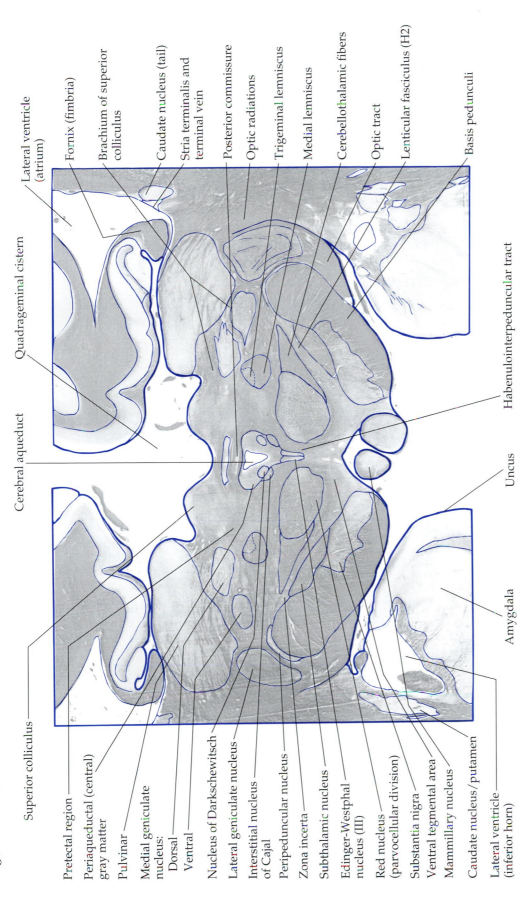

Lateral ventricle (atrium)
Fornix (fimbria)
Brachium of superior colliculus
Caudate nucleus (tail)
Stria terminalis and terminal vein
Posterior commissure
Optic radiations
Trigeminal lemniscus
Medial lemniscus
Cerebellothalamic fibers
Optic tract
Lenticular fasciculus (H2)
Basis pedunculi

Quadrageminal cistern
Cerebral aqueduct
Habenulointerpeduncular tract
Uncus
Amygdala

Superior colliculus
Pretectal region
Periaqueductal (central) gray matter
Pulvinar
Medial geniculate nucleus: Dorsal Ventral
Nucleus of Darkschewitsch
Lateral geniculate nucleus
Interstitial nucleus of Cajal
Peripeduncular nucleus
Zona incerta
Subthalamic nucleus
Edinger-Westphal nucleus (III)
Red nucleus (parvocellular division)
Substantia nigra
Ventral tegmental area
Mammillary nucleus
Caudate nucleus/putamen
Lateral ventricle (inferior horn)

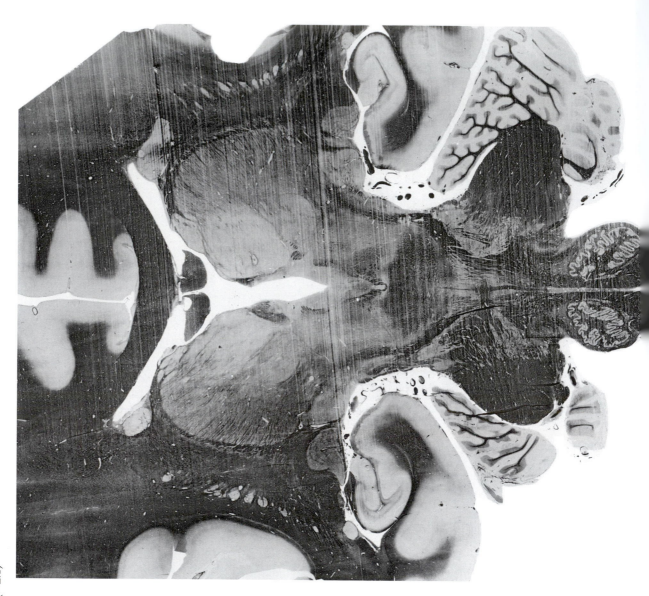

Figure AII–16. Coronal section of the dien-cephalon and cerebral hemisphere through the posterior limb of the internal capsule and the medial and lateral geniculate nuclei. The mid-brain and pontine tegmentum, lateral cerebel-lum, and ventral medulla are also shown. (×2.1)

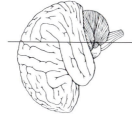

Figure AII–16 Continued.

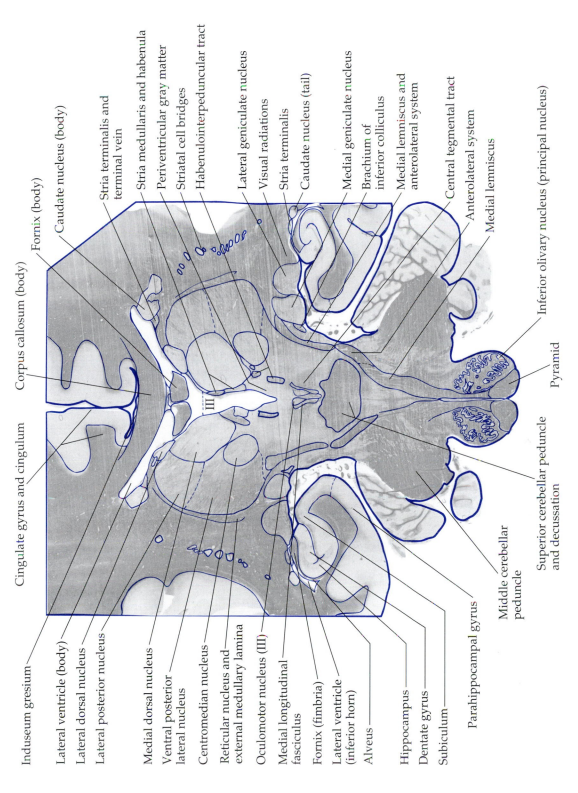

Induseum gresium

Lateral ventricle (body)

Lateral dorsal nucleus

Lateral posterior nucleus

Medial dorsal nucleus

Ventral posterior lateral nucleus

Centromedian nucleus

Reticular nucleus and external medullary lamina

Oculomotor nucleus (III)

Medial longitudinal fasciculus

Fornix (fimbria)

Lateral ventricle (inferior horn)

Alveus

Hippocampus

Dentate gyrus

Subiculum

Parahippocampal gyrus

Cingulate gyrus and cingulum

Corpus callosum (body)

Fornix (body)

Caudate nucleus (body)

Stria terminalis and terminal vein

Stria medullaris and habenula

Periventricular gray matter

Striatal cell bridges

Habenulointerpeduncular tract

Lateral geniculate nucleus

Visual radiations

Stria terminalis

Caudate nucleus (tail)

Medial geniculate nucleus

Brachium of inferior colliculus

Medial lemniscus and anterolateral system

Central tegmental tract

Anterolateral system

Medial lemniscus

Inferior olivary nucleus (principal nucleus)

Pyramid

Superior cerebellar peduncle and decussation

Middle cerebellar peduncle

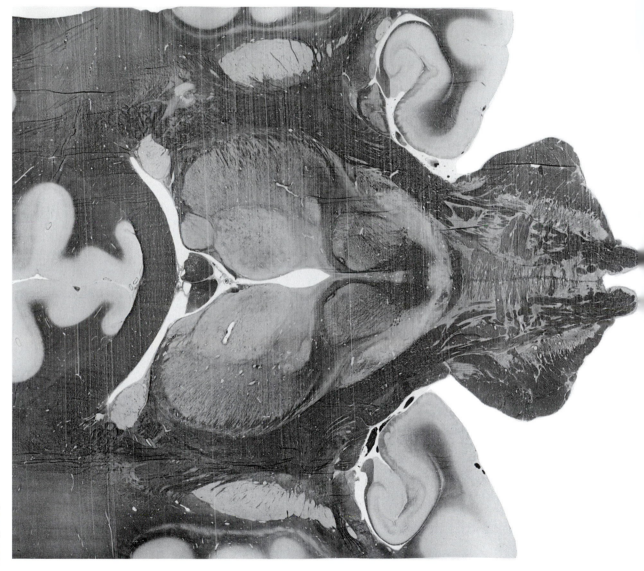

Figure AII–17. Coronal section of the diencephalon and cerebral hemisphere through the posterior limb of the internal capsule and ventral posterior nucleus. The midbrain tegmentum and base of the pons are also shown. (×2.3)

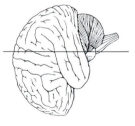

Figure AII–17 Continued.

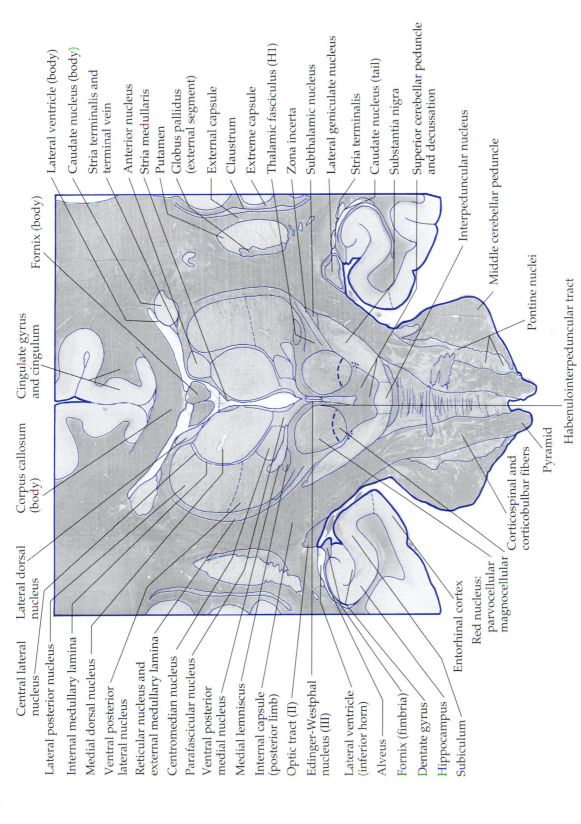

Central lateral nucleus

Lateral dorsal nucleus

Corpus callosum (body)

Cingulate gyrus and cingulum

Fornix (body)

Lateral ventricle (body)

Caudate nucleus (body)

Stria terminalis and terminal vein

Anterior nucleus

Stria medullaris

Putamen

Globus pallidus (external segment)

External capsule

Claustrum

Extreme capsule

Thalamic fasciculus (H1)

Zona incerta

Subthalamic nucleus

Lateral geniculate nucleus

Stria terminalis

Caudate nucleus (tail)

Substantia nigra

Superior cerebellar peduncle and decussation

Interpeduncular nucleus

Middle cerebellar peduncle

Pontine nuclei

Habenulointerpeduncular tract

Pyramid

Corticospinal and corticobulbar fibers

Red nucleus: parvocellular magnocellular

Entorhinal cortex

Subiculum

Hippocampus

Dentate gyrus

Fornix (fimbria)

Alveus

Lateral ventricle (inferior horn)

Edinger-Westphal nucleus (III)

Optic tract (II)

Internal capsule (posterior limb)

Medial lemniscus

Ventral posterior medial nucleus

Parafascicular nucleus

Centromedian nucleus

Reticular nucleus and external medullary lamina

Ventral posterior lateral nucleus

Medial dorsal nucleus

Internal medullary lamina

Lateral posterior nucleus

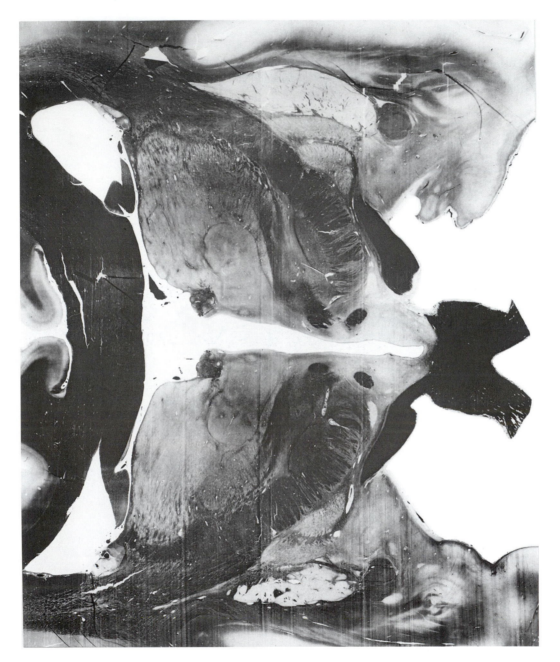

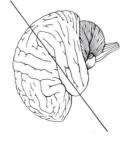

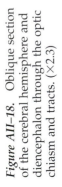

Figure AII–18. Oblique section of the cerebral hemisphere and diencephalon through the optic chiasm and tracts. (×2.3)

Figure AII–18 Continued.

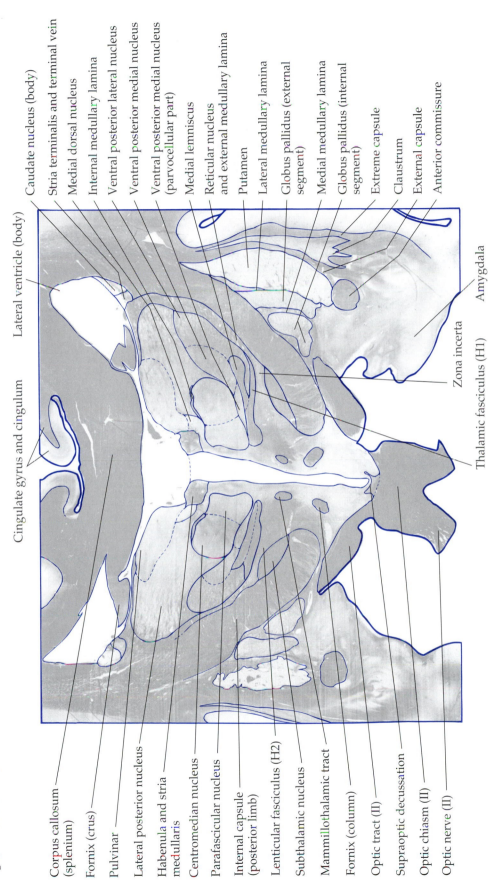

Caudate nucleus (body)

Stria terminalis and terminal vein

Medial dorsal nucleus

Internal medullary lamina

Ventral posterior lateral nucleus

Ventral posterior medial nucleus

Ventral posterior medial nucleus (parvocellular part)

Medial lemniscus

Reticular nucleus and external medullary lamina

Putamen

Lateral medullary lamina

Globus pallidus (external segment)

Medial medullary lamina

Globus pallidus (internal segment)

Extreme capsule

Claustrum

External capsule

Anterior commissure

Lateral ventricle (body)

Cingulate gyrus and cingulum

Zona incerta

Amygdala

Thalamic fasciculus (H1)

Corpus callosum (splenium)

Fornix (crus)

Pulvinar

Lateral posterior nucleus

Habenula and stria medullaris

Centromedian nucleus

Parafascicular nucleus

Internal capsule (posterior limb)

Lenticular fasciculus (H2)

Subthalamic nucleus

Mammillothalamic tract

Fornix (column)

Optic tract (II)

Supraoptic decussation

Optic chiasm (II)

Optic nerve (II)

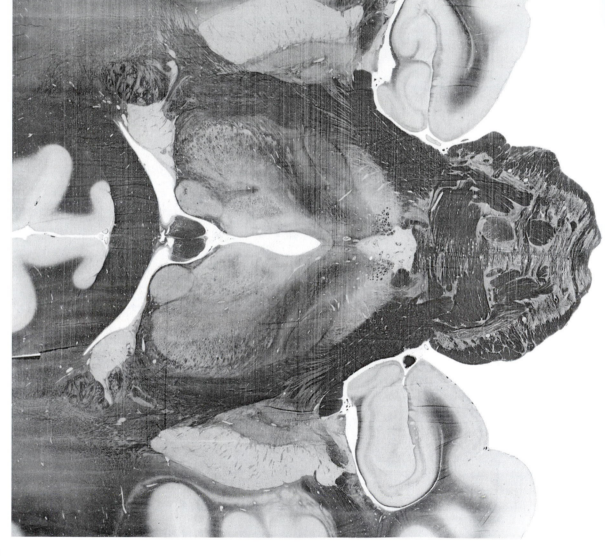

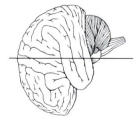

Figure AII-19. Coronal section of the diencephalon and cerebral hemisphere through the posterior limb of the internal capsule and anterior thalamic nuclei. The ventral midbrain and ventral pons are also shown. (×2.2)

Figure AII–19 Continued.

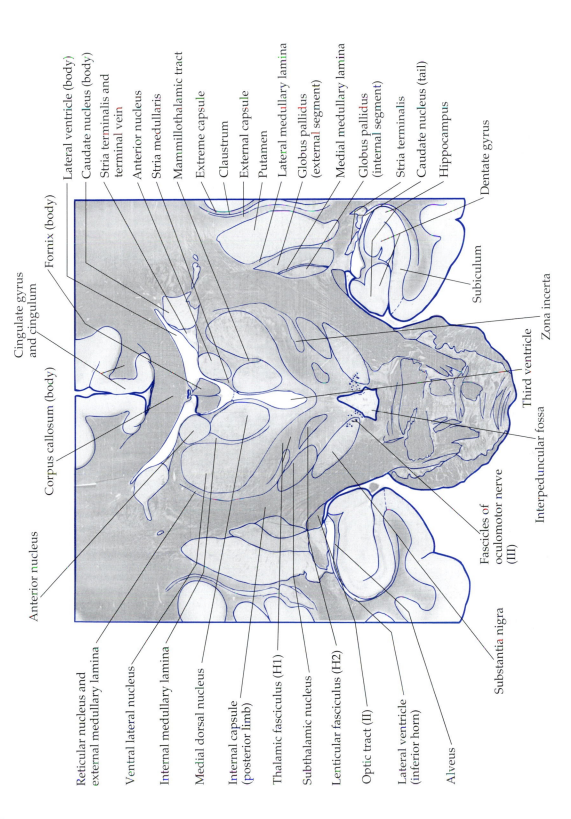

Cingulate gyrus and cingulum

Anterior nucleus

Corpus callosum (body)

Fornix (body)

Lateral ventricle (body)

Caudate nucleus (body)

Stria terminalis and terminal vein

Anterior nucleus

Stria medullaris

Mammillothalamic tract

Extreme capsule

Claustrum

External capsule

Putamen

Lateral medullary lamina

Globus pallidus (external segment)

Medial medullary lamina

Globus pallidus (internal segment)

Stria terminalis

Caudate nucleus (tail)

Hippocampus

Dentate gyrus

Subiculum

Zona incerta

Third ventricle

Interpeduncular fossa

Fascicles of oculomotor nerve (III)

Substantia nigra

Alveus

Lateral ventricle (inferior horn)

Optic tract (II)

Lenticular fasciculus (H2)

Subthalamic nucleus

Thalamic fasciculus (H1)

Internal capsule (posterior limb)

Medial dorsal nucleus

Internal medullary lamina

Ventral lateral nucleus

Reticular nucleus and external medullary lamina

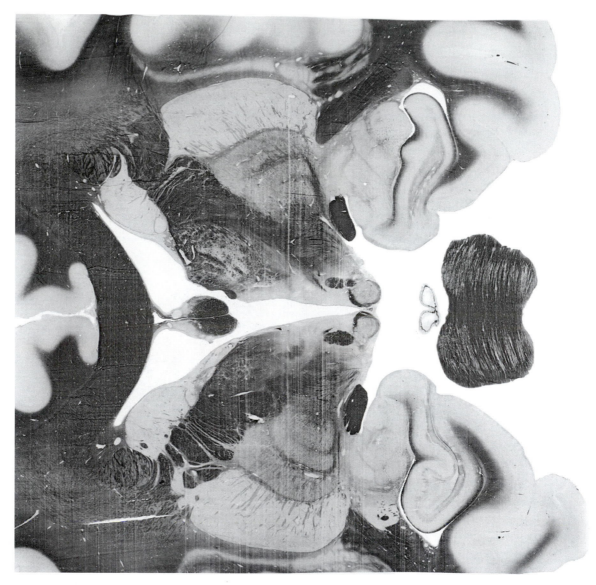

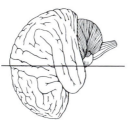

Figure AII–20. Coronal section of the cerebral hemisphere and diencephalon through the intraventricular foramen. The base of the pons is also shown. (×2.1)

Figure AII–20 Continued.

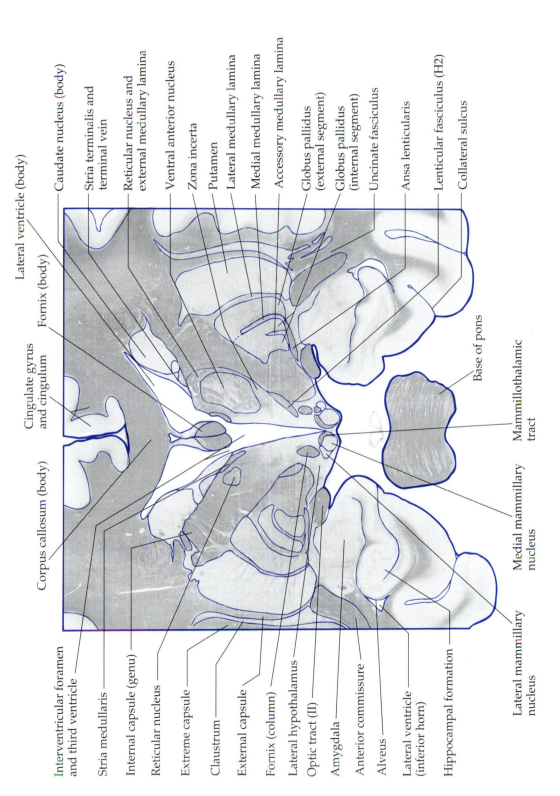

Lateral ventricle (body)

Caudate nucleus (body)

Stria terminalis and terminal vein

Reticular nucleus and external medullary lamina

Ventral anterior nucleus

Zona incerta

Putamen

Lateral medullary lamina

Medial medullary lamina

Accessory medullary lamina

Globus pallidus (external segment)

Globus pallidus (internal segment)

Uncinate fasciculus

Ansa lenticularis

Lenticular fasciculus (H2)

Collateral sulcus

Fornix (body)

Cingulate gyrus and cingulum

Corpus callosum (body)

Base of pons

Mammillothalamic tract

Medial mammillary nucleus

Interventricular foramen and third ventricle

Stria medullaris

Internal capsule (genu)

Reticular nucleus

Extreme capsule

Claustrum

External capsule

Fornix (column)

Lateral hypothalamus

Optic tract (II)

Amygdala

Anterior commissure

Alveus

Lateral ventricle (inferior horn)

Hippocampal formation

Lateral mammillary nucleus

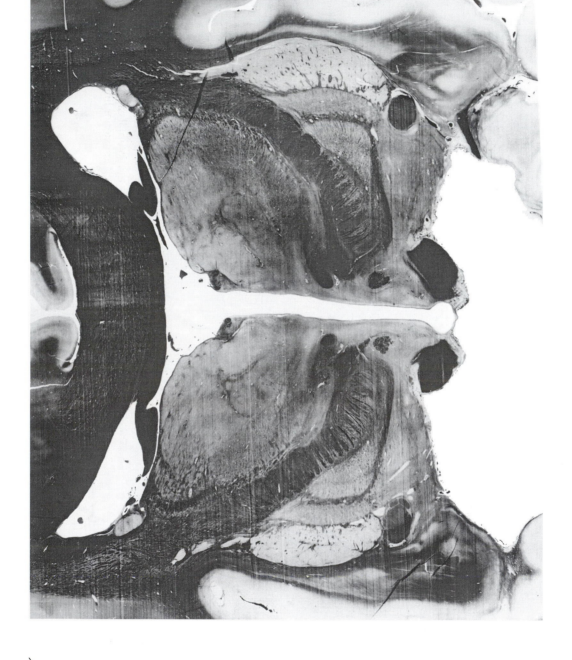

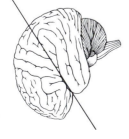

Figure AII–21. Oblique section of the cerebral hemisphere and diencephalon through the ansa lenticularis and optic tract. (×2.4)

Figure AII–21 Continued.

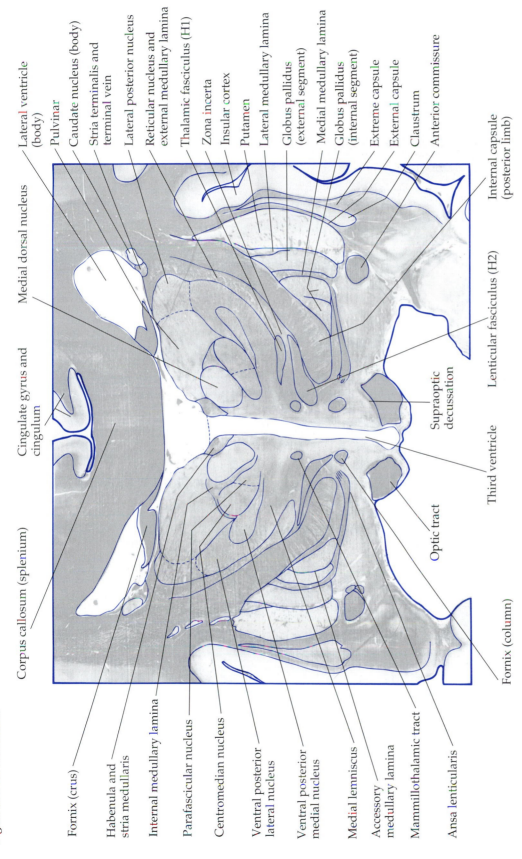

Lateral ventricle (body)

Pulvinar

Caudate nucleus (body)

Stria terminalis and terminal vein

Lateral posterior nucleus

Reticular nucleus and external medullary lamina

Thalamic fasciculus (H1)

Zona incerta

Insular cortex

Putamen

Lateral medullary lamina

Globus pallidus (external segment)

Medial medullary lamina

Globus pallidus (internal segment)

Extreme capsule

External capsule

Claustrum

Anterior commissure

Internal capsule (posterior limb)

Lenticular fasciculus (H2)

Supraoptic decussation

Third ventricle

Optic tract

Fornix (column)

Medial dorsal nucleus

Cingulate gyrus and cingulum

Corpus callosum (splenium)

Fornix (crus)

Habenula and stria medullaris

Internal medullary lamina

Parafascicular nucleus

Centromedian nucleus

Ventral posterior lateral nucleus

Ventral posterior medial nucleus

Medial lemniscus

Accessory medullary lamina

Mammillothalamic tract

Ansa lenticularis

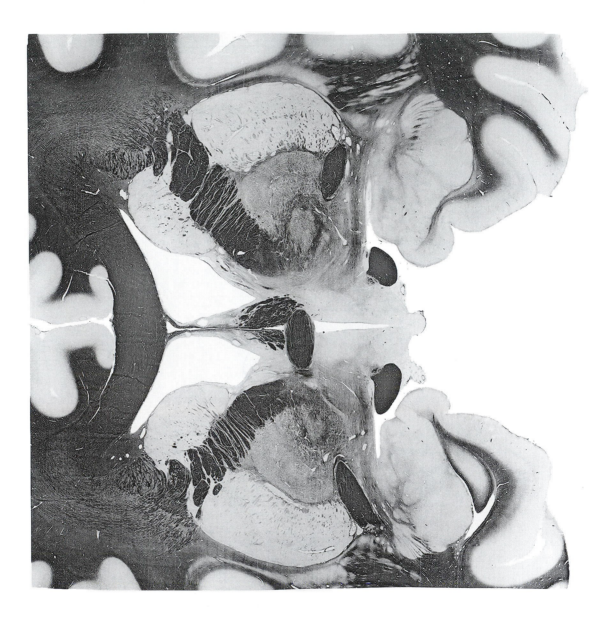

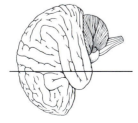

Figure AII–22. Coronal section of the cerebral hemisphere through the anterior limb of the internal capsule, column of the fornix, and amygdaloid complex. (×2.2)

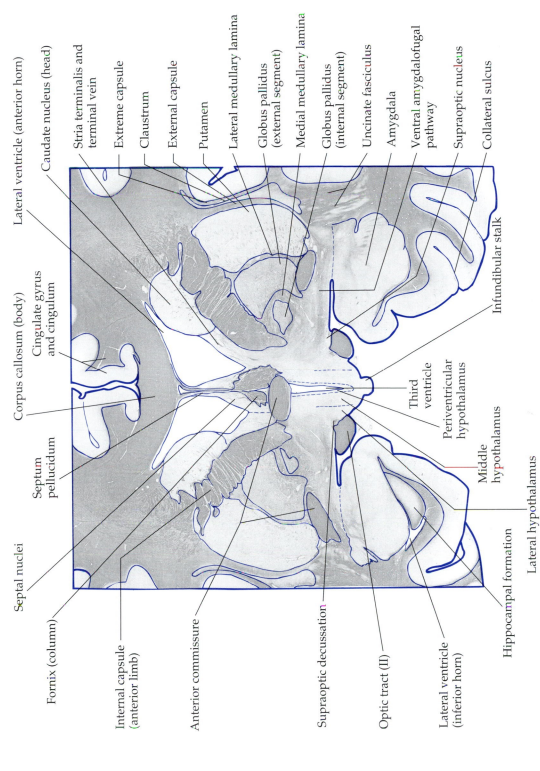

Figure AII–22 Continued.

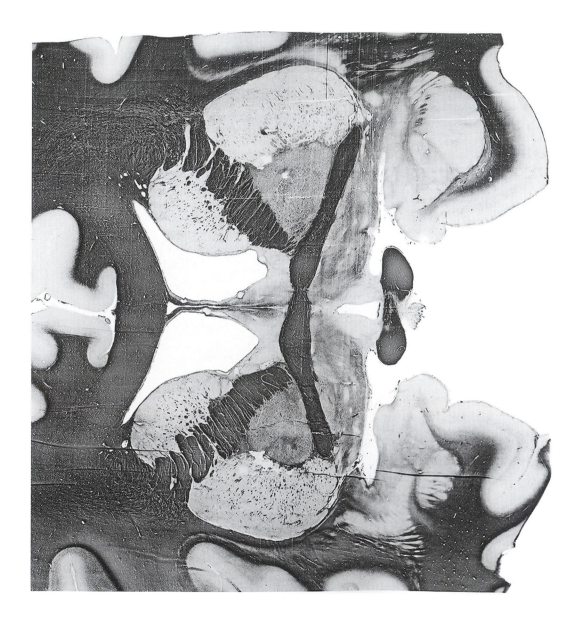

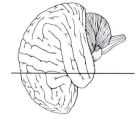

Figure AIII-23. Coronal section of the cerebral hemisphere through the anterior limb of the internal capsule, anterior commissure, and optic chiasm. (×2.2)

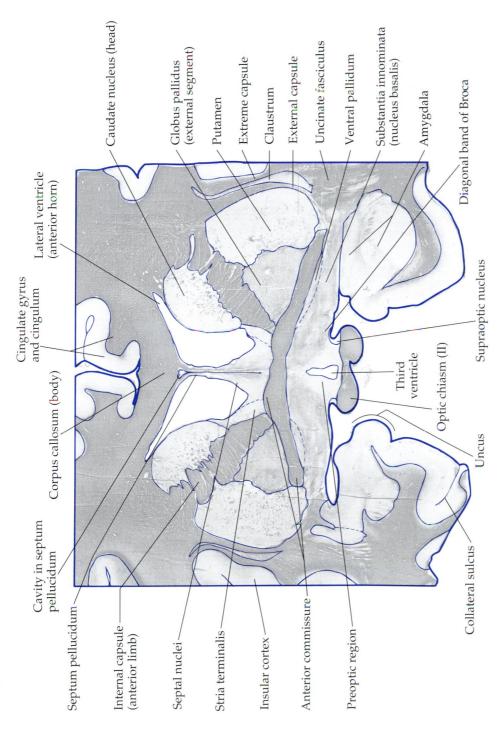

Caudate nucleus (head)

Globus pallidus (external segment)

Putamen

Extreme capsule

Claustrum

External capsule

Uncinate fasciculus

Ventral pallidum

Substantia inmominata (nucleus basalis)

Amygdala

Diagonal band of Broca

Lateral ventricle (anterior horn)

Cingulate gyrus and cingulum

Corpus callosum (body)

Cavity in septum pellucidum

Supraoptic nucleus

Third ventricle

Optic chiasm (II)

Uncus

Collateral sulcus

Septum pellucidum

Internal capsule (anterior limb)

Septal nuclei

Stria terminalis

Insular cortex

Anterior commissure

Preoptic region

Figure AII–23 Continued.

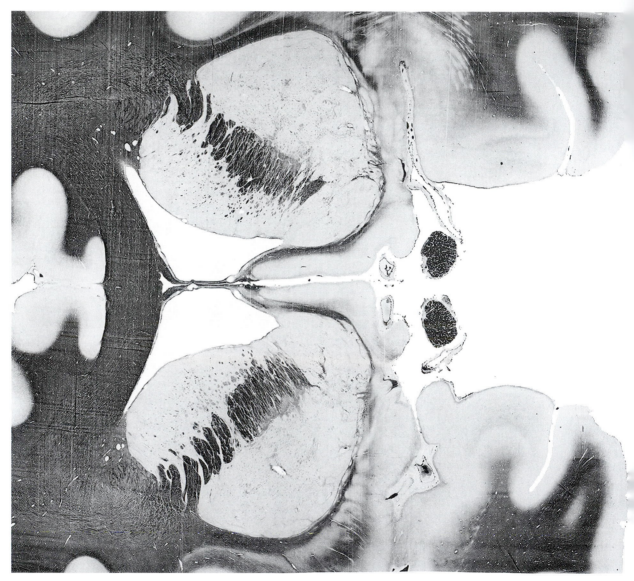

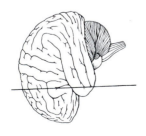

Figure AII–24. Coronal section of the cerebral hemisphere through the anterior limb of the internal capsule and the head of the caudate nucleus. (×2.4)

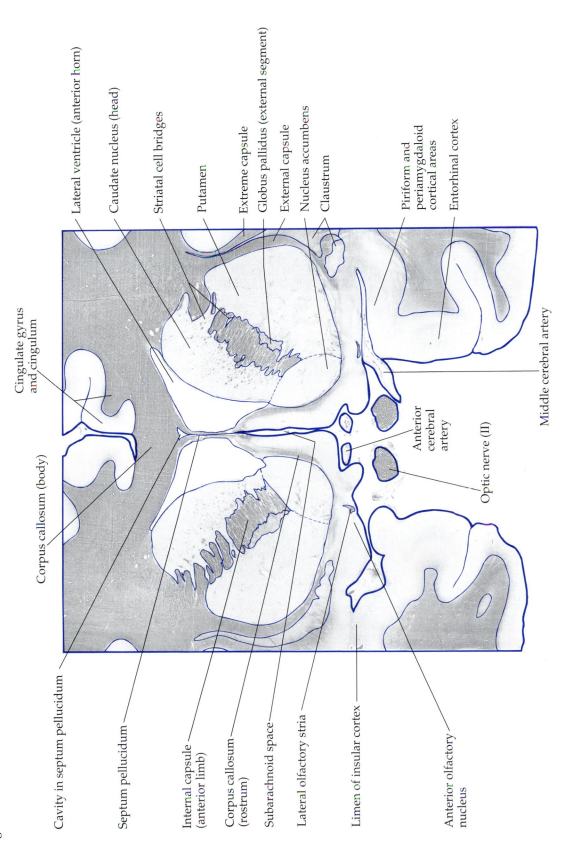

Figure AII–24 Continued.

Cingulate gyrus and cingulum

Corpus callosum (body)

Cavity in septum pellucidum

Septum pellucidum

Internal capsule (anterior limb)

Corpus callosum (rostrum)

Subarachnoid space

Lateral olfactory stria

Limen of insular cortex

Anterior olfactory nucleus

Lateral ventricle (anterior horn)

Caudate nucleus (head)

Striatal cell bridges

Putamen

Extreme capsule

Globus pallidus (external segment)

External capsule

Nucleus accumbens

Claustrum

Piriform and periamygdaloid cortical areas

Entorhinal cortex

Middle cerebral artery

Anterior cerebral artery

Optic nerve (II)

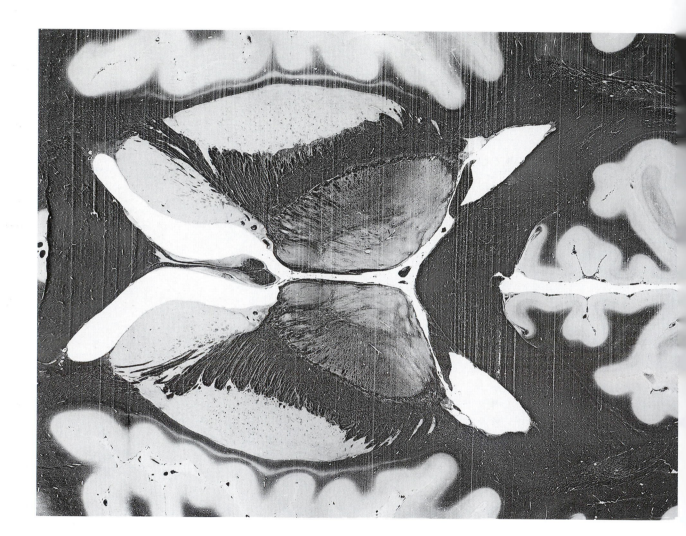

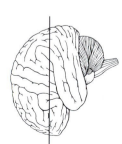

Figure AII–25. Horizontal section of the cerebral hemisphere and diencephalon through the anterior thalamic nuclei. (×1.9)

Figure AII–25 Continued.

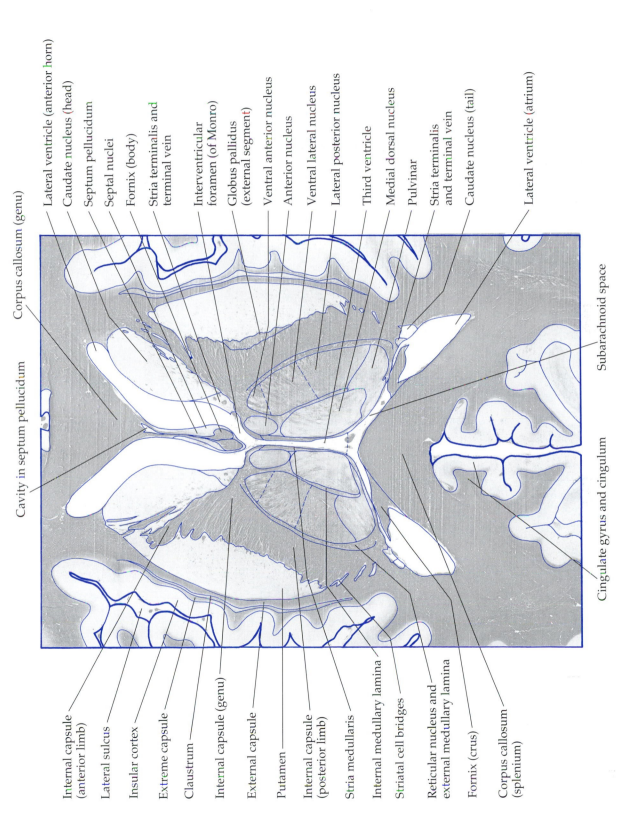

Corpus callosum (genu)

Cavity in septum pellucidum

Lateral ventricle (anterior horn)
Caudate nucleus (head)
Septum pellucidum
Septal nuclei
Fornix (body)
Stria terminalis and terminal vein
Interventricular foramen (of Monro)
Globus pallidus (external segment)
Ventral anterior nucleus
Anterior nucleus
Ventral lateral nucleus
Lateral posterior nucleus
Third ventricle
Medial dorsal nucleus
Pulvinar
Stria terminalis and terminal vein
Caudate nucleus (tail)
Lateral ventricle (atrium)

Subarachnoid space

Cingulate gyrus and cingulum

Internal capsule (anterior limb)
Lateral sulcus
Insular cortex
Extreme capsule
Claustrum
Internal capsule (genu)
External capsule
Putamen
Internal capsule (posterior limb)
Stria medullaris
Internal medullary lamina
Striatal cell bridges
Reticular nucleus and external medullary lamina
Fornix (crus)
Corpus callosum (splenium)

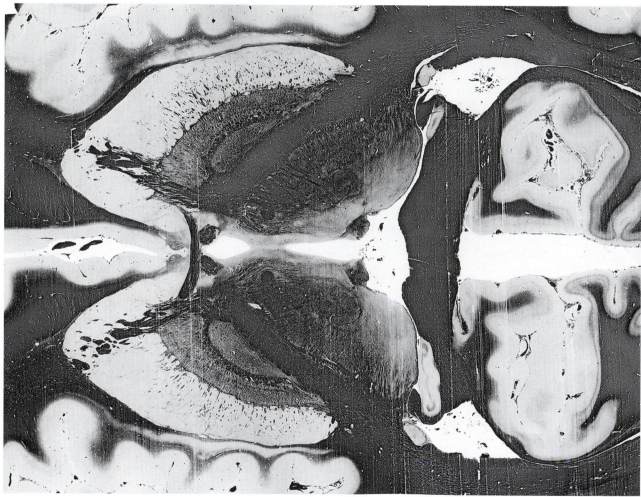

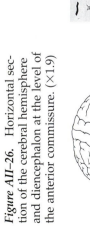

Figure AII–26. Horizontal section of the cerebral hemisphere and diencephalon at the level of the anterior commissure. (×1.9)

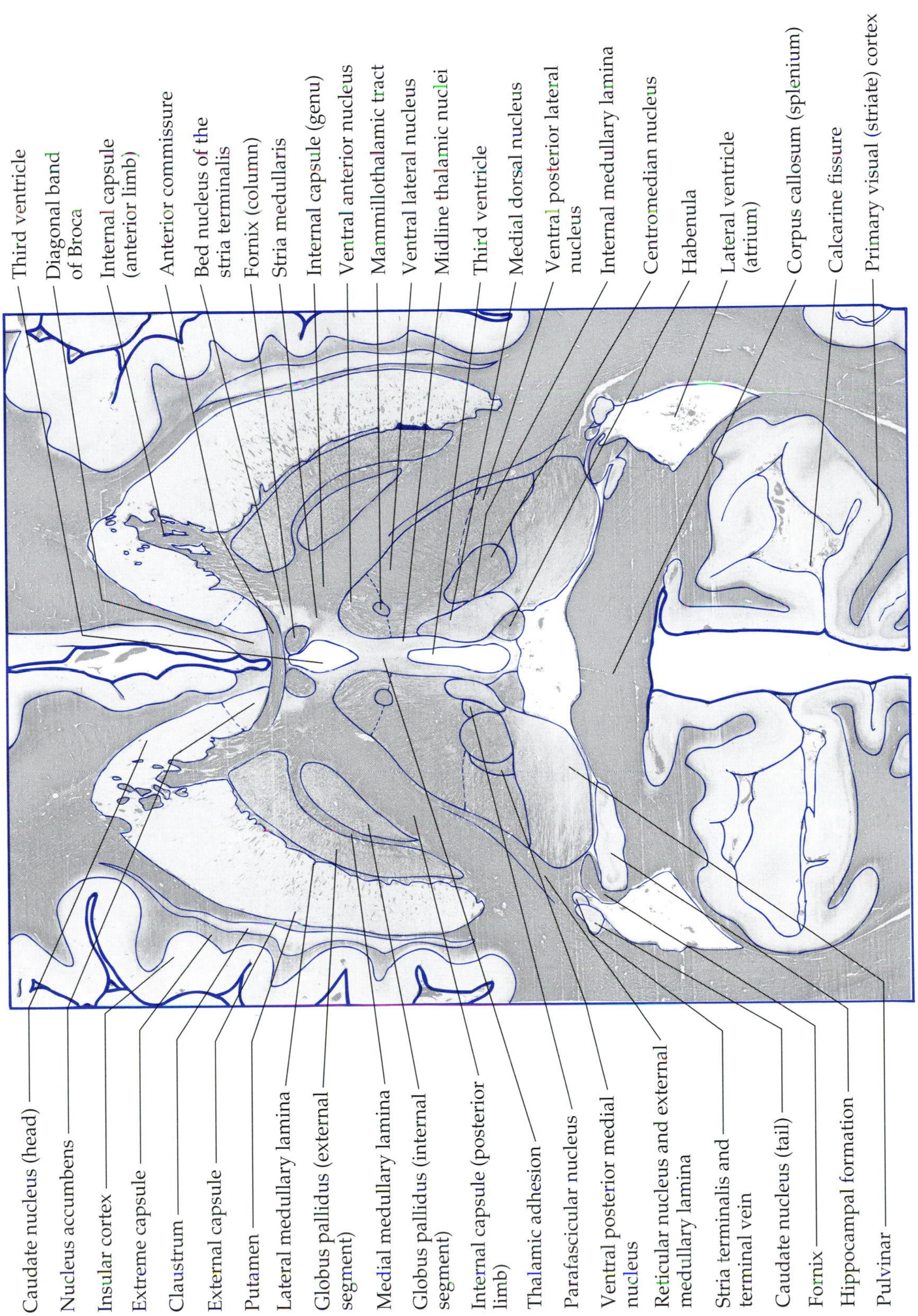

Figure AII–26 Continued.

Labels (top):
Third ventricle
Diagonal band of Broca
Internal capsule (anterior limb)
Anterior commissure
Bed nucleus of the stria terminalis
Fornix (column)
Stria medullaris
Internal capsule (genu)
Ventral anterior nucleus
Mammillothalamic tract
Ventral lateral nucleus
Midline thalamic nuclei
Third ventricle
Medial dorsal nucleus
Ventral posterior lateral nucleus
Internal medullary lamina
Centromedian nucleus
Habenula
Lateral ventricle (atrium)
Corpus callosum (splenium)
Calcarine fissure
Primary visual (striate) cortex

Labels (bottom):
Caudate nucleus (head)
Nucleus accumbens
Insular cortex
Extreme capsule
Claustrum
External capsule
Putamen
Lateral medullary lamina
Globus pallidus (external segment)
Medial medullary lamina
Globus pallidus (internal segment)
Internal capsule (posterior limb)
Thalamic adhesion
Parafascicular nucleus
Ventral posterior medial nucleus
Reticular nucleus and external medullary lamina
Stria terminalis and terminal vein
Caudate nucleus (tail)
Fornix
Hippocampal formation
Pulvinar

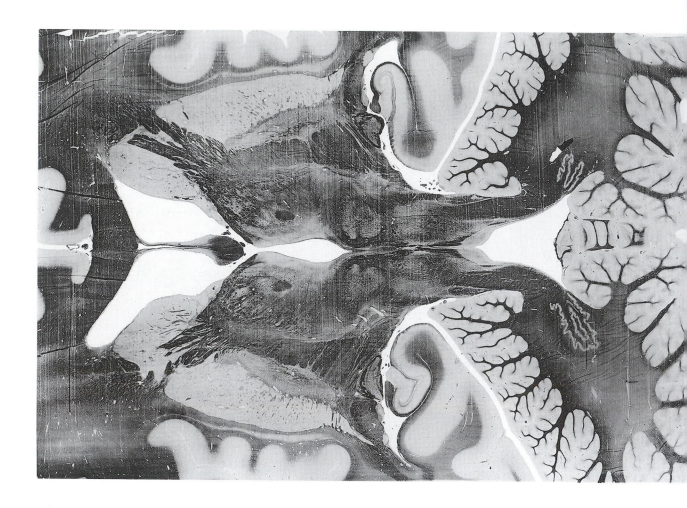

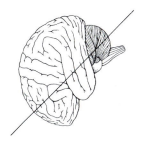

Figure AII-27. Oblique section of the cerebral hemisphere, diencephalon, brain stem, and cerebellum. (×1.6)

Figure AII-27 Continued.

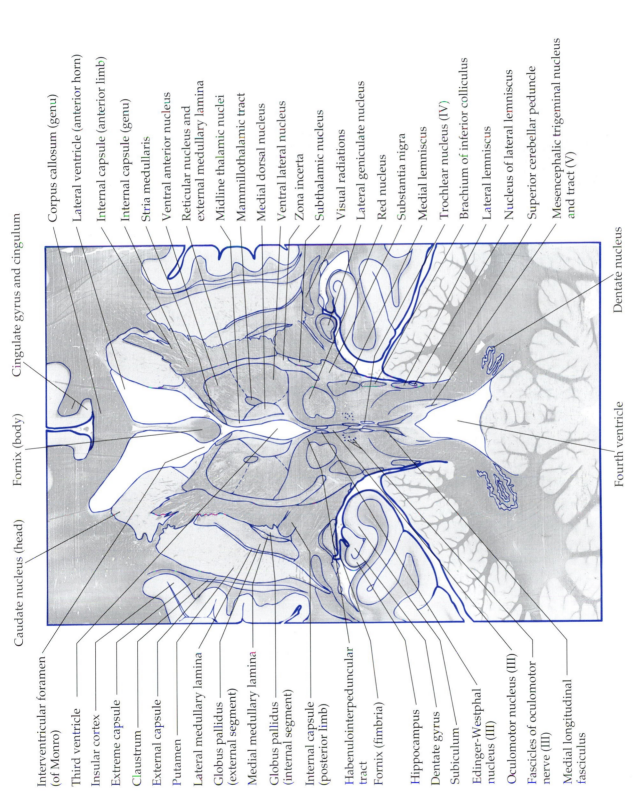

Cingulate gyrus and cingulum

Fornix (body)

Caudate nucleus (head)

Corpus callosum (genu)
Lateral ventricle (anterior horn)
Internal capsule (anterior limb)
Internal capsule (genu)
Stria medullaris
Ventral anterior nucleus
Reticular nucleus and external medullary lamina
Midline thalamic nuclei
Mammillothalamic tract
Medial dorsal nucleus
Ventral lateral nucleus
Zona incerta
Subthalamic nucleus
Visual radiations
Lateral geniculate nucleus
Red nucleus
Substantia nigra
Medial lemniscus
Trochlear nucleus (IV)
Brachium of inferior colliculus
Lateral lemniscus
Nucleus of lateral lemniscus
Superior cerebellar peduncle
Mesencephalic trigeminal nucleus and tract (V)

Dentate nucleus

Fourth ventricle

Interventricular foramen (of Monro)
Third ventricle
Insular cortex
Extreme capsule
Claustrum
External capsule
Putamen
Lateral medullary lamina
Globus pallidus (external segment)
Medial medullary lamina
Globus pallidus (internal segment)
Internal capsule (posterior limb)
Habenulointerpeduncular tract
Fornix (fimbria)
Hippocampus
Dentate gyrus
Subiculum
Edinger-Westphal nucleus (III)
Oculomotor nucleus (III)
Fascicles of oculomotor nerve (III)
Medial longitudinal fasciculus

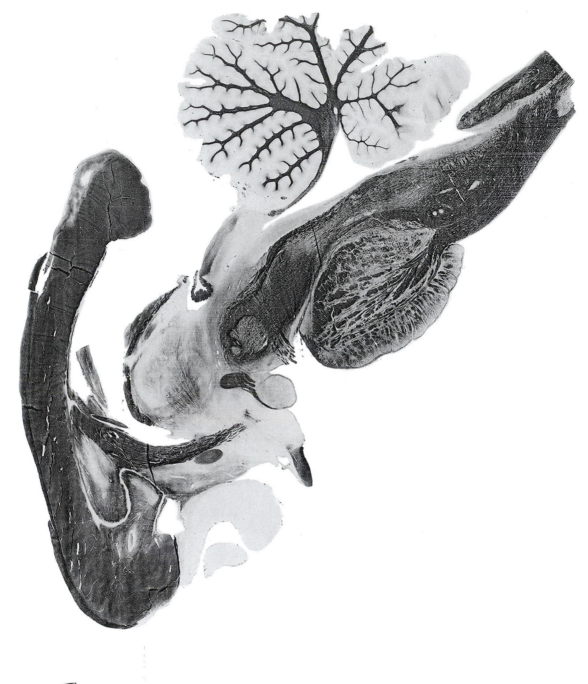

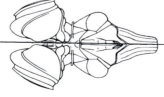

Figure AII–28. Sagittal section of the cerebral hemisphere, diencephalon, brain stem, and cerebellum close to the midline. (×1.9)

Figure AII–28 Continued.

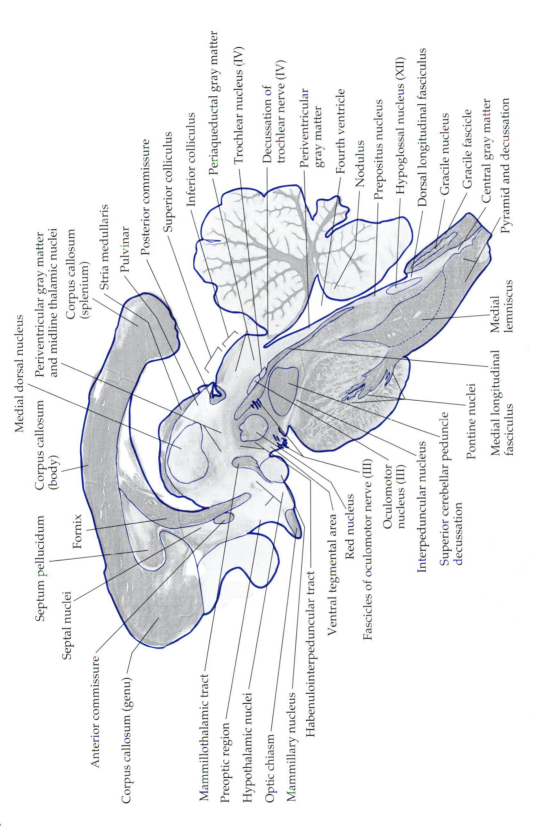

Medial dorsal nucleus

Periventricular gray matter
and midline thalamic nuclei

Corpus callosum
(splenium)

Stria medullaris

Pulvinar

Posterior commissure

Superior colliculus

Inferior colliculus

Periaqueductal gray matter

Trochlear nucleus (IV)

Decussation of
trochlear nerve (IV)

Periventricular
gray matter

Fourth ventricle

Nodulus

Prepositus nucleus

Hypoglossal nucleus (XII)

Dorsal longitudinal fasciculus

Gracile nucleus

Gracile fascicle

Central gray matter

Pyramid and decussation

Medial
lemniscus

Septum pellucidum

Septal nuclei

Anterior commissure

Corpus callosum (genu)

Mammillothalamic tract

Preoptic region

Hypothalamic nuclei

Optic chiasm

Mammillary nucleus

Habenulointerpeduncular tract

Ventral tegmental area

Red nucleus

Fascicles of oculomotor nerve (III)

Oculomotor
nucleus (III)

Interpeduncular nucleus

Superior cerebellar peduncle
decussation

Pontine nuclei

Medial longitudinal
fasciculus

Corpus callosum
(body)

Fornix

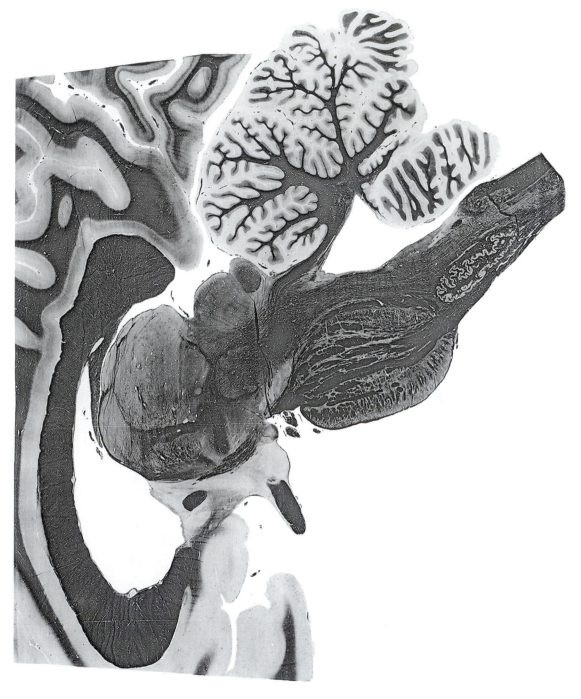

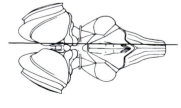

Figure AII–29. Sagittal section of the cerebral hemisphere, diencephalon, brain stem, and cerebellum through the mammillothalamic tract and anterior thalamic nucleus. (×1.8)

Figure AII–29 Continued.

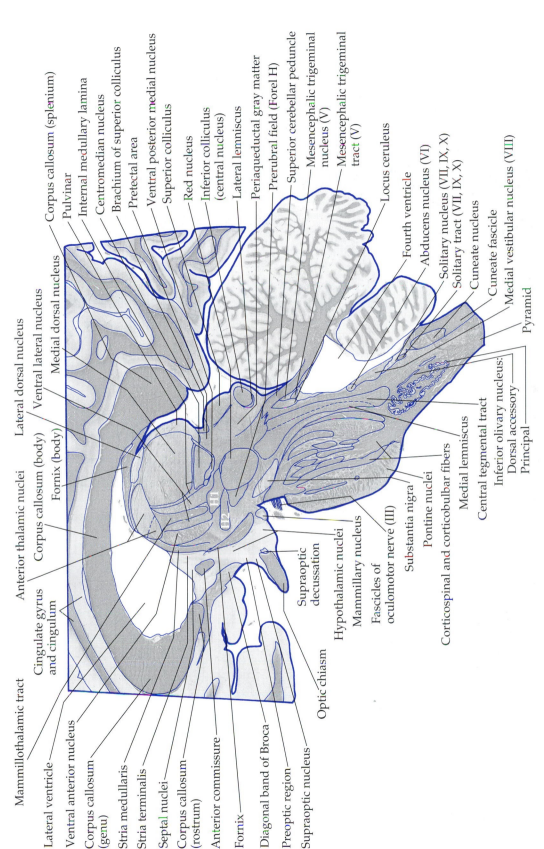

Mammillothalamic tract

Lateral dorsal nucleus

Anterior thalamic nuclei

Cingulate gyrus and cingulum

Lateral ventricle

Ventral anterior nucleus

Corpus callosum (genu)

Stria medullaris

Stria terminalis

Septal nuclei

Corpus callosum (rostrum)

Anterior commissure

Fornix

Diagonal band of Broca

Preoptic region

Supraoptic nucleus

Ventral lateral nucleus

Medial dorsal nucleus

Corpus callosum (body)

Fornix (body)

Corpus callosum (splenium)

Pulvinar

Internal medullary lamina

Centromedian nucleus

Brachium of superior colliculus

Pretectal area

Ventral posterior medial nucleus

Superior colliculus

Red nucleus

Inferior colliculus (central nucleus)

Lateral lemniscus

Periaqueductal gray matter

Prerubral field (Forel H)

Superior cerebellar peduncle

Mesencephalic trigeminal nucleus (V)

Mesencephalic trigeminal tract (V)

Locus ceruleus

Fourth ventricle

Abducens nucleus (VI)

Solitary nucleus (VII, IX, X)

Solitary tract (VII, IX, X)

Cuneate nucleus

Cuneate fascicle

Medial vestibular nucleus (VIII)

Pyramid

Inferior olivary nucleus:
Dorsal accessory
Principal

Medial lemniscus

Central tegmental tract

Corticospinal and corticobulbar fibers

Pontine nuclei

Substantia nigra

Fascicles of oculomotor nerve (III)

Mammillary nucleus

Hypothalamic nuclei

Supraoptic decussation

Optic chiasm

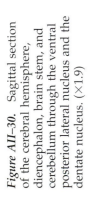

Figure AII–30. Sagittal section of the cerebral hemisphere, diencephalon, brain stem, and cerebellum through the ventral posterior lateral nucleus and the dentate nucleus. (×1.9)

Figure AII-30 Continued.

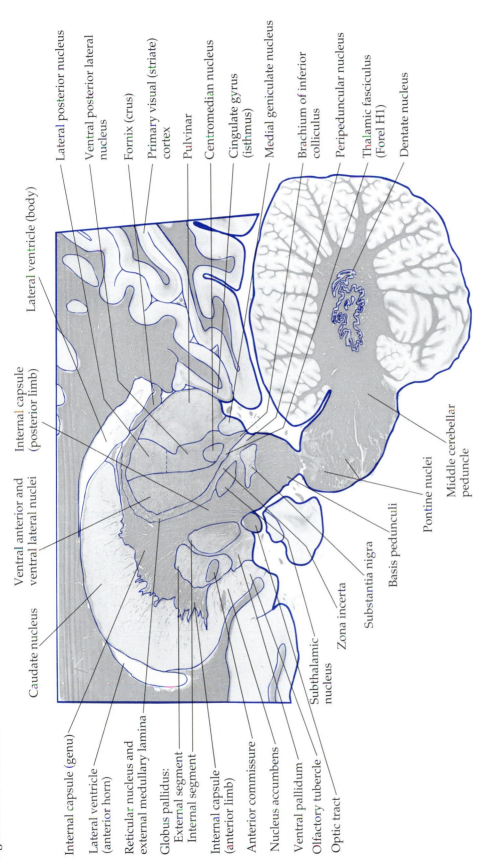

Lateral posterior nucleus

Ventral posterior lateral nucleus

Fornix (crus)

Primary visual (striate) cortex

Pulvinar

Centromedian nucleus

Cingulate gyrus (isthmus)

Medial geniculate nucleus

Brachium of inferior colliculus

Peripeduncular nucleus

Thalamic fasciculus (Forel H1)

Dentate nucleus

Lateral ventricle (body)

Internal capsule (posterior limb)

Ventral anterior and ventral lateral nuclei

Caudate nucleus

Internal capsule (genu)

Lateral ventricle (anterior horn)

Reticular nucleus and external medullary lamina

Globus pallidus:
External segment
Internal segment

Internal capsule (anterior limb)

Anterior commissure

Nucleus accumbens

Ventral pallidum

Olfactory tubercle

Optic tract

Subthalamic nucleus

Zona incerta

Substantia nigra

Basis pedunculi

Pontine nuclei

Middle cerebellar peduncle

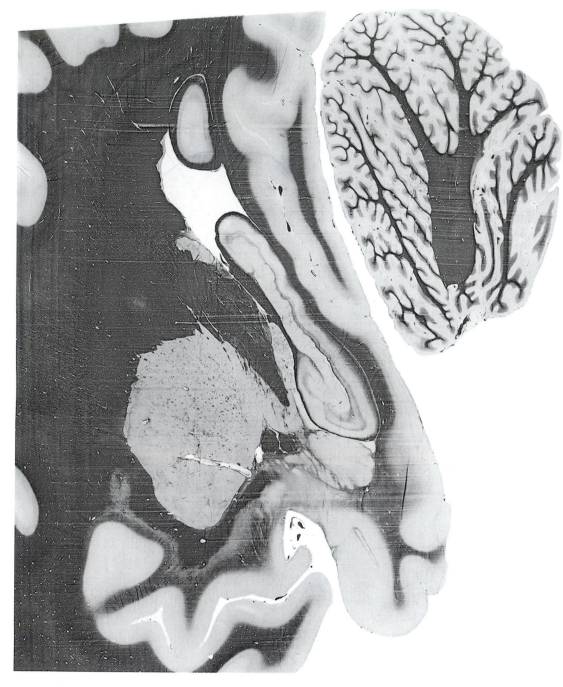

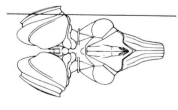

Figure AII–31. Sagittal section of the cerebral hemisphere and cerebellum through the amygdaloid complex and hippocampal formation. (×1.9)

Figure AII–31 Continued.

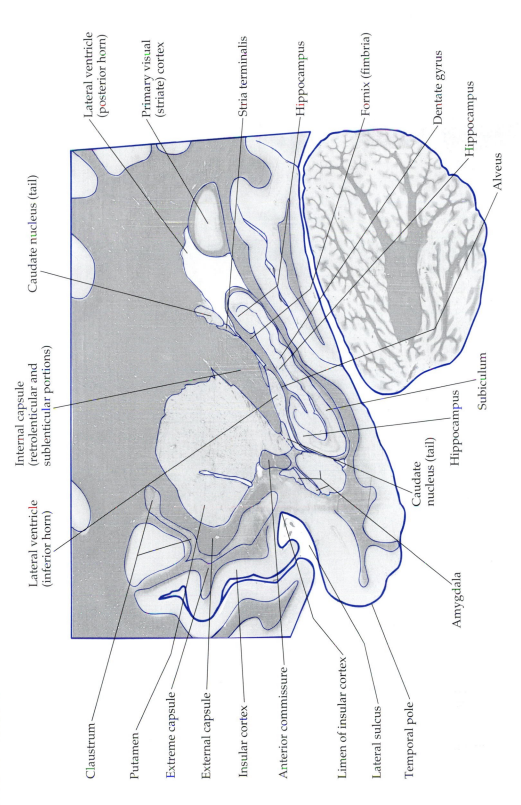

Lateral ventricle (posterior horn)

Primary visual (striate) cortex

Stria terminalis

Hippocampus

Fornix (fimbria)

Dentate gyrus

Hippocampus

Alveus

Caudate nucleus (tail)

Internal capsule (retrolenticular and sublenticular portions)

Subiculum

Hippocampus

Caudate nucleus (tail)

Lateral ventricle (inferior horn)

Amygdala

Claustrum

Putamen

Extreme capsule

External capsule

Insular cortex

Anterior commissure

Limen of insular cortex

Lateral sulcus

Temporal pole

References

Alheld GF, Heimer L, Switzer RC III: Basal ganglia. In Paxinos G (editor): The Human Central Nervous System. Academic Press; 1990:483–582.

Amaral DG, Insausti R: Hippocampal formation. In Paxinos G (editor): The Human Central Nervous System. Academic Press; 1990:711–755.

Andy OJ, Stephan H: The septum of the human brain. J Comp Neurol 1968;133:383–410.

Bruce A: A Topographical Atlas of the Spinal Cord. Williams & Norgate, 1901.

Carpenter MB, Sutin J: Human Neuroanatomy. Williams & Wilkins, 1983.

Crosby EC, Humphrey T, Lauer EW: Correlative Anatomy of the Nervous System. Macmillan, 1962.

DeArmond SJ, Fusco MM, Dewey MM: Structure of the Human Brain. Oxford University Press, 1976.

De Olmos JS: Amygdala. In Paxinos G (editor): The Human Central Nervous System. Academic Press, 1990.

Haines D: Neuroanatomy: An Atlas of Structures, Sections, and Systems. Urban & Schwarzenberg, 1983.

Hirai T, Jones EG: A new parcellation of the human thalamus on the basis of histochemical staining. Brain Res Rev 1989;14:1–34.

Martin GF, Holstege G, Mehler WR: Reticular formation of the pons and medulla. In Paxinos G (editor): The Human Central Nervous System. Academic Press, 1990.

Nathan PW, Smith MC: Long descending tracts in man. I. Review of present knowledge. Brain 1955;78:248–303.

Nathan PW, Smith MC: The rubrospinal and central tegmental tracts in man. Brain 1982;105:223–269.

Olszewski J, Baxter D (editors): Cytoarchitecture of the Human Brain Stem. Vol. I: Head, Neck, Upper Extremities. S. Karger, 1982.

Paxinos G, Törk I, Halliday G, Mehler WR: Human homologs to brainstem nuclei identified in other animals as revealed by acetylcholinesterase activity. In Paxinos G (editor): The Human Central Nervous System. Academic Press; 1990:149–202.

Price JL: Olfactory system. In Paxinos G (editor): The Human Central Nervous System. Academic Press; 1990:979–998.

Riley HA: An Atlas of the Basal Ganglia, Brain Stem and Spinal Cord. Williams & Wilkins, 1943.

Schaltenbrand G, Wahren W: Atlas for Stereotaxy of the Human Brain. Georg Thieme, 1977.

Williams PL, Warwick R: Functional Neuroanatomy of Man. W. B. Saunders, 1975.

Glossary

abducens (VI) nerve: cranial nerve; axons innervate the lateral rectus muscle

abducens nucleus: contains lateral rectus motor neurons and internuclear neurons; located in pons

accessory cuneate nucleus: relays somatic sensory information from upper trunk, arm, and neck to the cerebellum; located in medulla

accessory optic system: transmits visual information to brain stem nuclei for eye movement control

accommodation-convergence reaction: a complex response that prepares the eyes for near vision by (1) increasing lens curvature, (2) constricting the pupils, and (3) coordinating convergence of the eyes

accommodation reflex: increase in lens curvature that occurs during near vision

acetylcholine: neurotransmitter used by motor neurons and neurons in several nuclei, including the basal nucleus and the pedunculopontine nucleus

acetylcholinesterase: enzyme that inactivates acetylcholine

acousticomotor function: motor behavioral response triggered or controlled by sound such as orienting towards a sound

adrenergic: neuron that uses adrenalin as a neurotransmitter or neuromodulator

afferent: axons that transmit information toward a particular structure; *afferent* is not synonymous with *sensory,* which means related to processing information from a receptor sheet (eg, body surface or retina)

airway protective reflex: closure of the larynx to prevent fluid and food from entering the trachea

akinesia: impairment in initiating voluntary movement

alar plate: dorsal portion of the neuroepithelium that gives rise to sensory nuclei of the spinal cord and brain stem

allocortex: cortex having a variable number of layers, but always fewer that six

alveus: thin sheet of myelinated axons covering hippocampal formation; axons of pyramidal neurons in the hippocampus and subiculum

Alzheimer disease: presenile dementia

amacrine cells: retinal interneuron

amygdala: telencephalic structure that plays an essential role in emotions and their behavioral expression; has three component nuclear divisions: basolateral, central, and corticomedial

amygdaloid nuclear complex: another name for the amygdala

anastomosis: a network of interconnected arteries

anencephaly: developmental disorder in which certain cerebral structures fail to develop

angiogram: radiological image of vasculature

anosmia: absence of the sense of smell

ansa lenticularis: output pathway of the internal segment of the globus pallidus; axons terminate in the thalamus

anterior: toward the abdomen; synonymous with *ventral*

anterior cerebral artery: supplies blood to the medial frontal lobes and underlying deep structures

489

anterior choroidal artery: supplies blood to the choroid plexus in the lateral ventricle and several deep structures

anterior cingulate gyrus: portion of the cingulate important for emotions; activated while experiencing painful stimuli; a major target of the limbic loop of the basal ganglia

anterior circulation: arterial supply provided by the internal carotid artery

anterior commissure: tract that interconnects the anterior temporal lobes and olfactory structures on the two sides of the brain

anterior communicating artery: interconnects anterior cerebral arteries on the two sides of the brain; part of the circle of Willis

anterior inferior cerebellar artery (AICA): supplies the caudal pons and parts of the cerebellum

anterior limb of the internal capsule: subcortical tract between the anterior portions of the caudate nucleus and putamen; rostral to the thalamus

anterior lobe of the pituitary gland: contains epithelial cells that release hormones for controlling a variety of target glands in the periphery

anterior nuclei of the thalamus: receive input from the mammillary bodies and project to the cingulate gyrus

anterior olfactory nucleus: relays information from the olfactory nucleus to other parts of the central nervous system

anterior perforated substance: basal forebrain region where branches of the anterior and middle cerebral arteries (lenticulostriate) penetrate and supply deep structures

anterior temporal lobes: involved in emotions, especially during anxiety states

anterior thalamic nuclei: participate in aspects of learning and memory; principal target of the mammillary bodies

anterograde: away from a neuron's cell body and toward the axon terminal; typically related to the pattern of degeneration (*see* Wallerian degeneration) or axonal transport

anterograde amnesia: failure to remember new events

anterolateral system: spinal pathways for pain, temperature, and itch; includes spinothalamic, spinomesencephalic (spinotectal), and spinoreticular tracts

anteroventral cochlear nucleus: portion of the cochlear nucleus important for sound localization in the horizontal plane; located in the rostral medulla

antidiuretic hormone: released by the posterior lobe of the pituitary; acts on the kidney to concentrate urine

anxiety: an emotional state characterized by nervousness or agitation, often about what might happen

aortic arch: site of arterial blood pressure sensor

arachnoid granulations: unidirectional valves for cerebrospinal fluid to flow from the subarachnoid space to the circulatory system

arachnoid mater: middle meningeal layer

arachnoid villi: *see* arachnoid granulations

arbor vitae: appearance of cerebellar white matter on sagittal section

archicortex: primitive three-layered cortex; primarily in hippocampal formation

arcuate nucleus: hypothalamic nucleus important for control of neuroendocrine function and feeding

area postrema: portion of caudal medulla where there is no blood-brain barrier; important for sensing blood-borne toxins and in control of vomiting

Argyll Robertson pupils: pupil sign characterized by a small diameter and unreactive to light but which gets smaller to accommodation; associated with neurosyphilis

ascending pathway: pathway transmitting information from lower levels of the central nervous system to higher levels; typically used to describe somatic sensory pathways of the spinal cord and brain stem

association cortex: areas of cortex that serve diverse mental processes but that are not engaged in basic stimulus processing or control of muscle contractions; formally those areas that associate sensory events with motor responses and perform mental processes that intervene between sensory inputs and motor outputs

astrocytes: class of glial cell that serve diverse support functions, including axonal guidance during development and helping to maintain the blood-brain barrier

ataxia: uncoordinated and highly inaccurate movements; typically associated with cerebellar damage

athetosis: slow, writhing involuntary movements

atrium: portion of the lateral ventricle at the confluence of the body, posterior horn, and inferior horn

autonomic motor column: formation of sympathetic and parasympathetic preganglionic neurons into rostrocaudal columns in the spinal cord and brain stem

autonomic nervous system: part of peripheral nervous system engaged in the control of body organs; consists of separate sympathetic and parasympathetic divisions

axial muscles: muscles located close to the body midline; control neck and back

axon: portion of neuron specialized for conducting information encoded in the form of action potentials

axon terminal: presynaptic component of the synapse; where neurotransmitters are released

β-endorphin: an endogenous opiate cleaved from the large peptide proopiomelanocortin; plays a role in opiate analgesia

Babinski's sign: extension (also termed dorsiflexion) of the big toe in response to scratching the lateral margin and then the ball of the foot (but not the toes); associated with lesions of the corticospinal system in adults; present normally in children until about two years of age

ballistic movement: movement with high initial velocity

bare nerve endings: sensitive to noxious and thermal stimuli as well as itch-producing agents

baroreceptor: blood pressure receptor

basal cells: cells that differentiate to become taste receptor cells; thought to be stem cells

basal forebrain: portion of the ventral telencephalon caudal to the frontal lobes; contains the basal nucleus (of Meynert) and structures for emotions and olfaction

basal ganglia: telencephalic nuclei with strong interconnections with the cerebral cortex; serve diverse motor, cognitive, and emotional functions

basal hair cells: auditory hair cells located near the cochlear base

basal nucleus (of Meynert): contains neurons that use acetylcholine as their neurotransmitter and project widely throughout the cerebral cortex; neurons are among the first to degenerate in Alzheimer disease

basal plate: portion of the ventral neuroepithelium that gives rise to motor nuclei of the spinal cord and brain stem

base of the pons: ventral portion of the pons; contains primarily pontine nuclei and descending cortical axons

basilar artery: supplies pons and parts of the cerebellum and midbrain

basilar membrane: component of the organ of Corti that oscillates in response to sounds; mechanical displacement of the membrane stimulates auditory hair cells

basis pedunculi: ventral portion of the midbrain; contains descending cortical axons

basket cells: class of cerebellar inhibitory interneuron; makes very strong synapse on Purkinje cell body

basolateral nuclei (of the amygdala): division of amygdala that receives information from sensory systems and cortical association areas

bed nucleus of the stria terminalis: C-shaped component of the amygdala; related in function to the central nucleus

bilateral control: form of somatic or visceromotor control in which a cranial nerve or spinal motor nucleus receives projections from both sides of the cortex; typically provides a measure of redundancy, so that if one projection becomes damaged, the other projection can provide basic control

bilateral projection: one structure sends axons to both sides of the central nervous system

bilateral temporal visual field defect: *see* bitemporal heteronymous hemianopia

bipolar cells: neuronal morphology in which processes are located at opposite poles of the cell body; most commonly a class of sensory neuron

bitemporal heteronymous hemianopia: loss of peripheral vision; common with lesions involving the optic chiasm

blind spot: blind portion of visual field; corresponds on the retina to the exit point of the optic nerve, where there are no photoreceptors

blobs: location of color-sensitive neurons in primary visual cortex; primarily in layers II and III

blood-brain barrier: cellular specializations that prevent blood-borne materials from gaining access to the central nervous system

blood–cerebrospinal fluid barrier: specializations that prevent blood-borne materials from gaining access to the cerebrospinal fluid

border zone infarct: loss of arterial supply at the peripheral borders of the territories supplied by major cerebral vessels

border zones: peripheral borders of the territories supplied by major cerebral vessels

brachium of inferior colliculus: output pathway from the inferior colliculus to the medial geniculate nucleus

brachium of superior colliculus: input pathway to the superior colliculus from the retina

bradykinesia: movement disorder in which movements are slowed or absent

brain: cerebral hemispheres, diencephalon, cerebellum and brain stem

brain stem: medulla, pons, and midbrain

branchial arches: also known as gill arches; territory of developing head and neck; many cranial nerves develop in association with the branchial arches

branchiomeric: derived from the branchial arches

branchiomeric motor column: motor neurons that innervate muscles that develop from the branchial arches

branchiomeric skeletal motor fibers: *see* branchiomeric motor column

Broca's area: portion of the inferior frontal lobe important for articulation of speech

Brodmann's areas: divisions of the cerebral cortex based on the size and shapes of neurons in the different laminae and their packing densities; named after Korbinian Brodmann, a German neuroanatomist who worked during the late 19th and early 20th centuries

Brown-Séquard syndrome: set of signs associated with spinal cord hemisection; include ipsilateral loss of motor functions, ipsilateral loss of mechanical sensations, and contralateral loss of pain, temperature, and itch; all caudal to the lesion

bulb: archaic term for medulla and pons; commonly used to describe a cortical projection system (*see* corticobulbar tract)

C-shaped: description of the shape of many telencephalic structures

calcarine fissure: located in the primary visual cortex; occipital lobe

callosal connections: connections made by callosal neurons

callosal neurons: class of cortical projection neuron

capillary endothelium: inner layer of a capillary in brain and spinal cord contributes to the blood brain barrier

carotid circulation: *see* anterior circulation

carotid sinus: blood-pressure-sensing organ

carotid siphon: segment of the internal carotid artery

cataplexy: transient loss of muscle tone without loss of consciousness

cauda equina: spinal nerves within the vertebral canal caudal to the last spinal segment

caudal: toward the tail or coccyx

caudal nucleus (of the spinal trigeminal nucleus): important for facial pain, temperature sense, and itch; located in the caudal medulla; rostral extension of the dorsal horn

caudal solitary nucleus: important for viscerosensory function; located in the caudal medulla

cell body: where the nucleus is located and from which the axon and dendrites emerge

cell bridges: *see* striatal cell bridges

cell stains: method of revealing neuronal cell bodies; an example is the Nissl stain

central canal: portion of the ventricular system located in the spinal cord and caudal medulla

central nervous system: division of the nervous system located within the skull and vertebral column

central nucleus (of the amygdala): nuclear division of the amygdala important for the visceral expression of emotions, such as changes in blood pressure and gastrointestinal function during anxiety

central sulcus: separates frontal and parietal lobes

central tegmental tract: contains the ascending gustatory projection from the solitary nucleus to the thalamus and descending axons from the parvocellular red nucleus to the inferior olivary nucleus

centromedian nucleus: thalamic diffuse-projecting nucleus with widespread projections to the frontal lobe and striatum

cephalic flexure: bend in neuraxis at the level of the midbrain

cerebellar glomerulus: basic processing unit of the cerebellum; comprises one mossy fiber axon terminal (presynaptic), and many granule cell dendrites and several Golgi axons (postsynaptic)

cerebellar tentorium: rigid dural flap dorsal to the cerebellum; separates the cerebellum from the cerebral cortex and defines the posterior fossa

cerebellopontine angle: where the cerebellum joins the brain stem

cerebellothalamic tract: output pathway from the deep cerebellar nuclei to the thalamus

cerebellum: portion of the hindbrain; important for automatic control of movements and thought to play a role in automating many complex sensory and cognitive functions

cerebral angiography: radiological technique for imaging brain vasculature

cerebral aqueduct (of Sylvius): portion of the ventricular system in the midbrain

cerebral cortex: portion of the telencephalon; important for diverse sensory, motor, cognitive, emotional, and integrative functions

cerebral hemispheres: major brain division

cerebral peduncle: ventral portion of midbrain, formally corresponds to the tegmentum and base

cerebrocerebellum: comprises the lateral cerebellar cortex and dentate nucleus; important for motor planning

cerebrospinal fluid: watery fluid contained within the ventricular system and subarachnoid space

cervical: spinal cord segment; there are eight in total

cervical flexure: bend in the developing nervous system; located in the midbrain; persists into maturity

cholinergic: a neuron that uses acetylcholine as its neurotransmitter

chorda tympani nerve: a branch of cranial nerve VII; carries taste afferents

chorea: disordered movement characterized by involuntary rapid and random movements of the limbs and trunk

choroid epithelium: cells of the choroid plexus specialized to secrete cerebrospinal fluid

choroid plexus: intraventricular organ that contains cells that secrete cerebrospinal fluid

ciliary ganglion: peripheral ganglion containing parasympathetic postganglionic neurons

ciliary muscle: intraocular muscle that increases lens curvature

cingulate gyrus: C-shaped gyrus on medial brain surface spanning the frontal and parietal lobes

cingulate motor areas: premotor cortical area located in the cingulate gyrus

cingulum: C-shaped tract located within the white matter of the cortex beneath the cingulate gyrus

circle of Willis: anastomotic network of arteries on the ventral surface of the diencephalon

circumventricular organs: a set of eight structures lying near the ventricular surface that do not have a blood-brain barrier

cisterna magna: the portion of the subarachnoid space, dorsal to the medulla and caudal to the cerebellum, where cerebrospinal fluid pools

cisterns: portions of the subarachnoid space where cerebrospinal fluid pools

Clarke's nucleus: contains neurons that project to the ipsilateral cerebellum via the dorsal spinocerebellar tract

claustrum: telencephalic nucleus located beneath the insular cortex

climbing fibers: axons of the inferior olivary nucleus that synapse on Purkinje neurons in the cerebellar cortex; forms one of the strongest excitatory synapses in the central nervous system

cochlea: inner ear organ for hearing

cochlear apex: portion of the cochlea sensitive to low-frequency tones

cochlear division (of the vestibulocochlear nerve): cranial nerve sensitive to sounds

cochlear nuclei: first relay site for axons of the cochlear division of the vestibulocochlear nerve; located in the medulla

collateral circulation: redundant arterial supply for a given structure

collateral sulcus: separates the parahippocampal gyrus from more lateral temporal lobe regions

colliculi: set of four structures on the dorsal midbrain; superior colliculi are important for saccadic eye movement control, and inferior colliculi are important for hearing

color columns: collections of neurons in the primary visual cortex, predominantly located in layers II and III; also termed color blobs

columnar organization (of the cerebral cortex): vertical arrays of neurons that serve similar functions

commissural neurons: class of cortical neuron that contains an axon that projects to the contralateral cortex via the corpus callosum

commissure: tract through which axons cross the midline

computerized tomography: a technique for producing images of a single plane of tissue

conditioned taste aversion: rapid and very robust form of learning in which an individual avoids foods that made it ill

cone bipolar cells: class of retinal interneuron that transmits control signals from cone cells to ganglion neurons

cones: photoreceptor class sensitive to light wavelength (ie, color)

constrictor muscles of the iris: produce pupillary constriction

contralateral: relative spatial term related to the opposite side of the body

contralateral homonymous hemianopia with macular sparing: visual field defect in which there is a loss of vision in the contralateral visual field but preservation of foveal (or macular) vision; can be produced with visual system lesions affecting a portion of the primary visual cortex

contralateral homonymous hemianopia: visual field defect characterized by the loss of sight of the contralateral visual field; can be produced with visual system lesions affecting the optic tract, lateral geniculate nucleus, optic radiations, or primary visual cortex

cornea: transparent avascular portion of the sclera

corona radiata: portion of the subcortical white matter superior (or dorsal) to the internal capsule

coronal: plane of section or imaging plane; parallel to the coronal suture; equivalent to transverse plane for cerebral hemispheres and diencephalon

corpus callosum: commissure connecting the two cerebral hemispheres; contains four major subdivisions: rostrum, genu, body, and splenium

corpus striatum: subcortical telencephalic nuclei comprised of the caudate nucleus, putamen, and nucleus accumbens; generally synonymous with the striatum

cortex: thin sheet of neuronal cell bodies and afferent and efferent axons

cortical column: collection of radially oriented neurons that have similar functions and anatomical connections; basic functional unit of the cerebral cortex

corticobulbar tract: cortical projections that terminate on cranial nerve motor nuclei in the medulla and pons

corticocortical association connections: connections between cortical areas on the same side

corticocortical association neurons: cortical neurons that project axons to cortical areas on the same side

corticomedial nuclei: nuclei of the amygdala that play a role in visceral motor control

corticopontine pathway: descending projection from the cerebral cortex to the pontine nuclei; major input to the cerebrocerebellum

corticoreticular fibers: axons that originate from neurons in layer V of the cortex that project to the reticular formation

cortico-reticulo-spinal pathway: indirect cortical pathway to the spinal cord via neurons of the reticulospinal tract

corticospinal tract: projection from the cerebral cortex to the spinal cord

cranial and spinal roots: nerves that enter and exit the spinal cord and brain stem

cranial nerve II: optic nerve; contains axons of retinal ganglion cells; major targets are the lateral geniculate nucleus, rostral midbrain, nuclei at the midbrain-diencephalon junction, and hypothalamus

cranial nerve motor nuclei: location of motor neurons whose axons are located in the cranial nerves

cranial nerves: sensory and motor nerves containing axons that enter and exit the brain stem, diencephalon, and telencephalon; analogous to the spinal nerves

cribriform plate: part of the ethmoid bone; contains tiny foramina through which olfactory nerve fibers course from the olfactory epithelium to the olfactory bulb

cuneate fascicle: tract containing ascending axons of dorsal root ganglion neurons that innervate the upper trunk (rostral to T6), arm, neck, and back of the head; mediates mechanosensations

cuneate nucleus: termination of axons in the cuneate fascicle; neurons project axons to contralateral ventral posterior nucleus of the thalamus; mediates mechanosensations

cuneocerebellar tract: pathway from the lateral cuneate nucleus to the cerebellum; courses through the inferior cerebellar peduncle

cytoarchitecture: characterization of the morphology of the cerebral cortex based on the density of neuronal cell bodies

cytochrome oxidase: mitochondrial enzyme; marker for neuronal metabolism

declarative memory: memory such as the conscious recollection of facts

decussate: crossing the midline

decussation: a site where axons cross the midline

deep cerebellar nuclei: sets of nuclei located beneath the cerebellar cortex; fastigial, interposed (comprising the globose and emboliform), and dentate nuclei

deep cerebral veins: veins that drain the diencephalon and parts of the brain stem

Deiters' nucleus: lateral vestibular nucleus; origin of the lateral vestibulospinal tract

dendrites: receptive portion of a neuron

dentate gyrus: component of the hippocampal formation; receives input from the entorhinal cortex and contains neurons that project to the hippocampus proper

dentate nucleus: one of the deep cerebellar nuclei; transmits the output of the lateral cerebellar hemisphere

depression: a psychiatric disorder characterized by the persistent feeling of hopelessness and dejection; can be associated with poor concentration, lethargy, and sometime suicidal tendencies

dermatome: area of skin innervated by sensory axons within a single dorsal root

descending motor pathways: connections between the cerebral cortex or brain stem to the spinal cord; densest to the intermediate zone and ventral horn

descending pain inhibitory system: neural circuit for modulating transmission of information about pain from nociceptors, through the dorsal horn, and to the brain stem; primarily originates from serotonergic neurons in the raphe nuclei and noradrenergic neurons in the reticular formation; projects to the spinal cord dorsal horn

descending projection neurons: neurons that give rise to descending pathways

detached retina: pathological condition in which portions of the retina separate from the pigment epithelium

diabetes insipidus: condition in which the kidneys are unable to concentrate urine because of the absence of vasopressin (or antidiuretic hormone); the individual produces copious amounts of urine

diencephalon: one of the secondary brain vesicles; major brain division in maturity, containing primarily the thalamus and hypothalamus; means "between brain"

diffuse-projecting neurons: thalamic neurons that project widely to several cortical areas

diffuse-projecting nuclei: location of thalamic diffuse-projecting neurons

diffusion-weighted magnetic resonance imaging: type of magnetic resonance imaging that can distinguish axonal orientation, especially axons within tracts

direct path: pathway through the basal ganglia from the striatum to the internal segment of the globus pallidus; promotes the production of movements

disinhibition: removal of inhibition; net effect is similar to excitation

distal muscles: muscles that innervate the limbs, especially distal to the elbow; controlled principally by the lateral descending motor pathways

dopamine: neurotransmitter

dopaminergic: neurons that use dopamine as their neurotransmitter

dorsal: close to the back; also termed posterior

dorsal cochlear nucleus: auditory relay nucleus located in the pons; receives input from primary auditory receptors and projects to the contralateral inferior colliculus; implicated in vertical localization of sounds

dorsal column nuclei: cuneate and gracile nuclei; receive input from mechanoreceptor axons in the dorsal columns

dorsal column–medial lemniscal system: tracts, nuclei, and cortical areas collectively involved in mechanosensations (touch, vibration sense, pressure, and limb position sense)

dorsal columns: located on the dorsal spinal cord surface; contain ascending axons of mechanoreceptors; gracile fascicle (or tract) carries axons that originate from receptors on the leg and lower back, whereas the cuneate tract carries axons that originate from receptors on the upper back, arm, neck, and back of the head

dorsal horn: laminae I–VI of the spinal gray matter; processes incoming somatic sensory information, especially about pain, temperature, and itch

dorsal intermediate septum: separates the cuneate and gracile fascicles

dorsal longitudinal fasciculus: pathway to and from the hypothalamus; located in the periventricular and aqueductal gray matter

dorsal median septum: divides the dorsal columns into right and left halves

dorsal motor nucleus of the vagus: contains parasympathetic preganglionic neurons whose axons course in the vagus nerve (cranial nerve X); located in the medulla

dorsal raphe nucleus: located in the rostral pons and caudal midbrain; most neurons in the nucleus use serotonin as their neurotransmitter; projects widely to telencephalic and diencephalic structures

dorsal root: spinal sensory root

dorsal root ganglia: contains cell bodies of primary sensory neurons that innervate skin and deep tissues of the back of the head, neck, limbs, and trunk

dorsal root ganglion neurons: cell bodies of primary sensory neurons that innervate skin and deep tissues of the back of the head, neck, limbs, and trunk

dorsal spinocerebellar tract: an ipsilateral pathway to the cerebellum; originates in Clarke's nucleus

dorsolateral prefrontal cortex: cortical region important for organizing behavior, working memory, and a variety of higher mental processes

dorsoventral axis: between the back and abdomen

dura mater: outermost and toughest meningeal layer; contains an outer periosteal layer and an inner meningeal layer

dural sinus: channel for returning venous blood to the systemic circulation; also a path for flow of cerebrospinal fluid into the venous circulation

dural sinuses: channels within the meningeal layer of the dura, through which venous blood and cerebrospinal fluids are returned to the systemic circulation

dynorphin: neurotransmitter/neuromodulator

dysphagia: impairment in ability to swallow

ectoderm: outermost layer of the embryo

Edinger-Westphal nucleus: contains parasympathetic preganglionic neurons that innervate smooth muscle in the eye to control pupil diameter and lens curvature

efferent: axons transmit information away from a particular structure, *efferent* is not synonymous with *motor*, which means related to muscle or glandular function

electrical synapses: site of communication between neurons that does not use a neurotransmitter; usually associated with a gap junction, where ions and other small and intermediate-sized molecules can pass

emboliform nucleus: one of the deep cerebellar nuclei; together with the globose nucleus is termed the interposed nucleus

encapsulated axon terminals: specialized tissue surrounding the terminal of certain mechanoreceptors; helps to determine the sensitivity and duration of the response of the receptor to a mechanical stimulus

endocrine hormones: biologically active chemicals released by endocrine cells into the blood; regulate metabolism, growth, and other cellular and bodily functions

endoderm: innermost layer of the embryo

endolymph: fluid that fills most of the membranous labyrinth; resembles intracellular fluid in its ionic constituents; has a high potassium concentration and low sodium concentration

enkephalin: neurotransmitter

enteric nervous system: nervous system division that controls the functions of the large intestine

entorhinal cortex: portion of the medial temporal lobe; major input to the hippocampal formation

ependymal cells: epithelial cell type that lines the ventricles

epiglottis: pharyngeal structure that, during swallowing, helps to prevent passage of fluids and food into the trachea

episodic memory: memory of events that have a specific spatial and temporal context (such as meeting a friend last week)

ethmoid bone: cranial bone; contains the cribriform plate, through which olfactory sensory axons course en route from the olfactory mucosa to the olfactory bulb

explicit memory: conscious recollection of facts; also termed declarative memory

external capsule: white matter region between the putamen and the claustrum; contains primarily cortical association fibers

external nucleus: component of the inferior colliculus that participates in ear reflexes in animals, such as when a cat orients its ears to a sound source

external segment of the globus pallidus: contains neurons that project to the subthalamic nucleus; part of the indirect basal ganglia path

extrastriate cortex: visual cortical areas excluding the primary (or striate) cortex

extreme capsule: white matter region between the claustrum and insular cortex; contains primarily cortical association fibers

facial (VII) nerve: contains axons of motor neurons that innervate muscles of facial expression, as well as the stapedius muscle and part of the digastric muscle; exits from the pontomedullary junction

facial colliculus: surface landmark on ventricular (dorsal) surface of the pons; overlies the genu of the facial nerve and the abducens nucleus

facial nucleus: contains motor neurons that innervate muscles of facial expression, as well as the stapedius muscle and part of the digastric muscle; located in the pons

falx cerebri: dural flap between the two cerebral hemispheres; extension of the meningeal layer of the dura

fastigial nucleus: one of the deep cerebellar nuclei; transmits the output of the vermis to the medial descending motor pathways

fenestrated capillaries: contain pores through which substances can diffuse from within the capillary to surrounding tissue

fimbria: portion of the fornix that covers part of the hippocampal formation

fissure: groove in the cortical surface; more consistent in shape and depth than a sulcus

flaccid paralysis: inability to contract a muscle, together with a profound loss of muscle tone

flexure: bend in the axis of the central nervous system or axis of the embryo

flocculonodular lobe: portion of the cerebellar cortex involved in eye movement control and balance

flocculus: *see* flocculonodular lobe

floor plate: ventral surface of the developing central nervous system; key site for organizing the dorsoventral patterning of the spinal cord during development

folia: thin folds of the cerebellar cortex

foramen of Magendie: opening in the fourth ventricle where cerebrospinal fluid can pass into the subarachnoid space; located on the midline

foramina of Luschka: openings in the fourth ventricle where cerebrospinal fluid can pass into the subarachnoid space; located at the lateral recesses of the ventricle

forebrain: most rostral primary brain vesicle; divides into the telencephalon and diencephalon

Forel's field H2: another name for the lenticular fasciculus; region of the white matter though which axons from the internal segment of the globus pallidus course en route to the thalamus

fornix: a major output tract from the hippocampal formation

fourth ventricle: portion of the ventricular system located in the brain stem; separates medulla and pons from the cerebellum

fovea: portion of the retina with the greatest visual acuity, where only cone receptors are located; located in the center of the macula

fractionate movements: ability to isolate one movement from another, such as move one finger while keeping the other fingers still

fractured somatotopy: characteristic of a central sensory or motor representation in which the somatotopic plan is disorganized and a single body part becomes represented at multiple sites

frontal: close to the forehead

frontal eye fields: portion of the lateral frontal lobe important in the control of eye movements

frontal lobe: one of the lobes of the cerebral hemisphere

functional localization: identification of brain regions that participate in particular functions

functional magnetic resonance imaging (fMRI): a form of magnetic resonance imaging that can monitor blood oxygenation, which correlates with neuronal activity

functional neuroanatomy: examines those parts of the nervous system that work together to accomplish a particular task

GABA: γ-aminobutyric acid; principal inhibitory neurotransmitter in the central nervous system

gag reflex: stereotypic contraction of pharyngeal muscles in response to stimulation of the posterior oral cavity; the afferent limb is the glossopharyngeal nerve, and the efferent limb is the vagus nerve primarily

ganglion: collections of neuronal cell bodies outside the central nervous system

ganglion cell layer: innermost retinal cell layer; contains cell bodies of ganglion cells

ganglion cells: retinal projection neurons; axons course in the optic nerve and terminate in the diencephalon and midbrain

geniculate ganglion: location of cell bodies of primary sensory neurons that project in the intermediate nerve (cranial nerve VII)

genu: Latin for knee; used to describe structures with an acute bend, such as the corpus callosum and facial nerve

genu of the internal capsule: separates the anterior and posterior limbs of the internal capsule

ghrelin: protein secreted by enteroendocrine cells of the stomach; promotes food intake

girdle muscles: striated muscles that insert proximally and attach on parts of the shoulder or hip

glial cells: major cell type in the nervous system; outnumber neurons about 10 to 1; also termed glia

globose nucleus: deep cerebellar nucleus; together with the emboliform nucleus comprise the interposed nuclei, which transmit information from the intermediate cerebellar hemisphere

globus pallidus: basal ganglia nucleus; comprises distinct internal and external divisions

glomerulus: collection of neuronal cell bodies and processes surrounded by glial cells; structures within the glomerulus are physically isolated from surrounding neurons; typically corresponds to a basic functional processing unit

glossopharyngeal (IX) nerve: cranial nerve; located in the medulla

glutamate: principal excitatory neurotransmitter of neurons in the central nervous system

Golgi cells: cerebellar cortical interneuron; inhibitory

Golgi tendon receptor: mechanoreceptors sensitive to active force generated by contracting muscle

gracile fascicle: medial component of the dorsal column; transmits mechanoreceptive information from the legs and lower trunk to the ipsilateral gracile nucleus

gracile nucleus: target of the axons of the gracile fascicle; transmits information to the contralateral thalamus via the medial lemniscus

granular layer: innermost cell layer of the cerebellum; primarily contains granule and Golgi neurons and the axon terminals of mossy fibers

granule cell: cerebellar excitatory interneuron; cell of origin of parallel fibers

gray matter: portions of the central nervous system that contain predominantly neuronal cell bodies

great cerebral vein (of Galen): major vein; carries venous drainage from the diencephalon and deep telencephalic structures

gyri: grooves in the cerebral cortex

gyrus rectus: located on the inferior frontal lobe; runs parallel to the olfactory tract

habenula: portion of the diencephalon; located lateral and ventral to the pineal gland; part of a circuit with the midbrain medial dopaminergic and the serotonergic systems

hair cells: auditory receptor neurons

hearing: one of the five major senses

hemiballism: movement disorder produced by damage to the subthalamic nucleus; characterized by involuntary rapid (ballistic) limb movements

hemorrhagic stroke: condition following the rupture of an artery; tissue around the hemorrhage can become damaged because blood leaks out of the artery under high pressure

Heschl's gyri: location of primary auditory cortex

hierarchical organization: property of neural systems in which individual components comprise distinct functional levels with respect to one another

hindbrain: most caudal portion of the brain; includes the medulla, pons, and cerebellum

hippocampal formation: telencephalic structure located primarily within the temporal lobe; comprises the dentate gyrus, hippocampus, and subiculum; involved in learning and memory

hippocampal sulcus: separates the dentate gyrus from the subiculum; largely obscured in the mature brain

hippocampus: component of the hippocampal formation

histamine: neuroactive compound; generally excitatory; important in hypothalamic circuits for regulating sleep and wakefulness

Hoffmann's sign: thumb adduction in response to flexion of the distal phalanx of the third digit; an upper limb equivalent of the Babinski sign

horizontal cells: retinal interneuron

Horner syndrome: constellation of neurological signs associated with dysfunction of the sympathetic innervation of the head

Huntington disease: genetic autosomal dominant disorder; produces hyperkinetic motor signs

hydrocephalus: buildup of cerebrospinal fluid within the brain

hyperkinetic signs: set of abnormal involuntary motor behaviors characterized by increased rate of occurrence and inability to control; examples include tremor, tics, chorea, and athetosis

hypoglossal motor neurons: innervate intrinsic tongue muscles

hypoglossal (XII) nerve: cranial nerve located in the medulla

hypoglossal nucleus: location of hypoglossal motor neurons

hypokinetic signs: set of abnormal involuntary motor behaviors characterized by decreased rate of occurrence or slowing; examples include bradykinesia (slowing of movements) and failure to initiate a motor behavior in a timely manner

hypothalamic sulcus: roughly separates the hypothalamus and thalamus on the medial brain surface

hypothalamus: major brain division; part of diencephalon

immunocytochemistry: process in which antibodies to a particular molecule are used to label that molecule in tissue

implicit memory: memory of procedures and actions; also termed nondeclarative memory

incus: one of the middle ear ossicles (bones); essential for conducting changes in air pressure from the tympanic membrane to the oval window; located between the other two ossicles

indirect cortical pathways: motor pathway from the cerebral cortex that synapses first in the brain stem before synapsing on spinal neurons

indirect path: pathway through the basal ganglia from the striatum, to the external segment of the globus pallidus, to the subthalamic nucleus, and then to the internal segment of the globus pallidus; functions to retard the production of movements

infarction: death of tissue because of cessation of blood flow

inferior cerebellar peduncle: predominantly an input pathway to the cerebellum

inferior colliculus: located in the caudal midbrain, on its dorsal surface; contains neurons that are part of the ascending auditory pathway

inferior ganglia: location of primary somatic sensory cell bodies of vagus and glossopharyngeal nerves that innervate visceral tissues

inferior oblique muscle: extraocular muscle that depresses the eye, mostly when the eye is adducted

inferior olivary nucleus: origin of the climbing fibers; comprises several component nuclei

inferior parietal lobule: located dorsal to the lateral sulcus; important for a variety of higher brain functions, including language and perception

inferior petrosal sinus: major dural sinus

inferior rectus muscle: extraocular muscle that depresses the eye, especially when eye is abducted

inferior sagittal sinus: major dural sinus

inferior salivatory nuclei: location of parasympathetic preganglionic neurons that innervate cranial glands

inferior temporal gyrus: important in visual form perception

inferior vestibular nucleus: receives direct input from the vestibular organs; projects to various brain stem and spinal targets for eye movement control and balance

infundibular stalk: interconnects hypothalamus and pituitary gland; also termed the infundibulum

initial segment: junction of the neuronal cell body and axon; important site for integration of electrical signals and for initiating action potentials conducted along the axon

inner hair cells: principal auditory receptor neuron

inner nuclear layer: retinal layer that contains the cell bodies and proximal processes of the retinal interneurons: bipolar, horizontal, and amacrine cells

inner synaptic (or plexiform) layer: where synaptic connections between the bipolar cells and the ganglion cells are made

insular cortex: portion of the cerebral cortex buried beneath the frontal, parietal, and temporal lobes; several sensory representations are located there, including those for taste, balance, and pain

insulin: hormone secreted by the pancreatic islet cells; can inhibit food intake through hypothalamic circuits

interaural intensity difference: a mechanism for determining the horizontal location of high-frequency sounds

interaural time difference: a mechanism for determining the horizontal location of low-frequency sounds

interlaminar neurons: neurons in the lateral geniculate nucleus that are sensitive to color; project to the color columns (or blobs) in primary visual cortex located between the principal cell layers

intermediate hemisphere: portion of the cerebellar cortex involved in limb and trunk control

intermediate horn: the lateral intermediate zone of the spinal cord; location of sympathetic preganglionic neurons

intermediate nerve: sensory and parasympathetic branch of cranial nerve VII

intermediate zone: portion of spinal gray matter located between the dorsal and ventral horns

intermediolateral cell column: *see* intermediolateral nucleus

intermediolateral nucleus: location of sympathetic preganglionic neurons; present from about T1 to about L2

internal arcuate fibers: decussating fibers of the dorsal column nuclei

internal capsule: location of axons coursing to and from the cerebral cortex; present between the thalamus and parts of the basal ganglia

internal carotid artery: major cerebral artery; supplies blood to the cerebral cortex and many deep structures excluding the brain stem and cerebellum

internal medullary laminae: bands of white matter that divide the thalamus into several nuclear divisions

internal segment of the globus pallidus: one of the principal output nuclei of the basal ganglia

internuclear neurons: neurons located in the abducens nucleus that project to the contralateral oculomotor nucleus to transmit control signals for horizontal saccadic eye movements

internuclear ophthalmoplegia: produced by lesion of the medial longitudinal fasciculus between the levels of the abducens and oculomotor nuclei; interrupts axons of internuclear neurons; inability to adduct the ipsilateral eye when looking to the side opposite the lesion

interpeduncular cistern: where cerebrospinal fluid collects between the cerebral peduncles

interpeduncular fossa: space between the cerebral peduncles

interpolar nucleus: component of the spinal trigeminal nucleus; important for facial pain, especially within the mouth and teeth

interposed nuclei: deep cerebellar nuclei; comprises the globose and emboliform nuclei

intersegmental neurons: spinal interneurons that interconnect neurons in different segments; also termed propriospinal neurons

interstitial nucleus of Cajal: involved in eye and head control; located in rostral midbrain; gives rise to a small descending motor pathway

interstitial nucleus of the MLF: center for control of vertical eye movements; located in rostral midbrain

interventricular foramen (of Monro): conduit through which cerebrospinal fluid and choroid plexus passes from the lateral ventricles to the third ventricle

interventricular foramina: *see* interventricular foramen

intracavernous segment: portion of internal carotid artery as it passes through the cavernous sinus

intralaminar nuclei: set of thalamic nuclei that have diffuse cortical projections and may play a role in regulating the level of cortical activity and arousal

intrapetrosal segment: portion of the carotid artery as it travels through the petrous bone

intrasegmental neurons: local spinal interneurons; their axons remain with the segment of the cell body

ipsilateral: on the same side; term used relative to a particular landmark or event

ischemia: decreased delivery of oxygenated blood to the tissue

ischemic stroke: occlusion of an artery that results in downstream cessation of blood flow

isthmus: narrow portion of the developing brain stem between the pons and midbrain; in maturity the isthmus is typically included as part of the rostral pons

itch: sensory experience produced by histamine

jaw-jerk (or closure) reflex: automatic closure of the jaw upon stimulation of muscle spindle afferents in jaw muscles; analogous to the knee-jerk reflex

jaw proprioception: the ability to sense jaw angle; more commonly used to describe the sensory events signaled by primary sensory neurons whose cell bodies are located within the mesencephalic trigeminal nucleus

juxtarestiform body: efferent pathway from the cerebellum to the caudal brain stem; principal location of axons from the fastigial nucleus to vestibular and other brain stem neurons

knee-jerk reflex: automatic extension of the leg upon stimulation of the patella tendon; the stimulus stretches muscle spindle receptors in the quadriceps muscle

Korsakoff syndrome: a form of memory loss in patients with alcoholism or thiamine deficiency; produced by degeneration of the mammillary bodies and parts of the medial thalamus

lacrimal gland: tear gland

lamina terminalis: most rostral portion of the ventricular system

laminated: morphological feature in which neuronal cell bodies or axons form discrete layers

large-diameter axon: mechanoreceptive sensory axons

large-diameter fiber entry zone: site at which large-diameter axons enter the spinal cord; located medial to Lissauer's tract

laryngeal closure reflex: automatic contraction of laryngeal adductor muscles to prevent food and fluids from entering the trachea

lateral column: portion of the spinal white matter; contains diverse somatic sensory, cerebellar, and motor control pathways

lateral corticospinal tract: pathway in which descending axons for voluntary limb control descend; originates primarily from the motor areas of the frontal lobe

lateral descending pathways: motor pathways for controlling limb muscles

lateral gaze palsy: *see* internuclear ophthalmoplegia

lateral geniculate nucleus: thalamic visual relay nucleus

lateral hypothalamus: portion of hypothalamus involved in several integrative functions, including sleep and wakefulness regulation and control of feeding

lateral intermediate zone: portion of spinal gray matter that plays a role in limb muscle control

lateral lemniscus: ascending brain stem auditory pathway

lateral medullary lamina: band of axons that separates the external segment of the globus pallidus and the putamen

lateral medullary syndrome: set of neurological signs associated with occlusion of the posterior inferior cerebellar artery; signs include difficulty in swallowing, vertigo, loss of pain and temperature sense on the ipsilateral face and contralateral limbs and trunk, ataxia, and Horner syndrome

lateral olfactory stria: pathway by which axons from the olfactory tract project to the olfactory cortical areas

lateral posterior nucleus: thalamic nucleus with projections to the posterior parietal lobe

lateral rectus muscle: ocular abductor muscle; moves eye laterally

lateral reticular nucleus: precerebellar nucleus; transmits information from the cerebral cortex and spinal cord to the intermediate cerebellum

lateral septal nucleus: telencephalic nucleus; part of limbic system

lateral sulcus: separates the temporal lobe from the frontal and parietal lobes

lateral superior olivary nucleus: contains neurons sensitive to interaural intensity differences; plays role in horizontal localization of high-frequency sounds

lateral ventral horn: contains motor neurons that innervate limb muscles

lateral ventricle: telencephalic component of the ventricular system; bilaterally paired, with four components (anterior horn, body, atrium, posterior horn, and inferior horn)

lateral vestibular nucleus: key brain stem nucleus for control of proximal muscles; important in balance; gives rise to the lateral vestibulospinal tract

lateral vestibulospinal tract: ipsilateral pathway; component of the medial descending pathways

laterality: pertains to one side or the other

L-dopa: precursor to dopamine; used in the treatment of Parkinson disease

lenticular fasciculus: region of the white matter through which axons from the internal segment of the globus pallidus course en route to the thalamus

lenticular nucleus: globus pallidus (both internal and external segments) and putamen

lenticulostriate arteries: branches of the middle cerebral artery and anterior cerebral artery that supply deep structures of the cerebral hemispheres, including parts of the internal capsule and basal ganglia

leptin: hormone produced by adipocytes in proportion to the amount of body fat; suppresses feeding

levator palpebrae superioris muscle: principal eyelid elevator

limb position sense: ability to judge the position of one's limbs without using vision

limbic association cortex: diverse regions of primarily the frontal and temporal lobes; involved in emotions, learning, and memory

limbic loop of the basal ganglia: circuit of the basal ganglia that comprises the ventral striatum, ventral pallidum, and medial dorsal nucleus of the thalamus

limbic system: brain structures and their interconnections that collectively mediate emotions, learning, and memory

Lissauer's tract: location of central branches of small-diameter afferent fibers prior to termination in the superficial dorsal horn

lobe: major division of the cerebral cortex

lobule: a division of a lobe

locus ceruleus: principal noradrenergic brain stem nucleus; located in the rostral pons

long circumferential branches: brain stem arterial branches that supply the most dorsolateral portions; also supply the cerebellum

longitudinal axis: the head-to-tail (or head-to-coccyx) axis of the nervous system

lumbar: spinal cord segment; there are five in total

lumbar cistern: space within the vertebral canal where cerebrospinal fluid pools; commonly used for withdrawing cerebrospinal fluid from patients

lumbar tap: process of removing cerebrospinal fluid from the lumbar cistern; needle is inserted into the intervertebral space between the third and fourth (or the fourth and fifth) lumbar vertebrae

M cell: retinal ganglion neuron with a large dendritic arbor; plays a preferential role in sensing of visual motion; magnocellular

macroglia: glial cell class that comprises oligodendrocytes, Schwann cells, astrocytes, and ependymal cells; serve a variety of support and nutritive functions; contrast with microglia

macula lutea: portion of the central retina that contains the fovea

macular region: portion of the retina surrounding the macula lutea

macular sparing: maintenance of vision around the fovea after visual cortex damage that produces a loss of parafoveal and peripheral vision

magnetic resonance angiography: application of magnetic resonance imaging to study vasculature by monitoring motion of water molecules in blood vessels

magnetic resonance imaging: radiological technique to examine brain structure; uses primarily the water content of tissue to provide a structural image

magnocellular division (of red nucleus): component of the red nucleus that contains large neurons that project to the spinal cord as the rubrospinal tract

magnocellular neurosecretory system: hypothalamic neurons in the supraoptic and paraventricular nuclei that project their axons to the posterior lobe of the pituitary, where they release oxytocin and vasopressin

main (or principal) trigeminal sensory nucleus: brain stem relay nucleus for mechanosensory information from the face and oral cavity

malleus: one of the middle ear ossicles (bones); essential for conducting changes in air pressure from the tympanic membrane to the oval window; attaches to the tympanic membrane

mammillary bodies: hypothalamic nuclear complex; contains the medial and lateral mammillary nuclei; the mammillary bodies give rise to the mammillothalamic and mammillotegmental tracts

mammillotegmental tract: originates from the lateral mammillary nucleus; terminates in the pontine tegmentum

mammillothalamic tract: originates from both the medial and lateral mammillary nuclei; terminates in the anterior thalamic nuclei

mandibular division: trigeminal sensory nerve root that innervates primarily the lower face and parts of the oral cavity

marginal zone: outermost layer of the dorsal horn

mastication: chewing

maxillary division: trigeminal sensory nerve root that innervates primarily the lips, cheek, and parts of the oral cavity

mechanoreceptive afferent fibers: sensory axons that have mechanoreceptive terminals

mechanoreceptors: sensory receptors sensitive to mechanical stimulation

medial descending pathways: motor pathways for controlling axial and other proximal muscles

medial dorsal nucleus (of the thalamus): principal thalamic nucleus projecting to the frontal lobe

medial forebrain bundle: pathway that carries functionally diverse brain stem pathways to subcortical nuclei and the cerebral cortex, including the monoaminergic pathways

medial geniculate nucleus: thalamic auditory relay nucleus

medial lemniscus: brain stem tract that contains axons traveling from the dorsal column nuclei to the thalamus

medial longitudinal fasciculus: brain stem tract that contains axons from the vestibular nuclei, extraocular motor nuclei, and various brain stem nuclei; primarily for control of eye movements

medial mammillary nucleus: principal nucleus of the mammillary body; projects to the anterior nuclei of the thalamus

medial medullary lamina: band of myelinated axons that separates the internal and external segments of the globus pallidus

medial olfactory stria: small tract that contains axons from other brain regions that project to the olfactory bulb

medial orbital gyri: *see* medial orbitofrontal gyri

medial orbitofrontal gyri: part of the limbic association cortex

medial prefrontal cortical areas: portion of the prefrontal cortex one function of which is object recognition

medial preoptic area: portion of the anterior hypothalamus that contains parvocellular neurosecretory neurons; sexually dimorphic

medial rectus muscle: extraocular muscle that adducts eye (ie, moves toward the nose); innervated by the oculomotor nerve (cranial nerve III)

medial septal nucleus: telencephalic nucleus; important projections to the hippocampal formation; gives rise to cholinergic and GABA-ergic projections

medial superior olivary nucleus: contains neurons sensitive to interaural timing differences; plays role in horizontal localization of low-frequency sounds

medial ventral horn: contains motor neurons that innervate proximal limb and axial muscles; controlled by the medial descending pathways

medial vestibular nucleus: part of the vestibular nuclear complex; gives rise to the medial vestibulospinal tract for head and eye coordination

medial vestibulospinal tract: motor pathway for coordinating head and eye movements

median eminence: contains the primary capillaries of the hypophyseal portal system; located in the proximal portion of the infundibular stalk; lacks blood-brain barrier

medium spiny neurons: major class of striatal neuron; projects to the globus pallidus

medulla: major brain division; part of hindbrain

medullary dorsal horn: extension of dorsal horn into the medulla; also termed caudal nucleus

Meissner's corpuscle: mechanoreceptor

melanin-concentrating hormone: peptide that affects food intake

membranous labyrinth: cavity within which the vestibular apparatus are located; contains endolymph

meninges: membranes that cover the central nervous system; comprises dura, arachnoid, and pia

Merkel's receptor: mechanoreceptor

mesencephalic trigeminal nucleus: contains cell bodies of jaw muscle stretch receptors; only site in the central nervous system that contains cell bodies of sensory receptor neurons; more similar to a ganglion than a nucleus

mesencephalic trigeminal tract: contains the axons of jaw muscle stretch receptors

mesencephalon: secondary brain vesicle; major brain division; also termed midbrain

mesocorticolimbic dopaminergic system: dopaminergic projection to the frontal lobe and ventral striatum; primarily originates from the ventral tegmental area

mesoderm: middle layer of the embryo

metencephalon: secondary brain vesicle; gives rise to the pons and cerebellum

Meyer's loop: component of the optic radiation from the lateral geniculate nucleus to the occipital lobe that courses through the rostral temporal lobe; axons transmit visual information from the contralateral upper visual field

microglia: class of glial cell that subserves a phagocytic or scavenger role; responds to nervous system infection or damage; contrasts with macroglia

midbrain: major brain division

midbrain dopaminergic neurons: correspond to dopaminergic neurons in the substantia nigra pars compacta and the ventral tegmental area

midbrain tectum: region dorsal to the cerebral aqueduct; corresponds to the superior and inferior colliculi

middle cerebellar peduncle: major input pathway to the cerebrocerebellum; consists of axons of pontine nuclei

middle cerebral artery: supplies blood to the lateral surface of the cerebral cortex and deep structures of the cerebral hemisphere and diencephalon

middle ear ossicles: three bones that conduct sound pressure waves from the tympanic membrane to the oval window

midline thalamic nuclei: diffuse-projecting nuclei; one of its major targets is the hippocampal formation

midsagittal: anatomical or imaging plane through the midline that is parallel both to the longitudinal axis of the central nervous system and to the midline, between the dorsal and ventral surfaces

miosis: pupillary constriction

mitral cells: projection neuron of the olfactory bulb

mixed nerve: peripheral nerve composed of somatic sensory and motor axons

modality: sensory attribute that corresponds to quality (eg, pain)

molecular layer: outermost cerebellar layer; contains stellate and basket neurons, Purkinje cell dendrites, climbing fibers, and parallel fibers

mossy fiber terminal: enlarged axon terminal; one of the principal components of the cerebellar glomerulus

mossy fibers: in the cerebellum, major input to the cortex that originates from diverse structures, including the spinal cord and pontine nuclei; in the hippocampus, axon branch of granule cells in the dentate gyrus that synapse on neurons in the CA3 region

motor cranial nerve nuclei: contain cell bodies of somatic and branchiomeric motor neurons; nuclei containing parasympathetic preganglionic motor neurons are typically termed autonomic motor nuclei or columns

motor homunculus: representation of body musculature in the primary motor cortex; organization is similar to the form of the body

motor neurons: central nervous system neurons that have an axon that projects to the periphery, to synapse on striated muscles (somatic or branchiomeric motor neurons) or autonomic postganglionic neurons and adrenal cells (autonomic motor neurons)

Müller cell: retinal glial cell that stretches from the outer to the inner limiting membranes; have important structural and metabolic functions

multipolar neurons: neurons with a complex dendritic array and a single axon; principal neuron class in the central nervous system

muscarinic receptors: membrane proteins that transduce acetylcholine into neuronal depolarization; named for agonist muscarine

muscle spindle receptor: stretch receptor in muscle; has efferent sensitivity control

myelencephalon: secondary brain vesicle; forms the medulla of the mature brain

myelin: fatty substance that contains numerous myelin proteins

myelin sheath: covering around peripheral and central axons to speed action potential conduction; formed by Schwann cells in the periphery and oligodendrocytes in the central nervous system

myelin stains: methods to reveal the presence of the myelin sheath

myotatic reflexes: mechanoreceptors in muscle excite or inhibit motor neurons at short latency with only one or just a few synapses (eg, the knee-jerk [stretch] reflex)

narcolepsy: disease in which the patient experiences persistent daytime sleepiness; often associated with cataplexy, which is the transient loss of muscle tone without a loss of consciousness

nasal hemiretina: portion of the retina medial to a vertical line that runs through the macula

neocortex: phylogenetically most recent portion of the cerebral cortex; most abundant form of cortex; has six or more layers

neural crest: collection of dorsal neural tube cells that migrate peripherally and give rise to all of the neurons whose cell bodies are outside of the central nervous system; also gives rise to Schwann cells and the arachnoid and pial meningeal layers

neural degeneration: deterioration in neuron structure and function

neural groove: midline region of the neural tube where neurons and glial cells do not proliferate; where the floor plate forms

neural induction: process by which a portion of the dorsal ectoderm of the embryo becomes committed to form the nervous system

neural plate: dorsal ectoderm region from which the nervous system forms

neural tube: embryonic structure that gives rise to the central nervous system; cells in the walls of the neural tube form neurons and glial cells, whereas the cavity within the tube forms the ventricular system

neuraxis: principal axis of the central nervous system

neuroactive compounds: chemicals that alter neuronal function

neuroectoderm: portion of the ectoderm that gives rise to the nervous system; corresponds to the neural plate

neurohypophysis: portion of the pituitary that develops from the neuroectoderm; where vasopressin and oxytocin are released into the systemic circulation

neuromelanin: polymer of the catecholamine precursor dihydroxyphenylalanine (or dopa), which is contained in the neurons in the pars compacta

neuromeres: segments of the developing hindbrain

neuron: nerve cell

neurophysins: protein that derives from the prohormone that gives rise to oxytocin and vasopressin; coreleased with oxytocin and vasopressin

neurotransmitter: typically small molecular weight compounds (eg, glutamate and γ-aminobutyric acid, and acetylcholine) that excite or inhibit neurons

nigrostriatal dopaminergic system: originates from the substantia nigra pars compacta and terminates primarily in the dorsal and lateral portions of the putamen and caudate nucleus

nigrostriatal tract: pathway in which nigrostriatal axons course

nociceptors: somatic sensory receptors that are selectively activated by noxious or damaging stimuli

nodulus: portion of the cerebellum critical for vestibular control of eye and head movements

nondeclarative memory: memory of procedures and actions

noradrenalin: neurotransmitter; also termed norepinephrine

noradrenergic: neuron that uses noradrenalin as a neurotransmitter

notochord: releases substances important for organizing the ventral neural tube, such as determining whether a developing neuron becomes a motor neuron; located ventral to the developing nervous system

noxious: tissue damaging

nucleus: collection of neuronal cell bodies within the central nervous system

nucleus accumbens: component of the striatum located ventrally and medially; key structure in drug addiction

nucleus ambiguus: contains primarily motor neurons that innervate the pharynx and larynx; also contains parasympathetic preganglionic neurons; located in the medulla

nucleus of the diagonal band of Broca: cholinergic telencephalic nucleus with diverse cortical projections; located in the basal forebrain

nucleus of the lateral lemniscus: auditory projection nucleus; located in the rostral pons

nucleus of the trapezoid body: contains inhibitory neurons that receive input from the anteroventral cochlear nucleus and project to the lateral superior olivary nucleus; may participate in shaping the interaural timing sensitivity of neurons in the lateral superior olivary nucleus located in the pons

nucleus proprius: contains neurons that process somatic sensory information; corresponds to laminae III–IV of the dorsal horn

nystagmus: rhythmical oscillations of the eyeball

occipital lobe: one of the lobes of the cerebral hemisphere

occipital somites: somites from which neck and cranial structures develop

ocular dominance columns: clusters of neurons in the primary visual cortex that receive and process information predominantly from either the ipsilateral or the contralateral eye

oculomotor (III) nerve: motor cranial nerve; contains axons that innervate the medial rectus, superior rectus, inferior rectus, inferior oblique, and levator palpebrae muscles, as well as axons of parasympathetic preganglionic neurons

oculomotor loop: basal ganglia circuit that engages frontal eye movement control areas

oculomotor nucleus: contains motor neurons that innervate the medial rectus, superior rectus, inferior rectus, inferior oblique, and levator palpebrae muscles

odorants: chemicals that produce odors

olfactory bulb: telencephalic structure that receives input from olfactory sensory neurons and projects to the olfactory cortical areas

olfactory discrimination: ability to discriminate one odorant from another

olfactory epithelium: portion of the olfactory mucosa that contains olfactory sensory neurons

olfactory (I) nerve: central branches of olfactory sensory neurons; travels the short distance between the olfactory mucosa, through the cribriform plate, to synapse in the olfactory bulb

olfactory receptor: transmembrane protein complex in an olfactory sensory neuron; transduces a particular set of odorants into a neural potential; any given olfactory sensory neurons contains a single (or just a few) olfactory receptor types

olfactory sulcus: groove on the inferior frontal lobe surface in which the olfactory bulb and tract course

olfactory tract: contains axons that interconnect the olfactory bulb with the other olfactory nuclear regions of the brain

olfactory tubercle: region on the ventral brain surface that receives input from the olfactory tract; may play a role in emotions in addition to olfaction

oligodendrocytes: class of glial cell that forms the myelin sheath around axons within the central nervous system

olive: landmark on ventral surface of the medulla under which the inferior olivary nucleus is located

olivocochlear bundle: efferent projection from the inferior olivary nucleus to hair cells in the cochlea

olivocochlear projection: *see* olivocochlear bundle

operculum: portions of frontal, parietal, and temporal lobes that overlie the insular cortex

ophthalmic artery: supplies the eye; can be a pathway for collateral brain circulation after occlusion of the internal carotid artery

ophthalmic division: trigeminal sensory nerve root that innervates primarily the upper face

optic chiasm: site of decussation of ganglion cell axons from the nasal hemiretinae

optic disk: site on retina where ganglion cell axons exit from the eye

optic (II) nerve: sensory cranial nerve that contains axons of retinal ganglion cells; major projections are to the lateral geniculate nucleus, superior colliculus, and pretectal nuclei

optic radiations: pathway from the lateral geniculate nucleus to the primary visual cortex; forms the lateral wall of the posterior horn of the lateral ventricle

optic tectum: also termed the superior colliculus

optic tract: retinal ganglion cell axon pathway between the optic chiasm and the lateral geniculate nucleus

optokinetic reflexes: ocular reflexes that use visual information; supplements the actions of vestibulo-ocular reflexes

oral nucleus: rostral component of the spinal trigeminal nucleus

orbital gyri: gyri on the inferior surface of the frontal lobes; overlie the bony orbits

orbitofrontal cortex: portion of the inferior frontal lobe that contains the orbital gyri

orexin: peptide that is essential for the proper maintenance of the aroused state; loss of orexin is implicated in the sleep disorder narcolepsy; may also participate in feeding; also termed hypocretin

organ of Corti: component of the inner ear for transducing sound into neural signals

organum vasculosum of the lamina terminalis: one of the circumventricular organs; region in which the blood-brain barrier is absent; axons project to magnocellular neurons of the paraventricular nucleus

orientation column: cluster of neurons in the primary visual cortex that processes information about the orientation of a visual stimulus

otic ganglion: contains parasympathetic postganglionic neurons that innervate the parotid gland, which secretes saliva

otolith organs: the utricle and saccule; sensitive to linear acceleration

outer hair cells: class of auditory receptor neurons; may be more important in regulating the sensitivity of the organ of Corti than in auditory signal transduction

outer nuclear layer: retinal layer that contains the cell bodies of photoreceptors (rods and cones)

outer synaptic (or plexiform) layer: retinal layer in which connections are made between photoreceptors and two classes of retinal interneurons (horizontal cells and bipolar neurons)

oxytocin: peptide released by magnocellular neurons in the paraventricular and supraoptic nuclei

P cell: retinal ganglion neurons with a small dendritic arbor; plays a preferential role in sensing of form and color; parvocellular

pacinian corpuscle: rapidly adapting mechanoreceptor sensitive to high-frequency vibration

pain: sensation evoked by noxious stimulation

palate: arch-shaped portion of the superior oral cavity

paleocortex: type of cerebral cortex with fewer than six layers; commonly associated with processing of olfactory stimuli; located on the basal surface of the cerebral hemispheres, in part of the insular cortex, and caudally along the parahippocampal gyrus and retrosplenial cortex

pallidotomy: therapeutic lesion of a portion of the globus pallidus to alleviate dyskinesias

parabrachial nucleus: transmits viscerosensory information from the solitary nucleus to the diencephalon; located in the rostral pons

parafascicular nucleus: thalamic diffuse-projecting nucleus with widespread projections to the frontal lobe and striatum

parahippocampal gyrus: located on medial temporal lobe; contains cortical association areas that project to the hippocampal formation

parallel fibers: axons of cerebellar granule cells that course along the long axis of the folia; a single parallel fiber makes synapses with many Purkinje cells

parallel organization: property of neural systems in which pathways with similar anatomical organizations serve distinct functions

parallel sensory pathways: two or more sensory pathways that have similar anatomical projections and overlapping sets of functions

paramedian arterial branches: supply the most medial portions of the brain stem; originate primarily from the basilar artery

paramedian pontine reticular formation: transmits control signals from the contralateral cerebral cortex to brain stem centers for controlling horizontal saccades; major target of neurons in this structure is the abducens nucleus

parasagittal: anatomical or imaging plane off the midline that is parallel both to the longitudinal axis of the central nervous system and to the midline, between the dorsal and ventral surfaces

parasympathetic nervous system: component of the autonomic nervous system; originates from the brain stem and the caudal sacral spinal cord

parasympathetic preganglionic neurons: autonomic neurons located in the central nervous system; project to parasympathetic postganglionic neurons, which are located in the periphery

paraterminal gyrus: located anterior to the rostral wall of the third ventricle and ventral to the rostrum of the corpus callosum

paraventricular nucleus: hypothalamic nucleus that contains magnocellular neurosecretory neurons, parvocellular neurosecretory neurons, and descending projection neurons that regulate the functions of the autonomic nervous system

paravertebral ganglia: contain sympathetic postganglionic neurons

parietal lobe: one of the lobes of the cerebral hemisphere

parietal-temporal-occipital association area: association cortex at the junction of the parietal, temporal, and occipital lobes; important for linguistics, perception, and other higher brain functions

parietooccipital sulcus: separates the parietal and occipital lobes

Parkinson disease: results from loss of dopaminergic neurons in the substantia nigra pars compacta; characterized by slowing or absence of movement (bradykinesia) and tremor

parotid gland: salivary gland; innervated by axons of the glossopharyngeal (IX) nerve

parvocellular division (of red nucleus): component of the red nucleus that contains small neurons that project to the inferior olivary nucleus as the rubroolivary tract

parvocellular neurosecretory system: hypothalamic neurons, predominantly in the periventricular zone, that project their axons to the median eminence

peduncles: a large collection of axons

pedunculopontine nucleus: a pontine nucleus that receives a projection from the internal segment of the globus pallidus; participates in diverse functions, including regulating arousal and movement control; contains cholinergic neurons

perforant pathway: projection from the entorhinal cortex to the dentate gyrus

periamygdaloid cortex: one of the olfactory cortical areas; receives a direct projection from the olfactory tract; located on the rostromedial temporal lobe

periaqueductal gray matter: central region of the midbrain that surrounds the cerebral aqueduct; participates in diverse functions, including pain suppression

periglomerular cell: an inhibitory interneuron in the olfactory bulb that receives input from olfactory sensory neurons and inhibits mitral cells in the same and adjacent glomeruli

perilymph: fluid that fills the space between the membranous labyrinth and the temporal bone; resembles extracellular fluid and cerebrospinal fluid

peripheral autonomic ganglia: clusters of sympathetic and parasympathetic postganglionic neurons

peripheral nervous system: contains the axons of motor neurons, the peripheral axons and cell bodies of dorsal root ganglion neurons, the axon of autonomic preganglionic neurons, and the cell body and axon of autonomic postganglionic neurons

periventricular nucleus: contains parvocellular neurosecretory neurons; located in the hypothalamus, beneath the walls of the third ventricle

periventricular zone: portion of the hypothalamus that contains most of the parvocellular neurosecretory neurons; located beneath the walls and floor of the third ventricle

pharynx: the portion of the digestive tube between the esophagus and mouth; the throat

pheromones: a chemical produced and secreted by an animal that influences the behavior and development of other members of the same species

pia mater: inner meningeal layer; adheres closely to the surface of the central nervous system

pigment epithelium: external to the photoreceptor layer; it serves a phagocytic role during renewal of rod outer segment disks

pineal gland: functions in the diurnal secretion of melatonin; receives a sympathetic nervous system innervation

piriform cortex: one of the olfactory cortical areas; receives a direct projection from the olfactory tract; located on the rostromedial temporal lobe

pons: one of the major brain divisions; Latin for bridge

pontine cistern: site of accumulation of cerebrospinal fluid at the pontomedullary junction

pontine flexure: bend in the developing nervous system at the pons

pontine nuclei: relay information from the ipsilateral cerebral cortex to the contralateral cerebellar cortex and deep nuclei, principally the lateral cerebellar cortex and the dentate nucleus

pontomedullary junction: where the pons and medulla join

portal circulation: contains two capillary beds joined by portal veins; present in the pituitary gland and the liver

portal veins: join the two capillary beds of a portal circulation

positron emission tomography: functional imaging technique based on the emission of positively charged unstable subatomic particles (positrons); PET

postcentral gyrus: important for mechanical sensations, including position sense; located in the parietal lobe

postcommissural fornix: principal division of the fornix; contains axons principally from the subiculum that terminate in the mammillary bodies

posterior: toward the abdomen

posterior cerebellar incisure: shallow groove in the posterior lobe of the cerebellum

posterior cerebral artery: supplies portions of the occipital and temporal lobes as well as the diencephalon

posterior circulation: arterial supply provided by the vertebral and basilar arteries

posterior commissure: interconnects midbrain structures in the two halves of the brain stem; axons that mediate the pupillary light reflex in the nonilluminated eye course within the anterior commissure

posterior communicating artery: branch of the internal carotid artery that joins the posterior cerebral arteries; connects the anterior and posterior circulations, thereby providing a pathway for collateral circulation; part of the circle of Willis

posterior inferior cerebellar artery (PICA): supplies the dorsolateral medulla and portions of the inferior (posterior) cerebellum

posterior limb of the internal capsule: component of the internal capsule that lies lateral to the thalamus; carries axons from various sources including those coursing to and from the primary motor and somatic sensory cortical areas

posterior parietal cortex: contains higher-order somatic sensory area and association cortex; involved in diverse functions including stereognosis, forming of a sense of body image, sensing of visual motion and use of visual stimuli to guide movements, and a general awareness of the relative locations of objects

posterior spinal arteries: supply blood to the dorsal columns and dorsal horn predominantly

posterolateral fissure: separates the posterior and flocculonodular cerebellar lobes

posteroventral cochlear nucleus: contributes to a system of connections that regulate hair cell sensitivity

postganglionic neuron: autonomic neuron that projects to a peripheral motor target, such as a smooth muscle or a gland

postsynaptic neuron: component of a synapse; contacted by a presynaptic neuron

precentral gyrus: contains the primary motor cortex and the caudal portion of the premotor cortex; located in the frontal lobe

precommissural fornix: small division of the fornix that contains axons primarily from the hippocampus that terminate in the septal nuclei

prefrontal association cortex: involved in diverse functions, including thought and working memory

prefrontal cortex loop: circuit of the basal ganglia that projects to the prefrontal cortex; involved in higher brain functions, such as thought and working memory

prefrontal cortex: *see* prefrontal association cortex

preganglionic neuron: autonomic neuron located in the central nervous system

premotor areas: participate in the planning of movements; located in the frontal lobe, in areas 6, 23, and 24

premotor cortex: specific premotor region located in the lateral portion of area 6

preoccipital notch: surface landmark that forms part of the boundary between the temporal and occipital lobes on the lateral surface

preoptic area: serves diverse functions including the control of sex hormone release from the anterior pituitary gland and regulation of sleep and wakefulness; located in the most rostral part of the hypothalamus

prepositus nucleus: participates in eye position control; receives abundant inputs from the vestibular nuclei; located in the medulla

presynaptic neuron: component of the synapse; transmits information to the postsynaptic neuron

presynaptic terminal: axon terminal

pretectal nuclei: involved in pupillary light reflex; located in the junction between the midbrain and diencephalon

prevertebral ganglia: sympathetic ganglia that lie along the vertebral column

primary auditory cortex: first cortical processing site for auditory information; located in the transverse temporal gyri (of Heschl) in the temporal lobe; corresponds to cytoarchitectonic area 41

primary fissure: separates the anterior and posterior lobes of the cerebellum

primary motor cortex: contains neurons that participate in the control of limb and trunk movements; contains neurons that synapse directly on motor neurons; consists of area 4

primary olfactory cortex: defined as the target areas of olfactory tract axons; located in the rostromedial temporal lobe and the basal surface of the frontal lobes; corresponds to the paleocortex

primary olfactory neurons: transduce odorant molecules into neural signals; located within the olfactory epithelium

primary sensory (or afferent) fibers: somatic sensory receptor; dorsal root ganglion neuron

primary somatic sensory cortex: participates in somatic sensations, principally mechanical sensations and limb position sense; corresponds to cytoarchitectonic areas 1, 2, and 3; located in the postcentral gyrus

primary vestibular afferents: innervate vestibular hair cells; terminate primarily in the vestibular nuclei and cerebellum

primary visual cortex: participates in visual perceptions; located in the occipital lobe

projection neurons: cortical pyramidal neurons that project their axons to subcortical sites

proopiomelanocortin: a large peptide from which β-endorphin is cleaved

propriospinal neurons: spinal interneurons that interconnect neurons in different segments; also termed intersegmental neurons

prosencephalon: most rostral brain vesicle; gives rise to the telencephalon and diencephalon, which are the forebrain structures

prosopagnosia: inability to recognize faces

proximal limb muscles: muscles that innervate the shoulder or hip

pruritic: related to itch

pseudoptosis: partial dropping of the eyelid

pseudounipolar neurons: neuron type that has a single axon and few or no dendrites in maturity (eg, the dorsal root ganglion neuron)

pulmonary aspiration: the presence of food or consumed fluids in the lungs

pulvinar nucleus: major thalamic nucleus that has diverse projections to the parietal, temporal, and occipital lobes; involved in perception and linguistic functions

pupillary constriction: reduction in pupil diameter

pupillary dilation: increase in pupil diameter

pupillary light reflex: closure of the pupil with visual stimulation of the retina; used to test midbrain function in comatose patients

pupillary reflexes: changes in pupil diameter that occur without voluntary control; usually occur together with other ocular reflexes

Purkinje cell: output neuron of the cerebellum; GABA-ergic

Purkinje layer: location of Purkinje cell bodies

putamen: component of the striatum; important in limb and trunk control

pyramidal cells: a major cerebral cortex neuron class

pyramidal decussation: where pyramidal cell axons from the motor and premotor areas cross the midline; located in the medulla

pyramidal signs: motor impairments that follow lesion of the corticospinal system

pyramidal tract: location of descending motor control pathway that originates in the motor and somatic sensory areas

quadrigeminal bodies: another name for the superior and inferior colliculi

quadrigeminal cistern: portion of the subarachnoid space that overlies the superior and inferior colliculi

radial glia: type of astrocyte that plays a role in organizing neural development; form scaffold for neuron growth and migration

radicular arteries: segmental arteries that supply the spinal cord, together with anterior and posterior spinal arteries

radicular pain: pain localized to the distribution of a single dermatome or several adjoining dermatomes

raphe nuclei: contain serotonin; located along the midline throughout most of the brain stem

rapidly adapting: response characteristic of neurons to a sudden stimulus in which a brief series of action potentials decrement rapidly to few or no action potentials

Rathke's pouch: an ectodermal diverticulum in the roof of the developing oral cavity from which the anterior and intermediate lobes of the pituitary develop

receptive membrane: portion of a neuron's membrane that contains receptors sensitive to neuroactive compounds or a particular stimulus

red nucleus: plays a role in limb movement control; gives rise to the rubrospinal and rubroolivary tracts

reduced myotatic reflexes: a condition in which the strength of muscle stretch or tendon reflexes are diminished

regional neuroanatomy: examines the spatial relations between brain structures within a portion of the nervous system

relaxation times: in magnetic resonance imaging, the times it takes protons to return to the energy state they were in before excitation by electromagnetic waves

relay nuclei: contain neurons that transmit (or relay) incoming information to other sites in the central nervous system

release-inhibiting hormones: chemicals that inhibit the release of a hormone from the anterior pituitary gland; usually neuroactive compounds secreted into the portal circulation at the median eminence

releasing hormones: chemicals that promote the release of a hormone from the anterior pituitary gland; usually neuroactive compounds secreted into the portal circulation at the median eminence

reproductive behaviors: relatively stereotypic behaviors between members of the same species that lead to a reproductive act; in animals, the hypothalamus plays an important role in promoting reproductive behaviors, often in response to pheromones

reticular formation: a diffuse collection of nuclei in the central (medial) portion of the brain stem that play a role in a variety of functions, including regulation of arousal, motor control, and vegetative functions

reticular nucleus: a thalamic nucleus that projects to other thalamic nuclei; plays a role in regulating thalamic neuronal activity

reticulospinal tract: descending motor pathway that originates from the reticular formation, primarily in the pons and medulla, and synapses in the spinal cord

retina: peripheral portion of the visual system that contains photoreceptors as well as interneurons and projection neurons for the initial processing of visual information

and transmission to several brain structures; develops from the diencephalon

retinitis pigmentosa: disease in which breakdown products accumulate at the pigment epithelium of the retina

retinohypothalamic tract: axons of retinal ganglion cells that project to the suprachiasmatic nucleus; information in this tract is used to synchronize circadian rhythms to the day-night cycle

Rexed's laminae: thin sheets of neurons in the spinal cord, which are clearest in the dorsal horn; they are significant because neurons in different layers receive input from different afferent and brain sources and, in turn, project to different targets

rhinal sulcus: rostral extension of the collateral sulcus, which separates the parahippocampal gyrus from more lateral temporal lobe regions

rhodopsin: photopigment in rod cells

rhombencephalon: most caudal primary brain vesicle; gives rise to the pons and medulla

rhombic lip: portion of the developing pons that gives rise to most of the cerebellum

rhombomeres: segments in the developing pons and medulla; eight in total

rigidity: condition in patients with Parkinson disease in which there is resistance to passive movement about a joint; sometimes there are phasic decreases in this resistance, termed cog-wheel rigidity

rod bipolar cells: retinal interneurons that transmit signals from rod cells to ganglion cells

rods: photoreceptors; important in low light conditions

rostral: toward the nose

rostral interstitial nucleus of the medial longitudinal fasciculus: plays a role in control of vertical saccades

rostral spinocerebellar tract: transmits information about the level of activation in cervical spinal interneuronal systems to the cerebellum; thought to relay internal signals from motor pathways, via spinal interneurons, to the cerebellum

rostrocaudal axis: from the nose to the coccyx; the long axis of the central nervous system

rubrospinal tract: projection from the magnocellular portion of the red nucleus to the spinal cord

Ruffini's corpuscle: type of mechanoreceptor; distal process of large-diameter myelinated afferent fibers (A-β)

saccades: rapid, darting movements of the eye from one site of gaze to another

saccadic eye movements: *see* saccades

saccule: vestibular sensory organ (or otolith organ) sensitive to linear acceleration

sacral: spinal cord segment; there are five in total

sagittal: anatomical or imaging plane that is parallel both to the longitudinal axis of the central nervous system and to the midline, between the dorsal and ventral surfaces

scala media: inner ear fluid compartment

scala tympani: inner ear fluid compartment

scala vestibuli: inner ear fluid compartment; conducts pressure waves from the tympanic membrane to the other fluid compartments

Schaefer collaterals: collateral axon branch of neurons in the CA3 region of the hippocampus that synapse on neurons in the CA1 region

schizophrenia: psychiatric disease characterized by disordered thoughts, often associated with hallucinations

Schwann cells: glial cells that form the myelin sheath around peripheral axons

sclera: nonneural cover over the eye

scotoma: blind spot

seasonal affective disorder (SAD): form of depression during periods when days are short and nights are long

secondary auditory areas: cortical areas that process auditory information from the primary area

secondary somatic sensory cortex: cortical areas that process somatic sensory information from the primary area

segmental interneurons: neurons whose axons remain within a single spinal cord segment

segmental: pertaining to the segmental organization of the spinal cord

semantic memory: memory and knowledge of facts, people, and objects, including new word meaning

semicircular canals: vestibular organs sensitive to angular acceleration; there are three semicircular canals, each sensitive to acceleration in a different plane

semilunar ganglion: contains cell bodies of primary trigeminal sensory neurons

sensory: related to any of a wide range of stimuli from the environment or from within the body

sensory cranial nerve nuclei: process sensory information from the cranial nerves

sensory homunculus: form of somatic sensory representation in the postcentral gyrus (primary somatic sensory cortex)

septal nuclei: may participate in assessing the reward potential of events; receives input from the hippocampus and projects to the hypothalamus and other areas; located in rostral portion of the cerebral hemispheres

septum pellucidum: forms the medial walls of the anterior horn and part of the body of the lateral ventricle

serotonergic: neurons that use serotonin as a neurotransmitter

serotonin: neuroactive compound; also termed 5-HT (5-hydroxytryptamine)

short circumferential branches: supply ventral portions of the brain stem away from the midline; primarily from the basilar artery

sigmoid: S-shaped

six layers: describes laminar pattern of neocortex

skeletal somatic motor: neuron class in which axons synapse on skeletal muscle that derives from the somites

skeletomotor loop: basal ganglia circuit that engages the motor and premotor areas

slowly adapting: response characteristic of neurons to an enduring stimulus in which a prolonged series of action potentials decrement slowly or not at all

small-diameter axons: afferent fibers that are sensitive to pain, temperature, and itch (ie, histamine)

smell: one of the five major senses

smooth pursuit eye movements: slow eye movements that follow visual stimuli

soft palate: caudal, arch-shaped, portion of superior oral cavity formed by muscle

solitary nucleus: contains neurons that receive and process gustatory and viscerosensory information and project to other brain stem and diencephalic nuclei, including the parabrachial nucleus and the thalamus

solitary tract: where the central branches of gustatory and viscerosensory axons collect before synapsing in the solitary nucleus

somatic: related to the body

somatic motor systems: pathways and neurons that participate in limb and trunk muscle control

somatic sensory: body sense; includes pain, temperature sense, itch, touch, and limb position sense

somatic skeletal motor column: motor nuclei in the spinal cord that contain motor neurons that innervate somatic skeletal muscle

somatotopy: organization of central sensory and motor representations based on the shape and spatial characteristics of the body

somites: para-axial mesoderm that organizes development of muscles, bones, and other structures of the neck, limbs, and trunk

spastic paralysis: condition in which the presence of spasticity produces an inability to voluntarily control striated muscle

spasticity: velocity-dependent increase in muscle tone; occurs after damage to the corticospinal system during development or in maturity

spina bifida: neural tube defect; failure of the caudal neural tube to close, producing impairments in lumbosacral spinal cord functions

spinal accessory (XI) nerve: cranial motor nerve that innervates the sternocleidomastoid muscle and parts of the trapezius muscle

spinal accessory nucleus: contains motor neurons whose axons course in the spinal accessory (XI) nerve to innervate the sternocleidomastoid muscle and parts of the trapezius muscle

spinal border cells: neurons that contribute axons to the ventral spinocerebellar tract

spinal cord: major division of the central nervous system

spinal nerves: mixed nerves present at each spinal segment

spinal trigeminal nucleus: portion of the trigeminal sensory nuclear complex within the medulla and caudal pons; contains the caudal, interposed, and oral subnuclei; involved in diverse trigeminal functions, the most important of which are pain, temperature, and itch

spinal trigeminal tract: pathway in which trigeminal afferent fibers course before synapsing in the spinal trigeminal nucleus

spinocerebellar tracts: paths transmitting somatic sensory information from the limbs and trunk to the cerebellum for movement control

spinocerebellum: portion of the cerebellum that plays a key role in limb and trunk control; includes the vermis and intermediate hemisphere of the cortex and the fastigial and interposed nuclei

spinomesencephalic tract: transmits somatic sensory information from the limbs and trunk to the midbrain

spinoreticular tract: transmits somatic sensory information from the limbs and trunk to the reticular formation

spinotectal tract: transmits somatic sensory information from the limbs and trunk to the dorsal midbrain; term often used interchangeably with spinomesencephalic tract

spinothalamic tract: transmits somatic sensory information from the limbs and trunk to the thalamus

spiral ganglion: where the cell bodies of auditory primary sensory neurons are located

stapes one of the middle ear ossicles (bones); essential for conducting changes in air pressure from the tympanic membrane to the oval window; attaches to the oval window

stellate cells: in the cerebellum, inhibitory interneurons located in the molecular layer; more generally, a class of small multipolar neuron in the central nervous system

stem cells: multipotential cell that can develop into nerve, glial, or other cell types

stria (or stripe) of Gennari: band of myelinated axons in layer 4B of the primary visual cortex; axons interconnect local areas of cortex for visual stimulus processing

stria medullaris: pathway that courses along the lateral walls of the third ventricle; contains axons from the septal nuclei to the habenula

stria terminalis: C-shaped pathway from the amygdala to portions of the diencephalon and cerebral hemispheres; also contains neurons

striatal cell bridges: places of continuity of the caudate nucleus and putamen that span the internal capsule

striate cortex: another term for the primary visual cortex based on the location of the stria of Gennari

striatum: component of the basal ganglia; comprises the caudate nucleus, putamen, and nucleus accumbens

subarachnoid space: between the outer portion of the arachnoid and the pia; where cerebrospinal fluid accumulates over the surface of the brain and spinal cord

subcommissural organ: a circumventricular organ; located near the posterior commissure

subdural hematoma: hemorrhage of blood into the potential space between the dura and the arachnoid

subdural space: potential space between the dura and the arachnoid

subfornical organ: one of the circumventricular organs; region in which the blood-brain barrier is absent; axons project to magnocellular neurons of the paraventricular nucleus

subiculum: component of the hippocampal formation

submodality: category of a sensory modality, such as color vision, bitter, or pain

substance P: neuroactive compound; present in neurons that process painful stimuli

substantia gelatinosa: laminae II and III of the dorsal horn; process pain, temperature, and itch

substantia nigra pars compacta: portion of the substantia nigra where neurons contain dopamine and project widely to the striatum

substantia nigra pars reticulata: portion of the substantia nigra where neurons contain GABA and project to the thalamus primarily

substantia nigra: component of the basal ganglia; comprises the pars reticulata and the pars compacta

subthalamic nucleus: basal ganglia nucleus involved in limb control; when damaged, can produce hemiballism; part of the indirect basal ganglia circuit

sulci: grooves

sulcus limitans: groove that separates developing sensory and motor structures in the spinal cord and brain stem

sulcus: groove

superior cerebellar artery: supplies rostral pons and cerebellum; long circumferential branch of the basilar artery

superior cerebellar peduncle: tract that primarily carries axons from the deep cerebellar nuclei to the brain stem and thalamus

superior colliculus: plays a key role in controlling saccades; located in the rostral midbrain

superior ganglion: of the vagus and glossopharyngeal nerves, contains cell bodies of somatic sensory afferent fibers

superior oblique muscle: depresses the eye when the eye is adducted and intorts the eye when it is abducted

superior olivary nuclear complex: involved in processing incoming auditory signals; especially important for horizontal localization of sounds

superior parietal lobule: important for spatial localization

superior petrosal sinus: dural sinus; drains into the sigmoid sinus

superior rectus muscle: elevates the eye

superior sagittal sinus: dural sinus; drains into the straight sinus

superior salivatory nucleus: contains parasympathetic preganglionic neurons whose axons course in the intermediate (VII) nerve

superior temporal gyrus: involved in hearing and speech

supplementary motor area: portion of the medial frontal lobe important in the control of eye movements

supporting cells: provide structural and possibly trophic support for taste buds

suprachiasmatic nucleus: hypothalamic nucleus important for circadian rhythms; center of the biological clock

supraoptic nucleus: contains magnocellular neurosecretory neurons; secretes oxytocin and vasopressin into the systemic circulation in the posterior pituitary gland

Sylvian fissure: separates the temporal lobe from the parietal and frontal lobes; also termed the lateral sulcus

sympathetic nervous system: component of the autonomic nervous system

sympathetic preganglionic neurons: sympathetic nervous system neurons that are located in the central nervous system and synapse on sympathetic postganglionic neurons and cells in the adrenal medulla

synapses: specialized sites of contact where neurons communicate and where neurotransmitters are released; comprise three components—presynaptic axon terminal, synaptic cleft, and postsynaptic membrane

synaptic cleft: narrow intercellular space between the neurons at synapses

syringomyelia: cavity

T1 relaxation time: proton relaxation time related to the overall tissue environment; also termed spin-lattice relaxation time

T2 relaxation time: proton relaxation time related to interactions between protons; also termed spin-spin relaxation time

tabes dorsalis: degenerative loss of large-diameter mechanoreceptive fibers; associated with end-stage neurosyphilis

tarsal muscle: a smooth muscle that assists the actions of the levator palpebrae muscle; under control of the sympathetic nervous system

tastants: chemicals that produce tastes

taste: one of the five major senses

taste buds: gustatory organ, which consists of taste receptor cells, support cells, and basal cells, which may be stem cells for replenishing taste receptor cells

taste receptor cells: component of taste buds; transduce oral chemicals into gustatory signals

tectorial membrane: component of the organ of Corti; stereocilia of hair cells embed within the tectorial membrane

tectospinal tract: projection from the deep layers of the superior colliculus to the spinal cord

tectum: most dorsal portion of the brain stem; present only in midbrain in maturity

tegmentum: portion of the brain stem between the tectum and the base; present throughout the brain stem; Latin for cover

telencephalon: secondary brain vesicle that gives rise to structures of the cerebral hemisphere; derives from the prosencephalon

temporal hemiretina: temporal half of the retina

temporal lobe: one of the lobes of the cerebral hemisphere

temporal pole: most rostral portion of the temporal lobe

tentorium cerebelli: dural flap between the occipital lobes and the cerebellum

terminal ganglia: parasympathetic ganglia that contain postganglionic neurons; receive input from the vagus nerve; located on the structure their axons innervate

thalamic adhesion: site of adhesion of the two halves of the thalamus; said to be present in approximately 80% of individuals; in humans, no axons decussate in the thalamic adhesion

thalamic fasciculus: tract in which axons from the deep cerebellar nuclei and part of the internal segment of the globus pallidus course to the thalamus

thalamic radiations: axons of thalamic nuclei that project to the cerebral cortex

thalamus: major site of relay nuclei that transmit information to the cerebral cortex; component of the diencephalon

thermoreceptors: primary sensory neurons sensitive to thermal changes

third ventricle: component of the ventricular system; located between the two halves of the diencephalon

thoracic: spinal cord segment; there are 12 in humans

tonotopic organization: organization of central auditory representations based on the frequency sensitivity of the organ of Corti

touch: one of the five major senses

tract: collection of axons within the central nervous system

transverse plane: perpendicular to the longitudinal axis of the central nervous system, between the dorsal and ventral surfaces

transverse sinus: dural sinus that carries blood into the systemic circulation

trapezoid body: site of decussation of auditory fibers

tremor: trembling or shaking movement

trigeminal lemniscus: tract in which axons from the main trigeminal sensory nucleus ascend to the thalamus

trigeminal mesencephalic nucleus: contains cell bodies of primary sensory neurons innervating stretch receptors in jaw muscles

trigeminal motor nucleus: contains motor neurons that innervate jaw muscles

trigeminal (V) nerve: mixed cranial nerve containing sensory axons that innervate much of the head and oral cavity and motor axons that innervate jaw muscles

trigeminocerebellar pathways: projection from spinal trigeminal nuclei to the cerebellum

trigeminothalamic tract: projection from spinal trigeminal nuclei to the thalamus

trochlear (IV) nerve: cranial nerve that contains the axons of trochlear motor neurons, which innervate the superior oblique muscle

trochlear nucleus: contains motor neurons that innervate the superior oblique muscle

tufted cells: olfactory bulb projection neurons

tympanic membrane: ear drum; oscillates in response to environmental pressure changes associated with sounds; coupled to middle ear ossicles

uncal herniation: displacement of the uncus medially due to an expanding space-occupying lesion above the cerebellar tentorium

uncinate fasciculus: association pathway interconnecting frontal and anterior temporal cortical areas

uncus: bulge on the medial temporal lobe; overlies the anterior hippocampal formation and amygdala

unipolar neuron: neuron with a cell body and axon but few dendrites

urination: release of urine from the bladder

utricle: vestibular sensory organ (or otolith organ) sensitive to linear acceleration

vagus (X) nerve: mixed cranial nerve; contains axons of branchiomeric motor neurons that innervate laryngeal and pharyngeal muscles, parasympathetic preganglionic fibers, gustatory and visceral afferent fibers, and somatic sensory afferents; located in the medulla

vascular organ of the lamina terminalis: a circumventricular organ; located in the rostral wall of the third ventricle

vasopressin: neuroactive peptide that also acts on peripheral structures, including promoting fluid reabsorption in the kidney; also termed antidiuretic hormone (ADH)

venogram: radiological image of veins

ventral: toward the abdomen; synonymous with anterior

ventral (anterior) commissure: *see* ventral spinal commissure

ventral (or anterior) corticospinal tract: pathway for control of axial and proximal limb muscles of the neck and upper body

ventral amygdalofugal pathway: output pathway from the basolateral and central nuclei of the amygdala

ventral anterior nucleus: thalamic nucleus that transmits information from the basal ganglia to the motor and premotor areas

ventral column: portion of spinal cord white matter medial to the ventral horn; contains primarily descending fibers for controlling axial and proximal limb musculature

ventral horn: laminae VIII and IX of the spinal gray matter; location of neurons for somatic motor control

ventral pallidum: output nucleus of the limbic circuit of the basal ganglia; located ventral to the anterior commissure

ventral posterior lateral nucleus: division of the ventral posterior nucleus where information from the dorsal column nuclei is processed

ventral posterior medial nucleus: division of the ventral posterior nucleus where trigeminal information is processed

ventral posterior nucleus: thalamic nucleus for processing somatic sensory information; projects to the primary somatic sensory cortex

ventral root: where motor axons leave the spinal cord

ventral spinal commissure: where axons of the anterolateral system decussate; located ventral to lamina X and the central canal

ventral spinocerebellar tract: transmits information about the level of activation in thoracic, lumbar, and sacral spinal interneuronal systems to the cerebellum; thought to relay internal signals from motor pathways, via spinal interneurons, to the cerebellum

ventral striatum: consists of the ventromedial portions of the caudate nucleus and putamen and the nucleus accumbens

ventral tegmental area: contains dopaminergic neurons that project to the ventromedial portion of the striatum and the prefrontal cortex; located in the rostral midbrain

ventricles: dilated channels within the ventricular system; contain choroid plexus

ventricular system: cavities within the central nervous system that contain cerebrospinal fluid

ventricular zone: innermost layer of the developing central nervous system; layer from which nerve cells are generated

ventrolateral medulla: contains neurons that participate in blood pressure regulation through projections to the intermediolateral cell column

ventrolateral nucleus: principal motor control nucleus of the thalamus; receives cerebellar input and projects to primary and premotor cortical areas

ventrolateral preoptic area: important in promoting REM and non-REM sleep, through inhibitory connections with other hypothalamic nuclei and brain stem nuclei that promote wakefulness

ventromedial hypothalamic nucleus: important in regulating appetite and other consummatory behaviors; receives input from limbic system structures

ventromedial posterior nucleus: thalamic nucleus important for processing noxious stimuli; projects to the posterior insular cortex; caudal to the thalamic region that processes viscerosensory information

vergence movements: convergent or divergent eye movements; ensure that the image of an object of interest falls on the same place on the retina of each eye

vermis: midline portion of the cerebellar cortex; plays a role in axial and proximal limb control

vertebral canal: cavity within the vertebral column within which the spinal cord is located

vertebral-basilar circulation: arterial supply to the brain stem and parts of the temporal and occipital lobes

vertigo: the sense of the world spinning around or that of an individual whirling around

vestibular ganglion: location of cell bodies of primary vestibular neurons; also termed Scarpa's ganglion

vestibular labyrinth: fluid-filled cavities within the temporal bone within which the vestibular organs are located

vestibular nuclei: major termination site of vestibular sensory fibers

vestibulocerebellum: portion of the cerebellum that receives a monosynaptic projection from primary vestibular axons; processes this information for eye movement control and balance; includes primarily the flocculonodular lobe

vestibulocochlear (VIII) nerve: contains afferent fibers that innervate the auditory and vestibular structures of the inner ear

vestibuloocular reflex: automatic control of eye position by vestibular sensory information

vestibulospinal tract: axons that originate from the vestibular nuclei and project to the brain stem

vibration sense: the capacity to detect and distinguish mechanical vibration of the body

visceral: related to the internal organs of the body

visceral (autonomic) motor fibers: axons of autonomic preganglionic or postganglionic neurons as they course in the periphery

visceral motor nuclei: contain autonomic preganglionic neurons

viscerosensory: related to the sensory innervation of the internal organs of the body

vision: one of the five major senses

visual field: the total area that is seen

visual field defect: loss of vision within a portion of the visual field

visual motion pathway: originates primarily from the magnocellular ganglion cells of the retina and projects to V5 and ultimately to regions of the posterior parietal cortex

Wallenberg syndrome: *see* lateral medullary syndrome

Wallerian degeneration: deterioration of the structure and function of the distal portion of an axon, when cut; also termed anterograde generation

Wernicke's area: important for understanding speech; located in the posterior superior temporal gyrus (area 22)

white matter: location of predominantly myelinated axons

working memory: the temporary storing of information used to plan and shape upcoming behaviors

zona incerta: contains GABA-ergic neurons that project widely to the cerebral cortex; nuclear region of the diencephalon

Index

Page numbers followed by *t* and *f* indicate tables and figures, respectively. Page numbers in italics indicate Atlas figures.